FOOD, PEOPLE AND NUTRITION

FOOD, PEOPLE AND NUTRITION

Eleanor F. Eckstein, Ph.D., R.D.

Associate Professor
Keene State College

AVI PUBLISHING COMPANY, INC.
Westport, Connecticut

Library of Congress Cataloging in Publication Data

Eckstein, Eleanor F
    Food, people, and nutrition.

    Includes bibliographies and index.
    1. Nutrition.   2. Food.   3. Diet.   I. Title.
TX354.E33   641.1   80–15575
ISBN 0–87055–355–0

Printed in the United States of America
by Eastern Graphics, Inc., Old Saybrook, Connecticut

Preface

The American mainstream diet is acknowledged to have its faults in relation to providing the nutrition everyone needs. Many foods that are not very nutritious individually are considered by nutrition experts to have considerable value. This seeming inconsistency is irrelevant. A nutritious diet is one that supplies the right assortment of nutrients in the right quantity at the right time in response to metabolic demands. Nutritive quality of the diet is independent of food source. An immense number of natural and/or formulated foods can be combined in providing a nourishing diet. But, knowledge of nutrient contributions of individual foods and an estimate of nutrient needs are both necessary prerequisites of informed decision-making.

An understanding of human nutrition involves knowledge of each of the nutrients and respective quantities necessary, the functions of each of the nutrients in metabolic processes, and the effects of variation in levels of supply and demand for each in the context of the food and people interactions that determine what and how much is eaten. Thus, a functional knowledge requires a blending of information from the various disciplines involved in foods and nutrition.

Most people do not have the opportunity to take three courses in nutrition, i.e., whole body nutrition, cellular level nutrition, and life cycle nutrition, plus three courses in foods, i.e., introductory food technology, meal management, and the cultural aspects of foods, in order to develop a functional understanding. Recognizing this fact, I was confronted with a need for a new approach in teaching nutrition. The concepts that make this textbook different were developed and tested in the classroom. This textbook is only a vehicle for sharing.

Most scientists are cautious, being aware of the limits of the extent of their knowledge. In writing scientific papers for an audience of scientists like themselves, the discussion of findings is often limited and inferences with respect to the implications and ramifications are left to the reader.

In the context of a scientific journal, such a procedure is all right. The intended reader should be knowledgeable enough to have demonstrated competence at the higher levels of learning, namely analysis and synthesis.

Unfortunately, in today's world this is no longer true. Many "scientific writers" routinely extract findings from context. Out of context, the points are picked up and used by the unscrupulous. Interesting, if not sensational, they form the basis for food and nutrient fads. This is an unwanted outcome. Therefore, I do not feel comfortable in leaving the tasks of analysis and synthesis to the reader. So, I have attempted to write this textbook in a style that deals with the problem of misinterpretation.

A number of style features have been used to alert the reader. Paragraph structure is deliberately designed to focus attention on the point. IF . . . THEN . . . logic is utilized for identification of accepted relationships. Qualifiers are used deliberately for specific delineation, e.g., ". . . from limited research using human subjects . . . ," ". . . inferred from animal studies . . . ," "Although some species differences have been observed, all species so far . . . ," etc. All of these lead to a statement that starts with "The findings suggest . . . ." Throughout, an attempt has been made to identify unknowns and points that are unknowable. Lists are used throughout for emphasis. The reader should note the deliberate and systematic use of the phrase, ". . . includes, but is not limited to . . ." It may imply that all factors may not be known or that a limited number of the more important items have been selected from an extensive array. I invite reader comment and suggestions for additions to content and corrections for clarity.

The universal true definition of a nutritious diet is unknown and unknowable. Under the controlled conditions of an experimental study, some limited information is obtained. From epidemiologic and other surveys, additional information is obtained. But, even taken together these kinds of information do not add up to the complete answer. They provide only an approximation that can be used as a working definition in making recommendations. Therefore, when a correction is recommended and implemented and results are assessed, some improvement will be demonstrated and so will unanticipated effects that require additional adjustments. These unanticipated effects are due to interactions that had been obscured previously by more pressing nutrient needs. Therefore, a new approximation, new recommendations, and new adjustments will be necessary on a continuing basis.

The disciplines of foods and nutrition are in a rapid growth phase, so data and concepts are updated frequently. The enduring portions form the basic content of this textbook. New evidence that creates another view is indicated when presented. There are many gaps and these I have tried to identify.

One of my major interests is information processing. This involves (a) on-going monitoring of the technical literature in foods and nutrition, which includes but is not limited to research reports, conference proceedings, and government documents, (b) information retrieval, (c) classification, and (d) analysis, interpretation, and integration of new information into an evolving understanding of and philosophy with respect to contemporary events and issues related to the discipline. Understandings and appreciations that are generally accepted are acknowledged to come from the work of myriad unknown researchers. Other contributions are credited in the lists of references.

I gratefully acknowledge the assistance and cooperation of numerous book and journal editors in granting permission to quote. Credit lines provide specific information.

Government documents are in *the public domain,* so they cannot be copyrighted. Thus, permission to quote is unnecessary. I gratefully acknowledge frequent quotations from proceedings and reports of the Senate Select Committee on Nutrition and Human Needs. Hearings publications document the complete proceedings, including oral testimony of witnesses, questions by committee members, discussions among committee members that may include outside participation, written statements submitted for the record, other materials admitted as evidence during testimony, and correspondence and material submitted as a matter of record by committee members and staff. *Committee prints* are published internal reports of staff research, investigative and/or oversight hearings. As such, they may contain background historical and/or statistical information, situation reports, and legislative analyses. Committee reports are published reports to members of the Senate and House that summarize committee findings and make recommendations for legislative action. I am indebted to the USDA for tables and figures from some of these.

Further, I would like to express my appreciation to Dr. Norman W. Desrosier and Ms. Karen L. Carter of The AVI Publishing Company for their encouragement and assistance in bringing this book into being.

Errors of omission and commission are mine alone to bear. Your understanding is solicited.

ELEANOR F. ECKSTEIN
Keene, New Hampshire

December 1979

Dedication

This book is dedicated to those individuals who desire to assume personal responsibility for monitoring and controlling their nutrient intake via adjustments in food and people interactions.

Contents

Food Consumption and Life Expectancy

Food consumption patterns of Americans have changed greatly during this century, especially since World War II. The effects of these changes on health and various aspects of life-style are unclear. A growing public awareness that major changes have occurred and lack of explanation of expected effects or reassurance have undermined public confidence. So, many questions are being asked, e.g., What is the relationship between food consumption patterns and life expectancy?

The relationship between food consumption and life expectancy appears to be as follows:

(a) IF one rules out accidents as a cause of death, THEN life expectancy, or the probability of living X years, depends on physical health and well-being.

(b) IF one rules out malfunction and injury, THEN physical health depends on nutritional status, other conditions such as exercise being equal.

(c) Nutritional status is a result of the cumulative and aggregate intake of nutrients; it usually depends on food consumption.

The effects of extreme malnutrition of two types, i.e., deficiency or under-nutrition and excess or over-nutrition, on life expectancy have long been recognized. But, many cases coexist in all segments of the American population—a recently recognized finding.

Nutritionists can state only approximations of truth based on limited current knowledge, since all of the implications and ramifications are unknowable. This much is clear: (a) optimal nutritional status is a prerequisite to good health and (b) individual adults must take personal responsibility for control of their own nutrient intake and to monitor and adjust food consumption to changing physical needs.

The evidence accumulated to date demonstrates that food consumption by many Americans is not adjusted to supply nutrients for optimal nutritional status, given physiological needs. So, malnutrition has been implicated in the etiology of six out of ten leading causes of death in the

United States. For some of these conditions, the nature of the food consumption problem is known. The extent of the problem is unknowable; it is only approximated by population statistics and summarized as a mean, based on data collected at a certain point in time. However, the indications are that most of the health problems underlying the leading causes of death could be modified by adjustment of food consumption. Potential benefits from improved diets cannot be quantified. But, available evidence suggests that risk of developing a clinical condition can be reduced. The nature of the food consumption problems and what is known of the resulting effects on nutritional status and life expectancy will be summarized.

THE AMERICAN SITUATION

As of 1975, probably the best estimate of American health was contained in the "Report of the President's Biomedical Research Panel." This report stated:

> . . . the state of general physical health in this country is considerably better than at any earlier period in history. There are . . . serious problems for concern: perinatal mortality in impoverished sectors of the population is unacceptably high; the morbidity and mortality rates for cardiopulmonary disease, stroke, and cancer are slowly but steadily increasing; and chronic illness, especially in the aged, is a formidable problem. Nonetheless, the total mortality for the United States population in 1974 was less than 1 percent . . . and the average life expectancy had risen to 72 years, the longest in the country's history.[1]

As of July, 1977, another approximation became available. It showed a somewhat different picture. Life expectancy had increased to 81 years for females and 72 years for males, according to a report released by the Census Bureau. The increased life expectancy was attributed to reduction in death rate from major cardiovascular disease, especially myocardial infarctions. Information on whether the decrease in mortality rate was due to improved medical techniques or low cholesterol diets was not available.

An earlier 1977 report, "Dietary Goals for the United States," prepared by the staff of the Select Committee on Nutrition and Human Needs—the so-called "McGovern Committee"—contained some interesting statements:

---

[1]From Anon. (1975).

The over-consumption of fat, generally, and saturated fat in particular, as well as cholesterol, sugar, and salt, and alcohol have been related to six of the ten leading causes of death: heart disease, cancer, cerebrovascular disease, diabetes, atherosclerosis and cirrhosis of the liver . . .

The over-consumption of food in general has become a major public health problem . . .

At the same time, current dietary trends may also be leading to malnutrition through under-nourishment. Fats and sugar are relatively low in vitamins and minerals. Consequently, diets reduced to control weight and/or save money, but which are high in fat and sugar, are likely to lead to vitamin and mineral deficiencies . . . low-income people may be particularly susceptible to inducements to consume high-fat/high-sugar diets. . .

During this century, the composition of the average diet in the United States has changed radically. Complex carbohydrates—fruit, vegetables and grain products—which were the mainstay of the diet, now play a minority role. At the same time, fat and sugar consumption have risen to a point where these two dietary elements alone now comprise at least 60 percent of total calorie intake, up from 50 percent in the early 1900's . . .

The diet of the American people has become increasingly rich—rich in meat, other sources of saturated fat and cholesterol, and in sugar. . . It has been pointed out repeatedly that total sugar use has remained relatively constant for a number of years. We would emphasize, however, that our total food consumption has fallen even though we still eat too much relative to our needs. Thus, the proportion of the total diet contributed by fatty and cholesterol-rich foods and by refined foods has risen. We might be better able to tolerate this diet if we were much more active physically, but we are a sedentary people.[1]

Until recently, medical efforts largely were directed to treating the major diseases after they became clinically manifest. But, to undo the effects is difficult if not impossible. So, emphasis has shifted to detection of a developing pattern of risk and intervention with preventive measures, especially in relation to the following diseases: coronary heart disease, hypertension, cancer of breast and colon, obesity, diabetes, and cirrhosis of the liver. Each will be discussed briefly.

Coronary Heart Disease (CHD)

Excessive intakes of the following have been implicated as etiologic factors in the development of CHD: total fat, saturated fat, cholesterol, salt, sugar, and alcohol. Intakes of fat, saturated fat, and cholesterol have been correlated positively with serum cholesterol levels and so with

---

[1]From Select Comm. on Nutrition and Human Needs, U.S. Senate (1977).

incidence of myocardial infarctions. Salt intake is related to blood pressure and hypertension, which aggravate a heart condition. Sugar and alcohol are low nutrient density foods that may displace foods containing needed minerals and vitamins, and have some not-clearly-defined effects of their own. In regard to CHD, the "Report of the President's Biomedical Research Panel" stated,

There are no proven ways to prevent atherosclerosis. In a few cases of congenital hyperlipidemia the course of the disease can be improved by dietary and other measures to reduce blood cholesterol and lipid, but these are the exception. The ordinary, common type of atherosclerosis—probably the most common life-threatening disorder in our society—is still without a satisfactory explanation for the arterial lesions . . . Elaborate studies are planned or underway to learn whether a reduction in animal fat, or drugs to reduce cholesterol, will reduce the incidence or severity of atherosclerosis . . . Even so, if diet regulation proves to be partially effective, there will still be the crucial question whether the population at risk is willing to undergo radical changes in lifelong habits of eating.[1]

Because dietary factors are clearly implicated, the Inter-Society Commission for Heart Disease Resources and the American Heart Association have issued recommendations. The Prudent Diet, which incorporates the recommended preventive diet modifications, is detailed in Chapter 24.

Hypertension

About one-third of the American population is susceptible to high blood pressure or hypertension when sodium intake is elevated. Table salt is the main source of sodium. Consumption ranges from 6 to 18 g, but only about 1 g is necessary to supply sodium.

Cancer of Breast and Colon

Dietary intake of fat has been correlated with incidence of breast and colon cancer. Incidence of colon cancer also has been correlated with low bulk diets. Speculation is that a high fat intake causes increased secretion of prolactin which induces breast tumors. Some evidence indicating that normal colon bacteria can produce carcinogens, perhaps from fat fragments, has been presented. Current speculation is that IF one consumes a low bulk diet and thus becomes constipated, so that the passage rate is

---

[1]From Anon. (1975).

slower than normal, THEN carcinogens could be formed and absorbed. A return to a normo-bulk diet is advocated.

Obesity

A 1976 review, "Report of the President's Biomedical Research Panel," states the magnitude of the problem: "According to current estimates one-fourth to one-third of the American adult population and at least ten percent of American children are overweight or obese." A variety of health problems are created by or aggravated by obesity. So major efforts have been made to understand its etiology and to develop effective strategies for weight control.

Recent research has provided a basis for understanding and controlling obesity. According to the same report,

Both the number and size of fat cells (adipocytes) determine the fat content of the body. While the size of fat cells appears to be variable throughout life, the number of these cells apparently is not . . . the number of adipocytes in the organism stabilizes relatively early, certainly before adulthood, and remains a fixed quantity thereafter. Thus, it is suggested that the eventual weight pattern is set by early nutritional history, in infancy or during adolescence. Later in life, only cell size can be modulated.[1]

Both fat and sugar are concentrated sources of energy and little else. Since they are preferred, they displace fruits, vegetables, and cereals in the diet. The latter are relatively low in calories and high in bulk; increased intake of these would ease the problem of weight control. Weight control is an important factor in increasing life expectancy of many people. Major changes in food consumption are necessary. See Chapter 24.

Diabetes

Testimony given at the 1973-1974 hearings of the "McGovern Committee" on diabetes and the daily diet supported the position that there is a definite connection. Some points made in the hearings were:

(a) Over-nutrition leads to diabetes in those predisposed to it because more insulin is necessary than can be produced. When insulin is insufficient to control blood sugar levels within normal ranges, the person is considered to be diabetic. Thus, overeating precipitates diabetes. This

---

[1]From Anon. (1975).

occurs in about 85% of the more than 5 million cases of diabetes that exist.

(b) Diabetics are more vulnerable to cardiovascular disease since increased blood sugar leads to increased blood lipid levels. The result is progressive deposition of lipids in vascular tissue until occlusion occurs somewhere. If it occurs in the large blood vessels that supply the heart, heart tissue dies (myocardial infarction), which may disrupt or prevent heart muscle action and result in death.

(c) Diabetics are vulnerable to gangrene, especially of the toes. When the blood vessels become occluded, circulation is reduced. IF the tissue becomes infected, THEN the tissue dies.

(d) Diabetes is the leading cause of blindness—increased pressure in small blood vessels results in ruptures, formation of scar tissue, and blindness when light cannot penetrate the tissue.

(e) Diabetes also leads to kidney failure. Juvenile type diabetics develop kidney failure after 20 to 25 years of the disease due to a combination of the stress of filtering out the excess sugar and development of scar tissue resulting from occlusion and/or rupture of small blood vessels.

Management of diabetes usually involves a modified diet. The American Diabetes Association issued new guidelines for diet management in 1972. Important concepts for mild and moderately severe cases are:

(a) The most important objective is to attain and maintain "ideal" weight.

(b) Decrease fat intake to approximately 35% kcal.

(c) Increase carbohydrate intake to approximately 45% of kcal; consume these primarily as complex carbohydrates from starch, since it is broken down to glucose slowly and will not produce high blood sugar peaks.

(d) Food intake should be spaced in relation to exercise (and insulin activity peaks, if applicable) in order to avoid intermittent periods of low blood sugar.

IF dietary measures were followed, THEN the dependence on insulin and/or oral drugs might be reduced. Many cases can be controlled by diet alone.

Cirrhosis of the Liver

Immoderate consumption of alcohol is the major cause of cirrhosis. There is limited but conflicting evidence concerning the role of diet in its etiology. One study reported that the typically deficient teenage diet fed to rats seemed to predispose them to alcoholism. There is abundant evidence that alcoholics do not regularly consume a nutritionally adequate diet. And, there is some evidence that metabolism of alcohol by liver cells inflates the need for thiamin and a few other vitamins.

U.S. DIETARY GOALS

Malnutrition resulting from inappropriate food consumption is related to six of the leading causes of death, and modified intake is regarded as the solution to some major health problems. Therefore, as a result of the testimony heard by the "McGovern Committee," a set of dietary goals was developed. After additional testimony, a second set was developed (Select Comm. on Nutrition and Human Needs, U.S. Senate 1977). These are:

(a) To avoid overweight, and to consume only as much energy (calories) as is expended; if overweight, decrease energy intake and increase energy expenditure.

(b) Increase the consumption of complex carbohydrates and "naturally occurring" sugars from about 28% of energy intake to about 48% of energy intake.

(c) Reduce the consumption of refined and processed sugars by about 45% to account for about 10% of total energy intake.

(d) Reduce overall fat consumption from approximately 40% to about 30% of energy intake.

(e) Reduce saturated fat consumption to account for about 10% of total energy intake; balance with polyunsaturated and mono-unsaturated fats, which should account for about 10% of energy intake each.

(f) Reduce cholesterol consumption to about 300 mg per day.

(g) Limit the intake of sodium by reducing the intake of salt to about 5 g per day.

Attaining these dietary goals will require major changes in food consumption habits and practices on the part of a significant number of Americans. The ecological effects cannot be predicted because of the magnitude of the changes required and uncertainty regarding the degree to which changes can or will be made. The definitions of food/poison, the eating experience, and food and people interactions will all be affected. New strategies will need to be devised to help people make appropriate adjustments.

Simplified food group systems do not seem feasible because of the number of nutrients and foods involved as well as the need for individualization. A monitoring/feedback control system may work for those who come to value consumption of a nutritious diet that is designed to meet personal needs. Such a system is described in Chapter 19.

In 1948 Ms. Stiebeling, then chief of the Bureau of Human Nutrition and Home Economics in the USDA, made a statement that still holds:

We do not yet understand the dynamics of modifying food habits well enough to apply . . . laws (of nutrition) in a fully effective way. But we are all aware of the bewilderment that household food buyers feel over much of the current advertising—advertising that attempts to push to the maximum of human capacity the consumption of every separate commodity—indiscriminately. Surely in the education of the public and in the orientation of food production and trade for bettering consumption patterns, we should look at the physiological research, and at the relative economy and usefulness of various foods to serve these needs. And science should speak with one voice in broad over-all terms about food choice and food use. This will have to be done if we are to progress at a pace in keeping with scientific knowledge and potentialities.[1]

In 1979, "Healthy People, The Surgeon General's Report on Health Promotion and Disease Prevention" was published. It listed the six major causes of death for persons aged 25 to 64 years as heart disease, cancer, stroke, cirrhosis of the liver, all other accidents, and motor vehicle accidents (USNCHS 1976). Heart disease, cancer, stroke, influenza and pneumonia, arteriosclerosis, and diabetes mellitus were listed as the six major causes of death for adults aged 65 and older (USNCHS 1976). This report discussed the need for nutrition as part of a preventive health program and stated that Americans probably would be healthier if they consumed a diet low in calories, lower in saturated fat, cholesterol, salt, and sugar, with more complex CHO, and relatively more fish, poultry, and legumes, and less red meat.

In early 1980, "Nutrition and Your Health" was issued jointly by the USDA and the Department of Health, Education and Welfare. It was a set of general guidelines that are similar to the dietary goals in principle: eat a variety of foods; maintain ideal weight; avoid too much fat, saturated fat, cholesterol, sugar, and sodium; eat foods with adequate starch and fiber; if you drink alcohol, do so in moderation. The notation that, "These represent a nutritional consensus by scientists in the government's food and health agencies," adds the weight of authority in efforts of persuasion.

THE FOOD AND NUTRITION "TRIP"

Food and nutrition education programs are costly and are always at issue, provoking strong feelings on both sides. The real problem in relation to funding is that, "We can't afford to and we can't afford not to." We cannot afford to fund the programs enough to aid everybody, updating and upgrading information and skills to keep pace with our growing understanding of nutrition and its many impacts. So, persons with an accounting mentality can always create a crisis in confidence regarding

---

[1]From Select Comm. on Nutrition and Human Needs, U.S. Senate (1977).

program accomplishments. We cannot afford not to fund programs. In democracy, people must be educated to do voluntarily what they cannot be coerced into, and some people are slow learners. So, idealistic goals are retargeted to realistic objectives, given resources.

Good nutrition for the American population is probably an impossible dream that can be achieved only by a people's movement. Food and nutrition education programs can be designed to develop awareness, some knowledge of symbols and terms, some understanding of relationships, and some appreciation for the values associated with good nutritional status. A people's movement is needed to remind people of facts and give support for appropriate and spontaneous control of their own food habits and practices. Motivation that sustains self-discipline comes from within a person. In this society, nobody has the power to force people to consume an appropriate diet, but social pressure can provide strong reinforcement.

There is power in a "people's" movement—it can do what is seemingly impossible. A people's movement appeals and takes hold when people are ready because they can relate to it as it meets a felt need(s). IF a people's movement for good nutrition is rooted in science and other contemporary forces come together in support of it, THEN it can overcome traditions, inertia, and fear as a positive force in extending life expectancy.

BIBLIOGRAPHY

ANON. 1975. Report of the President's Biomedical Research Panel. DHEW Publ. (05)76-501.

ANON. 1979. Healthy People, The Surgeon General's Report of Health Promotion and Disease Prevention. DHEW (PHS) Publ. 79-55071. Public Health Service, Office of the Assistant Secretary for Health and Surgeon General. GPO, Washington, D.C.

SELECT COMM. ON NUTRITION AND HUMAN NEEDS, U.S. SENATE. 1977. Dietary Goals for the United States (Committee Print). GPO, Washington, D.C.

SELECT COMM. ON NUTRITION AND HUMAN NEEDS, U.S. SENATE. 1977. Dietary Goals for the United States. Second edition. (Committee Print). GPO, Washington, D.C.

USDA and DHEW. 1980. Nutrition and Your Health. Off. Govt. & Public Affairs, USDA, Washington, D.C.

USNCHS. 1976. Mortality trends for leading causes of death. Vital and Health Statistics Series. U.S. National Center for Health Statistics, Public Health Service, Dep. Health, Education, and Welfare, Washington, D.C.

2

Foods as Sources of Nutrients

Foods are the natural and usual source of nutrients. But, since they are highly variable in nutrient content, one cannot take it for granted that an uncontrolled intake will meet nutritional needs. To assure consumption of a nutritionally adequate diet, informed control is necessary. Competence and confidence in evaluation of alternate foods as sources of nutrients form the basis for informed control.

WHAT IS A NUTRIENT?

Strictly speaking, a nutrient is a chemical substance that is necessary for human life and growth/repair of tissues. This is a seemingly simple statement, but its implications and ramifications are far-reaching. Definition of some key terms will clarify some points and provide the basis for an initial understanding. Key terms related to the concept of nutrient are:

(a) necessary—absolutely needed; required in human nutrition

(b) essential—indispensable and must be provided by an exogenous supply, i.e., by dietary intake, ingestion of supplements, injection, or intravenous feeding. Essentiality may be partial or total. When used with respect to trace element needs, "essential" has a different meaning, as discussed in Chapter 10.

(c) fundamental—a substance that is a constituent or cofactor without which the human organism would fail to function

(d) vital—necessary to continued existence

(e) cardinal—a substance on which a functional outcome depends.

Today, more than 50 substances are known, or presumed, to be nourishing to humans.

More than 100 chemical elements are known at the present time; not all are recognized as nutrients at this time. Functionally, elements with nutriment roles interact as:

(a) inorganic ionic elements *per se*, e.g., Na^+, K^+, Cl^-

(b) inorganic ionic radicals, e.g., sulfur, oxygen, and phosphorus are constituents of sulfates (SO_4^{--}) and phosphates (PO_4^{---})

(c) inorganic molecules, e.g., hydrogen and oxygen are constituents of water (H_2O) molecules

(d) organic ionized radicals, e.g., carbon and oxygen are constituents of carbonate (CO_3^{--})

(e) organic molecules, e.g., glucose and fatty acids contain carbon, hydrogen, and oxygen whereas protein also contains nitrogen and may contain sulfur

For purposes of discussion, roles of many of the elements and radicals traditionally have been subsumed under discussion of various classes of molecules. Thus, discussion has been organized around carbohydrates, proteins, fats, and vitamins. The remaining elements then were aggregated and discussed as "minerals."

Thirty-one substances are currently recognized by the Food and Nutrition Board of the National Academy of Sciences, the American authority on nutrition, as essential nutrients. For other purposes, the essential and nonessential amino acids that comprise proteins, the essential and nonessential fatty acids that comprise fats and oils, the various sugars, and some polysaccharides also may be classified as nutrients. Water fits the technical definitions of both food and nutrient. Energy is a nutrient, as are three of its four sources— (a) carbohydrate, as glucose, fructose, and galactose; (b) protein as amino acids; and (c) fatty acids.

Alcohol is not a nutrient since it is not necessary to life. Oxygen is necessary to life, but because it is supplied by respiration and as a constituent of many organic radicals and molecules, in and of itself, it is not essential from diet or supplements, so it is not considered to be a nutrient.

WHAT IS FOOD?

Food sources of nutrients include natural foods (plant and animal tissues); food mixtures made from natural food ingredients; formulated foods, i.e., items created according to new food concepts to simulate natural foods; food mixtures made from a combination of natural food and synthetic food ingredients; and food supplements or some combination thereof. For purposes of this discussion, all of the above will be considered as food since they are consumed by some Americans—either as food or in place of food.

Given this definition of food, there are many thousand items. A given individual may consume some 2,000 of these. However, the particular subset of items depends on the individual's personal definition of what is food.

RELIABILITY OF FOODS AS SOURCES OF NUTRIENTS

Most natural food is perishable; when spoiled, it is considered to be inedible so all of its nutrients are wasted. Processing preserves, i.e., keeps food safe so that it does not injure the consumer, keeps the food itself safe from decomposition (physical and nutritional), and makes it available for future use. Although processing may reduce the relative nutrient content, it usually preserves a substantial quantity. Whether a greater percentage of nutrients might be retained by alternate processing methods is a moot question; the discussion is beyond the scope of this book.

The practices of restoring or enriching processed foods raise the relative nutrient content of selected nutrients. Since trace minerals and unknown nutrients are not added, natural foods need to be the predominant kinds of foods consumed as sources of nutrients.

There are many sources of variation in the nutrient content of food. These generally can be categorized as inherent factors, environmental effects, or the effects of processing. Abbreviated descriptions follow.

Inherent factors are those belonging to the raw animal or plant tissues used as food; they are in its constitution or essential character as determinants of composition. These include, but are not limited to:

(a) genetics—Variation is due to species differences, varietal differences, or inbreeding.

(b) portion of the plant or animal consumed—Tissues that are nutrient sources for embryos, e.g., eggs or seeds, or those that are metabolically active, e.g., liver, brain, leaves, or muscles are good sources of minerals and vitamins. Tissues that are used to store energy are good sources of fat or starch. Muscle tissue, blood, and milk are good sources of protein.

(c) age or maturity—Veal is a less concentrated source of all nutrients than is beef since it is from a younger animal. Fruits are usually starchy when unripe, and sweet when ripe due to degradation of the starch to sugars. Vegetables are sweet when young and starchy when mature.

(d) stage of lactation—At freshening, the fat content of the cow's milk is greater than later.

(e) rumen or intestinal synthesis of nutrients by bacteria—The absolute quantity produced and absorbed by animals of the same species is highly variable. The relative quantity of a nutrient also varies among species.

(f) quantity of degradative enzymes and conditions for activation—Fresh foods have more nutrients than ones harvested too soon. Temperature, pH, and moisture content affect the rate of breakdown. Food stored at high temperatures becomes rancid, putrid, etc., faster than that stored at refrigerator temperatures because of the effect on reaction rate.

Environmental effects comprise a cluster of factors which affect the growth, harvesting, handling, and service of food. Together these determine the food yield per unit (acre, pound, portion, etc.) as well as its nutritional quality. Environmental factors include, but are not limited to:

(a) soil content of nutrients and availability to plants—The kind of plants and the number of crops per year determine the rate at which nutrients are extracted from the soil and are used in plant nutriture. Plant growth rate is determined by the availability of necessary nutrients. IF the soil is poor, i.e., depleted in even one essential nutrient, THEN food production yield will be low, i.e., tissue growth will be stunted and the quantity of that nutrient will be low. The natural soil content of various nutrients varies widely in the United States, and different crops require and deplete the soil of the various nutrients to various degrees. Therefore, to sustain profitable food production yields, all of the nutrients known to be depleted by a crop are systematically replaced. Fertilizers, i.e., non-food plant tissues, manure, nitrogen and/or mineral compounds (natural or synthetic) are used in replenishment. Therefore, in the United States, since very high yields are customary and sufficient fertilizer is used to sustain yields, the nutrient content of plant and animal tissues used for food will approximate the maximum.

In the United States, the natural variation of iodine and other nutrients in soil content is not of great importance in human nutrition for another reason. Few people consume a diet composed of locally produced foods. Therefore, the probability of a deficient intake is greatly reduced.

(b) climatic effects on length and quality of the growing season— These include daylength and amount of sunlight, temperature, relative humidity, windflow, and rainfall. The mean levels, the timing, the variation within and among days, as well as the cumulative and aggregate effects of the variations determine the yield per acre of crops and lean-to-fat ratio in animals.

(c) cultural techniques—The frequency and degree of loosening the soil have effects on moisture absorption and evaporation rate, given soil type.

(d) climatic effects on harvesting efficiency—These include temperature, relative humidity, and windflow. All of these affect yield per acre and resultant concentration of nutrients. When harvested in hot, dry windy weather, the food will be somewhat desiccated and relatively concentrated, whereas in damp weather the food will take up moisture and swell, reducing the relative nutrient concentration.

(e) animal husbandry methods employed—Diet, exercise, etc., have a major effect on the lean-to-fat ratio.

(f) handling during transport and short-term storage—Plant tissues that are chilled immediately after harvest and are kept moist will retain freshness and vitamins longest because the metabolic progress toward the peak and beyond is retarded. Animal tissues bled and stored in a cool, dry, bacteria-free atmosphere after slaughter will retain freshness and nutrients longest since degradation is retarded.

(g) service of food—Loss of thiamin and ascorbic acid is related to length of hot holding time and exposure to air and are progressive. Loss of vitamin A by oxidation of cut surfaces is progressive. Minerals are lost by leaching into juices, soaking water, etc., and is progressive. If the liquid is hot, the rate of leaching is enhanced. The shorter the interval between preparation and service, the greater the probability that nutrients have been retained.

Effects of processing vary with the type and degree of processing. Minerals are added as catalysts in some processes such as hydrogenation of oils and as contaminants from processing equipment and water. Other changes are related to specific factors and/or processes that include, but are not limited to, conditions of ingredient handling, storage, and transport; washing, soaking, and blanching; peeling; refining; drying; salting; smoking; pickling; canning; freezing; freeze-drying; extrusion; foam mat drying; agglomerating; and aseptic packaging. Effects of each of these are indicated briefly:

(a) conditions of ingredient handling, storage, and transport—Continued storage at low temperatures with controlled humidity is essential in retarding the rate at which nutrients are destroyed during extended storage periods. Packaging, in some cases with oxygen excluded and addition of an inert gas, is usually necessary to prevent fat breakdown and destruction of vitamin A. CO_2 is used to retard the metabolic processes in fruits. As a result, some fruits can be available and approximately equal to newly harvested ones in eating quality almost throughout the year.

(b) washing, soaking, and blanching—Washing has a negligible effect on nutrient content. Soaking results in progressive leaching out of minerals and water-soluble vitamins. These are lost when the soaking water is discarded. Blanching reduces the ascorbic acid content of vegetables, especially leafy ones, but it also inactivates enzymes that would result in inedibility. It also loosens skins of fruits, facilitating their removal with minimal loss of pulp.

(c) peeling—Conventional lye peeling raises the sodium content. It also reduces the water-soluble vitamin content, especially of thiamin, by alkaline degradation. The mineral content is reduced by leaching in the rinse removal of the lye. Abrasion peeling reduces the content of all nutrients. The degree is highly variable, depending on the length of processing. Fortunately, for economic reasons the processor minimizes peeling time.

(d) refining—Sugar refining results in some loss of minerals and vitamins; however, cane and beet juice are not naturally rich sources of these nutrients. IF the sugar intake exceeds about 10% of the caloric intake, THEN this nutrient loss may be significant. However, displacement of more nutritious foods accounts for a much greater nutrient loss. Whole wheat flour is a crude product in the sense that refining is incomplete, which has nutritional merit since loss of vitamins and minerals is trivial. By comparison, white flours are refined or more pure depending on the level of extraction. Cake flour is the most refined and is almost pure wheat starch. In producing all-purpose white flour, about 25% of the wheat kernel is removed, including the bran and endosperm. These contain fiber, fat, vitamins, and minerals—hence, the observed processing losses. Enrichment and fortification are legal procedures used to replace and/or augment quantities of stipulated nutrients. Not all of the vitamins and minerals that are removed in processing are replaced by enrichment, fortification, or restoring. Those of concern and not presently replaced include folic acid, Zn, Mn, Cu, and Mo.

(e) drying—The protein, fat, and carbohydrate content of dry foods is relatively high since the water has been removed. The nutrient content on a reconstituted basis is lower due to processing losses. The vitamin A content is reduced 5%. The thiamin content is reduced 15% if the food is blanched prior to drying and 75% if it is not. Ascorbic acid destruction is highly variable among foods. Destruction is total in meat and milk, which are naturally low in ascorbic acid. Destruction is partial in fruits and vegetables.

(f) salting—Progressive drying is achieved by drawing water from the tissues to dissolve the salt. In the process, water-soluble vitamins and minerals are leached out. In addition, soaking or parboiling to decrease the saltiness to a palatable level further reduces the water-soluble vitamin and mineral content.

(g) smoking—Progressive drying is achieved by evaporation. Comments on nutrient losses in (e) pertain.

(h) pickling—Dehydration in salt brine is accompanied by fermentation of natural or added sugar. The carbohydrate content is reduced by degradation to acid. Minerals and vitamins are leached out in the brine.

(i) canning—This process involves cooking and commercial sterilization. The cumulative and aggregate losses of peeling, soaking, particulation—dicing, slicing, waffling, cutting julienne style—and cooking are approximately 25% for minerals and most vitamins, except thiamin and ascorbic acid. Losses of these vitamins may be 50% or more. Storage periods greater than one year, especially at 70°F or above, result in progressive losses of protein and vitamins.

(j) freezing—Individually quick frozen foods, e.g., blueberries, peas, or cut green beans, when processed in the field, have an average vitamin content that is greater than that reported for store purchased "fresh" counterparts. The thiamin and ascorbic acid content of plate frozen foods, i.e., those frozen as a solid block such as spinach or mustard greens, is greatly reduced. Most other foods are frozen by blast freezing. Losses of nutrients are highly variable among foods.

(k) freeze drying—Losses are less than from conventional drying since freezing causes the process of drying to proceed at a lower temperature.

(l) extrusion—Little data on nutrient losses are available.

(m) foam mat drying—Puréed food is first foamed to increase its surface area so that it will dry faster. The foamed food is spread in a layer or "mat" to dry. The increased surface area may result in high losses of vitamin A and ascorbic acid.

(n) agglomerating or instantizing—A liquid food or a solid food that has been puréed is dried and ground to a powder, rewet, and sprayed as a mist into a heated chamber. It dries as it falls, and large irregular particles that will not pack are formed. The extra processing plus the increased surface area result in an additional 10% decrease in the vitamin A and ascorbic acid content.

(o) aseptic packaging using form, fill, and seal systems—The food is cooked rapidly in batches and is portioned into sterile containers and sealed. This procedure greatly reduces processing time. The amount of thiamin and ascorbic acid retained is greater than that achieved by conventional canning methods. Since air is excluded from the package, vitamin A and ascorbic acid are retained longer during storage.

Home storage and preparation procedures can maintain or reduce the nutrient content of foods. Home storage of most fruits and vegetables in an air-tight/moisture-proof container in the refrigerator retains vitamins as well as crispness. Even so, IF fresh dark leafy greens and broccoli are stored more than five days, THEN more than half of their ascorbic acid content will be lost. Intact cell walls protect vitamin and mineral content; cut surfaces result in loss. So, foods should be diced, sliced, etc., as close to cooking time as possible. Then, in order to minimize cooking losses, the items should be cooked as rapidly and in as little water as possible. As it contains dissolved minerals, cooking water from vegetables should be saved and used as the liquid in soups, stews, casseroles, and the like. Toasting destroys thiamin. IF bread and cereals are customarily consumed in toasted form, THEN supplementation of thiamin may be necessary.

Each of the factors that can affect the nutrient content of food has been discussed briefly. All do not, but more than one may, affect the nutrient content of a particular food. Some may increase the natural content and others may decrease it. For a particular specimen, the relative effects are unknown and unknowable. All that can be determined is the end result. But, the analytical procedures destroy the food, so for most purposes a table value is used as the best approximation.

Another way to evaluate the nutritional quality of foods as sources of nutrients is to assess the stability of the various nutrients, primarily vitamins, in processed foods. IF nutrient stability is reasonable, i.e., good manufacturing procedures have been implemented to minimize destruction and/or protect nutrient potency, THEN foods are the best sources of nutrients they can be unless enriched or fortified. Recent research findings related to nutrient stability in processed foods are summarized below:

(a) vitamins A and D—Pre-formed vitamin A, β-carotene, and vitamin D are unstable in the presence of oxygen, oxidizing agents, mineral pro-oxidents such as iron and copper, and ultraviolet light. High temperature storage increases the rate of decomposition and, hence, loss of vitamin function. Also, vitamin A is partially transformed from all *trans* to *cis* form at pH of 4.5 or less, which diminishes vitamin activity in proportion to the extent of transformation.

Therefore, potency of these vitamins in foods must be protected. Common methods are processing in pro-oxident-free equipment, addition of food-use-approved antioxidants such as BHA, BHT, and/or propyl gallate; packaging to minimize exposure to oxygen and ultraviolet light; and attempting to control home storage length and conditions through public education. When these common procedures are followed, at least two-thirds of the original vitamin activity is retained. Table values reflect normal retention levels for the various foods. Potency of added vitamins in dry foods is stabilized by use of encapsulated beadlets or granules that are dispersed throughout, as in a powdered product, or by use of an antioxidant-stabilized emulsion that will dry as a coating.

The potency of β-carotene in fruits and vegetables is not greatly reduced by processing methods except dehydration. It is stable to blanching, canning, freezing, and frozen storage. Dehydration losses tend to be high and complete destruction may occur unless the food is packed in an inert gas.

(b) vitamin E—α-tocopherol is unstable in the presence of oxygen, especially at room temperature and above. Processing by cooking methods other than deep fat frying does not destroy vitamin potency. Protection of naturally occurring tocopherols from oxidation is accomplished by addition of food-use-approved antioxidants. Stability of added tocopherol content is achieved by use of the acetate form.

(c) thiamin—Destruction of potency is highly variable among foods and for the same food under various conditions of processing and storage.

Generalizations about degree of destruction are unwarranted. Destruction is caused by low acid to alkaline pH, oxidation, ultraviolet and gamma radiation, presence of sulfites, and high temperature processing. Thiaminases in vegetables and seafoods also destroy thiamin during storage. Potency is protected by processing in pro-oxidant-free equipment, addition of food-use-approved acidulents to adjust pH, addition of food-use-approved antioxidants, minimization of heat processing times, packaging to minimize exposure to oxygen and ultraviolet light, and consumer education on preparation and storage procedures for conservation of thiamin.

(d) ascorbic acid—The vitamin is unstable in the presence of moisture, oxygen, oxidizing agents, and ultraviolet and gamma radiation. Presence of pro-oxidant metal ions and rising temperature or pH increase the rate of destruction of potency. Stability is determined by the inherent characteristics of the food, method of processing used, and packaging type. Potency is protected by processing in pro-oxidant-free equipment, i.e., not containing black iron, brass, bronze, cold rolled steel, or copper; addition of food-use-approved antioxidants, minimization of heat processing time, packaging to minimize exposure to oxygen and ultraviolet light, and consumer information on recommended storage conditions. Table values are based on normal retention levels. Potency of ascorbic acid added to dry foods is stabilized by use of sodium ascorbate (the sodium salt form) and packaging to control moisture uptake. Ascorbic acid is also added to many foods as a reducing agent to improve color, palatability, clarity, or keeping quality. In addition to the procedures noted above, to conserve ascorbic acid potency for intended function as a reducing agent, the vitamin is added as late in processing as possible.

(e) vitamin B_6—Pyridoxine is more stable in foods than are the pyridoxal or pyridoxamine forms. Heat is the main destroyer. Retention of vitamin potency is highly variable among foods. In flours and cereal products, retention appears to be 90% or more. In milk products, heating and storage losses are high, so evaporated milk contains about one-third to one-half that of fresh milk, which is halved again after storage at room temperature for six months. Canning losses are approximately 50% for many foods.

(f) vitamin B_{12}—The vitamin is normally stable to processing in meat, fish, and egg products due to presence of iron salts (80 to 100% potency is retained), but labile in milk exposed to sunlight, oxidizing agents, or high temperature processing.

(g) folic acid—The vitamin and its polyglutamate forms are unstable below pH 5 and in the presence of oxygen or sunlight and riboflavin. Even short cooking times reduce potency 50%.

The nutritive values reported for foods are not necessarily the same as the amount absorbed and available for metabolic use. Bioavailability is reduced by factors which include, but are not limited to:

(a) variable absorption efficiencies in the presence of other nutrients—For example, a high calcium content reduces the proportion of amino acids and magnesium that are absorbed. A high ascorbic acid content increases the percentage of iron absorbed.

(b) binding of metal ions to form insoluble salts—Calcium and magnesium form insoluble compounds with the free radicals of oxalic and phytic acids so that these minerals cannot be absorbed. Normally, for American omnivores, this is unimportant as the ratio of minerals to these free radicals leaves much free mineral when all of the free radical is bound. But for vegetarians with a low calcium (no dairy products) and high phytic acid (high whole grain cereal) diet this may be critical.

(c) relative percentage of nutrient liberated and absorbed—The efficiency of absorption of some minerals such as calcium and iron is determined partly by metabolic need.

Analytical values are obtained primarily by chemical analysis. These are the best estimates available regarding the nutrient composition. Still, these values are imperfect. Variable estimates are obtained for a variety of reasons that include, but are not limited to:

(a) method of analysis—The various methods do not measure exactly the same fraction or with the same accuracy and/or precision, so norms vary.

(b) sample selected—When possible, the food is puréed so that aliquot samples will be identical. Otherwise, obtained values tend to be randomly distributed. Replications are used to derive a mean value, which is reported.

(c) contamination—Laboratory contamination of food samples with minerals absorbed from equipment, water, or chemicals is controlled when relevant to a particular analysis, to the extent possible.

(d) number of samples—Values are obtained from a variable number of samples of the various foods. Availability, not need for accuracy, is often the determining factor. Values for the various nutrient in the same food are obtained from a variable number of samples. Again, the number of samples is often unrelated to the need for accuracy.

A particular group of foods may be relied on to supply particular nutrients. If the food is not inherently a good source, too low or unreliable, it may be used as a vehicle for providing the nutrient(s). In this case, the level(s) of the nutrient(s) must be standardized by enrichment, fortification, or restoration.

Cereal products are relied upon for their contributions of calories, protein, iron, thiamin, niacin, and riboflavin. When flour and cereal enrichment decisions were first made in the 1940s, Americans consumed an average of four to six servings per day. The loss of nutrients by refining was significant because of the quantity consumed. Moreover, diets of many Americans were shown to be low in thiamin, riboflavin, and niacin. So, these were added.

By the 1970s, consumption of breads and cereals had dropped to an average of two servings per day. Therefore, the loss of nutrients by refining was less important to total intake. However, the Food and Nutrition Board of the NAS has provided evidence of potential risk of deficiency of vitamin A, thiamin, iron, calcium, magnesium, and zinc. Therefore, in 1974 the NAS submitted a proposal to fortify cereals with the following nutrients: thiamin, riboflavin, niacin, iron, calcium, vitamin A, pyridoxine, folic acid, magnesium, and zinc. Feasibility of bread and cereal fortification with these nutrients is under study. To date, research has demonstrated that these nutrients are stable in flour for storage periods of up to 6 months at room temperature and for 4 months at 113°F, except when stored in a moist atmosphere. They are also stable in bread stored five days at room temperature, by which time bread is usually consumed in the typical American household.

TABLES OF FOOD COMPOSITION

The actual nutrient content of foods as consumed is unknown and unknowable. A table of food composition (see Appendix) contains a selected array of foods that are consumed by a large number of people (which justifies the costs of analysis and reporting of values), but is by no means complete. More than 50 nutrients are known to be required in human nutrition. Tables of food composition list nutrients for which values are in demand for assessment calculations because they are listed in the Recommended Dietary Allowances or are necessary for specialized nutrition research controls and for which reliable values are available for most of the foods listed. This means that nutritive values are available for about 30 nutrients for some foods.

The printed values are an approximation of the nutrient contributions of a food, based on what is known of its composition. The values are deliberately weighted or adjusted for varietal differences, breed, stage of maturity, seasonal or geographic differences, etc., according to estimated proportions in the American food supply at the time the values are compiled. They are adjusted also for known losses in storage, trimming, manufacturing, home preparation, and handling. As a result, values are regarded as the best estimate country-wide, year-round.

Table values are only approximations; still, they are useful. A table value is useful for two purposes:

   (a) as a *standard* for comparison—The nutritive values of foods b, c, d

. . .n can be compared with the nutritive value of food a. For example, the mean ascorbic acid value for oranges is only an approximation; however, one can easily see the differences in magnitude between the mean value for oranges and the means for apples, bananas, and grapes.

(b) as a *basis* for assessing nutritional adequacy of intake—Small differences in absolute sums must be ignored. The relative difference between the expected intake (or standard such as the RDA) and the observed (or obtained sum) is what is important. For example, the obtained estimate of caloric intake is considered accurate only to the nearest 50 kcal, since reported table values are rounded to the nearest 10 kcal. Thus, intakes of 1960 and 2010 are taken as 2000, and one becomes concerned that someone whose RDA is 2000 consumes a mean of only 1000 kcal.

In the United States, a number of tables of food composition are available. Those commonly available are USDA Handbook *8*, Composition of Foods—raw, processed, prepared; Bowes and Church, Food Values of Portions Commonly Used; Home and Garden Bulletin *72*; Short Dietary Tables; and USDA Handbook *456*, Nutritive Value of American Food in Common Units. A brief description of each follows:

(a) USDA Handbook *8*—Was first published in 1963 and is the base data on which the other tables described here were developed. Data are no longer regarded as valid due to changes in varieties, breeds, processing practices, and proportions of the food supply. Moreover, the array of foods available has changed so that many reported values are irrelevant and no values are available for many foods commonly consumed.

In 1972, a national Nutrient Data Base was created at the USDA to remedy the acknowledged problem. New data have been solicited and are being accumulated and compiled for approximately 100 nutrients and related components as well as for 215 other constituents (Hertzler and Hoover 1977).

Starting in late 1976, revised sections of USDA Handbook *8* were released, beginning with No. 8-1 "Dairy and Egg Products." The 1963 data form the base; updated values replace earlier ones, where available. The records carry the date of when updating occurred as an aid to the user in assessing the weight given the value in interpreting findings. The revised food composition data are available in printed, punched card, and magnetic tape forms.

(b) Bowes and Church—Using the 1963 USDA Handbook *8* data, which are reported per 100 g portion, and information on the weight to volume relationship for the various foods as reported in USDA Home Economics Report *41*, nutritive values were recalculated for portions commonly used. Thus, values are for items listed in slices, quarts, cups, teaspoons, etc. New editions are available every few years.

(c) USDA Home and Garden Bulletin 72—The 1977 edition has been reproduced as the Appendix.

(d) Short Dietary Tables—These were developed by Leichsenring and Wilson. These use grouped data for similar items. Accuracy approximates that achieved by the long calculations using Handbook 8. Values were derived from the 1963 edition of Handbook 8.

(e) USDA Handbook 456—This was published in 1975. It contains data on approximately 1500 foods in common portions. Like Bowes and Church, its values are based largely on the 1963 Handbook 8 values. These were recalculated using the weight to volume relationships reported in USDA Home Economics Report 41. Fatty acid values are more complete than those listed in the 1963 edition of Handbook 8.

The nutrient values in the tables of food composition are useful in determining the contribution(s) of a particular food and the total intake in a given time period. However, the comparison of foods of the same caloric value in terms of the other nutrients contained is tedious and beyond the interests and ability of most people. When caloric values vary as well, the amount of calculation necessary is discouraging, even to the professional. So, a method of scoring relative nutrient density has been sought. A number of proposals are under investigation.

A NUTRITIOUS FOOD IS . . .

The available data on the nutrient contribution(s) of the various foods demonstrate that *no one food can supply all of the nutrients necessary in human nutrition*, even when consumed in large quantity. Therefore, a varied diet is necessary. And, in order to balance intake according to needs, items must be selected for their complementary contributions.

Together, the foods consumed on a given day are expected to provide (a) energy, (b) protein and minerals necessary to build and maintain body tissues, and (c) minerals and vitamins to regulate body processes. Sufficient water to replace losses should be ingested also. Nearly all foods are nourishing, i.e., they supply one of the nutrients, if only energy. A smaller but variable number of foods are considered "nutritious" or not, depending on the definition used.

The Index to Nutritional Quality (INQ) is a score used to describe the relative adequacy of a food as a source of a nutrient. The INQ represents the nutrient density of a food, i.e., the ratio of each reported nutrient to the number of calories per 100 g portion. An INQ greater than 1.0 means that the food is a significant source of that nutrient. INQs have been computed for every food in USDA Handbook 8; data from this handbook were used to derive the scores. The percentages of foods in the various food groups with INQs greater than 1.0 are shown in Table 2.1.

TABLE 2.1. PERCENTAGE OF FOODS FROM HANDBOOK 8 WITH INDEX OF NUTRITIONAL QUALITY OF 1.0 OR HIGHER

Food Classification	Number of Foods	Protein[1]	Calcium	Phosphorus	Iron	Vitamin A	Thiamin	Riboflavin	Niacin[2]	Vitamin C
Fruits	307	3.0	14.2	11.9	41.7	44.7	38.0	20.9	22.6	79.5
Vegetables	414	81.3	60.3	92.2	86.3	63.9	82.8	73.7	79.0	93.0
Grains and grain products[3]	547	36.3	10.3	47.1	28.6	2.8	40.7	12.2	26.7	2.7
Nuts, soybeans and seeds	65	73.9	32.2	86.2	56.9	6.2	58.6	32.3	33.7	9.1
Meat, fish and egg products	921	91.7	8.2	87.1	57.2	13.8	36.5	58.0	82.4	6.3
Milk products	57	84.2	85.8	85.8	0.0	61.4	20.9	84.1	0.0	5.3
Sweets and sugars	80	12.5	18.6	30.8	21.1	0.0	2.6	15.0	11.3	1.3
Fats and oils	35	9.1	11.3	11.2	2.7	22.8	0.0	8.6	0.0	8.7

Source: A.J. Wittwer, A.W. Sorenson, B.W. Wyse, and R.G. Hansen (1977). Reproduced with permission of R.G. Hansen.
[1]Protein calculated on a standard of 45 g for milk, meat, fish and egg products, 65 g otherwise.
[2]Preformed niacin.
[3]Includes pies, cakes and cookies.

The nutrient:calorie benefit ratio (NCBR) is another index that can be used to estimate how "nutritious" a food is. Other simplified tools also have been devised to assist in assessment.

There is a quantitative aspect to intake that often is given token consideration. The amount of food that a person ingests is largely determined by the intrinsic desire for food, which is called hunger. The type of food that is ingested is largely a matter of preferences which is determined by appetite for a food. Spacing of food intake is also important. A state of incipient starvation exists 12 hours after ingestion of food. This results in hunger pangs. The most recent explanation is that when blood sugar falls, stored fat in adipose tissue is mobilized and degraded to replenish blood sugar. Hunger pangs are generated as long as adipose tissue fat stores are below their customary level.

A NUTRITIOUS DIET IS . . .

A nutritious or well-balanced diet supplies needed nutrients in needed quantities from a variety of foods. A vast number of combinations of foods can be selected that will be adequate to meet the specific needs of any individual. It is both unnecessary and unwise to develop a fixed combination of foods that is adequate because, no matter how well the items are liked, the combination will become monotonous and will be rejected. And, the individual will not have developed good food habits, leaving him vulnerable when the "diet" fails because of rejection.

Most people select combinations of foods because they like the items and/or the combinations, not with regard to nutritional needs. Since nutrient intake is not controlled, it may be relatively invariate or highly variable in quality and quantity, depending on the individual's eating habits. IF it turns out that the uncontrolled intake is inadequate, THEN the individual is confronted with a need to retrain habits. But, this is difficult. People make deliberate changes in their eating habits only as a result of necessity, although unconscious changes are made continually.

The first habit that needs to be established is to consume a diet that is balanced to the extent that it contains foods from each of the Basic 4 food groups in recommended quantities. For adults, these are: milk and dairy products (2 servings), meat or meat substitute (2 servings), breads and cereals (4 servings), and fruits and vegetables (4 servings). IF people can identify the foods that belong to these food groups, THEN this most simplified model of what is necessary provides some limited assurance of nutritional balance. Some nutrients generally occur together in the plant/animal tissues commonly consumed as food, because these nutrients are necessary to the plant/animal tissue in order for it to perform its function(s) in tissue life. Fortunately, man's needs are qualitatively similar. So, until now, man's main problem just has been to get enough food. But, now that formulated foods that do *not* contain nutrients in natural proportions are available, many deficiencies can occur because of selection errors.

Since the nutrients occur together naturally in foods from the same class of natural foods, one nutrient can be selected to represent the group of nutrients that occur together. This nutrient is designated a key nutrient. IF the key nutrient is present in an adequate or planned quantity, THEN the other nutrients are expected to be present in expected quantities. This is the basis on which a simplified model such as the Basic 4 can be used. The key nutrients expected to be contributed by the Basic 4 food groups are shown in Table 2.2.

TABLE 2.2. KEY NUTRIENTS EXPECTED TO BE PROVIDED BY THE BASIC 4 FOOD GROUPS, GIVEN THE RECOMMENDED NUMBER OF SERVINGS FOR ADULTS

| Food Group | Nutrients Provided | | | |
	10-25%	25-50%	50-75%	75+%
Milk	calories vitamin A thiamin	riboflavin protein	calcium	
Meat	calories vitamin A (if liver)	protein thiamin iron riboflavin	niacin	
Fruits & Vegetables	calories calcium iron thiamin riboflavin niacin			vitamin A (if green or yellow) vitamin C (if citrus)
Bread	calories protein iron riboflavin niacin	thiamin		

Source: Adapted from USDA (1956).

A recent study of 1500 homemakers has investigated the popular definition of a well-balanced diet. The report revealed the percentages of respondents that consider each food group necessary to the definition of a well-balanced diet: vegetables/fruit (65.6%), meat/poultry/fish/eggs/beans (58.3%), milk/cheese (39.7%), and bread/cereal (26.7%). Clearly, many do not even recognize the necessity of consuming foods from each of the Basic 4 food groups. So, even this simplified concept is not well accepted. Therefore, the basic habit is not well established.

TABLE 2.3. REPORTED RESULTS' OF HOMEMAKERS' RESPONSE TO WHETHER OR NOT MILK, BEEF, GREEN PEAS, OR BREAD IS A PARTICULARLY GOOD SOURCE OF SELECTED NUTRIENTS

Key Foods[2]	Vitamin A	Thiamin	Riboflavin	Niacin	Vitamin C	Vitamin D	Protein	CHO	Fat	Kcal	Fe	Ca
Milk	26.0	6.2	6.8	4.2	7.8	42.5	41.5	10.8	34.1	27.9	12.1	76.0
Beef	7.2	10.1	12.6	6.4	2.8	4.7	83.2	12.6	46.8	30.9	46.9	6.7
Green peas	22.9	12.3	9.4	7.0	12.4	9.9	18.7	23.6	3.8	20.8	17.3	5.9
Enriched bread	19.3	32.3	32.6	23.5	9.3	15.0	24.2	44.5	21.2	49.2	15.6	19.5

[1] Adapted from detailed tabulations for the *Consumer Nutrition Knowledge Survey:* Report I 1973-74. Division of Consumer Studies, Bureau of Foods, Food and Drug Administration, Princeton, N.J. Response Analysis Corp., Contract #FDA 23-247. Adapted and included by permission. Div. Consumer Studies, Ms. Alice E. Fusillo.
[2] Indicator foods, one from each of the Basic 4 food groups.

In the same study, homemakers were asked to indicate which of a list of nutrients were provided by indicator or key foods from the Basic 4. Results are shown in Table 2.3. Then they were asked to select other listed foods that had similar composition. Results are shown in Table 2.4. Obviously, homemakers are not well informed about foods as sources of nutrients, so failure to understand and apply the Basic 4 concept is to be expected.

TABLE 2.4. REPORTED RESULTS' OF HOMEMAKERS' RESPONSE TO WHICH OTHER FOODS (LISTED ON A CARD) HAVE A LOT OF THE SAME BENEFITS TO THE BODY THAT MILK, BEEF, GREEN PEAS, BREAD HAVE

Other Foods	Milk[2] %	Beef %	Green Peas %	Enriched Bread %
Oatmeal	17.4	6.6	6.0	58.5
Fish	21.7	58.8	4.4	3.0
Rice	9.9	6.0	9.7	43.4
Navy beans	8.8	29.2	35.4	15.7
Chicken	12.9	56.2	2.6	1.8
Potatoes	9.8	5.2	17.4	55.3
Eggs	51.2	46.9	4.9	7.5
Macaroni	10.2	5.9	7.8	67.0
Pork and lamb	7.4	63.4	1.7	1.4
String beans	4.2	6.1	66.2	1.9
Carrots	7.6	4.8	49.7	2.6
Bananas	6.2	3.8	7.1	7.8
Peanut butter	23.3	46.0	5.6	11.9
Cottage cheese	83.5	18.9	3.1	7.2

[1] Adapted from detailed tabulations for the *Consumer Nutrition Knowledge Survey*: Report I 1973-74. Division of Consumer Studies, Bureau of Foods, Food and Drug Administration, Princeton, N.J. Response Analysis Corp., Contract #FDA 23-247. Adapted and included by permission, Div. Consumer Studies, Ms. Alice E. Fusillo.
[2] Indicator foods, one from each of the Basic 4 food groups.

The second habit that needs to be established is for the individual to be personally responsible for his/her nutrient intake. In general, people do not want to be responsible, so they attempt to shift responsibility by asking "Is it OK for me to eat X?" or "Should I take a vitamin/mineral supplement?" The appropriate response is to help the individual decide by supplying information and/or reminding the person of what he/she knows and of providing encouragement and support as each step of the think-through process is addressed. People also feel guilty for having given in to desire. So, they say, "I know I shouldn't eat X, but ..." or "I ate an ice cream cone today." The appropriate response is to help the individual accept the need to compensate by supplying information on expected outcomes of various alternative ways of dealing with the fact and by providing encouragement and support as each part of the think-through process is addressed.

Whether a person should or should not or did or did not eat X is *not* a moral issue. It is not bad or good in some absolute sense. It is only good or bad as a part of a pattern in relation to need for specific nutrients, given what else the person has eaten, is eating, or is likely to eat that day. Some choices are wiser than others, some are less expensive, some result in an excess of unwanted nutrients, and some are good in theory only as they are likely to be unacceptable.

IF a person will find out what nutrients he/she is likely to be short of, given usual food habits, and will get a list of good sources of these, THEN he/she can know what alternatives are available in selecting for them. People vary in the amount of effort they will make to improve the nutritional quality of their diet. The details of the process are outlined in Unit IV. However, everybody can do the minimum.

The minimum involves a quick label check prior to selection—it takes almost no time and does not require changes in eating habits or life-style. IF nothing else, THEN they can improve by deliberate selection as follows:

(a) milk and butter or margarine that are *fortified* with vitamins A and D

(b) bread and cereal products that are *enriched* with B vitamins and iron

(c) salt that is *iodized*.

Probably less than 16% of the population is so lacking in interest and/or ability as to be unable to exceed this minimum.

Probably about 50% can and will do more. An instructional program should create an awareness, understanding, and appreciation of (a) the normal changing needs of people at different stages of the life cycle, (b) increased needs associated with normal expected stresses such as pregnancy, injury, illness, etc., and (c) dietary modifications for prevention and treatment of common chronic diseases, so that the individual will be receptive to specific instruction should it become necessary or desirable. The Basic 4, the need to monitor and control intakes of vitamins A and C, and the need for consumption of a variety of natural foods—these concepts form the basis for an average program of nutrient intake control.

Probably another 16% will show extraordinary interest in food, nutrition, and life expectancy. In addition to the above topics, an instructional program should create awareness, understanding, and appreciation of (a) the roles of all nutrients in human nutrition, (b) common sources of the various nutrients, (c) use of nutrition labeling in food selection, (d) nutrient conservation through good food handling and preparation techniques, and (e) monitoring and controlling strategies.

Clearly, since people differ in levels of interest and ability in relation to shaping their food ecology to achieve control of their nutrient intake, a graduated series of presentations is needed. Both depth and breadth need to be expanded progressively in order to meet the needs of those with greater interest and ability in understanding food as a source of nutrients. Until now, presentations have seemed to remain at the lowest common denominator, and breadth was added by scheduling presentations of whatever topics were in vogue. What is needed is a master plan with a matrix of topics and levels. Perhaps a series of certificates could be issued for each section of topics. By making these graduated series, they might be effective in rewarding people and motivating them to continued development.

DELIBERATE DESIGN

At the present time, in the United States we have the technological capability of producing whatever array of plant, animal, and/or formulated foods is necessary to satisfy the desires of the American people. The array of alternatives offered is and will continue to be determined by the variability in underlying values that determine which characteristics are critical variables in food selection. The foods available will have the characteristics that make them sell. IF nutrient contribution is a determining characteristic, all other things being equal, THEN at least it will be controlled. Ideally, nutrient contribution would be controlled at the desired level and other attributes, e.g., color, flavor, texture, cost, would be optimized to encourage selection of nutritious foods.

At the present time, in the United States we also have the technological capability of producing food that contains food additives included by deliberate design to reduce the unwanted effects of self-indulgence. For example, a cariostatic can be added to pre-sweetened cereals. A 1% sodium diacid phosphate content significantly reduces the incidence of decayed, missing, or filled surfaces of teeth. Proponents accept human weakness and support the position that cereal manufacturers should deal with its effects. Opponents accept human weakness and support the position that cereal manufacturers should not create/maintain a situation that rewards it. Which do we want?

BIBLIOGRAPHY

ADAMS, C.F. 1975. Nutritive value of American foods in common units. USDA Agric. Handb. *456*. Washington, D.C.

CHURCH, C.F., and CHURCH, H.N. 1975. Bowes & Church Food Values of Portions Commonly Used. 12th edition. J.B. Lippincott Co., Philadelphia.

CONSUMER AND FOOD ECONOMICS INST. 1976. Composition of foods—raw, processed, prepared. USDA Agric. Handb. *8* (rev. sections). Washington, D.C.

CORT, W.M. *et al.* 1976. Nutrient stability of fortified cereal products. Food Technol. *30*, 52-53, 56, 58, 60, 62.

COUNCIL ON FOODS AND NUTRITION, AMA. 1971. Symposium on Vitamins and Minerals in Processed Foods. Tulane University, New Orleans. March 22-24, 1971. Am. Med. Assoc.

DE RITTER, E. 1976. Stability characteristics of vitamins in processed foods. Food Technol. *30* (1) 48-50, 52.

HANSEN, R.G., WYSE, B.W., and SORENSEN, A.W. 1979. Nutritional Quality Index of Foods. AVI Publ. Co., Westport, Ct.

HERTZLER, A.A., and HOOVER, L.W. 1977. Development of food tables and use with computers. Review of nutrient data bases. J. Am. Dietet. Assoc. *70*, 20-31.

USDA. 1956. Essentials of an adequate diet . . . facts for nutrition programs. ARS-62-4. USDA, Washington, D.C.

USDA. 1977. Average weight of a measured cup of various foods. USDA Home Econ. Res. Rept. *41*. GPO, Washington, D.C.

USDA. 1977. Nutritive value of foods. USDA Home & Garden Bull. 72. GPO, Washington, D.C.

WITTWER, A.J., SORENSON A.W., WYSE, B.W., and HANSEN, R.G. 1977. Nutrient density—evaluation of nutritional attributes of foods. J. Nutr. Educ. *9*, 26-30.

3

Control of Nutrient Supply and Demand

Nutrients may be supplied to the tissues of the human body, from external or exogenous sources, by four basic methods: (a) ingestion, digestion, and absorption from the gastrointestinal (GI) tract, (b) intestinal production and absorption, e.g., vitamins such as vitamin K, (c) intravenous drip, and (d) periodic injection, e.g., vitamin B_{12}. Of these, only the ingestion/digestion/absorption method is of nutritional importance to normal healthy people. Intestinal production is highly variable within and among people, depending on the nature of the bacterial culture and its growth conditions, so it cannot be relied on to produce nutrients other than vitamin K in any significant quantity. Intravenous drip is reserved for treatment of hospitalized patients. Injection is usually used only in treating those who are in grave need or, in the case of vitamin B_{12}, either vegetarians who have no dietary source of supply or those with pernicious anemia who are unable to absorb it. Therefore, subsequent discussion of exogenous sources will be limited to the ingestion/digestion/absorption sequence.

Nutrients may be supplied to tissues of the human body from internal or endogenous sources. Provision is by removal from stores or by synthesis. Which method will predominate, in a given instance, depends on supply/demand status.

Nutrient supply to the tissues of the body is maintained by an elaborate transport system that is controlled by a monitoring and control system. This system is linked to nutrient conservation and excretion subsystems. As a result, the circulating level of most nutrients is regulated within established ranges as long as supply is adequate but not excessive. Outside of these ranges, compensatory actions may result in abnormal responses.

REGULATION OF FOOD INTAKE

Regulation of food intake is a very complex phenomenon that can be viewed from several levels of organization. The emotional and psychological components that interact with aesthetic, cultural, socioeconomic, and other parameters are discussed in Chapters 16 through 18. The means of assessing their effects and determining whether adjustments are necessary are discussed in Chapters 18 through 21. An overall model of the physiologic processes involved is presented here. Details of selected aspects are discussed in other chapters in relation to nutrient supply/demand at cellular and tissue levels.

The mechanism by which food intake is regulated is unknown. However, a two-component model has been developed by Van Itallie, Smith, and Quartermain (1977).

The short-term component limits the nature and quantity of food ingested at a feeding according to physical capacity of the organs of the gastrointestinal tract. Capacity is determined to some extent by the nature and quantity of customary intake. Stated another way, this is the historical usage of muscles of the gastrointestinal tract, enzymes and hormones secreted during the process of digestion and absorption, and perhaps the quantities of enzymes and hormones used in processing the incoming nutrient flow. Thus, IF one habitually sparingly consumes a low-fat, high-carbohydrate diet and for once consumes a rich, full meal, THEN one will experience discomfort. This is because the short-term capacity is limited due to the habitual historical usage associated with sparing intake. One could become habituated to the rich type of meal, but other effects might be observed, since the will would be overruling the food intake regulatory mechanism.

For purposes of discussion, the regulatory activities associated with the short-term component may be conceptualized as occurring in two different phases. During the "pre-absorptive phase," the stretch receptors of the stomach are activated and produce a signal acknowledging food intake. In the small intestine, presence of fat results in secretion of two hormones that signal satiety and ultimately inhibit appetite. Osmoreceptors respond to the presence of electrolytes and other small molecules and send signals to inhibit gastric emptying rate. During the "absorptive phase," in some unknown way, signals from absorbed nutrients appear to affect the onset of feelings of satiety and also their duration.

The long-term component controls the nature and quantity of food and eating frequency. Desires are regulated according to the need to replenish nutrient stores. Desires are determined to some extent by the nature and quantity of customary intake. Stated another way, this is the historical usage by muscles in physical activity, metabolic processing that sustains life, including tissue maintenance, etc. Thus, IF one habitually consumes a diet adjusted to needs, THEN balance will be maintained by an accommodating eating frequency and food selection. Otherwise, food seeking may become urgent or frantic and will overrule the dictates of the nutrient supply/demand based food regulatory mechanism.

At the present time, obesity is a major problem of Americans. So, regulation of food intake has been investigated solely with respect to regulation of caloric intake. Only the limited fragments of the regulatory mechanism related to caloric intake have begun to emerge. Since there are interrelationships with respect to uptake and/or metabolism between and among several, if not all, nutrients, current models represent only a limited first approximation.

INGESTION

At the present time, the eating habits of Americans present a tremendous challenge to the GI tract because (a) we eat in a hurry with the result that the bolus of food that is swallowed is often a lumpy mass of marginally chewed food, (b) a large proportion of the food consumed is highly refined to uniform small particles that pack in a solid lump unless quickly dispersed during chewing by a large volume of fluid, (c) the proportion of deep fat fried foods consumed is high and these are characterized by a thick fat coating around a mixed cereal casing that retards the rate of penetration by digestive juices, and (d) we eat "busy" foods such as salty sunflower seeds and dry cereals that stimulate the flow of saliva and gastric juice but provide little substance for them to work on. The result is that digestion is unnecessarily difficult.

DIGESTION

The processes of digesting food facilitate (a) the liberation of nutrients from their food matrix, (b) presentation of the nutrients to the absorptive surface, and (c) removal of indigestible portions. Digestion is complex due to the diversity of food material to be digested and the number of actions involved. A food's structure determines the complexity of the process involved in digesting it. Physical and/or chemical bonds have to be broken in order to liberate the various nutrients from their food matrix so that they can be absorbed.

The simple structures of food emulsions, foams, and gels are easily broken. Milk is a food emulsion in which fat droplets are dispersed in a watery mixture of protein, carbohydrate (sugar), minerals, and vitamins;

the emulsion is broken by the action of the digestive juices in coagulating the protein. A fruit whip is an example of a food foam in which air is trapped within a protein film containing carbohydrate (sugar), minerals, and vitamins; the foam is broken by compression during swallowing and mixing in the stomach. A gelatin dessert is a gel in which a solid structure of protein holds a watery solution of carbohydrate (sugar); the gel structure is broken by heat (body temperature is above the refrigeration storage temperature) and mixing in the stomach. Even the more complex food foams such as angel food cake or puffy omelets and food gels such as puddings are broken more easily than the structures of plant and animal tissues.

In plant and animal tissues, nutrients are located in one of three places according to the functions they serve in the life of the tissue. Some nutrients may be in the spaces between tissues, as in the case of electrolytes such as sodium which are dissolved in the extracellular fluid; when the tissue walls are broken by a combination of cooking, mastication, and/or penetration by digestive juices, these are liberated. Other nutrients may be an integral part of the cell structure itself, as in the case of lipoproteins and glycoproteins; the cell wall itself must be degraded by the digestive juices in order to begin liberation of these nutrient complexes. Nutrients such as starch and fat are found inside storage cells whereas many proteins, minerals, and vitamins are part of enzymes in the active parts of cells, and mineral ions may be free in the intracellular fluid. To begin liberation of these nutrients, the cell walls must be broken by cooking, mastication, and/or penetration by digestive juices.

Once the food structures have been broken down, further processing usually is necessary because most nutrients normally can be absorbed only in their free form. Thus, NaCl, which is present in the watery digestive mixture as the Na^+ and Cl^- ions, is in a form that allows immediate absorption. In contrast, the majority of nutrients exist as complex molecules containing several nutrients or are polymers, so the chemical bonds must be broken. On the other hand, the watery digestive mixture also allows nutrients to come together and form insoluble complexes that cannot be absorbed; iron and calcium complex with phytic acid in this way.

The alimentary canal is a long, elastic tubular passage of irregular dimensions, extending from the mouth where digestion and absorption may begin to the anus where residual wastes are expelled (Fig. 3.1). Within the confines of this passageway, food structures are broken down and nutrients are liberated by a combination of mechanical and chemical actions. The mechanical aspects of digestion include normal muscle tone, a low level force that keeps the mass in motion, and peristalsis, a strong periodic force that propels the mass along. These are under neural control

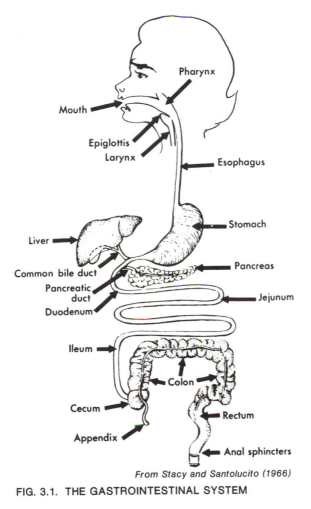

From Stacy and Santolucito (1966)

FIG. 3.1. THE GASTROINTESTINAL SYSTEM

Note the relative position of the successive parts.

and determine the rate of GI motility which, under normal conditions, is a rate that allows normal digestion and absorption efficiencies. The chemical aspects of digestion include actions by enzymes, strong acids and bases, and wetting agents—all of which are solutions secreted by specialized cells and glands. Both mechanical and chemical aspects are facilitated by the secretion of (a) mucus, which is a lubricant and provides a physical barrier that prevents digestion of the walls of the GI tract and (b) water, which is a solvent and dispersing medium that facilitates interaction of enzymes and food substrates.

Digestion in the Mouth and Esophagus

The role of the mouth and esophagus in converting food to absorbable nutrients is almost limited to pre-treatment to facilitate safe delivery to the first processing center. Both mechanical and chemical forces are involved. In addition, a small amount of starch is degraded to maltose, but this conversion is not nutritionally important.

Mechanical Aspects.—The degree of mastication, which mechanically divides solids, determines whether the bolus that is swallowed can move easily down the esophagus, which is like a gravity chute. A solid, a semi-solid, or a pasty mass can be swallowed but the consistency is important. Smaller particles are (a) more easily moved along by peristalsis and are unlikely to get caught (a particle caught in the esophagus causes choking and one caught in a diverticulum causes an ulcer), (b) more easily dispersed in the watery gastric juices, and (c) have a greater surface area available for chemical attack in the stomach and small intestine.

Chemical Aspects.—Saliva is secreted by the salivary glands in the mouth. It contains mucus which is a lubricating and binding agent and a starch-splitting enzyme, *ptyalin*. Psychological, physical, and chemical stimuli are involved in control of the secretion of saliva. When no stimulation occurs, a fairly constant but low volume of dilute but viscous saliva is secreted. The thought of tasty food stimulates a copius flow of a somewhat thinner consistency. The flow may continue or not, depending on whether the thought is pursued or repressed or followed with food-getting actions and food consumption. The presence of food introduces both physical stimuli (the wetness of the oral tissues is decreased) and chemical stimuli (pepper bites and leads to swallowing to remove the irritant, salt dries, etc.); as a result, the flow is varied to maintain effective swallowing activity. Strong emotions such as fear, anger, and worry may decrease the volume of saliva, impairing the capacity to swallow.

Digestion in the Stomach

The stomach is the first processing center involved in the actual conversion of food to absorbable nutrients. The functions of the stomach are to (a) store the ingested food mass temporarily, (b) mix and disperse it in liquid, and (c) extrude it into the small intestine for further processing. Both mechanical and chemical forces are involved in these processing actions.

Mechanical Aspects.—The muscles in the walls of the stomach are arranged to facilitate its three basic functions of temporary storage, mixing, and controlled emptying. The walls are elastic and stretch so as to accommodate what otherwise would be an excessive volume of food, as well as mix it and move it into the small intestine. The mixture entering from the esophagus is thick and nearly solid. By means of a series of contractions, gastric juice is gradually mixed with it, progressively diluting portions at the leading edge to a semi-fluid consistency as they move toward the pyloric end. The pressure of the contractions moves portions in both directions from the area of contraction. The portion moved back mixes into the remainder and the portion moved forward extrudes into the small intestine. Liquids and carbohydrates, which are hydrophilic or water-loving, are easily dispersed and diluted to a suitable consistency for emptying. Large particles as well as proteins and fats, which are hydrophobic or water-hating, are less easily dispersed.

Emptying of the stomach is controlled by the receptivity of the duodenum to an influx of additional material to be digested and the consistency of the mixture. The receptivity of the duodenum depends on the amount, the acidity, and the composition of material already there.

In the stomach, a large mass of food reduces the efficiency of mixing and moving it to the pyloric end. This allows a longer period of time for contact with the gastric secretions which increases the likelihood of adequate action. But, when the contact time with the mucosa is increased, some irritation occurs, which results in increased force and frequency of contractions in order to remove the irritant. This increases efficiency somewhat.

IF the mass is small, or low acid, or mainly carbohydrate, THEN the processing required in the duodenum and subsequent segments of the small intestine is not great, so an additional quantity can be accepted for processing. As a result, the muscles of the duodenum are relaxed compared to those of the stomach. So, peristalsis propels an additional quantity into the small intestine, if it is fluid enough to move easily. Proteins require greater than normal contact with gastric secretions in order for digestion to be complete. If the mixture is hypertonic then it will draw fluid into the alimentary tract in order to equalize osmotic pressure, but at the same time this would dangerously disturb electrolyte and water balance in surrounding tissues. For these reasons, gastric peristalsis is temporarily inhibited until duodenal readiness to process an additional portion is achieved. In this way, the rate of stomach emptying is regulated so that the small intestine's efficiency in liberation and absorption of nutrients is controlled.

As noted above, when the mixture is irritating to the gastric mucosa, gastric peristalsis is increased to remove the irritant by propelling it toward the small intestine. But, at the same time the duodenum is non-receptive, which adds a force to inhibit gastric peristalsis. When this force is greater, stasis or a slowing/stoppage of normal movement occurs. If this results in prolonged contact of the irritant with the mucosa, a localized ulceration results.

Chemical Aspects.—Gastric secretions from several types of glands in the mucosal lining of the stomach include (a) thick mucus for coating and binding food particles and lubricating actions; (b) a concentrated solution of hydrochloric acid (HCl) for attacking some chemical bonds and for reducing the pH to allow activation of some enzymes; and (c) enzymes such as the inactive *pepsiongen* that is activated in acid medium to its active enzyme form *pepsin*. Pepsin attacks the chemical bonds that maintain protein structure in raw and properly cooked foods; it is ineffective with proteins that have been denatured at very high temperatures, e.g., the frizzled edges of improperly fried eggs. A tributyrinase is also secreted. Its purpose is to degrade tributyrin in butter fat, but its activity is insignificant nutritionally since butterfat consumption is low. Glands at the pyloric end secrete an additional quantity of thin mucus for lubrication, and other specialized cells secrete a very thick mucus to protect the lining from the corrosive effects of HCl.

Psychological, physical, and chemical stimuli are involved in control of the volume and composition of gastric secretions. When no stimulation is present, the secretion of dilute gastric juice is continuous at a low level. Psychological responses cause nerve stimulation of the gastric glands: the thought of a tasty meal, anger, and hostility result in increased flow whereas fear and depression result in decreased flow. The physical presence of food in the stomach creates tactile stimulation of the mucosa and distension excites nerve reflexes; both stimulate secretion. Chemical stimulation by gastric secretogogues, i.e., coffee, alcohol, and meat extractives, causes release of the hormone *gastrin* which increases the quantity of HCl secreted, until the pH drops to 2.0. When this happens, the cells of the duodenum respond to the low pH of the incoming mixture by stimulating secretion of the hormone *enterogastrone*, which inhibits secretion of HCl. When irritation of the gastric mucosa occurs, for any reason, the quantity of mucus secreted is markedly increased.

Digestion in the Small Intestine

The small intestine is the major center for converting partially degraded food to absorbable nutrients. Several kinds of mechanical and chemical actions are involved in the digestive processes.

Mechanical Aspects.—Five types of mechanical action are produced by several kinds of muscles in the wall of the small intestine. Stretch pressure from the undigested mass and hormones activates the nerves that control the intensity and regularity of the mechanical action. The types of mechanical action are: (a) segmentation, a result of contraction and relaxation of alternate segments of the circular muscles forming rings, is the mechanism by which digestive secretions are cut in; (b) spiral movement by the long muscles that run in a long counterclockwise spiral around the passageway mixes the mass and brings additional molecules close to the wall for absorption; (c) pendular movements by small local muscles, in which the mass is moved back and forth in a rocking motion that mixes the mass; (d) peristalsis, which is a series of waves of contraction and relaxation that propel the undigested mass analward a short distance, as a result of major contractions of the circular muscles; and (e) villi movement, an alternate extension and retraction of the finger-like projections on the surface of the intestinal wall that is controlled by the hormone *villikinen*, which mixes the layer next to the wall, bringing it into contact with the absorptive sites.

The rate at which the partially digested mass is moved along the small intestine is regulated by the rate of entry from the stomach. Distension in the duodenum results in greater intensity of peristaltic waves in order to spread the mass along the alimentary canal. Irritation, hypertonicity, and too large a volume can cause a massive propulsion to remove the entire mass.

The combination of the five basic types of continuous movement is necessary to facilitate substrate-reagent interactions, since several hours elapse during passage along the alimentary canal. The particles to be broken down are of variable density, so some will settle out and some will float, reducing contact with the digestive secretions. Moreover, the quantity of nutrient to be liberated is large. When a reaction is complete, the products must be removed and a new set of substrate and reagents brought together. The constant motion facilitates this action. And, finally, when the material to be digested is spread out in a continuous mass over a considerable area, the digestive actions proceed more rapidly than when the mass is packed into a small area. This is because mixing with the digestive secretions is more efficient, thus facilitating the substrate-reagent interactions. Moreover, the spreading also facilitates dispersal for absorption. Sufficient liquid and indigestible fiber aid mechanical action by diluting the mass and preventing packing.

Chemical Aspects.—Intestinal secretions, bile, and pancreatic secretions are involved in the digestion of chyme, the semi-fluid mass of partially digested food that has been expelled by the stomach into the small intestine. A combination of tactile, neural, and hormonal stimuli regulates the composition and flow of the intestinal secretions (Fig. 3.2). Bile secretion is under hormonal control alone, whereas the pancreatic secretions are regulated by both neural and hormonal stimulation.

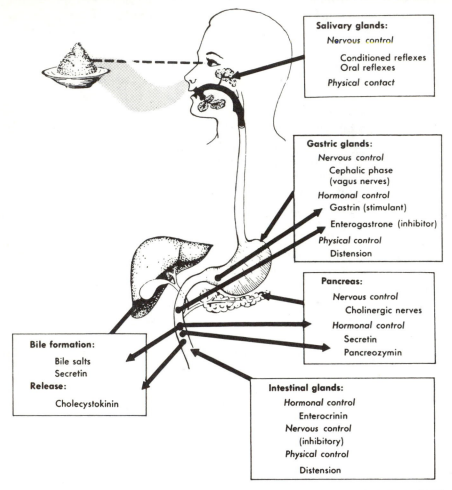

From Stacy and Santolucito (1966)

FIG. 3.2. SUMMARY OF FACTORS INFLUENCING SECRETIONS OF THE GASTROINTESTINAL GLANDS

Mucosal glands located at the upper end of the duodenum produce large quantities of mucus to protect the mucosa from corrosion (ulceration) by the acid chyme which is extruded from the stomach at this point. Other mucosal glands, throughout the length of the small intestine, secrete additional mucus when tactile stimulation or irritation occurs.

The epithelial cells of the mucosa contain the digestive enzymes, and appear to complete digestion during absorption *through* the epithelium. The classes of enzymes contained within the epithelial cells are:

(a) *intestinal lipase*—This enzyme degrades fats to a variety of mono- and diglycerides as well as saturated mono- and polyunsaturated fatty acid fragments. Attached lecithin, choline, and the various fat-soluble vitamins also are liberated.

(b) *intestinal peptidases*—These enzymes degrade peptides. *Amino peptidase* breaks the peptide bond, removing terminal amino acids from peptides. A *nucleosidase* splits nucleosides into their component purine or pyrimidine bases and a 5-carbon sugar. A specialized protease, *enterokinase*, converts inactive *trypsinogen* into active *trypsin*.

(c) *disaccharidases*—These split the four double sugars maltose, sucrose, isomaltose, and lactose to their single sugar components.

(d) *intestinal amylase*—A small amount is available for splitting carbohydrate polymers into disaccharides.

(e) *intestinal phosphatase*—This splits off phosphate.

Bile is an alkaline fluid containing bile salts, bile acids, bile pigments, and cholesterol. It is produced continuously in the liver, is stored in the gallbladder, and is emptied into the upper end of the small intestine via the common bile duct. The presence of fat in the chyme causes the intestinal mucosal glands to secrete the hormone *cholecystokinen-pancreozymin*. This is the major stimulus that causes the gallbladder to contract, emptying the bile into the common bile duct. The function of bile is to emulsify fats and their hydrophobic or water-hating breakdown products. Emulsification is necessary because the fats and their breakdown products must be dispersed as fine particles in the watery medium so that the lipase can penetrate and progressively degrade them. Emulsification of the final fragments also is necessary for absorption. Most of the bile salts are reabsorbed from the large intestine, which is important in maintaining the normal flow of bile.

The pancreatic secretions are produced outside the small intestine and are secreted into the upper end via the pancreatic ducts. These secretions contain a number of enzymes, are of variable alkalinity, and provide additional mucus to protect the intestinal wall from alkaline corrosion. The kinds of enzymes secreted are:

(a) *pancreatic lipase*—This augments the actions of the intestinal lipase.

(b) *proteases*—These degrade proteins. *Trypsin* causes initial breakdown of proteins and polypeptides and initiates the conversion of inactive *chymotrypsinogen* to active *chymotrypsin*. Carboxypeptidases remove terminal amino acids from peptides by attacking the carboxyl group that links the last two amino acids. Nucleases convert nucleic acids to nucleosides.

(c) *pancreatic amylases*—α-amylase hydrolyzes the interior bonds of (a) amylose randomly yielding a mixture of glucose and maltose, and (b) amylopectin randomly yielding a mixture of branched and unbranched polysaccharides of variable chain length. β-amylase hydrolyzes polysaccharides from the nonreducing end of the chain: (a) amylose is broken down to maltose and (b) amylopectin yields maltose and highly branched dextrins, since it can act only on the α-1,4 linkages up to between two and three residues of the α-1,6 linkages.

The hormone *secretin*, which is produced in the mucosal cells of the duodenum, is released in response to the presence of chyme. It stimulates the release of the pancreatic secretions and regulates their pH by varying the quantity of sodium bicarbonate, which dissociates into carbon dioxide and water. The carbon dioxide is absorbed and the sodium combines with the chloride ion to form sodium chloride—a neutral salt. This reaction corrects the pH of the entering chyme to 8.0 by neutralizing the HCl. As a result of the alkaline pH, the action of pepsin is attenuated, which protects the mucosa from corrosion. Also, this pH is optimal for activation of the pancreatic enzymes. However, it destroys some of the vitamins so that if they have not been previously absorbed, they become unavailable.

Within 4 hours of ingestion, the first portion of chyme has traversed the approximately 21-foot length of the small intestine and digestion of this portion is complete, although some digestible material may remain. Nutrients have been liberated from their food matrix by a combination of mechanical and chemical actions. These have been presented to the absorptive surfaces by constant mechanical action. When the residue passes into the large intestine at this point, digestion ends, since no additional enzymes are available for participation in the reactions.

ABSORPTION

Nutrients are absorbed *into* the body through the cells of the walls of the alimentary canal. The term *absorb* means to suck up, which is an active process such as active transport, or take in, which is a passive process such as diffusion. Absorption of nutrients occurs in the small and large intestine. Only alcohol and some fat-soluble substances, primarily drugs, can be absorbed from the stomach.

Absorption from the Small Intestine

The small intestine is the primary site of nutrient absorption. Its structure is uniquely fitted for the various tasks involved. It provides a maximum external surface area for contact with the chyme as well as integral internal units involved in its functions which include induction, processing, transport, storage, packaging, and distribution.

Structure.—The area of the mucosal surface, which forms the walls of the alimentary canal, is about 600 times as great per segment as is the area of its corresponding serosal surface. This increase is a result of (a) convoluted folds which extend the basic area inward, (b) a covering of the surface with villi, and (c) a covering of the surface of the villi with microvilli which resemble bristles of a brush so are referred to as the brush border.

Within the intestinal wall is a vascular network that includes arterial capillaries, venous capillaries, and lacteals, which are small lymph vessels. The arterial capillary flow is involved in the control of the uptake of several nutrients because the circulating level of some nutrients, e.g., iron, calcium, and vitamin D in its active form, provides feedback that determines the efficiency with which these nutrients will be absorbed. The venous capillaries are involved in removal of absorbed nutrients; the gradient between absorption rate and removal rate acts as brakes on absorption. The lacteals are involved in removal of absorbed fats and fat-soluble nutrients, via the lymphatic system.

Functions.—Induction is the first step in absorption. The continuous movement of the chyme maintains a surface layer of liberated nutrients in contact with the absorptive surface. The brush border is covered with a variety of specialized absorptive sites that can accept and process a particular kind, or at most a few kinds, of molecules. The concentration of a particular nutrient depends on its proportion in the food ingested and its liberation rate. IF the concentration is greater than the absorption rate, THEN the effect is similar to that observed with waiting lines anywhere. As the lines build up, pressure develops at the processing unit. At this point, it becomes inefficient due to problems in supply of other materials involved in the processing and in removal of processed products. Irritation results and reject signals are sent to relieve the pressure. At the same time, retardation of the absorption rate has a negative feedback effect which temporarily reduces the liberation rate.

In general, those nutrients that are absorbed by an active transport process are absorbed more rapidly and more completely than those absorbed by diffusion. The active process requires an energy input and involves a carrier(s) in an exchange process. Some competition for carriers exists, which allows for a selectivity that increases the efficiency in uptake of those nutrients that historically have been scarce. Lines move fastest in inducting these. The diffusion process allows nutrients whose concentration is greater in the alimentary tract than in the venous flow to migrate along the gradient. Since the capillary exchange provides and removes a liquid that is usually of a lower concentration, the diffusion process is important in nutrient induction.

Processing differs for each class of nutrients absorbed. A brief sketch will be presented here with elaboration of details in subsequent chapters concerning each of the nutrients.

Carbohydrates are absorbed by an active transport process which selects some monosaccharides for preferential and rapid transport into the mucosal cell. There is competition among the various monosaccharides, so an excess of one that is transported preferentially may preclude uptake of others because the mass moves past the absorption area before the carriers are free.

Proteins are *not* absorbed as such, except rarely. They must be degraded to amino acids; dipeptides are absorbed to a very limited extent. Both selectivity and competition are characteristic. Absorption is very rapid and depends on the liberation rate.

Fats are usually degraded to fatty acids and monoglycerides prior to absorption. The absorption mechanism has been explained as follows: the fatty acid or monoglyceride is dissolved in the lipid portion of the cell wall and diffuses through it to the interior where it is used in synthesis of new triglycerides which are then coated with a protein envelope and discharged into the lacteals for transport via the lymphatic system. The fat-soluble vitamins are absorbed along with the fats.

Minerals are absorbed in the upper areas of the small intestine. The monovalent ions, e.g., sodium, potassium, and chlorine, are more readily absorbed than the polyvalent ions, e.g., calcium, magnesium, zinc, chromium. Similarly, nitrates, bicarbonates, etc., are absorbed more readily than sulfates, citrates, etc. Sodium, calcium, and iron are definitely known to be actively absorbed; whether others are actively absorbed is unknown.

The site of absorption of the water-soluble vitamins is known, but the mechanism is not, except for B_{12}. The water-soluble vitamins, except for B_{12}, are absorbed at the upper end of the small intestine. B_{12} is absorbed from the lower end of the small intestine.

Water flows back and forth across the intestinal wall by osmosis in order to maintain osmotic equilibrium between the body fluids and intestinal fluids. Therefore, when salty foods are consumed, water is drawn into the intestine and remains until the sodium is absorbed. When glucose and electrolytes are actively absorbed, the osmolality of the chyme is progressively decreased, so water is progressively absorbed.

Transport of glucose and amino acids within the cells of the intestinal wall is effected by means of exchange of sodium carriers. The mechanism is referred to as the sodium pump because the exchange provides the energy for moving the glucose and amino acids through the cell. Three different systems have been identified for the three different classes of amino acids. The importance of and need for these separate systems is not known.

A storage mechanism in the cells of the intestinal wall has been identified for iron. Whether storage mechanisms exist for other nutrients is unknown. The details of the storage mechanism are under investigation, but some points are accepted as true. Iron is stored in a storage compound, ferritin. When the oxygen carrying capacity of the arterial blood that supplies the mucosal cell is low, iron is released from the ferritin for incorporation into hemoglobin to correct the problem. This special mechanism is compensatory in nature. Since dietary iron supply is usually low as well as irregular, this mechanism allows augmented uptake when available, which increases the efficiency of absorption. Details will follow in the chapter on iron.

As of now, it seems that the packaging function is limited to fats, fatty acids, and fat-soluble vitamins. Since these are hydrophobic, and blood is a water-based fluid with both dissolved and suspended materials, they would not be compatible and would float. If fats were to float, this would interfere with transport efficiency. So, packaging is used to overcome the problem. By packaging the fats with a lipoprotein (or fat-protein) in which the lipid portion binds to the fat and the protein portion binds to the water of the blood, fats can be dispersed in a fine emulsion that facilitates transport and subsequent processing at their destination.

The main distribution system for incoming nutrients is via the portal blood flow. The blood is collected from the capillary bed associated with the intestinal tract into the portal vein which carries the blood from the digestive organs to the liver. This flow is a rapid current that picks up and carries away loose items in its path, e.g., minerals and sugars which dissolve, amino acids and water-soluble vitamins which are dispersed, and short- and medium-chain fatty acids which are dispersed as an emulsion.

A second system is used for distribution of long-chain fatty acids, lecithin, cholesterol, and fat-soluble vitamins. These are packaged droplets called chylomicrons. They are picked up from the lacteals, pumped through the thoracic duct, and emptied into the main veins of the neck and proceed from there.

Absorption from the Large Intestine or Colon

The large intestine is a secondary site of nutrient absorption. Its structure allows limited kinds of absorption throughout the first half of its length, which is called the absorbing colon. Absorption is the first step in preparation for the colon's main function, formation of feces. Fecal loss of nutrients varies with nutrient density of the chyme and inversely with absorption efficiency of the small intestine. Discussion is limited to the function of the absorbing colon, since this is the function that is most pertinent to nutritional status of man.

When the chyme reaches the ileocecal valve, which regulates emptying of the intestinal contents into the colon, it backs up until another meal is consumed. Then, peristalsis in this area is intensified and gradually forces the chyme through into the colon where it is now called feces. Distension in the absorbing colon or an irritant in the colon, other portions of the GI tract, or kidneys can delay or prevent passage of the chyme into the colon. Thus, instead of a reflex rejection, the passage of chyme is retarded. This promotes maximum absorption of nutrients that may be needed for repair. Moreover, movement in the absorbing colon is sluggish, which further facilitates absorption.

Mechanical Aspects.—Two classes of mechanical action are involved in moving the contents of the absorbing colon: mixing and propulsion. The rate of passage, controlled by the intensity of the mechanical action, determines absorption efficiency and, therefore, the consistency of the feces.

The mixing movements involve localized contraction of both circular and longitudinal muscles. Intense contraction in one small area forces the contents to turn over into an adjacent area, ballooning it out in order to accommodate the additional material. Then, the action is repeated in a nearby area. The effect is to continually expose a new surface of the mass to the absorptive surface. By this means nutrients are progressively removed and are carried away on the inside by the portal blood flow.

The propulsive movements in the colon differ from the peristaltic waves in the rest of the GI tract. They are mass movements and are so called. Mass movements are initiated primarily in the duodenum, although a gastric reflex is also involved. Muscle stimulation in response to the presence of chyme in the duodenum travels to the colon. Frequency and intensity are greatest after a period when no food is consumed. Thus, for those who consume daily meals, the observed action follows the first meal of the day. Intensive sustained contraction in a localized area that is distended moves the mass ahead of this point analward about 8 in. before relaxation occurs.

Chemical Aspects.—Mucus, water, and electrolytes are secreted by the cells of the colonic mucosa. Mucus secretion is regulated by tactile stimulation of localized nerves in response to irritation and general nerve stimulation of emotional-psychological origin. Here again, the functions of mucus are protection of the mucosal cells from the corrosive actions of the alkaline feces and variable acidity produced by colon bacteria, lubrication, and binding of the mass. Water and electrolytes are secreted in response to irritation. The water dilutes the feces and the electrolytes retain it in the feces. The increased volume of the feces causes a mass movement which removes the cause of irritation by a flushing action.

Nutrients absorbed from the colon are:

(a) sodium—It is absorbed by an active and highly efficient process which absorbs almost all present. As in the small intestine, osmotic pressure then causes water and negative mineral ions such as chloride to be absorbed.

(b) glucose—It is produced in small quantity by bacterial degradation of cellulose.

(c) vitamin K, thiamin, and riboflavin—These are produced to support bacterial life and become available when bacteria die and decompose.

This completes discussion of the ingestion/digestion/absorption sequence by which nutrients are supplied to the body from external sources. Discussion will now proceed to internal supply system.

PROVISION

Good nutrition at the cellular level means supply of the correct assortment of nutrients in the proper ratio and quantity at the right time in relation to need. Since the body has an uncountable number of cells, the cumulative and aggregate effect is a continuous but variable demand for each of the various nutrients. The external supply is regulated by eating habits rather than need. So, it is an unreliable supply source. That is, it is potentially too highly variable, which makes the cells nutritionally vulnerable. To achieve gross control of supply, mechanisms exist for recycling, storage, and excretion. To achieve fine control of supply, a system exists for monitoring and control of the circulating levels of the various nutrients.

Nutrient Transport and Circulating Levels

The liver is a master processing center that largely controls the possibility of supply to the cells by monitoring and controlling the circulating levels of nutrients. The process of absorption brings an input of nutrients from an external source of supply to a connection with the liver. With the exception of long chain fatty acids, cholesterol, and fat-soluble vitamins, all nutrients that are absorbed go directly to the liver via the portal blood. Eventually, the long-chain fatty acids, etc., also reach the liver via the systemic circulation. Leftover, recycled, and newly synthesized nutrients are also a part of the input from the systemic circulation. Thus, blood circulation is the mechanism for translocation between points of supply and demand.

The cells of the liver monitor the incoming flow of nutrients. In effect, the liver compares the inflow level with predetermined circulating levels (Table 3.1) and directs the nutrients for transport, synthesis, conversion, degradation, storage or detoxification in order to control circulating levels. Whether the incoming nutrients come from external or internal sources is irrelevant to the liver cells; they are identical molecules in any case. Disposition is a simple function of supply and demand, as determined by circulating level. Some examples of class representative processing will be identified for each class of nutrients in order to illustrate the concept:

TABLE 3.1. NORMAL CIRCULATING LEVELS

Nutrient	Level/100 ml	
	Minimum	Maximum
Ascorbic acid	0.4	1.5 mg
Calcium	9	11 mg
Carotenoids	100	300 IU
Chloride	355	376 mg
Copper	70	140 mcg
Glucose	60	100 mg
Iodine, protein-bound	3.5	8 mcg
Iron	75	175 mcg
Lipids, total	450	850 mg
Magnesium	1.8	3 mg
Nitrogen, non-protein	15	35 mg
Phosphate	3	4.5 mg
Potassium	14	20 mg
Proteins	6	8 g
Sodium	313	334 mg
Sulfates	0.5	1.5 mg
Vitamin A	30	100 IU

(a)   amino acids—IF the circulating level is low, THEN the amino acids follow the route for transporting out. IF need is for non-essential amino acids, THEN conversion by transamination results, i.e., amino acid X + keto acid Q interact to form non-essential amino acid Z and keto acid R. IF need is for enzymes or plasma proteins such as albumins or globulins, THEN synthesis results; IF the circulating level of amino acids is adequate AND amino acids are not needed by liver cells to produce other products, THEN they are degraded by a deamination process in which urea is formed.

(b) carbohydrate as glucose, fructose, or galactose—IF the circulating level of glucose is low, the fructose or galactose present is converted to glucose, THEN glucose follows the route for transporting out; IF it is still low, THEN liver glycogen is degraded and/or amino acids are degraded by a process of deamination and the resulting glucose follows the route for transporting out. IF the circulating level is high, THEN glycogen is synthesized and any excess glucose that remains is used to synthesize triglycerides, the basic form of fat.

(c) fatty acids—IF an excess of fatty acids is present, THEN they are processed to form very low density lipoproteins (fat-proteins) the transport form, and THEN follow the route for transport out. IF the circulating level of cholesterol is low, THEN fatty acids will be used as building blocks to synthesize cholesterol which will be used in production of bile.

(d) minerals—IF the circulating level is low, THEN they will be linked to their transport protein (e.g., iron will be incorporated into transferrin, copper will be incorporated into ceruloplasmin, manganese will be incorporated into transmanganin) and will follow the route for transport out. IF the circulating level is still low, THEN the storage compound will be degraded (e.g., ferritin, the iron storage compound will be split so as to separate the iron and protein portions) and the mineral will be incorporated into the transport compound prior to following the route for transporting out. IF need is for enzymes and hormones, THEN the appropriate minerals will be incorporated.

(e) vitamins—IF the circulating levels of vitamins A, D, and E are low, THEN they follow the route for transport out. IF the circulating level of vitamin A is low and a supply of carotene is present, THEN it will be converted to vitamin A by degradation and follow the route for transporting out. IF the circulating level of vitamins A, D, E, and K is still low, THEN they will be removed from storage and will follow the route for transporting out. IF the circulating level of vitamins A, D, E, K, and B_{12} is all right, THEN these can be incorporated into other molecules such as enzymes or stored in the liver. IF the supply of water-soluble vitamins is all right, THEN these will be incorporated into enzymes and will follow the route for transporting out.

(f) all nutrients, at toxic levels—IF circulating level is high, THEN the maximum circulating level may be reset at a higher level (e.g., the addiction of ascorbic acid), OR the excess may be disposed of by conversion to a compound that is excreted by the kidney, i.e., the nutrient is detoxified (e.g., ascorbic acid is converted to oxalic acid, trace elements are combined to form insoluble salts, etc.), OR an additional storage compound that is insoluble and will precipitate out may be synthesized (e.g., iron is incorporated into hemosiderin).

After processing in the liver cells, the nutrients follow the route for transport out. The blood with its load of nutrients and other compounds is collected in the capillary tubes and merges with progressively larger tubes to join the systemic circulation which supplies the other organs of the body.

Nutrient utilization by the cells of other tissues is of three types: (a) continuous use of nearly all nutrients in minute quantities for growth or repair/replacement, (b) intermittent use of large quantities of selected nutrients in support of special functions, and (c) processing and release of large quantities of selected nutrients as a result of specialized functions. Use of large quantities of selected nutrients in special functions occurs in such tissues as (a) bones—calcium, phosphate, magnesium, fluorine, amino acids, and vitamins A and D—these are involved in tissue formation; (b) muscles—amino acids, B vitamins, calcium, magnesium, iron, glucose, fatty acids, and vitamin E are incorporated into the muscle tissue in order to support muscle contraction; (c) eyes—amino acids and vitamin A are incorporated into retinal tissue in order to elicit the visual response; (d) thyroid—amino acids and iodine are combined in order to produce several hormones.

Storage and subsequent discharge of nutrients into the blood stream is a specialized function of tissues such as (a) bones—whenever the circulating levels of calcium or phosphate are low, bone tissue is degraded by a process called resorption and (b) adipose tissue—whenever the circulating level of glucose is low, fatty acids are released. Thus, the circulating level will be variable at various points in the body depending on whether withdrawal or release of nutrients predominates. At the same time, the liver will be monitoring and making continuous adjustments.

Nutrient Conservation: Recycling and Storage

The demand for nutrients is continuous. The external supply is variable within and among days according to the assortment of foods consumed, which is determined by food habits. Moreover, the liberation/absorption rate causes differences in supply. Some nutrients peak quickly and fall off; others are absorbed at a low level over a relatively long period of time. To avoid the effects of fluctuation in supply, nutrient conservation systems for recycling and storage exist.

Recycling is the mechanism for conservation of those nutrients that are likely to be scarce and are necessary to meet a fixed maintenance demand. The need for recycling iron will illustrate this concept. The mean dietary intake of iron is low, approximately 10 to 15 mg/day. Of this, only 1.0 to 1.5 mg is absorbed. It is necessary to replace the 0.5 to 1.0 mg lost per day. Iron is a critical nutrient because of its functional role as part of the hemoglobin molecule, the oxygen-carrying component of the red blood cells. Approximately 3 million red blood cells are produced per second, which requires supply of 21 mg iron for incorporation in hemoglobin in a 24-hour period. Intake is only slightly above that needed to replace losses and is far below that needed to produce hemoglobin. Therefore, recycling of iron from the 3 million red blood cells that die each second is necessary in order for supply to meet a fixed maintenance demand.

In another sense, all nutrients can be recycled to some degree. Amino acids are secreted into the GI tract, which prevents degradation and loss of functional value, and are reabsorbed with newly liberated ones. Amino acids, glucose, and fatty acids can be used and reused many times until they become involved in degrading or energy-producing reactions. Minerals are used as catalysts and can be reused so long as they do not complex to form insoluble compounds. Vitamins also function as catalysts and can be reused as long as their functional group remains intact.

The kidney is also involved in conservation of nutrients. It performs three interrelated functions that modify the circulating levels of some nutrients: (a) filtration to remove the end-products of protein metabolism; (b) control of the circulating levels of electrolytes, amino acids, water-soluble vitamins, and glucose; and (c) control of blood volume. Recycling is involved in implementing these functions. For example, implementation of the filtering function involves removal of urea and reabsorption of about half, removal of creatine and reabsorption of a variable fraction, removal of uric acid and nearly total reabsorption, and removal of ammonia and reabsorption of a variable quantity. These end-products can then be reused in production of nonessential amino acids and non-protein nitrogen compounds. Implementation of the control function in relation to electrolytes involves reabsorption of sodium when the circulating levels of potassium are high, i.e., sodium is recycled in order to increase its availability and rebalance the sodium-to-potassium ratio. Maintenance of the lower circulating levels for the amino acids, glucose, B vitamins, and ascorbic acid involves active reabsorption when their level is low to normal. Otherwise, these are lost in the urine. When blood volume is low to normal, water and sodium are reabsorbed and reused to restore blood volume.

Storage is a mechanism used to (a) reduce vulnerability due to scarcity and (b) remove excesses. Storage roles in stabilizing the supply of nutrients will be illustrated using iron and vitamin A.

Recycling of iron provides a mechanism for meeting a fixed maintenance need. It is necessary and sufficient as long as need for replacement of red blood cells is fixed. However, there is a variable component to the need for iron. It results from blood loss. This need cannot be met by recycling since recycling cannot increase the quantity available. The probability is low that a dietary intake high enough AND increased efficiency in absorption will be sufficient to overcome the blood loss-related decrease in iron available for red blood cell formation. To meet this contingency, a mechanism that allows for controlled but gradual accumulation of iron in a stable form that can be released on demand is a more reliable mechanism for meeting a sharp, discrete and occasional need. The storage of iron in ferritin serves this function.

The usual dietary iron intake is low and normal control fixes absorption slightly above the quantity lost. However, there is a variable component to intake since the iron content of foods is not evenly distributed, i.e., beef liver contains 8.8 mg/100 g whereas milk contains 0.04 mg/100 g, and intake is related to food choices not need. Thus, intake is likely to be variable among days, and could be deficient or excessive on the average, which would create vulnerability. To meet this contingency, a mechanism that allows for a sharp but temporary expansion in capacity to absorb and retain iron as well as a mechanism for removal of excess is needed. The storage of iron in ferritin serves the first function. The storage of iron in the relatively insoluble compound hemosiderin serves the second.

The usual dietary intake of vitamin A tends to be low and absorption efficiency is affected by fat intake. Intake tends to be highly variable among days because the vitamin A content of foods is not evenly distributed, i.e., liver contains 43,900 IU/100 g, carrots and dried apricots contain more than 10,000 IU/100 g, other commonly consumed green and yellow vegetables contain between 1,000 IU/100 g, and 4,000 IU/100 g, and other foods contain almost none. Moreover, the quantity consumed has been highly variable among seasons—being very low except during the harvest season. Thus, the external supply variations would create vulnerability. To meet this contingency, a mechanism to allow accumulation during periods of surplus is needed. Liver and adipose cell storage serve this function.

EXCRETION

The human body has only one important mechanism for excretion of excess nutrients. This is via the urine. The quantity of a given nutrient that can be reabsorbed by kidney cells is limited. When the circulating level of a given nutrient exceeds a threshold, the excess is excreted by the kidney. Excess water also may be excreted in order to adjust the circulating level of other nutrients. For example:

   (a) IF the circulating level of sodium is high (hypernatremia), THEN sodium and water are excreted.

(b) IF the circulating level of chloride, phosphate, sulfate, or magnesium ions is high, THEN the respective ion is compounded to a salt and is excreted.

(c) IF the circulating level of glucose is high (hyperglycemia), THEN glucose and water are excreted (glucosuria and polyuria, respectively).

(d) IF the circulating levels of any of the B vitamins or ascorbic acid is high, THEN it is excreted. (Excess ascorbic acid is converted to oxalate for excretion.)

Two less important excretion mechanisms allow limited excretion of specific substances. Calcium is secreted into the small intestine. Since absorption is fixed in relation to need, any excess from exogenous and/or endogenous sources is excreted in the feces. Cholesterol, which is synthesized from fat, is itself a precursor for bile acids and salts. The higher the fat intake, the greater the quantity of bile that is secreted to deal with it. Since reabsorption of bile acids and salts is only partial, cholesterol is excreted in the feces.

FOOD, PEOPLE, AND NUTRIENT SUPPLY

In addition to presenting a challenge to the digestive system, food and people interactions can interfere with nutrient supply in spite of adequate intake. Some common examples follow:

(a) Busy foods such as sunflower seeds, popcorn, and chips are consumed a few at a time over an extended period of time such as an hour. Increased and continued secretion of gastric HCl, as well as inhibition of gastric emptying in order to allow adequate mixing, results in extrusion of a hyperacid chyme. This requires that extraordinary quantities of sodium bicarbonate be secreted in the small intestine in order to neutralize the acid. In the meantime, the pH is not optimal for digestion, so efficiency is reduced and malabsorption of some nutrients is likely. Thus, consumption of busy foods is a poor habit nutritionally.

(b) Anger, tension, and anxiety have the same effects on HCl secretion and gastric emptying time. Therefore, the value of creating a pleasant, relaxed meal climate is supported by physiological as well as sociopsychological imperatives.

(c) The presence of dietary fat causes secretion of the hormone enterogastrone which retards gastric emptying so as to allow a prolonged time for digestion of the fat already present in the small intestine. The amount, kind, and distribution of fat in foods determine digestion rate and, therefore, continuation of release of enterogastrone. Food fats are liquid at body temperature, which facilitates digestion. IF *not* enclosed with a vegetable or muscle cell wall or intimately mixed with other components as is the case with pastry and foods that have soaked up frying fat, THEN emulsification, penetration, and degradation are relatively rapid. However, insufficient chewing or poor cooking techniques are common, so rate of digestion is frequently slow. Often, this problem is compounded by the presence of acrolein, a fat breakdown product that results when foods are fried at high temperatures. Acrolein is an irritant. Irritation causes peristalsis and removal of the irritant. Malabsorption of nutrients in incompletely digested chyme results. Thus, frequent consumption of very high fat, and especially improperly fried foods is a poor habit nutritionally.

(d) Unfavorable intake ratios of some nutrients can interfere with absorption by favoring formation of insoluble compounds. For example, a high ratio of fatty acids to calcium or magnesium results in formation of soaps; phytic acid in cereal products can form an insoluble salt with all available iron; oxalic acid can tie up calcium by forming calcium oxalate; and a high ratio of phosphate to calcium and magnesium may tie them up by forming their phosphate salts.

(e) Fear and depression repress gastric and intestinal secretions and mucosal blood flow. Both liberation rate and absorption efficiency are reduced, so that unless peristalsis is inhibited, malabsorption may occur.

Approximately one-third of the population reports a problem of flatulence. In an attempt to minimize the problem people eliminate certain foods from their diets. Depending on the food(s) eliminated and the food(s) substituted, nutrient supply may be adversely affected.

Fads affect food and people interactions. The fiber fad can have good and bad nutritional effects. A reasonable fiber intake results in normal distension of the colon and normal transit time. A certain amount of fat, cholesterol, and other nutrients are usually trapped within the structure of the fibrous mass and excreted. Moreover, excessive fiber intake reduces transit time, which may result in malabsorption of other nutrients. For those whose supply is adequate, this is all right. For those whose intake is marginal, nutritional disaster may result.

Food ecology is also affected by routine and/or long-term use of many drugs. Many effect loss of taste or smell, resulting in loss of appetite. Others, even relatively innocuous over-the-counter drugs such as aspirin and antacids, can impair nutrient absorption by irritation which reduces transit time or changing the pH which affects enzymatic function. Awareness of common effects of drugs taken routinely and medical monitoring of the circulating level of nutrients likely to be affected can form the basis for appropriate intake adjustment. Diet instruction can be used to minimize disruption of the customary food and people interactions when implementing an adjusted intake. This supportive assistance facilitates the adjustments necessary for nutritional correction.

BIBLIOGRAPHY

STACY, R.W., and SANTOLUCITO, J.A. 1966. Modern College Physiology. The C.V. Mosby Co., St. Louis.

VAN ITALLIE, T.B., SMITH, N.S., and QUARTERMAIN, D. 1977. Short-term and long-term components in the regulation of food intake: evidence for a modulatory role of carbohydrate status. Am. J. Clin. Nutr. *30*, 742-757.

4

Lipids–Fatty Acids and Complex Compounds

The food and people interactions involving lipids have become critical to the health of many Americans. For many, the need to control intake is either a result of a decision to take preventive measures to reduce the risk of coronary heart disease (CHD) or part of a therapeutic regimen for reducing the rate of progress of manifest CHD. So intakes of saturated fats, unsaturated fats, and cholesterol have become important. In the United States, intakes of fat have changed in recent years, both in quantity and quality. There is no RDA for fat, but other groups have made recommendations. Is there a need to consume fat?

FOOD SOURCES OF LIPIDS

Fats, oils, waxes, phosphatides, cerebrosides, and related as well as derived compounds are included in the class of organic compounds designated as lipids. Plant and animal tissues naturally contain a variable mixture of lipids which serve as a reserve energy source or as a structural component. Food processing technology has enabled further modification of the composition of food lipid mixtures.

The basic component of a lipid is a fatty acid (Table 4.1), which may be combined with other fatty acids, proteins, carbohydrates, minerals, vitamins, or other compounds to form the various compounds in this class. The fatty acid composition of the various food lipids is highly variable. More than 50 fatty acids are known components. Even so, the fatty acid composition is characteristic for the source and one fatty acid may predominate. With few exceptions, natural food fats contain straight chain, even-numbered fatty acids of variable length. Major groups of food lipids are identified below.

TABLE 4.1. COMMON FATTY ACIDS

Common Name	Systematic Name	Structural Formula
		Saturated Acids
Butyric	*n*-Butanoic	$CH_3(CH_2)_2COOH$
Isovaleric	3-Methyl-*n*-Butanoic	$(CH_3)_2CHCH_2COOH$
Caproic	*n*-Hexanoic	$CH_3(CH_2)_4COOH$
Caprylic	*n*-Octanoic	$CH_3(CH_2)_6COOH$
Capric	*n*-Decanoic	$CH_3(CH_2)_8COOH$
Lauric	*n*-Dodecanoic	$CH_3(CH_2)_{10}COOH$
Myristic	*n*-Tetradecanoic	$CH_3(CH_2)_{12}COOH$
Palmitic	*n*-Hexadecanoic	$CH_3(CH_2)_{14}COOH$
Stearic	*n*-Octadecanoic	$CH_3(CH_2)_{16}COOH$
Arachidic	*n*-Eicosanoic	$CH_3(CH_2)_{18}COOH$
Behenic	*n*-Docosanoic	$CH_3(CH_2)_{20}COOH$
Lignoceric	*n*-Tetracosanoic	$CH_3(CH_2)_{22}COOH$
		Unsaturated Acids
Palmitoleic	Hexadec-9-enoic	$CH_3(CH_2)_5CH:CH(CH_2)_7COOH$
Oleic	Octadec-9-enoic	$CH_3(CH_2)_7CH:CH(CH_2)_7COOH$
Linoleic	Octadeca-9,12-dienoic	$CH_3(CH_2)_4CH:CH CH_2CH:CH(CH_2)_7COOH$
Linolenic	Octadeca-9,12,15-trienoic	$CH_3(CH_2)CH:CHCH_2CH:CHCH_2CH:CH(CH_2)_7COOH$
Arachidonic	Eicosa-5,8,11,14-tetraenoic	$CH_3(CH_2)_4CH:CHCH_2CH:CHCH_2CH:CHCH_2CH:CH(CH_2)_3COOH$

The simplest kind of lipid is a *monoacylglycerol* or monoglyceride (MG) in which one fatty acid is attached to a glycerol base (└ , ┠ , or ┌). Monoglycerides with a long chain fatty acid are added to many processed foods as an emulsifier because they are soluble in both fat and water so can bind the two together forming and stabilizing an emulsion.

Diacylglycerols or diglycerides (DG) are lipids in which two fatty acids are attached to a glycerol base (⊏ ⊏ or ⊢). These also are used as emulsifiers, often in conjunction with monoglycerides.

Triacylglycerols or triglycerides (TG) are lipids in which three fatty acids are attached to a glycerol base (⊟). Triglycerides are of two types: (a) simple, in which all of the fatty acids are the same and (b) mixed, in which they vary (⊟ , ⊨ , ⊟ , ⊟ , etc.). Natural triglycerides in foods are usually of the mixed type. Since there are over 50 fatty acids and 3 alternate positions, a vast array of distinct triglycerides is possible. The triglyceride composition of the various natural food lipids is highly variable, but is characteristic for the food and accounts for many of its physical properties.

Lipids in live plant and animal tissues exist largely as mixtures of triglycerides in liquid form, i.e., as oils. This is necessary in order to facilitate the chemical changes that are involved as the lipid is metabolized in performing its functional role(s). (Reaction rates in solids are greatly reduced.) When a lipid solidifies or crystallizes out, as when cholesterol is deposited in vascular tissue, it interferes with cellular function. Plant food lipids, with the exception of coconut and palm oil, are mostly polyunsaturated oils. This is because the structure of most of the component triglycerides are composed of fatty acids with mono- (e.g., ⊟ times n variations) or polyunsaturated bonds, i.e., contain several bonds that could have hydrogen or some other ion added to complete bonding (e.g., ⊟ times n variations). Polyunsaturated bonds create an unstable structure that is fluid. At ambient temperatures, animal lipids in meat are solid fats and in fish are primarily lipid oils. The lipids in meat solidify as the animal body cools because the structures of most of the component triglycerides include long-chain fatty acids with saturated bonds, i.e., the bonds are tied up with hydrogen or some other ion forming a relatively stable structure (e.g., ⊟ times n variations). The lipids in fish are oils because fish live in a cold medium. The polyunsaturated fatty acids (PUFA) form a structure that will not solidify until lower temperatures are reached (e.g., ⊟ times n variations).

Lipids in harvested plant tissues and in meat and fish also contain various percentages of malodorous breakdown fragments and products (e.g., 1,-,—,┠ etc.). Rancidity, i.e., the development of a disagreeable odor or flavor in a food lipid as a result of accumulation of these breakdown products, is progressive as storage time increases. Short-chain fatty acids are formed by two processes: lipolysis and oxidation. Lipolysis, i.e., hydrolytic breakdown by the action of a lipase, occurs in foods that are not subjected to high temperature processing, e.g., butter, cheese, chocolate. A variety of fragments are formed by oxidation, i.e., adding oxygen at the unsaturated bond. The currently accepted explanation is that development of oxidative rancidity is a three-stage process involving a free-radical chain mechanism in formation of hydroperoxides.

(a) initiation:

$$RH \text{ (lipid)} \xrightarrow{\text{activation}} R \cdot \text{(free radical)} + (H)$$

(b) propagation:

$$R \cdot + O_2 \longrightarrow RO_2 \cdot$$

$$RO_2 \cdot + RH \longrightarrow R \cdot + ROOH$$

(c) termination:

$$RO_2 \cdot + X \text{ (free radical or free radical inhibitor)} \longrightarrow \text{inactive end products}$$

Rancidity is retarded by added antioxidants. Antioxidants such as BHA, BHT, and propyl gallate are oxygen scavengers that function by binding the oxygen so that it is not free to combine with other chemicals present.

Waxes are mixtures of long-chain fatty acid esters with long-chain alcohols, free long-chain fatty acids, long-chain alcohols, and hydrocarbons. These are less greasy, harder, and more brittle than fats. They are found in the skins of fruits and vegetables.

Phosphatides or phospholipids are compound lipids containing phosphoric acid in addition to fatty acids, glycerol, a nitrogen base, and other substances (F_{PO_4}-nitrogen base). This class includes lecithin which is a natural constituent of egg yolk and is used as an emulsifier, wetting agent, and antioxidant in food preparation.

Cerebrosides or glycolipids are compound lipids containing carbohydrate in addition to fatty acids and a nitrogen base. These are present in some animal tissues. The compound 4-sphingenine (formerly called sphingosine) is prominent.

Derived lipids are products of hydrolysis of lipids, i.e., free fatty acids, glycerol, and sterols such as ergosterol and sitosterol in plant tissues and cholesterol in animal tissue and eggs. Fat-soluble vitamins A, D, E, and K are often grouped with this class. Many of these are *terpenoids*, i.e., they contain the "isoprenoid unit." Mevalonic acid, steroids, and carotenoids are terpenoids.

Food lipids also include fabricated fats designed for cooking. These are made from triglycerides of vegetable and/or animal origin. The vegetable oils are modified by *hydrogenation*, i.e., saturation of double bonds in the natural oils, to form fats that are almost as saturated, solid, and plastic as those of animal origin. Fats containing mixtures of fatty acids are produced by controlled hydrogenation and blending to make shortenings of varying melting point and plasticity, i.e., that can be spread and shaped.

Food lipids also include fabricated fats designed for eating, such as the margarines, which are blends of hydrogenated oils and skim milk. In general, IF margarine is sold in soft form THEN it contains two to four times as much polyunsaturated fatty acids as saturated fatty acids. Special "diet" margarines are produced by two processes: (a) partial hydrogenation of all of the oil to the desired consistency and (b) more complete hydrogenation of a portion of the oil to form a saturated, solid fat that is blended with the oil. This produces a margarine with almost twice the linoleic acid content of the first process. The first ingredient is the one in greatest quantity. So, IF the label declaration is "liquid corn oil plus hydrogenated corn oil," THEN the second process has been used in fabrication. Note: the caloric value of "diet" margarines is reduced by dilution with air (whipped products) or water.

LIPIDS: NORMAL SUPPLY AND NORMAL DEMAND

Lipids are consumed in a variety of food forms: some in free form, some as liquids embedded within plant or animal tissues, and some as films associated with cereals in breadings or batters and in bakery products. Nonetheless, nearly all of the fat is available for absorption.

Lipid metabolism includes, but is not limited to, reactions involving free fatty acids (FFA), triacylglycerols, cholesterol, phospholipids (PL), lipoproteins, and glycolipids. Discussion will be limited to those just named.

Digestion/Absorption

The normal mixed diet in the United States at this time contains about 160 g fat, which accounts for approximately 42% of the calories ingested. The current intake differs in nature and extent from the traditional intake, which undoubtedly has implications for the digestion/absorption process. In recent years, fat consumption has increased and the major sources have changed to meat fat, salad oils, and shortenings, in that order.

With the exception of a few cultures, meat has not been the main source of fat. Game animals yield lean meat, perhaps 10% of largely saturated fatty acids, because of high exercise levels. Domestic animals are obese and yield richly marbled meat, approximately 50% of largely saturated fatty acids because exercise is minimized in order to maximize muscle tenderness. Moreover, until the 1940s, meat was cooked to the well-done stage. Consequently, a large proportion of the embedded fat was rendered out. And, traditionally, what little finishing fat was available was carefully conserved for use in cooking. It was precious, so in many cultures it was used sparingly. Olive oil was the only vegetable oil in common use. Except in countries of origin, it was too expensive for extensive use.

In the last 75 years, fat consumption has been different. Margarine became available and has been used increasingly. Shortenings and vegetable oils from a number of grains, legumes, and seeds are newer yet. They have been available for about 35 years. Even now, safflower and sesame oils are not used commonly in the home. Traditionally, cereal consumption was high, accounting for about 80% of the calories ingested. Since cereals are 1 to 3% lipid, even when refined, the quantity of PUFA consumed as plant oils was significant. Today we eat less cereal but extract the oils for use in cooking.

Digestion/absorption of TG is accomplished by a combination of two procedures. Details are only partly known (Fig. 4.1):

(a) hydrolysis of about half of the ingested TG to MG, DG, and FFA—Emulsification of these by bile salts to form a mixed micelle that is soluble in the aqueous phase of chyme is the first step. Next, the micelles come in contact with the intestinal wall by muscular action, the fragments are released, and are immediately absorbed at the tip of the villi. Inside the mucosal epithelial cells, i.e., enterocytes, these fragments are activated by a synthetase and MG are converted to DG which are in turn converted to TG by means of specific transferases. IF the TG contains fatty acids of 14 or more carbons, THEN it may dissolve cholesterol, fat-soluble vitamins, etc., prior to encasement in a lipoprotein envelope. The lipoprotein complex is called a chylomicron. It is then excreted into the lacteals for transport to the liver via the lymphatic and systemic circulation.

(b) emulsification of intact TG, especially those with chain lengths of 12 to 14 carbons—These are absorbed as is into the enterocyte. IF the TG contains fatty acids of 12 carbons or less, THEN these are complexed with albumin to form a lipoprotein for transport via the portal blood flow to the liver. Those TG with fatty acids of chain length 14 or more are handled as above.

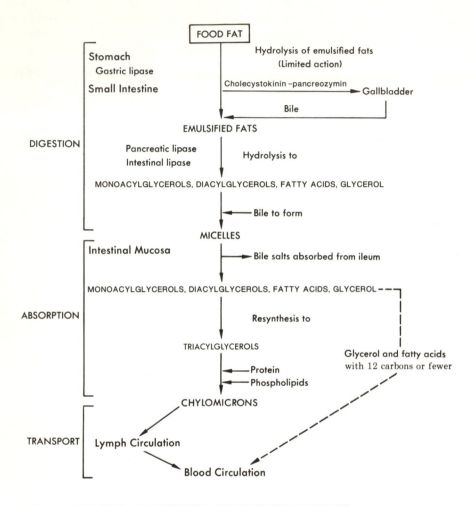

FIG. 4.1. DIGESTION, ABSORPTION, AND TRANSPORT OF FAT

Lecithin is absorbed as lysolecithin and is resynthesized to lecithin within the enterocyte. Then it is incorporated in the chylomicra for transport. *De novo* synthesis of lecithin also occurs within the enterocyte from DG and citidine diphosphate choline.

The details of the processes by which the fat-soluble vitamins are absorbed are described elsewhere. However, unless they are ingested in an aqueous dispersion, the presence of fat is necessary to absorption.

Absorption efficiency varies at different points along the GI tract. Lipid absorption is almost complete at the upper end, somewhat complete in the middle portions, and low at the distal or ileal portions. The distal portions are normally exposed to low-fat chyme because most of the fat will have been absorbed already. Therefore, this portion of the GI tract has low enzyme activity, which accounts for the low absorption efficiency. Consequently, the rate of passage of chyme is important to the degree of absorption achieved. In any case, long-chain saturated fatty acids are less readily absorbed than are long-chain PUFA. So, saturated fatty acids are more likely to be excreted than are PUFA. A fixed percentage of ingested fatty acids is excreted irrespective of the amount consumed.

The presence of acrolein, an irritating derived lipid, interferes with digestion/absorption. Acrolein is formed from cooking fats and oils or rendered fats by hydrolysis when they are used for long periods or are heated to the smoke point:

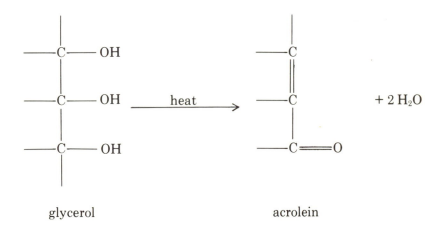

glycerol   acrolein

Because acrolein irritates, peristalsis is increased in order to remove the irritant. As a result, malabsorption is likely.

Metabolism of Lipids—in General

Lipids serve a number of roles. Each role is associated with different metabolic processes. Roles of lipids include, but are not limited to:

(a) source of energy

(b) structural component of membranes

(c) emulsifying agent

(d) precursor for prostaglandins and other derivatives.

All cells require a source of energy to fuel cellular processes, many of which are endergonic reactions. Two-thirds to three-fourths of this energy is derived from the oxidation of TG, since the carbon chains of both excess amino acids and glucose are conserved by conversion to TG. All cells contain a supply of stored TG and have additional access to a continuous supply from the circulating lipoprotein complexes. Energy is produced at the cellular level from TG as follows:

(a) TG are hydrolyzed to glycerol and FFA.

(b) The glycerol residue is converted to glyceraldehyde and is degraded via the phosphogluconate pathway, producing energy.

(c) Fatty acids are degraded by a stepwise procedure in which 2-carbon segments are removed as acetyl CoA, which enters the Krebs cycle for oxidation to CO_2, water, and energy. The Krebs cycle enzymes are located in the cellular matrix, whereas the enzymes for degradation for the fatty acid chain are located in the mitochondrial membrane. Fatty acids and fatty acyl-CoA require a carnitine shuttle to effect translocation. A carnitine acyl-CoA transferase is the effector. Four additional enzymes are involved in various steps of the degradation process.

The energy produced is in two forms, i.e., heat and a labile storage form (ATP), to be discussed in Chapter 7. The process of releasing energy from TG is long and of variable length, depending on the length of the fatty acid chain (e.g., repeated 8 times in degrading stearic acid which has an 18-carbon chain). Therefore, it is too slow as the immediate source of energy in rapidly metabolizing tissues such as muscles and the central nervous system. To compensate, muscles have a second supply system utilizing glycogen, to be discussed in a later chapter. However, the cells of the central nervous system lack a functional alternative so they require a continuous supply of glucose.

All cells require both intracellular and extracellular membranes to compartmentalize and isolate functions, substrates, intermediates, and end products. To *exist*, a membrane must be insoluble in the surrounding body fluids, it must be structurally stable, and it must degrade slowly. Only a few relatively insoluble compounds can serve as structural elements of cell membranes. These include phospholipids, TG, and cholesterol. The turnover rate for PL and cholesterol in membranes is very slow. Even fatty acids are not easily split off. Therefore, they provide the necessary structural stability. To *function*, a membrane must be permeable to water-soluble and/or fat-soluble substances. Phospholipids and cholesterol are somewhat water-soluble as well as somewhat fat-soluble. Therefore, they decrease the interfacial tension between the membrane and the surrounding fluid. This facilitates transport of lipids and lipid-soluble materials through the membrane. Thus, PL and cholesterol are produced by all cells to meet the demand for incorporation in membranes so as to ensure cell survival.

All cells require that non-structural substances be distributed in solution or suspension, i.e., they neither can settle out nor float. Since lipids are lighter than water, the base material of body fluids, emulsifying agents are necessary. Phospholipids, e.g., lecithin, form oil-in-water emulsions. So, PL are emulsifiers in the cell sap. Cholesterol forms water-in-oil emulsions. So, cholesterol would be the emulsifier in fat depots. Between these two kinds of molecules the lipids can be associated with other cellular components. Therefore, some quantity of these is produced on demand for this purpose.

All cells require a continuing supply of cholesterol for use in membrane synthesis and other functions. In the extrahepatic cells (i.e., other than liver), cholesterol supply needs can be met from liver and intestinal sources or by biosynthesis. In liver cells, the synthesis of cholesterol is affected by dietary cholesterol intake. In extrahepatic cells cholesterol synthesis is independent of dietary cholesterol intake and is related to demands created by the function(s) of the organ. IF the extrahepatic cellular supply of cholesterol is low, THEN the following occurs:

(a) cholesterol uptake is increased—The cells synthesize a specific plasma membrane receptor protein that binds LDL, which is the medium for transporting cholesterol from the liver and intestines. Regulation of the number of receptors controls the rate of cellular uptake of cholesterol from plasma. Cholesterol esters are taken up by endocytosis, translocated to the lysosome where they are hydrolyzed, and free cholesterol is liberated.

(b) cholesterol biosynthesis is initiated and continues until demand is met—According to Kandutsch, Chen, and Heiniger (1978), in extrahepatic tissues cholesterol biosynthesis is regulated by a feedback control mechanism in which a specific oxygenated sterol suppresses the rate-controlling enzyme 3-OH-3 methyl-glutaryl coenzyme A(HMG-CoA) reductase. Excess lipoprotein-derived free cholesterol is re-esterified by activating an acyl-CoA: cholesterol acyltransferase. And, synthesis of the LDL receptors is decreased. At this point, both uptake and synthesis are halted until demand again exceeds supply.

Prostaglandins (PG) are intermediaries with pharmacologic effects in target tissues that are produced via cAMP. Some of the effects have been identified and the mechanism of action is partially understood. PG mediate regulation of the blood supply to the various organs, mediate the inflammatory response, have roles in CNS function, and mediate control of the transport of water and electrolytes (Hinman 1972).

Linoleic acid, the recognized essential fatty acid, and four odd-numbered fatty acids are involved in the biosynthetic process for PG (Schlenk 1972). The four odd-numbered fatty acids of chain length C_{12}, C_{20}, and C_{21} with *cis* double bonds in positions 8, 11, 14, or 5, 8, 11, and 14 appear to function as essential fatty acids even though they can be synthesized. According to Schlenk (1972), these are:

(a) $8,11,14-19:3\omega5$
(b) $5,8,11,14-19:4\omega5$
(c) $8,11,14-21:3\omega7$
(d) $5,8,11,14-21:4\omega7$

Since these can be synthesized, given an adequate supply of linoleic acid, the essential fatty acid requirement has not been changed. These fatty acids are produced on demand for use in biosynthesis of PG.

Metabolism of Lipids in Specific Tissues

In order to perform normal specialized functions, some tissues have unique mechanisms for metabolizing lipids. These are outlined below.

(a) blood—One of the functions of blood is the translocation of lipids from the peripheral tissues to the liver and from the liver to the peripheral tissues. Therefore, a sample of blood or plasma can be used to obtain an index to the nature and extent of lipids available to the various tissues.

Blood lipids are of the following types: FFA, chylomicra, pre-β-lipoproteins, or very low density lipoproteins (VLDL) which contain somewhat less TG than chylomicra and negligible amounts of cholesterol; β or low density lipoproteins (LDL) which contain an intermediate proportion of TG and protein as well as free and esterified cholesterol; and α or high density lipoproteins (HDL) that contain the least TG and the most protein and most of the free cholesterol transported.

Fatty acids are released into the blood from adipose cells and from the action of lipoprotein lipase. Fatty acids are toxic, so they are immediately combined with albumin for transport. Normally, 3 molecules of fatty acid combine with one molecule of albumin, but as many as 30 may so combine. This ten-fold increase facilitates sharply increased transport to meet strong tissue demands. These fatty acid-albumin complexes are called free fatty acids (FFA) to distinguish them from the fatty acids esterified with glycerol, cholesterol, and other compounds.

For two to three hours after a meal, the plasma contains ingested chylomicra which are gradually removed via a two-step process. In the first step, lipoprotein lipase in blood vessels of adipocytes, cardiac, and skeletal muscle tissue hydrolyze the lipoprotein envelope of the chylomicron releasing the TG, cholesterol, or other lipids. In the second step, lipoprotein lipase further degrades the TG to fatty acids and glycerol. These diffuse into the adjoining cells for immediate use.

Between meals, i.e., in the postabsorptive state, the quantity of circulating fatty acids is low but highly variable. Although the normal resting level is approximately 15 mg/100 ml, the turnover rate is so fast that about half is replaced every 2 to 3 minutes. Therefore, more than half of the total resting body demand for energy is available by diffusion from circulation. Conditions that increase the rate of utilization of fatty acids for energy, e.g., a weight reduction diet or diabetes, increase the circulating level of fatty acids ten-fold or more in order to maintain an adequate energy supply.

In the postabsorptive state, more than 95% of the plasma lipids are lipoprotein mixtures of triglycerides, phospholipids, cholesterol, and protein. Two kinds of mixtures, the VLDL and the LDL, are produced in the liver for transport of the lipid, primarily triglycerides, to the peripheral tissues.

(b) liver—It is the main processing and regulatory organ for lipids. These two functions are interrelated.

Processing by liver or hepatic cells is of two types. *Degradation* is by the common stepwise decrease in chain length that produces energy by oxidation. This process is efficient, normally producing more energy than needed to meet local cell demand. Excess acetyl CoA that is formed is condensed to form acetoacetic acid, which diffuses into the blood for translocation to peripheral tissues. Skeletal muscle, brain, and cardiac cells remove it, which normally keeps the circulating level at less than 3 mg/100 ml. In the cells of these target tissues it is reconverted to acetyl CoA for oxidation via the Krebs cycle. *Synthesis* of TG and derived lipids is largely from carbohydrates and involves one or more of the following processes:

-*de novo* synthesis of a saturated fatty acid, i.e., palmitic acid, from acetyl CoA—Acetyl CoA and oxaloacetic acid are condensed by *citrate synthetase* to citrate in the mitochondrion. Citrate is then translocated to the cytosol where it is cleaved to acetyl CoA and oxaloacetate. In the cytosol acetyl CoA is converted to malonyl CoA. Then acetyl CoA and malonyl CoA are combined in a six-reaction sequence of steps to form palmitic acid. IF propionyl CoA is used instead of acetyl CoA, THEN the end product is an odd-numbered saturated fatty acid.

-increase in chain length, adding acetyl CoA or malonyl CoA to palmitic acid—When chain length has reached 14 to 18 carbons, TG are formed because the enzymes that enable the attachment of α-glycerophosphate specifically activate chains in this length range. Phosphatidic acid is formed by this union. Then the phosphate is removed, leaving a DG. Then, the third fatty acid is attached. The rate of synthesis by this method is dependent on availability of α-glycerophosphate, which is produced by carbohydrate metabolism. IF α-glycerophosphate is in short supply, THEN TG are degraded instead of being formed.

-desaturation of one bond, e.g., conversion of saturated stearic acid to monounsaturated oleic acid—Stearic acid is activated to stearyl CoA and, in the presence of oxygen, interacts with a membrane-bound enzyme system to form the oleyl CoA.

-desaturation to form PUFA—Linoleic acid (18-carbon chain with 2 double bonds) is converted to γ-linolenic acid (18-carbon chain with 3 double bonds). Then, it is elongated to homo-γ-linolenic acid (20-carbon chain with 3 double bonds). Finally, it loses $2\,H^+$ to form arachidonic acid (20-carbon chain with 4 double bonds).

-conversion of TG type A to TG type B—The type B form will have the same or different fatty acids in different positions.

The capacity to desaturate has important nutritional implications. First, this is a limited capacity. Monounsaturated fatty acids can be synthesized but a second double bond cannot. So, the fatty acid with two double bonds, i.e., linoleic acid, is essential, which means that it must be supplied by dietary intake. Second, the capacity to desaturate fatty acids is greater in hepatic than in other cells, so liver TG are less saturated than those of other cells. And, unsaturated fatty acids are available for translocation to other tissues for incorporation in structural lipoproteins of cell membranes.

Regulatory action by hepatic cells provides limited control over the circulating levels of FFA, TG, PL, and lipoproteins. IF the circulating level of any of these is high, THEN they will be removed from circulation by the hepatic cells and will be degraded. Conversely, IF the circulating level of any of these lipids is low and the precursor fragments are available, THEN these lipids can be synthesized. Feedback control mechanisms operate by means of reaction kinetics to control the direction between degradation and synthesis, all other things being equal. Details of regulation are incomplete at this time.

In addition to generalized lipid processing and regulatory functions, the liver also has specialized functions in processing cholesterol and its esters. These include synthesis of plasma and biliary cholesterol, degradation of cholesterol, and production of bile acids. These functions are interrelated and involve:

(a) exogenous cholesterol—This is cholesterol originating from dietary sources. Uptake is limited to 345 ± 75 mg/day (Krumdieck and Ho 1977). This is about 24% of the total amount turned over per day.

(b) endogenous cholesterol—This is cholesterol originating from hepatic biosynthesis and possibly from extrahepatic synthesis in intestinal, adrenal, epithelial, and other tissues.

Hepatic processing of cholesterol is a complex function and affects the concentrations of free cholesterol, cholesterol esters, bile acids, and a variety of intermediate compounds in bile acid production. After hepatic cell uptake of blood cholesterol, IF it is not needed immediately for bile acid production or some other function, THEN it will be disposed of by mechanisms that include, but may not be limited to:

(a) esterification and hepatic storage

(b) incorporation into a lipoprotein and secretion into the blood

(c) secretion into the intestine as such. Most of the free cholesterol is reabsorbed in the small intestine.

A large number of factors have been demonstrated to influence cholesterol biosynthesis in experimental animals. They are assumed to apply to human biosynthesis, although some species differences may exist. Dietary intake of cholesterol is believed to be the most important factor. However, Kandutsch, Chen, and Heiniger (1978) have pointed out that biosynthesis is also inhibited by a variety of other oxygenated sterols, and that the rate-limiting step is influenced by a number of hormones that include insulin, glucagon, testosterone, glucocorticoids, thyroxine, and adrenalin. Therefore, these authors concluded that the observed effect of dietary cholesterol intake in suppressing cholesterol synthesis was possibly a secondary effect related to rate of cholesterol catabolism or impact on the function of some other organ.

Cholesterol biosynthesis is a long and complex process; at least 26 steps have been identified. Acetyl CoA is the source of all of the carbon atoms in cholesterol. In the initial step, 3-hydroxy-3-methyl glutaryl CoA (HMG CoA) is formed from three acetyl CoA. In the second step, HMG CoA is converted to mevalonic acid by HMG CoA reductase. This is the critical step. IF the body set-point for cholesterol is reached by ingestion of dietary cholesterol, THEN HMG CoA reductase is suppressed and cholesterol biosynthesis is inhibited. The mechanism by which the suppression is effected is unclear. Alternatives are suppression of synthesis of HMG CoA reductase, increase in the rate at which it is degraded, or inactivation by some indirect mechanism. Kandutsch, Chen, and Heiniger (1978) have postulated repression by means of oxygenated sterols including cholesterol and additional inactivation by cholesterol.

The liver appears to be the only organ of the body that has the capacity to degrade cholesterol. Degradation yields cholyl CoA (a choline derivative).

Biliary secretion of cholesterol and its use in production of bile acids and salts is the mechanism for excretion of excess cholesterol. The cholesterol precursors of biliary cholesterol are free cholesterol (60%) and esterified cholesterol (10%) from plasma and newly synthesized cholesterol (30%). The free cholesterol is believed to originate from degradation of LDL in the peripheral tissues. It is transported to the liver by the HDL. Cholesterol esters are carried to the liver in chylomicra and LDL. The bile acids are produced from cholyl CoA that results from the degradation of cholesterol. Cholyl CoA conjugates with glycine and taurine to form glycocholic and taurocholic acids, respectively. These are converted to their sodium and potassium salts for excretion in the bile. Bile acid synthesis is regulated by a feedback control mechanism. IF the quantity of bile acids is high, THEN cholesterol synthesis is inhibited. IF the quantity of bile acids is low as when they are used to emulsify dietary fats, THEN liver cholesterol is used in meeting this need (biosynthesis is initiated as necessary).

(c)   adipose tissue—This is the storage unit for surplus lipids, primarily triglycerides but with some dissolved phospholipids and fat-soluble vitamins. Turnover time is three days for stored triglycerides, which results in total replacement in approximately two to three weeks; so metabolic activity is quite rapid.

Processing of lipids is regulated by hormonal action involving at least seven hormones. The hormones and their actions are shown in Table 4.2. Processing of lipids is of the following types:

-IF the circulating level of glucose and/or FFA is low, THEN hydrolysis of triglycerides occurs, releasing fatty acids into circulation where they are immediately complexed with albumin for transport. The glycerol residue is converted to glyceraldehyde and is degraded by the phosphogluconate pathway, producing energy.

-decrease in chain length of fatty acids by the same type of 2-carbon fragmentation process described above

-IF the circulating level of glucose is high and insulin is available to facilitate uptake by the adipose cell, THEN glucose migrates from circulation into the cell and is converted to acetyl CoA which combines with at least six molecules of malonyl CoA to form a fatty acid. When chain length has reached 14 to 18 carbons, the enzymes that enable attachment to α-glycerophosphate are activated, forming phosphatidic acid. Then the phosphate is removed, producing a diglyceride. Finally, the third fatty acid is added.

-IF the circulating level of any amino acid except leucine is high, THEN

TABLE 4.2. HORMONAL REGULATION OF FAT METABOLISM

Hormone	Action
Insulin	Lack—decreases fat synthesis and promotes tissue mobilization and increases the rate of utilization Excess—inhibits fat utilization, enhances fat synthesis, and increases rate of fat storage by facilitating entry of fatty acids
Glucocorticoids	Normal—increases rate of fat mobilization Lack—depresses rate of fat mobilization and usage Excess—ketogenic
Corticotropin	Normal—increases rate of fat mobilization and stimulates secretion of glucocorticoids
Growth hormone	Normal—causes increased rate of fat mobilization
Thyroxine	Normal—causes rapid mobilization of fats, indirectly by decreasing the intracellular acetyl CoA
Epinephrine	Normal—increases rate of fat mobilization by direct action on adipose cell Excess—causes sharp increase in rate of mobilization of fat, may result in 10- to 15-fold increase in circulating level of nonesterified fatty acids
Norepinephrine	Normal—increases rate of mobilization of fat by direct action on adipose cell

it will be converted to acetyl CoA or acetoacetic acid or β-hydroxy butyric acid and used in synthesis as outlined above.

-IF the circulating level of triglycerides or free fatty acids is high, THEN lipoprotein lipase will liberate the fatty acids close to the adipose cell for uptake and reattachment to α-glycerophosphate.

-IF a person is subjected to prolonged contact with a cold environment, THEN adaptation occurs by shortening chain length and desaturation of fatty acids in the stored triglycerides in order for the melting point to be shifted down so that the lipids will remain liquid. Both processes are the same as those occurring in the liver.

-IF mono- or diglycerides are freed from their lipoprotein envelopes and migrate into adipose cells, THEN they are processed just like locally produced ones.

(d) skin—Triglycerides and cholesterol are both metabolized in performing functional roles. Triglycerides are believed to have the following functional roles: individualization of body scent, retention of moisture, structural barrier to prevent penetration by bacteria, and barrier to uptake of water-soluble substances such as acids, alkalis, and various organic solvents. Skin triglycerides differ from those in other tissues in that they contain very short fatty acids, very long fatty acids, fatty acids containing an odd number of carbon atoms, and/or double bonds at different locations. All of these differences have been identified but the intracellular processing by which these differences are effected is presently unknown. Cholesterol is involved also in retention of moisture and as a barrier to the uptake of water-soluble substances. In addition, 7-dehydrocholesterol is converted to vitamin D by action of sunlight.

(e) nerve tissue—One of the phospholipids, sphingomyelin, is present in large quantity and functions as an insulator in the myelin sheath that surrounds nerve fibers. As an insulator, it prevents a flow of ions. Therefore, its function is to prevent diffusion of membrane potential or polarization in wrong directions. This controls the quality of nerve impulses transmitted.

(f) endocrine glands and brain—Secretion of steroid hormones creates a demand for cholesterol which is used in their production. In brain, the cholesterol supply must be sufficient to meet needs for cell division and for the myelination process. Again, oxygenated sterols regulate the cholesterol supply according to demand by suppressing HMG CoA reductase (Kandutsch, Chen, and Heiniger 1978).

LIPIDS: DEFICIENT SUPPLY OR INFLATED DEMAND

The basic functions and interactions of lipids under normal supply/demand conditions have been outlined above. Whenever deficient supply (absolute) or inflated demand (relative deficiency) occurs, interference with function and/or abnormal interactions occurs.

Digestion/Absorption

Low lipid intakes have several effects with important consequences. IF the lipid intake is low, THEN the quantity of triglyceride present in the duodenum may be insufficient to stimulate the secretion of cholecystokinin, which is the hormone that causes emptying of the gallbladder. Several unwanted outcomes may result. For example, since excretion of excess cholesterol is effected by incorporation in bile acids and salts, failure to empty the gallbladder may result in stasis, increased concentration and precipitation as gallstones requiring surgical removal of the gallbladder. The efficiency of absorption of the fat-soluble vitamins is also decreased and may result in deficiency. This is the result of lack of a fat carrier and lack of bile, which is needed for transport to the absorption site on the intestinal wall. This outcome can be overcome by use of a water-soluble emulsion, since bile is not necessary for transport.

Metabolism of Lipids, in General

The first observed effect of low dietary intake of fatty acids and/or cholesterol is a decrease in the quantity and/or proportionate fatty acid/cholesterol composition of the chylomicrons. As a result, fatty acid mobilization from adipose tissue will occur in the postabsorptive state in order to maintain normal circulating levels.

Another effect may also be observed. Linoleic acid is essential, i.e., it must be obtained by dietary intake. IF the supply is deficient, THEN cell membrane structure disintegrates, becoming permeable. This is manifested in skin as eczema, because permeability allows bacteria to invade and multiply.

Metabolism of Lipids, Effects in Specific Tissues

In addition to the general effects of deficient intake that affect the metabolism of all cells, there are effects on tissues with special functions. Tissues affected include, but are not limited to, blood, liver, adipose, and skin. Effects are as follows:

(a) blood—IF the circulating level of FFA and/or chylomicrons is low for any reason, THEN the transport of fat-soluble vitamins will be impaired. IF the circulating level of cholesterol is low, THEN the probability of massive precipitation in the vascular tissue is decreased. IF the circulating level of phospholipids and/or lipoproteins is low, THEN the number of molecules of fatty acid, etc., attached to the carrier is greater than normal and may destabilize the complex.

(b) liver—IF the circulating level of FFA is low AND a supply of acetyl CoA is available, THEN synthesis is initiated and continues until the normal circulating level is reached AND, in the meantime, synthesis of cholesterol, phospholipids, and lipoproteins is suppressed.

IF cholesterol intake is low AND saturated fatty acids are available, THEN cholesterol will be synthesized resulting in a 15 to 25% rise in the circulating level. This is explained as follows: an excess of saturated fatty acids leads to abundant production of acetyl CoA, which facilitates cholesterol production. IF cholesterol intake is low AND the available triglycerides contain PUFA, THEN cholesterol production may be reduced to some degree. IF cholesterol intake is low AND fatty acid intake is low, THEN fatty acids will be mobilized from adipose tissue and transported to the liver to enable synthesis. IF the circulating level of phospholipids and/or lipoproteins is low, THEN these will be produced.

(c) adipose—IF the circulating level of FFA is low, THEN the rate of lipolysis is increased. Weight is lost when the total energy supply is low and this process continues. IF the contents shrink rapidly and the cell wall remains the same, THEN the tissue will be flaccid since there is nothing to maintain the normal firmness.

(d) skin—IF the supply of FFA or cholesterol is chronically low, THEN the content of oil in the monolayer that protects the skin from dehydration is low so the skin becomes dry and scaly.

LIPIDS: EXCESS SUPPLY

Normal intake of lipids is highly desirable. The effect of a low intake is not that important but the effects of a chronically excessive intake of some of the lipids can be catastrophic.

Digestion/Absorption

There are two kinds of effects of excessive intake depending on whether the excess occurs on an occasional basis or is chronic. IF the fat intake is occasionally excessive, THEN a temporary digestive slowdown occurs. Nearly all ingested fat is absorbed, so because of the increased need to emulsify, penetrate, and breakdown the lipid materials coupled with a limited capacity to increase the quantity of lipases and bile, the overload creates what approximates waiting lines. Also, there is competition for carriers to move the lipid fractions through the mucosal wall, so again waiting lines occur. As a result, peristalsis is retarded and digestion is slowed so the bulk does not decrease at the normal rate and one feels stuffed.

IF the lipid intake is chronically large, THEN the gallbladder is stimulated to the point of stress and pathology in the form of gallstones is likely to result. This is because the excess supply of fatty acids allows for augmented production of cholesterol. Excess cholesterol is excreted in the bile, increasing its concentration to a point where it precipitates out.

Metabolism of Excess Lipids, in General

At present, no general metabolic effects of excess intake have been observed at the cellular level. IF a necessary and sufficient quantity of phospholipid has been incorporated in the cell membrane, THEN lipids can enter the cell and can be stored to what seems to be an unlimited degree. IF the quantity of phospholipid incorporated in the cell membrane is insufficient (absolutely or relative to the circulating level of FFA), THEN FFA remains in circulation until removed by adipose cells.

Metabolism of Excess Lipids, Effects in Specific Tissues

The effects of excessive lipid intake are observed in tissues where lipid metabolism is a major function. These tissues include, but are not limited to, the liver, adipose tissue, cardiovascular tissue, and skin. Present knowledge of effects is summarized below:

(a) the liver—IF lipid intake is in excess of needs, THEN the various metabolic subsystems will process the lipids up to capacity, at which point stress and functional failure occur. Phospholipid synthesis is the mechanism for clearing the liver of excess exogenous fatty acids, i.e., those from the chylomicrons. IF the phospholipid synthesis subsystem is normal and an excess of fatty acids is present, THEN phospholipids will be synthesized using some and the remainder will be transported to peripheral tissues via the newly made phospholipids. IF the phospholipid synthesis subsystem is inadequate (absolutely or relative to need), THEN the fatty acids will accumulate and interfere with cellular function. This condition is called fatty liver. Synthesis of lipoproteins is also a mechanism for clearing the liver of excess fatty acids. IF the supply of necessary amino acids is adequate, THEN lipoproteins will be made. IF the lipoprotein synthesis subsystem is inadequate (absolutely or relative to need), THEN the fatty acids will accumulate and interfere with function, producing a fatty liver. IF the dietary intake of cholesterol is in excess of immediate needs, THEN endogenous synthesis is reduced so that the circulating level is not usually increased by more than 15%.

(b) adipose tissue—Recent research indicates that the number of adipose cells is expanded during three rapid growth phases—prenatal, infancy, and adolescence—to provide a reserve energy supply. The cumulative total appears to determine an individual's propensity to gain weight because a greater number of cells has the potential of greater aggregate fat storage. IF the circulating level of FFA is abundant, THEN triglycerides will be synthesized. AND, IF there are many adipose cells as in hyperplasia, THEN the triglycerides will be distributed among them and the person will be a "fat fat-person." OR, IF there are few adipose cells but they are very full, i.e., a condition called hypertrophy, THEN when the adipose cells are well filled the excess will be distributed in other tissues and the person will be a "fat thin-person." IF triglycerides accumulate in adipose tissue, THEN the tissue will expand and require more protein to build vascular tissue in order to supply nutrients throughout. Also, IF triglycerides accumulate, THEN the subcutaneous fat layer will provide extra insulation, creating problems with heat dispersion and throwing the thermostat out of control.

There is a rate-limiting step in fatty acid processing in adipose tissue that becomes critical with excess supply. Adipose cells lack the enzyme glycerokinase, so α-glycerophosphate produced by carbohydrate metabolism must be supplied from Krebs cycle activity in other tissues. IF α-glycerophosphate is in short supply, THEN the circulating level of FFA will be high due to failure of adipose cells to process rapidly enough. This condition produces hyperlipidemia.

(c) cardiovascular system—Adipose tissue, like any other, must be supplied with nutrients via the cardiovascular system. The estimated requirement is one mile of capillaries per five pounds of adipose tissue or an extra five miles for a person twenty-five pounds overweight. Thus, IF triglycerides accumulate, THEN heart work is increased in order to provide necessary and sufficient mechanical force over extra distance AND fatigue/failure may result. Muscle tissue, like any other, must be supplied with nutrients. To carry excess weight around creates a nutrient supply problem which also creates work for the cardiovascular system. Here again, fatigue and failure may result.

Atherosclerosis is a disease of the cardiovascular system that results from deposition of cholesterol and cholesterol esters or phospholipids in the walls of these tissues. IF the circulating level of cholesterol, etc., exceeds its saturation point, THEN it will be precipitated in a local area of vascular tissue.

According to recent studies, when the cardiovascular tissue has been injured, cholesterol, etc., is precipitated at the point of injury as a part of the repair process and a plaque is formed. The rate of exchange of cholesterol, etc., between the plasma and a plaque is very low so plaque development is slow. It appears that, at first, liquid cholesterol migrates in. Then, when the saturation point is reached, some crystals are formed and a liquid-solid mixture results. Finally, fibrous tissue invades the vascular tissue associated with the plaque and as the proportion of crystals increases, a point is reached where the plaque is essentially solid. At this stage, the solid plaque may totally obstruct or occlude the blood flow, in which case the tissue supplied by this vascular tissue dies for lack of nutrients. IF this occurs in the heart, THEN myocardial infarction results. Or, IF the plaque expands along the vascular wall, narrowing the vessel, THEN the increased pressure of blood flow through a narrow tube may be sufficient to cause a weak segment to balloon and/or blow out; hemorrhage results. Both of these outcomes are life-threatening and combine to make CHD the number one killer. As of now, once crystals are formed, there is no way to dissolve them. Therefore, medical efforts have been directed to prevention by reducing the circulating level of various lipid fractions.

(d) skin—Fat people appear to have moister, smoother skin. Excess lipid intake is obviously involved but only limited explanation involving differences in chain length, saturation, etc., has emerged.

LIPIDS: FOOD ECOLOGY AND LIFE EXPECTANCY

Public education efforts have focused on the need to alter man's relation to his food as a preventive measure against development of CHD.

The goal is to improve quality of life as well as to lengthen life expectancy. In 1977, the "McGovern Committee" listed six Dietary Goals for the United States. Three of these relate to fat intake:

Goal 4. Reduce overall fat consumption from approximately 40 to 30% of energy intake. (Note: multiply calories by 0.30 and divide by 9 to obtain the number of grams of fat to be consumed.)

Goal 5. Reduce saturated fat consumption to account for about 10% of the total energy intake, and balance that with polyunsaturated and monounsaturated fats, which should account for about 10% of the energy intake each.

Goal 6. Reduce cholesterol consumption to about 300 mg a day.

These three Dietary Goals have been the focus of a heated controversy. Salient points of the two opposing arguments are:

(a) for—Proponents point out that CHD is the number one killer disease in the United States and that elevated circulating cholesterol levels are a major risk factor. Diet can influence cholesterol levels. Therefore, they contend that since an inappropriate diet appears to contribute to the prevalence of CHD, guidelines for intakes that offer hope of delay, prevention, and/or cure should be issued.

(b) against—Opponents point out that diet is not the only factor that affects the circulating levels of cholesterol, that the circulating cholesterol level is not the major risk factor although it is one that can be modified, and that an increased PUFA intake results in a decreased circulating level. This is a suggestive and provocative fact. But, there is no proof that decreasing the circulating cholesterol level prevents atherosclerosis. A moderate decrease in fat intake has, at most, a trivial effect on circulating lipid levels. And, decreased circulating lipid level has not been shown to decrease the incidence of CHD or the frequency of events in manifest cases. Ahrens (Select Comm. on Nutrition and Human Needs, U.S. Senate 1977), testifying at the U.S. Senate hearings on diet related to killer diseases, summarized the position:

Diet and coronary disease poses the same question: for which people is this dietary advice truly applicable? We must look at the population as being a group of different individuals who react in different ways to the food they eat and to the environmental situation in which they find themselves and to the different life styles they have adopted.

What we ought to be able to do, and can't yet do, is to identify the most appropriate modality of management for individual patients, based on the specific abnormalities each person has.

It is the objective in our research ... to single out those people for whom dietary changes are specifically demanded. To them we can give pointed advice in the most intelligent way, and spare the rest to whom that advice need not be given.

A recent review (Truswell 1978) has summarized what is known about diet and plasma lipids. Salient points made were:

(a) A positive correlation between the circulating plasma total cholesterol level and risk of CHD has been firmly established. Findings from 21 of 21 studies support this relationship.

(b) The circulating plasma HDL level is negatively related to risk of CHD. HDL removes deposited cholesterol from tissues.

(c) VLDL does not appear to be involved, since it carries a negligible amount of cholesterol. The TG carried in the VLDL is not a significant independent predictor of CHD.

(d) LDL level is positively correlated with circulating cholesterol levels.

(e) The dietary fatty acid pattern is the major dietary factor influencing the circulating cholesterol level. Myristic and palmitic acids increase it; linoleic decreases it.

(f) Whole milk contains a large quantity of myristic and palmitic acids so ingestion would be expected to result in an increase in the circulating cholesterol level. It does not; some unknown substance appears to neutralize their effect on the circulating cholesterol level.

(g) Pure cholesterol is poorly absorbed unless other lipids are present.

(h) Although eggs are a concentrated source of cholesterol, addition of or elimination of one egg per day has no effect on circulating levels. Increasing effects due to consumption of two to ten eggs per day have been demonstrated. Benefit of high protein quality and vitamins and minerals must be weighed against disadvantage of cholesterol content in deciding on a level of consumption.

(i) Consumption of sucrose up to and including 23% of calories had no measureable effect on circulating cholesterol levels. At the 34% level, TG were increased 11% and cholesterol 5%.

(j) When the protein intake was qualitatively and quantitatively adequate, cholesterol level was unaffected by intake.

(k) Dietary fiber intake is related to circulating cholesterol levels. Pectin reduces it but wheat fiber does not. The explanation of effect on absorption is incomplete.

(l) Nicotinic acid but not niacinamide in therapeutic doses will reduce the circulating cholesterol level.

(m) Vitamins C and E have no effect on circulating cholesterol level, irrespective of dose size.

(n) Some minerals may be involved in regulation of the circulating cholesterol level. Calcium, in 2 g doses, decreases it. The Zn-Cu ratio has not been proved to affect the circulating level. Vanadium affects the circulating level in animals but not in man. Silicon decreases the circulating level; perhaps this is what causes the effect with pectin since it is a constituent.

(o) Coffee drinking is not an independent risk factor for CHD.

(p) Alcohol has a highly variable effect on circulating cholesterol levels.

(q) Linoleic acid and some substance in onions decreases the circulating LDL level.

At this time, although much is known about some of the relationships between diet and plasma lipid levels, the picture is clearly fragmentary. To delay development of CHD susceptible individuals should decrease their circulating level of LDL, increase their circulating level of HDL and decrease the probability of developing a thrombosis.

Since there is a very complex interrelationship among protein, lipid, and carbohydrate metabolism, some imbalance among them may relate to development of atherosclerosis. A contemporary paper (Carroll 1978) reports that the amino acid pattern of proteins that comprise the intestinal mixture has an effect on the circulating level of cholesterol. Animal proteins tend to be associated with an increased level. Why and how is unknown. On the face of it, it makes no sense since the same pattern can be obtained from plant proteins. Perhaps it is the proportion of the various amino acids.

In ancient times, man's ability to convert carbohydrate to TG was important to survival. His diet was, and still is in many places, largely carbohydrate. About 2¼ times as much energy is stored in fat as in carbohydrate such as glycogen, gram for gram. And, carbohydrate is efficiently converted to TG; about 85% of the energy is recovered. Historically, this ability to convert was important, since it allowed a reduction in weight which increased mobility.

In the 1970s, man's ability to convert carbohydrate to TG again became important to survival. Excessive sugar intake and decreased starch intake was implicated in unwanted storage of TG and physiologic stress. Also, with respect to CHD, an unproved hypothesis that has some supporters but is not well accepted by experts is that the intake of sugar *per se* contributes to the risk of CHD. For these reasons, one of the goals listed by the "McGovern Committee" is to: "Reduce sugar consumption by about 40 percent to account for about 15 percent of total energy intake." (To compute quantity, multiply calories by 0.15 and divide by 4.)

BIBLIOGRAPHY

BOHLES, H., BIEBER, M.A., and HEIRD, W.C. 1976. Reversal of experimental essential fatty acid deficiency by cutaneous administration of safflower oil. Am. J. Clin. Nutr. *29*, 398-401.

BROWN, M.S., and GOLDSTEIN, J.L. 1977. Human mutations affecting the low density lipoprotein pathway. Am. J. Clin. Nutr. *30*, 975-978.

CARROLL, K.K. 1978. Dietary protein in relation to plasma cholesterol levels and atherosclerosis. Nutr. Rev. *36*, 1-5.

HINMAN, J.W. 1972. Prostaglandins. Ann. Rev. Biochem. *41*, 161-178.

KANDUTSCH, A.A., CHEN, H.W., and HEINIGER, H.J. 1978. Biological activity of some oxygenated sterols. Science *201* (4355) 498-501.

KRUMDIECK, C.L., and HO, K.J. 1977. Intestinal regulation of hepatic cholesterol synthesis: an hypothesis. Am. J. Clin. Nutr. *30*, 255-261.

MANSBACH, C.M., II. 1976. Conditions affecting the biosynthesis of lipids in the small intestine. Am. J. Clin. Nutr. *29*, 295-301.

SCHLENK, H. 1972. Odd numbered and new essential fatty acids. Fed. Proc., Fed. Am. Soc. Exp. Biol. *31*, 1430-1435.

SELECT COMM. ON NUTRITION AND HUMAN NEEDS, U.S. SENATE. 1977. Dietary Goals for the United States, 2nd Edition. (Committee Print). GPO, Washington, D.C.

SELECT COMM. ON NUTRITION AND HUMAN NEEDS, U.S. SENATE. 1977. Diet Related to Killer Diseases, III. Response to Dietary Goals of the United States: Re Meat (Committee Print). GPO, Washington, D.C.

TRUSWELL, A.S. 1978. Diet and plasma lipids—a reappraisal. Am. J. Clin. Nutr. *31*, 977-989.

5

Proteins and Amino Acids

The "protein problem" became a cause for popular concern in the mid-1970s. It first surfaced in conjunction with the World Food Crisis, grain sales abroad, and resulting higher domestic meat prices. For many, concern was expressed in fasting, meatless meals, and/or rejection of red meats. This phase was superceded by widespread belief that consumption of a vegetable protein supplement was necessary in order to meet protein needs. Then, dietary supplementation with digestive enzymes and "pre-digested" protein, i.e., amino acid mixtures, followed. Thus, the customary food and people interaction pattern involving consumption of red meat, especially beef, for dinner nightly was disrupted.

One may well ask, "How did this irrational sequence of events come about?" For some years, the protein problem has been a major research interest commanding top priority in allocation of time, energy, and money. Thousands of research reports have been produced as a number of alternative solutions were explored. The protein problem *does exist* as a world-wide problem, but not as an immediate problem for Americans, except for those who are destitute. Lack of understanding of the basis for the research emphasis led to misunderstanding and unwarranted public concern.

Supplementation with vegetable protein blends and amino acid mixtures is both unnecessary and undesirable. The RDA for protein is 45 to 65 g, depending on age-sex group; average American protein consumption is 125 g. Protein-rich foods are also relied upon to supply a variety of vitamins and minerals. Since the vegetable blends and amino acid mixtures are unlikely to contain these, deficiencies can result. For example, cases have been reported in which life-threatening cardiac arrest due to inadequate intake of potassium has been attributed to continued consumption of an amino acid mixture rather than a protein food. Clearly, mindless changes in food ecology can have dire consequences.

The RDA for protein was reduced recently. Why? Protein is a key nutrient. IF consumption of protein-rich foods changes in nature and/or extent, THEN will intakes of the other associated nutrients still be adequate?

FOOD SOURCES OF PROTEINS AND AMINO ACIDS

Plant and animal tissues are dietary sources of numerous proteins, each of which is a complex molecule composed of specific amino acids in fixed proportions, arranged in a predetermined sequence. The amino acid composition of a particular protein is nutritionally important, especially when only one protein-rich food is consumed at a feeding or as the predominant source in the diet.

Twenty amino acids are necessary and must be supplied in sufficient quantity to support tissue protein maintenance and/or increase. Of these, nine are essential, i.e., must be ingested (Tables 5.1 and 5.2). The others, simple straight-chain amino acids, are synthesized from the commonly available carbon skeleton plus amino groups. The explanation of essentiality is that some, like phenylalanine, contain a hexagonal ring (phenyl radical) that cannot be formed and some, like lysine, have a shape that does not allow attachment of the amino group.

The present recommended protein intake is 45 g for women and 60 g for men, with an essential amino acid profile equivalent to that of milk.

TABLE 5.1. AMINO ACIDS IN FOODS AND NUTRITION, ESSENTIAL AND NONESSENTIAL

Essential	Nonessential
Histidine[1]	Alanine
Isoleucine	Arginine[3]
Leucine	Asparagine
Lysine[2]	Aspartic acid
Methionine[2]	Citrulline[4]
Phenylalanine	Cysteine
Threonine	Cystine
Tryptophan	Glutamic acid
Valine	Glutamine
	Glycine
	Hydroxylysine
	Hydroxyproline
	Ornithine[4]
	Proline
	Serine
	Tyrosine

[1]Essential for growth during infancy; may be essential for maintenance and repair of tissue.
[2]Likely to be limiting because grains contain little.
[3]Formerly considered essential for growth during infancy.
[4]Not naturally occurring in proteins; metabolic intermediates in urea production.

Other foodstuffs meeting this criterion are meat, fish, poultry, and eggs (Table 5.2). The amino acid profiles of the various protein-rich vegetable foodstuffs reveal the fact that cereal proteins of wheat, rice, corn, rye, and oats are low in lysine, whereas the proteins of potatoes, nuts, and legumes are low in methionine and cystine. This limits their effectiveness in supporting tissue protein synthesis. Consumption of an additional 20 g of proteins from these foodstuffs provides sufficient quantities of the limiting amino acid(s), but also imbalances intake of the others. Such imbalance creates a side-effect: namely, a change in need for or utilization of some of the nonlimiting amino acids. Knowledge of the exact amino acid profile of a foodstuff enables one to plan combinations[1], mixtures[2], and/or blends[3] of food proteins for each meal that contain the necessary quantity of each of the essential amino acids.

TABLE 5.2. ESTIMATED AMINO ACID REQUIREMENTS AND HIGH QUALITY PROTEIN PATTERN

| Amino Acid | Requirement[1] | | | Pattern[2] |
	Infant (3-6 months)	Child (10-12 years)	Adult	
Histidine	33	?	?	17
Isoleucine	80	28	12	42
Leucine	128	42	16	70
Lysine	97	44	12	42
S-containing[3]	45	22	10	26
Aromatic[4]	132	22	16	73
Threonine	63	28	8	35
Tryptophan	19	4	3	11
Valine	89	25	14	48

Source: Adapted from Food and Nutr. Bd., Natl. Res. Counc. (1973).
[1]Listed as mg/kg body weight/day.
[2]Listed as mg/g protein.
[3]Methionine and/or cystine.
[4]Phenylalanine and/or tyrosine.

PROTEINS AND AMINO ACIDS: NORMAL SUPPLY AND NORMAL DEMAND

The proteins of foods and nutrition are complex and highly structured molecules. That is, they may contain 3 to 1,000 or more amino acids and

[1] Combination—Foods commonly served together; an association links them together because of compatible sensory attributes.
[2] Mixture—It is distinguished from a *compound* in that the ingredients are not present in absolutely fixed proportions, do not lose their individual characteristics, and can be separated by physical means.
[3] Blend—The ingredients are mixed thoroughly so that the attributes of the ingredients merge and are no longer distinct.

may have as many as 4 levels of molecular organization. Even so, they are not inert. Changes can occur at all four structural levels, for example:

(a) primary level—An amino acid can be deaminated or removed.

(b) secondary level—The fibrous or globular shape can be disrupted by breaking hydrogen bonds as in oxidation-reduction reactions.

(c) tertiary level—Functional capacity can be decreased due to cross-linking associated with denaturation.

(d) quarternary level—Functional capacity can be eliminated as when a subunit is removed.

Nutritionally, the aggregate effect of such changes is of theoretical importance. Ramifications affect the demand for one or more nutrients, e.g., those involved in replacement syntheses, in implementation of an alternate pathway, and inability to compensate. Practically, only the net effects of extensive changes of defined types have been evaluated.

Some changes related to degradation and synthesis are at least partially understood. The secondary structure of most proteins is known. The primary sequence of amino acid residues of some of the smaller proteins is known: this has enabled delineation of tertiary and quaternary structures of those proteins. Protein synthesis is known to be controlled genetically, and a model for DNA activity has been developed. And, changes in balance of plasma to labile tissue proteins are known to initiate/halt synthesis/degradation so as to restore equilibrium. The processes by which proteins are degraded during digestion and metabolism are clearly understood; not all steps are known in every case. Beyond this, there are many unknowns. Science is continually extending knowledge of detail that is important to a full explanation. Discussion is limited according to applicability.

Digestion/Absorption

Proteins are large macromolecules, so they are not normally absorbed intact. (IF absorbed, THEN they induce antibody formation and allergy results.) Therefore, the purpose of digestion is to liberate the individual amino acids by degrading the protein structure. In foods, proteins are bound to carbohydrate and lipids, both of which may need to be degraded before the protein can be attacked. When amino acid composition and the quantity present are approximately the same, biological value is a function of the degree of liberation.

The protein content of the normal mixed diet consumed in the United States at this time accounts for 12 to 15% of the calories ingested. Dietary protein is obtained from a combination of animal and vegetable sources that varies within and among days. Therefore, the quantity of each of the amino acids to be absorbed is highly variable. To deal with the range of normal variation, special absorption control mechanisms have evolved. These enable the selective absorption of those essential amino acids that historically have been in short supply. The mechanism by which selective absorption occurs is largely unknown at this time. Points related to nutritional aspects of digestion/absorption of proteins and amino acids include, but are not limited to, the following:

(a) Absorption is an active and a selective process, especially for methionine, since this amino acid is likely to be in short supply and has special metabolic roles. Vitamin B_6 is necessary for the active transport of amino acids through the mucosal cells of the intestinal wall.

(b) Competition for absorption sites exists among the amino acids. Therefore, IF an excess of one inhibits uptake of one that is short, THEN the expected effect is one of reducing overall utilization of amino acids in the interim. Moreover, anything that causes irritation and results in an increased rate of peristalsis will cause malabsorption of amino acids, as they will move beyond the absorption sites before they can be absorbed.

(c) Digestion and absorption require two to three hours. Even very large protein intakes, e.g., 500 g, can be tolerated with little observable effect. The quantity liberated at a given time is related to the rate of absorption; a larger quantity requires a longer processing time but ultimately approximately 92% is absorbed. As long as the quantity and quality are within the normal range, the circulating level of any of the amino acids does not rise significantly after a meal. This is because of the long timespan and cellular ability to remove circulating amino acids.

(d) Approximately two-thirds of the amino acids absorbed are derived from degradation of the protein from mucosal cells which are sloughed off when they become senescent. This conservation mechanism is important in balancing the mixture of amino acids absorbed.

Metabolism of Amino Acids—in General

The details of amino acid metabolism have been under investigation for many years. A recent review (Felig 1975) has summarized some of the newer findings that clarify the various aspects of the amino acid flow.

Skeletal muscle and liver tissue are the main organs that control the overall circulating level and turnover rate for individual amino acids. Skeletal muscle contains 50% of the total pool of free amino acids. The liver is the main organ for processing and degradation of amino acids. Salient points with respect to the overall flow are:

(a) Liver cells selectively remove nearly all of the circulating alanine, serine, threonine, and glycine. They also remove lesser amounts of the other essential amino acids *except* valine, isoleucine, and leucine. There-fore, these three must be catabolized elsewhere.

(b) Kidney cells remove glutamine, proline, and glycine from circula-tion and secrete serine and alanine into circulation. The kidney is con-sidered the source of circulating serine.

(c) Brain cells withdraw a greater quantity of valine, leucine, and isoleucine than do other cells.

(d) Mucosal cells catabolize glutamine, which provides a nitrogen source for synthesis of alanine. Alanine is released to circulation; 50% goes to the liver for metabolism.

(e) Liver cells utilize amino acid-derived carbon chains to form glucose. Alanine is present in abundance and may be the precursor for as much as 50% of the glucose that is derived from amino acids.

(f) Muscle cells withdraw branched chain amino acids and degrade these, liberating nitrogen for synthesis of alanine.

(g) Insulin stimulates protein synthesis and transport of amino acids. It also inhibits degradation of proteins, resulting in a decreased circulat-ing level of valine, leucine, isoleucine, methionine, tyrosine, and phenyl-alanine. In contrast, it stimulates alanine synthesis.

(h) Pharmacologic levels of glucagon decrease the circulating levels of all amino acids, especially alanine, increase the rate of conversion of ala-nine to glucose, increase the rate of oxidation of branched chain amino acids, and reduce the rate of incorporation of amino acids in protein. Be-cause of the action of glucagon, the rate of hepatic uptake of amino acids is greater than the rate of muscle release of the individual amino acids, so the circulating levels fall.

(i) When dietary protein is ingested, secretion of insulin, glucagon, and growth hormone is stimulated. Taken together with the preceding points, this finding suggests that increased glucose from alanine is what prevents the hypoglycemia that would otherwise result from the elevated insulin level.

(j) At present, there are no data from human studies on the interorgan exchange of amino acids as a result of consumption of protein. Moreover, there are no data on the exchange of amino acids between the intestinal mucosa and the liver.

Ten points concerning protein metabolism have been discussed. Clearly, many portions of the general metabolic process have not been char-acterized yet.

The general types of reactions that amino acids are involved in are:

(a) transamination—The reaction involves transfer of an amino group from an amino acid to a keto acid. A class of enzymes called trans-aminases effects the transfer. *Glutamate transaminase* specifically transfers the amino group from an amino acid to α-ketoglutaric acid forming glutamic acid. This transaminase has some capacity to effect this transfer in forming other amino acids. Similarly, *alanine transferase* specifically transfers an amino group from alanine to α-ketoglutarate forming pyruvic acid and glutamic acid. Together, these two reactions cause degradation products to converge in the form of glutamic acid.

(b) deamination—The reaction involves removal of an amine group with formation of a keto acid and NH_3, which must be disposed of via the urea cycle. *Glutamic dehydrogenase*, amino acid oxidase, ammonia lyases, specific deaminases, and deamidases can effect these reactions.

(c) decarboxylation—The reaction involves removal of CO_2; the remaining compound is an amine.

Amino acids are translocated throughout the body by the circulatory system in order to supply the cells of the various tissues (Fig. 5.1). Amino acids are withdrawn from circulation by the cells on demand and are actively transported into the cell by an as yet unclear mechanism involving the use of vitamin B_6. Then, the amino acids are conjugated to form

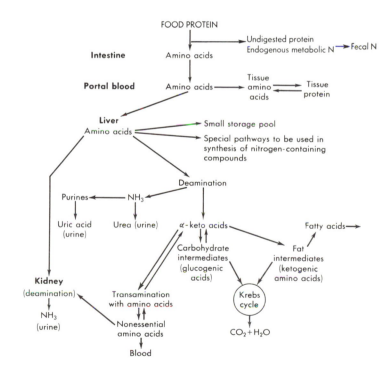

FIG. 5.1. PROTEIN METABOLISM

labile storage proteins, which keeps the intracellular concentration of amino acids low. When amino acids are needed, these labile storage proteins are degraded under the influence of intracellular enzymes called *kathepsins*. This mechanism stabilizes intracellular amino acid availability to some extent.

Whenever the circulating level of a plasma amino acid drops, the amino acid is liberated from the storage protein and is transported out to restore the circulating level. Under the influence of various hormones, the circulating level of each of the amino acids is maintained within narrow limits. The hormones involved are growth hormone and insulin, which increase the rate of tissue withdrawal, and the adrenocortical glucocorticoid hormones that increase the circulating level.

The mechanisms for synthesis and degradation of intracellular proteins, other than genes and structural proteins, allow a rapid exchange with those of the plasma. As a result, these proteins are in a dynamic state of equilibrium. So, if a particular tissue loses proteins by injury or other trauma, it can rapidly synthesize new protein from plasma protein-derived amino acids. These, in turn, are replenished by amino acids liberated from storage proteins in other tissues. In this way, the quantity of critical intracellular proteins is assured.

There is an upper limit to the quantity of storage proteins that a cell can generate. When all cells have reached their limit, the leftover amino acids are degraded. The carbon chain is used to produce energy and the nitrogen portion is used in synthesis of urea, as will be discussed.

All cells, except circulating red blood cells (RBC), which lack a nucleus so cannot reproduce themselves, synthesize a limited number of specified proteins. Twenty-two amino acids can be utilized. Of these, nine are essential, so normally are available for use as is. Available non-protein nitrogen and amino acids are used in production of the 13 nonessential amino acids by transamination and other processes. The steps in the protein synthesis process have become increasingly clear in recent years. Synthesis of a nucleoprotein such as DNA is commonly used for illustration. (See a biochemistry textbook for a description of the process.) Separate but similar processes are followed in synthesizing each of the other proteins produced by the cell.

The biosynthesis of proteins utilizes RNA in the process as indicated:

(a) Preliminary screening of the amino acid pool eliminates ornithine, citrulline, β-alanine, and diamino pimelic acid which are not used in protein synthesis.

(b) Amino acids are selected and activated as necessary. Each has its own amino acyl-tRNA synthetase system by which an amino acid-adenylate-enzyme complex is formed. This tRNA complex then functions as an adaptor and coordinator in sequencing the amino acids according to the mRNA pattern.

(c) Translation is a four-step process involving initiation or the binding of mRNA to a peptidyl site on the ribosome, elongation or repositioning over the next codon which is repeated $1 \ldots n$ times, and termination of the completed protein with the formation of the terminal formyl methional amino group. This terminal group must be removed before the folding of the protein is complete.

Tissue protein synthesis is initiated when a signal is received that there is need for a specific protein. There are three general classes of proteins: nucleoproteins, which are utilized for cell reproduction; structural proteins, which are used for tissue growth and cell wall repair; and enzymes for intracellular use. Two kinds of signals have been identified. The first is a hormonal induction which stimulates production 1000-fold. A second is derepression, as when the level of a particular endproduct is low, resulting in derepression.

Tissue protein synthesis is halted when a set-point is reached, all other things such as precursors being equal. There are two kinds of signals that modulate protein synthesis. Product inhibition is a mechanism whereby buildup of the end product slows production. A second is feedback inhibition of one type or another whereby buildup of the end product inhibits one or more of the enzymes that produce(s) one or more of the precursors.

Anabolism and catabolism are general processes of production and/or construction and destruction, respectively. They are continuous and in balance so that tissue integrity is maintained under normal circumstances. These processes appear to be under genetic control, i.e., the genes carry a master set of instructions that determine which proteins are replaced and in what order. In relation to structural proteins these processes have to be controlled; otherwise some parts might be replaced frequently and others not at all.

Anabolism is a production/construction process that is operative at several levels. For example, in order to make the protein necessary for an enzyme or structure or whatever, both amino acids and the protein need to be generated. IF the cytoplasmic pool of a nonessential amino acid is short and the labile storage protein is degraded but none becomes available, THEN production is initiated. IF there is a supply of keto acids and non-protein nitrogen, THEN nitrogen will be added to the keto acid. Or, IF there is a supply of keto acids and excess amino acids, THEN instead of degrading them, they will be diverted to this purpose and transamination or moving of the amino group from the amino acid to the keto acid will occur. When the necessary amino acids become available, they will be joined to make the protein.

Catabolism of proteins is a destructive process. Research studies have demonstrated that protein is replaced but whether the protein is removed, degraded, and replaced or amino acids are removed and replaced systematically along each protein molecule has not been determined.

Some tissues replace themselves by adding a new inner layer at a time and by sloughing off the outer layers. In tissues where this occurs, e.g., intestinal mucosa, skin, hair, nails, the nature and extent of protein catabolism may be a different process from that in tissues where systematic replacement is the mode.

Metabolism in Specific Tissues

In tissues where protein metabolism is involved in performing the special function(s) of that tissue, the normal processing activities are more vigorous. Although the processes of anabolism and catabolism are continuous, the protein turnover rate is variable among tissues. Research has demonstrated that turnover rate is highest in active tissues such as the intestinal mucosa, liver, pancreas, kidney, and plasma. It is lowest in tissues where function does not stress structure, e.g., muscle, brain, and skin. It is almost nonexistent in collagen. Metabolism in the following tissues will be discussed briefly: muscles; skin, hair, and nails; liver; and secretory cells.

Muscle.—The normal state for a muscle, once developed, is for it to maintain its strength and size by a continuous process of replacement and repair. On a continuous basis, as amino acids are released, the decision to reuse in protein synthesis or to deaminate, etc., depends on what is immediately available in the tissue pool as a result of the metabolic equilibrium. Historical usage determines muscle strength and size. Therefore, it determines the level of synthesis necessary for replacement and repair. A muscle tissue has potential for augmentation as a result of an increase in use; the set-point for the level of synthesis is shifted upward, increasing the rate of synthesis. Muscle wasting, as a result of non-use, is observed in the sedentary American who is not physically fit and in the elderly as a result of aging-related reduction in metabolic rate. Wasting occurs because the rate of catabolism exceeds that of anabolism. The nitrogen portion of the amino acid is diverted to urea production and the carbon chain is degraded or stored for energy.

Skin, Hair, and Nails.—These are composed largely of insoluble proteins. Cell proliferation occurs at the inside edge of the tissue, where new cells are contiguous with the immediately preceding layer. Metabolic rate of production of structural proteins is very rapid. Within the tissue, there is a progressive decrease in metabolic rate from the inner to the outer layer of cells. At some point it becomes so low that death occurs. Dead cells are sloughed off to some degree.

The Liver.—This is the organ for processing of amino acids from exogenous sources that arrive via the portal blood flow. Because it is a major processing center, the liver has a large capacity for storage of labile storage proteins. It is also the site of production of plasma proteins. It produces all of the plasma albumins and fibrinogen and at least half of the plasma globulins. Lipoproteins, glycoproteins, purines, and pyrimidines also are produced. Creatinine and urea are nitrogenous excretory products produced by hepatocytes.

Creatinine results from creatine metabolism. When creatine, in its phosphorylated form, is used as a high energy source in formation of ATP, creatinine is formed.

Urea is the endproduct of deamination of amino acids (Fig. 5.2). All amino acids participate in transamination reactions in one of which the amino acid and α-ketoglutarate react to form a keto acid and glutamic acid. Glutamic acid is the intermediate by which excess amino acid nitrogen, as ammonia, is disposed of. Ammonia is toxic so it must not accumulate in the free state; this mechanism utilizing formation of glutamic acid is the alternative. Glutamine, the acid amide form of glutamic acid, is formed as a temporary storage compound if the rate of urea synthesis is less than that of glutamic acid formation. Glutamic acid yields ammonia, which reacts with CO_2 to form a carbamyl phosphate. Two molecules of this compound combine with ornithine to form citrulline. Citrulline then combines with aspartic acid to yield arginosuccinic acid. The latter is split, yielding fumaric acid and arginine. Arginine is then hydrolyzed, yielding urea and ornithine. Thus, ornithine becomes available for a continued round of urea production.

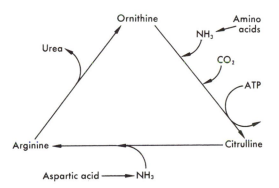

FIG. 5.2. THE KREBS-HENSELEIT CYCLE

A mechanism for disposing of ammonia by urea synthesis.

Secretory Cells.—These cells produce enzymes and/or hormones for distribution. IF the hormonal, pressure, or product-related signal to secrete an enzyme or hormone is received, THEN the action causes a sharp reduction in stored quantity, produces a signal to make, and resets the level for the production quantity. Enzymes are two-part molecules, the protein portion called an apoenzyme and the coenzyme which may be vitamin or mineral.

PROTEINS AND AMINO ACIDS: DEFICIENT SUPPLY OR INFLATED DEMAND

Kwashiorkor, the "protein deficiency disease," is a well defined syndrome resulting from chronic consumption of a low-protein, low calorie diet. Because of its prevalence in children of less developed countries, it has been studied extensively. However, for Americans it is interesting but irrelevant; it is a trivial public health problem limited to destitute families.

The problem of amino acid deficiency is somewhat different and probably much more extensive due to consumption of vegetarian diets. Protein synthesis requires a necessary and sufficient quantity of each of the amino acids to be incorporated in a particular protein. In some cases, a different amino acid can be substituted in, but the resultant protein will not be identical and will not be functionally equivalent. In other cases, lack of a specific amino acid halts protein synthesis; such an amino acid is called a limiting amino acid. Any of the essential amino acids can be a limiting amino acid.

Digestion/Absorption

A large proportion of the amino acids absorbed each day is derived from degradation of the dead mucosal cells that have been sloughed off. Mucus protects the lining as long as the cells are contiguous. When the cells become separated, a vulnerable surface is created and the cells are attacked by the digestive enzymes. IF the quantity or quality of protein intake is low, THEN there is a progressive decrease in the rate of replacement of mucosal cells due to impaired protein synthesis. Therefore, the quantity of essential amino acids from this source is greatly reduced, which continues the problem.

The effects of a low protein intake on the digestion/absorption function are insignificant. IF the quantity is low, THEN all are short to some degree and normal competition for carriers is absent. IF protein quality is low, THEN the nonessential amino acids may be absorbed more rapidly than usual since the carriers are free. Effects of this outcome are unknown.

Metabolism of Amino Acids—in General

On a temporary basis, a low quantity or a low quality protein intake is insignificant. Plasma proteins are withdrawn from circulation for intracellular synthesis. Storage proteins are degraded to replenish plasma proteins.

On a continuing basis, the effects are progressive. IF the low quantity continues, THEN since the proteins of most tissues are labile, a general slow down in repairs will result from a diversion to the lowest common level and will result in a general weakening of structure and decrease in function. This is most noticeable in muscle tissue. IF the intake quantity is adequate, but the quality or biologic value is low due to shortage of one or more of the essential amino acids, THEN synthesis will continue to the limit of the supply of the limiting amino acid. As a result, the lowest common level will usually be greater than when the quantity is low. However, the effects will be the same, if somewhat less. At the same time, the supply of other amino acids will be in excess since they cannot be utilized in synthesis. These will be deaminated. Both urea and keto acid (ketone body) formation will be abnormally high. The keto acids will be utilized for energy. In extreme cases where the body cannot cope uremia or acidosis may result.

Metabolism in Specific Tissues

The effects of continued deficient intake are observed first in those tissues where cell replacement is rapid and/or processing of amino acids is a major function. Tissues so affected include, but are not limited to, intestinal mucosa, liver, kidney, and muscles and skin, hair, and nails.

The cells of the intestinal mucosa are normally replaced every three days. IF the protein intake is quantitatively or qualitatively low, THEN reduced protein synthesis results in impaired replacement and leads to fragility, decreased functionality, and irritability. IF food is ingested, THEN since the mucosa cannot cope, it must be rejected and removed. Thus, nausea, vomiting, and diarrhea are the expected (and often observed) outcomes. Often plasma proteins must be given by IV to upgrade tissue integrity before feeding can be resumed.

A less than optimal intake of amino acids creates liver stress due to hyperactivity of an abnormal nature. When the intracellular supply of essential amino acids is low, then plasma proteins are transported in to make up the deficit. In order to maintain normal circulating levels of plasma albumins and globulins, these must be replenished by liver synthesis. This fails and the circulating level drops.

Recycling and conservation of limiting amino acids by immediate incorporation in protein have priority over transamination and deamination. Some nonessential amino acids continue to be necessary and synthesis continues at a low level. However, the majority of amino acids remain in excess and are processed by either transamination or deamination. Which predominates depends on whether the intake is quantitatively or qualitatively low, or both. IF intake is only quantitatively low, THEN transamination predominates in order to produce the nonessential amino acids necessary for some protein synthesis; urea production is also low. Some urea is reabsorbed and serves as a source of non-protein nitrogen in synthesis of nonessential amino acids. IF intake is qualitatively low, THEN deamination predominates and urea production increases because of excesses of some unusable amino acids. This may create a stress on the kidney.

Transamination and/or deamination results in formation of a large quantity of keto acids. Normally, these would be transported out to adipose tissue for processing. But, since the circulating level of plasma albumins is subnormal, transport is impaired. As a result, the keto acids are used for local triglyceride synthesis producing an abnormal condition known as fatty liver.

Muscular weakness results in lassitude and lethargy. Lassitude, i.e., fatigue resulting from poor health, is the effect of catabolism of muscle protein. Muscle proteins are degraded to the common level which is progressively lower as low intake continues. When there is insufficient protein to maintain contractile activity at normal functional levels, stamina decreases and fatigue is perceived. When even a small exertion causes fatigue, lethargy, i.e., an aversion to activity, results.

A deficient amino acid intake results in fragility of skin, hair, and nails. Cuts and other wounds heal less rapidly than normal; there is insufficient protein for repair. Hair breaks off. Nails are soft and bend or break due to overextension. All of these effects vary from mild to severe depending on the level of intake and its duration.

AMINO ACIDS: EXCESS SUPPLY

High protein diets have been customary for some peoples for centuries and recently have been advocated for weight reduction purposes. What are the expected outcomes?

Digestion/Absorption

The effects depend on whether the excess is of low quality or high quality protein. When intake provides an excess of nonessential amino acids, since these have lower transport carrier priority, they will form a crowd and result in an entry barrier to essential amino acids. This reduces absorption rate. When the intake provides an excess of essential amino acids, transport will be rapid but may be inadequate, resulting in long transport queues and an entry barrier that prolongs absorption time. In either case, the rate of liberation of amino acids by the digestive enzymes is retarded, so peristalsis is retarded in order to allow enough time for absorption. So, one feels "stuffed" and satiety value is high. Constipation may be perceived as another outcome. IF some other factor should intervene AND peristalsis is not retarded, THEN the incompletely digested protein will move on to the large intestine. Malabsorption is the result. Putrefaction in the colon may produce methane, sulfur dioxide, and other malodorous gases as well as carbon dioxide and hydrogen gases.

Metabolism of Amino Acids—in General

In general, an intracellular excess of amino acids does not occur. This is because any accumulated are immediately (a) incorporated into the labile storage proteins or (b) deaminated. Thus, effects are limited to specific tissues.

Metabolism in Specific Tissues

Generally speaking, the known effects of excess amino acid intake are not manifestly injurious or life-threatening. Some specific tissues are affected but not greatly stressed. These include, but are not limited to, the liver, muscles, kidney, and adipose tissue.

An excess intake of amino acids causes liver cells to be hyperactive. Absorbed amino acids are transported via the portal blood to the liver for disposal. Two types of activity are utilized in disposal of excess amino acids, namely (a) protein synthesis and (b) amino acid destruction. Enzymes, hormones, and plasma proteins are synthesized to the extent possible. The remainder of the amino acids are deaminated; urea and keto acids are produced in large quantity. IF the caloric intake is low, THEN the keto acids will be withdrawn rapidly from circulation and degraded, producing the needed energy. IF the caloric intake is adequate, THEN uptake of keto acids by adipose cells will result in triglyceride synthesis for energy storage. These are limited alternatives for processing amino acids. As a result, the only difference between an excess of one or all amino acids is in which enzymes, etc., can be produced to what extent and what proportion will be degraded to keto acids.

An excess amino acid intake ensures that the circulating level of one or more amino acids will remain high enough to result in sustained muscle cell uptake. IF the right assortment of amino acids is available intracellularly in necessary and sufficient quantity, THEN both structural and contractile proteins will be synthesized. This will allow both renewal and development within the framework of the historical usage record of the particular muscle, which sets the limits. Thus, a high use muscle will become larger and stronger in order to cope more efficiently with the inflated demands resulting from high use. A low use muscle will renew itself, but will not develop.

An excess amino acid intake, whether of one or several amino acids, results in increased urea production. A major function of the kidney is control of blood urea nitrogen (BUN) level. At normal levels of urea production, renal cells are accommodating, i.e., removal/reabsorption of urea is adjusted to control BUN within normal ranges. At somewhat elevated levels of urea production, renal cell removal of urea and elimination via the urine becomes urgent. At greatly elevated levels of urea production, renal cell removal of urea would become frantic in an attempt to control a rising BUN, which is associated with life-threatening outcomes. Fortunately, in biologically normal people, excess intake of amino acids has not resulted in greatly elevated levels of urea production. Still, hyperactivity on a continuing basis is undesirable because who is vulnerable is unknowable in advance.

An excess amino acid intake, whether of one or several amino acids, results in utilization of keto acids for triglyceride formation and storage when carbohydrate and/or lipid calories are adequate. Because average American intake is more than twice what is necessary and calories are abundant, many people must be adding to their weight control problem by overconsumption of protein (Fig. 5.3).

PROTEINS AND AMINO ACIDS: FOOD ECOLOGY AND LIFE EXPECTANCY

Because the average American protein intake is double the recommended quantity, and, since most of the protein consumed is of animal origin, the essential amino acid intake is more than adequate. Thus, most Americans' relation to protein-rich foods results in consumption at a level that supports health and does not interfere with life expectancy.

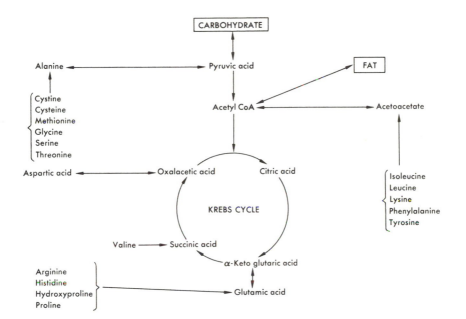

FIG. 5.3. AMINO ACIDS ENTER THE PATHWAYS COMMON TO CARBOHYDRATE AND FAT METABOLISM

Most amino acids are glucogenic; some are ketogenic; and a few may be either glucogenic or ketogenic.

However, when insecurity, anger, disgust, or other strong emotions are generated by some event or issue, the normal food and people interaction is changed and ecological balance is disturbed. A decision to change consumption can have unplanned nutritional effects, e.g., a decision to boycott red meat coupled with mindless substitution of other protein foods results in a change in amino acid intake. Those uninformed or misinformed about the amino acid composition of foods make unwitting errors. Fortunately, such changes in food and people interactions are usually short-lived, so for most people the impact on nutriture is unimportant. But, if the change occurs at a critical period for an individual, it can have unexpectedly large effects. Moreover, there are always some people who continue a practice developed in relation to a specific event or issue long after the cause has died. These people become nutritionally vulnerable. For these reasons, any faddish popular movement that affects the food and people interaction is a cause for concern.

The health food business is lucrative but hazardous for its customers. To maintain its market, this business introduces new pseudo-nutritional solutions to health problems at frequent intervals. New miracle foods are publicized in order to entice people into impulse purchases. The new foods are purported to correct unverified deficiencies of first one nutrient, then another. In the mid-1970s, the "protein problem" was exploited. Digestive enzymes and protein hydrolysates provided the solution.

As pointed out in Chapter 2, protein is a key nutrient. Therefore, when some people stopped eating protein-rich foods and substituted protein hydrolysates, the nutritional balance of their food-related ecosystem was disturbed. In some cases, both B-vitamin and mineral deficiencies, especially potassium, developed, creating life-threatening medical emergencies.

Vegetarianism creates a "protein problem" for uninformed or misinformed adherents. Soybean protein is the only complete vegetable protein, i.e., one that contains all of the essential amino acids in a significant quantity. Since one or more of the essential amino acids is lacking or is present only in very limited quantity in the other vegetable proteins, several must be consumed together in order to supply an adequate quantity of all. Thus, in order to meet essential amino acid needs on a daily basis, vegetarians, especially vegans, must (a) know the essential amino acid composition of the various vegetable proteins, (b) consciously select a combination of proteins with complementary essential amino acid patterns, and (c) adjust quantities consumed according to needs. Some people cannot or will not be consciously conscientious, so a protein problem develops.

When a diet is overly restrictive, such as the Zen Macrobiotic diet, there is no possibility of meeting essential amino acid needs. In this case beliefs affect man's relation to his food in such a way as to create a life-threatening deficiency of essential amino acids.

Awareness, understanding, and appreciation of the functions of proteins reinforce the concept of primacy of protein in human nutrition. A variety of functional proteins contributes to life-sustaining metabolic processes. These include, but are not limited to:

(a) enzymes, which must be replaced

(b) hormones, which are destroyed when they have served their function, must be replaced to maintain normal activity levels

(c) structural proteins of various tissues and organs, e.g., those of blood cells and blood vessels, heart muscle, musculature of the GI tract, skeletal muscle, brain and nerve tissues, pancreas, liver, skin, hair, nails, the base material of bones and teeth

(d) plasma proteins that serve as buffers to stabilize blood pH by neutralizing organic acids and bases produced in cellular metabolism, during transport to the kidneys for disposal

(e) plasma proteins bind plasma fluid, which contributes to maintenance of blood volume and blood pressure

(f) carrier proteins that bind various gases, minerals, and small molecules during transport via the circulatory system, e.g., hemoglobin (oxygen and carbon dioxide), transferrin (iron, chromium, and zinc), and albumin (fatty acids)

(g) storage proteins that bind precious minerals, e.g., ferritin and hemosiderin that retain iron in the intestinal wall and liver and thyroglobulin that retain iodine in the thyroid gland

(h) immunoglobulins, which are involved in the immune response

Clearly, tissue proteins have important functions in respect to physical well-being and longevity. Hence, dietary deviance by the uninformed can have unlooked-for effects.

BIBLIOGRAPHY

FELIG, P. 1975. Amino acid metabolism in man. Ann. Rev. Biochem. *44*, 933-955.

FOOD AND NUTR. BD., NATL. RES. COUNC. 1973. Improvement of protein nutriture. Natl. Acad. Sci., Washington, D.C.

Carbohydrates

For Americans, the food and people interactions involving carbohydrates (CHO) have changed in recent years. For some, it has taken a degenerate pathway. Four stages of progressive devaluing and decreasing consumption have been identified. The first stage is *disillusionment*—good foods such as bread and potatoes join pasta, cakes, refined sugar, and empty-calorie snack foods on a growing list of suspect and/or proscribed foods. The next stage is *erosion*—consumption goes into a decline. The value of consuming carbohydrate-rich foods as a class is undermined, with the result that portion sizes are reduced and the frequency of consumption drops. The third stage is *detachment*—since consumption of CHO is no longer valued, consumption is further reduced. The fourth stage is *separation*—CHO foods are assigned a negative value and are conscientiously avoided. For others, dietary intake of CHO also decreased, although not so drastically. In many cases the nature of the CHO changed from complex CHO such as starch to simple sugars. Thus, consumption of breads and potatoes decreased and consumption of table sugar (sucrose) continued to increase until 1974. Then, the use of sucrose decreased but use of other sugars and syrups increased so that the total intake of sweeteners remained the same. Is this change in food ecology important to health and/or life expectancy? There is no RDA for CHO; is there a need to consume a certain portion of calories as CHO?

FOOD SOURCES OF CARBOHYDRATE

Sugars, starch, cellulose, pectins, glycogen, and a number of other compounds containing carbon, hydrogen, and oxygen with hydrogen and oxygen in the same ratio as in water make up the class of organic compounds known as carbohydrates. With the exception of glycogen, these CHO compounds are produced by plants.

100

The simplest kinds of carbohydrates are sugars; there are two types of these. The first type are *monosaccharides* or single sugars. These may have between three and seven carbon atoms in their basic chain structure. The 5- (pentose) and 6- (hexose) carbon sugars are important physiologically and nutritionally. Common food sources of carbohydrate are predominantly 6-carbon sugars or are polymers of these. There are three hexose monosaccharides. Glucose or dextrose is the major monosaccharide of nutritional importance and is the class representative. Fructose, found in free form in honey and some fruits, is somewhat important. Galactose is not found in free form in foods.

Disaccharides or double sugars are made up of two monosaccharides, one of which is glucose. Common food disaccharides are:

(a) sucrose (glucose + fructose)—It occurs naturally in sugar cane, sugar beets, sorghum cane, maple syrup, pineapple, carrots, etc., in a partially refined form in molasses and brown sugar, and as a fully refined deliberate additive in beverages, baked goods, ice cream, etc.

(b) lactose (glucose + galactose)—It occurs naturally in milks of all species and most dairy products made from milks, in a processed form, i.e., usually dehydrated as non-fat dry milk solids, and as a deliberate additive in baked goods, mixes, etc.

(c) maltose (glucose + glucose)—It occurs naturally in germinating cereals and in malt beverages as a deliberate additive.

Sugars are contained in the cell sap of plants and are usually removed by crushing and grinding. They are refined by evaporation of the water until a supersaturated solution is formed. Then, the sugar precipitates out as pure crystals which are centrifuged out. The residue is molasses.

Polysaccharides are complex carbohydrates. The first class of these that is nutritionally important is the starches. There are three types of starches:

(a) amylose (a straight chain polymer of glucose that is degraded to maltose by digestive enzymes)—It occurs naturally as the predominant starch in baking potatoes, legumes, corn, wheat, and tapioca, in a partially refined state in white wheat or corn flour, in a fully refined state in cake flour, and as a deliberate additive in puddings and bakery products, etc.

(b) amylopectin (a branched chain polymer of glucose that is degraded to maltose and isomaltose by digestive enzymes)—It occurs naturally as the predominant starch in boiling potatoes, waxy maize, and waxy rice, and in a fully refined state in canned puddings and pie fillings and in frozen sauces and gravies.

(c) modified starches (a branched chain polymer of glucose that is degraded to maltose, isomaltose, and whichever of several substituent groups are used in modification)—It is a processed form of corn, wheat, or tapioca starch and is used in frozen sauces and gravies.

Starches are contained in storage granules inside cell walls. Raw starch is poorly digested. Cooking softens and ruptures cell walls. It also allows hydration of the starch molecules which increases the surface area, facilitating penetration by the starch-splitting digestive enzymes called amylases.

The second class of polysaccharides is the celluloses and hemicelluloses. There are three groups of these:

(a) cellulose (a straight chain polymer of glucose that cannot be degraded by digestive enzymes)—It occurs naturally in the cell walls of plant tissues, including the bran coat of cereal grains, and in a partially refined state in bran ready-to-eat cereals.

(b) cellulose ethers (cellulose derivatives called methylcellulose, hydroxypropylmethylcellulose, sodium carboxymethylcellulose (CMC), and microcrystalline cellulose)—These are indigestible processed forms used as synthetic food gums for their water-holding, thickening, and foam-stabilizing properties in ice cream and other frozen desserts, french dressings, and aerosol whips.

(c) hemicelluloses (polymers of unmodified pentose and hexose units or similar polymers that also include sugar acid units; these are water-insoluble)—They occur naturally in cell walls of plants and are degraded in hot alkaline cooking water.

The third class of polysaccharides is the pectic substances, a heterogeneous class of similar derivatives of galactose that contain other substituent groups. These substances are present in green fruits and soften as the fruits ripen. Also, they form a gel structure in jams and jellies when heated with acid and sugar.

The fourth class of polysaccharides is glycogen, a branched chain polymer of glucose. It occurs naturally in animal and fish muscle tissues as the storage form of glucose. The glycogen content of meat and fish is usually trivial.

The fifth class of polysaccharides and their derivatives is the vegetable gums. The term "food gums" applies to all members of this class that can be dispersed in water and swell to produce gels or viscous dispersions. There are three groups of natural food gums: (a) plant exudates, e.g., gum arabic, gum tragacanth, and gum karaya; (b) extracts from plant seeds, e.g., locust bean gum and guar gum; and (c) extracts of seaweeds, e.g., agar and carrageenan. The gums contain a complex and incompletely defined mixture of polysaccharides. The structures cannot be degraded by the digestive enzymes so they are non-caloric and are used to provide texture in dietetic foods. They are also used in puddings, mixes, ice cream, bakery products, french dressings, fruit drinks, chocolate milk, and whipped toppings.

The sixth class of polysaccharides contains only inulin, a polysaccharide of fructose. It occurs naturally in onions, garlic, and artichokes. Storage results in partial degradation to fructose. Inulin is only partially degraded by digestive enzymes but some further degradation by colon bacteria occurs.

Corn syrups are controlled, but variable mixtures of glucose, maltose, and higher glucose polymer fragment. They are produced by partial hydrolysis of corn starch.

CARBOHYDRATES: NORMAL SUPPLY AND NORMAL DEMAND

Although a variety of carbohydrates is consumed, unless they can be degraded to the three simple sugars glucose, fructose, and galactose, they cannot be used to nourish the human body. So, the polysaccharides except for starch and glycogen are regarded as non-nutritive. Since their fiber structures cannot be degraded, they provide bulk. So, they are referred to as bulking agents and are valued for that contribution.

Carbohydrate metabolism involves glucose, fructose, and galactose. However, fructose and galactose can be converted to glucose by cellular processing and the number of known functions for them *per se* is limited. Therefore, discussion of the expected effects of carbohydrate on generalized cells and specialized organs uses glucose, the class representative carbohydrate, for illustration.

Digestion/Absorption

The normal mixed diet, in the United States at this time, contains 250 to 375 g carbohydrate. The mean percentage of calories as carbohydrate is 46%. The particular mixture varies with the meal, among days, and with considerable variation among seasons. Variability has existed since the beginning. So the absorption control mechanisms, integral parts of the brush border of the intestinal wall where the disaccharidases are located, have been developed to deal with the expected variation.

The traditional diet of man, except for carnivores, has been predominantly starchy, with some sucrose and fructose from fruits and honey and little lactose after weaning. Therefore, the most abundant enzyme in the brush border is *maltase* for splitting maltose from starch. The supply of *lactase* is relatively low in adults. IF proportionate consumption is continued into adulthood, THEN the supply of lactase is continued in a compensatory way. THEREFORE, most adults can utilize lactose if their previous intake has been continuous; discrete or occasional intake creates an overload condition due to relative lactase deficiency. The usual symptoms of distress and irritation develop, i.e., gas and diarrhea. The *sucrase* supply is lower than the supply of maltase but it is necessary and sufficient to handle the traditional load of fruit sugar. IF consumption of sucrose is high, as when concentrated sweets are consumed, THEN a relative sucrase deficiency results in fatigue, irritation of the local villi, and symptoms of distress, i.e., nausea, gas, and diarrhea.

The traditional diet of man was variable with respect to fiber content, depending on whether peoples were vegetarian, carnivores, or omnivores. In general, man is adapted to a moderate fiber intake. This allows formation of an amorphous mass that is sufficiently loose that it can be moved, without creating muscle strain, by the combined efforts of the circular and longitudinal muscles of the GI tract. This looseness is necessary for efficient mixing in of acids, bases, and enzymes involved in digestion and absorption. IF the mass were compact, THEN mixing and penetration would be less efficient, thus retarding rate of and/or completeness of digestion/absorption. Moreover, in order to move a compact mass great mechanical pressure must be applied. A weak spot will give under the pressure, ballooning out into a sac (diverticulosis). Since sacs have narrow necks, the material is trapped and stagnates; a variety of unwanted outcomes can result. There is also some evidence that the intense muscle pressure itself involves venous flow in surrounding tissues and may lead to thrombosis or hemorrhoids.

An increase in stool volume is associated with increased fiber intake. It varies with the kind of fiber ingested. Wheat bran, hemicelluloses, and cellulose are more effective than other fibers in increasing the stool volume (Kelsay 1978). Particle size is not important to effectiveness.

Bile acid excretion is modified by fiber intake. Increased rates of excretion have been reported to result from corn, wheat, and vegetable mixtures, addition of cellulose, and wheat bran itself. Pectin is very effective in increasing bile acid excretion (Huang *et al.* 1978). Even so, the circulating levels of cholesterol, triacylglycerols, and other lipids are not affected.

A high fiber intake increases nutrient losses. Absorption of fat, nitrogen, and minerals such as calcium and iron is decreased when fiber content is increased.

Knowledge of human fiber needs is limited. Although many studies have been conducted, the subject is multifaceted and the number of studies per facet is not sufficient to support definitive statements and recommendations. Further investigation is necessary to establish the amount and kind of fiber necessary to provide benefits and to delineate the upper limit beyond which the adverse effects of nutrient losses outweigh benefits.

Metabolism of Carbohydrates in General

Glucose is the active fuel of the human body. All cells require it for energy production. It is stored in small quantities as glycogen, but dietary intake and local production are the main supply sources.

Glucose is translocated throughout the body via the circulatory system. The normal circulating level is between 70 to 90 mg/100 ml and 140 to 150 mg/100 ml. (The specific minimum and maximum criteria used in evaluation depend on the test used to obtain the measurement.)

The sources of supply of glucose are: (a) absorption, (b) breakdown of liver glycogen (glycogenolysis), (c) conversion of glucogenic amino acids, i.e., all except leucine which is degraded to the intermediate compounds β-hydroxybutyric acid and glycerol which may be metabolized as fat instead, (d) recycling of lactic and pyruvic acids which accumulate when the rate of production during heavy muscular exercise exceeds the rate of degradation due to lack of oxygen at the local level, and (e) conversion of the glycerol portion of fat to glycogen.

The demand for glucose is continuous. All cells withdraw glucose from circulation, under control of the hormone insulin, for use in producing energy via the Krebs cycle and the Embden-Meyerhof glycolytic pathway (Fig. 6.1). The end-products are CO_2, water, and energy (mechanical, chemical, or thermal). The conversion of matter to energy fuels the various chemical reactions involved in cellular processes. Energy must be released by a stepwise process to avoid waste or overheating. Insulin's role is in transport of glucose into cells. Therefore, it can initiate or speed up some reactions by augmenting the intracellular quantity of glucose. When death occurs, the production of heat ceases and the tissues become cold and solid. Thus, necessary reactions are prevented and the system stops.

The regulation of CHO metabolism is effected by means of (a) the intracellular energy charge and (b) several hormones. The intracellular energy charge is a function of the relative energy present, which is determined by the proportions of AMP, ADP, and ATP. When the proportion of ATP is high, some enzymes are induced and others are repressed. This determines the supply of nutrient substrates available and, therefore, whether reactions will go in the direction of glycogen synthesis or the opposite by which glucose is formed. The proportions of AMP, ADP, and ATP are in a dynamic state of change, so the direction of the reactions between glycogen and glucose are in a dynamic state of change.

Hormonal modulation is effected by varying enzyme activity levels. Thus, in muscle tissue *adrenalin* and in other tissues *glucagon* increase the rate of glycogen breakdown by phosphorylase and decrease glycogen

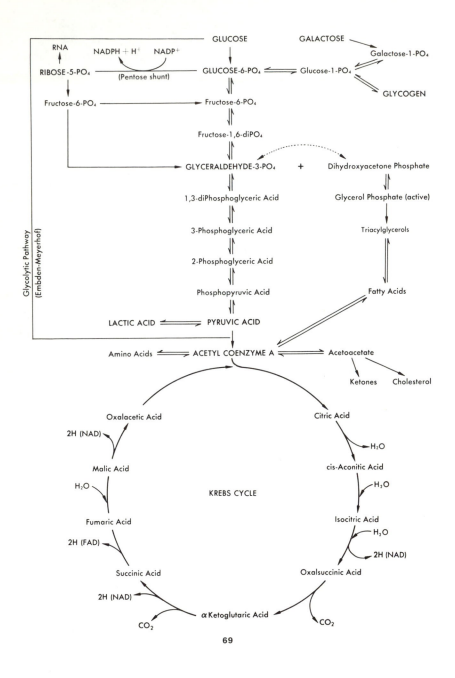

FIG. 6.1. LINKAGE OF PROTEIN, FAT, AND CHO METABOLISM

synthesis by inducing formation of the inactive phosphorylated glycogen synthetase D. By this means glycogenolysis is induced. In all tissues, *insulin* decreases the level of cAMP which results in a decreased rate of glycogen breakdown and formation of the active nonphosphorylated glycogen synthetase I. By this means glycogenesis is induced.

Galactose is a second simple sugar that is metabolically important. D-galactose amine is a major constituent of the polysaccharide of cartilage. Galactose is also a constituent of glycogen, cell wall components, and hyaluronic acid. Normally, glucose-1-phosphate and galactose-1-phosphate are interconvertable by means of a uridyl transferase which regulates supply.

Metabolism in Specific Tissues

The various tissues have unique uses for glucose. Muscle and liver tissue uses will be presented for illustration.

Muscle cell tissues have the common Krebs capacity for producing the basic quantity of energy necessary for resting cell processes PLUS extra capacity to enable muscle fiber contraction, which is the basis for muscular work. Complete explanation of the process(es) involved is not available, but the following summarizes what is known:

(a) IF actin and myosin, two muscle proteins, are given a stimulus (adrenalin activates phosphorylase to break glycogen to glucose) in the presence of glucose, 3 ATP, calcium, magnesium, heat (endergonic portion), and oxygen, THEN they will slide together or contract to form actomyosin and by-products ADP, heat (exergonic portion), and pyruvic acid.

(b) IF ADP is recycled to ATP and heat is removed by circulation, THEN the muscle will relax.

(c) IF pyruvic acid is formed at a rate that can be dealt with, THEN Krebs capacity degrades it, producing CO_2, water, and energy. Or IF pyruvic acid is formed more rapidly than it can be oxidized due to a physical limit to the supply of oxygen (the pigment myoglobin stores only a limited quantity and circulation supplies only a fixed quantity attached to hemoglobin), THEN pyruvic acid is converted to lactic acid. When lactic acid is formed, it is removed to the liver for oxidation via the Krebs cycle. When lactic acid is formed more rapidly than it can be removed, because of continuous contraction as in heavy muscular activity, THEN the pH decreases and the activity of enzymes is reduced, creating a slowdown which is perceived as fatigue.

(d) Most of the reaction is exergonic: IF heat is removed and dispersed throughout the body, THEN one feels hot all over and sweats.

(e) IF insulin is present and the muscle cell is not contracting, THEN it will cause glucose to be transported into the cell and stored as glycogen for future use.

Liver (hepatic) cells have the common Krebs capacity for producing energy for resting cell processes PLUS capacity for processing glucose and galactose in performing special cell functions:

(a) glucose-buffer function—Glucose can rapidly cross in and out of hepatic cells without assistance from insulin. The postulated mechanism for control of the circulating levels of glucose are via feedback mechanisms and hormonal override. IF the circulating level of glucose is high, THEN glucokinase is activated and causes increased use or storage of about two-thirds of the excess glucose as glycogen, which reduces the circulating level. IF the circulating level of glucose is low because insulin has caused rapid transport of glucose into peripheral cells, THEN the pancreas secretes glucagon which causes glycogen to be degraded AND glucose is dephosphorylated by glucose-6-phosphatase which enables it to diffuse out into circulation, which raises the circulating level. During the interdigestive period, glucose is produced from the carbon chain of excess amino acids and/or glycerol so as to maintain circulating levels. In times of stress brain and retinal tissues work overtime; adrenalin causes the degradation of glycogen to increase glucose supply needs of these tissues. Moreover, glucose is preferentially metabolized by other cells for energy, so an adequate supply must be sustained.

Details of glycogen degradation are emerging. Phosphorylase cleaves the α-1,4 linkage at the nonreducing end of glycogen, forming α-D-glucose-1-phosphate and glycogen with one less glucose unit. This is an iterative process that continues up to four glucose units from the α-1,6 branch. The branched residue is called a *limit dextrin*, since four glucose units from the branch is as far as this enzyme can degrade. Other enzymes further degrade the limit dextrins.

Details of glycogen synthesis are also emerging. The straight chain portions are formed by adding 1-UDP-glucose to a preformed acceptor portion by means of glycogen synthetase. The branches are formed by adding a 6- to 7-carbon residue. An *amylo* $(1,4 \rightarrow 1,6)$ transglycosylase effects this addition.

(b) conversion of glucose to ribose and deoxyribose—This is the course of the sugar moiety necessary for production of RNA and DNA.

(c) conversion of lactic acid back to pyruvic acid—IF surplus, THEN pyruvic acid is converted to glycogen.

(d) conversion of glucose to mannose, glucosamine, and galactoseamine—This supplies the precursors for production of mucopolysaccharides and glycoproteins such as heparin. Normally, fetal and infant liver tissue contains a uridyl transferase to effect these syntheses. Galactose is abundant in the infant diet from milk so it is used as is. Through a metabolic error, some infants lack this enzyme. UDP-galactose pyrophosphorylase is not present until puberty. Since galactose is necessary for formation of basic compounds, growth and development is halted and galactose accumulates. The condition is evident from the high circulating levels of galactose, i.e., galactosemia is manifest.

(e) conversion of glucose to galacturonic acid—Its main function is to combine with some compounds so as to detoxify them. These compounds are excreted because they cannot be reabsorbed.

(f) conversion of the glucose skeleton to the precursor of a nonessential amino or fatty acid—This provides for interconversion among energy sources, which decreases vulnerability to energy deficit.

CARBOHYDRATES: DEFICIENT SUPPLY OR INFLATED DEMAND

The basic functions and interactions of carbohydrates under normal supply/demand conditions have been outlined above. Whenever deficient supply (absolute) or inflated demand (relative deficiency) occurs, interference with function and/or abnormal interactions occurs.

Digestion/Absorption

Low intakes of sucrose and starch seem to have no discernible effects. Low intakes of lactose can result in a conditioned lactase deficiency with accompanying intestinal distress on challenge with a load of lactose. The greatest effect, however, is produced by chronic low intake of bulk.

(a) IF a low bulk diet is consumed, THEN a greater than normal density of chyme results. THEREFORE, the surface area is less and mixing with acids, bases, and enzymes is retarded. THEREFORE, the rate of release of absorbable sugars and other nutrients is decreased. THEREFORE, given the normal rate of passage, the percentage of absorption is decreased and the percentage of residue that can be fermented in the colon is increased.

(b) IF a low bulk diet is consumed AND the rate of passage is decreased, THEN increased bacterial action results in putrefaction of proteins, producing indole and skatole which are foul smelling odors and fermentation of sugars producing CO_2, hydrogen gas, and methane which are odorless.

(c) IF a very low bulk diet is consumed, THEN a dense solid mass is produced AND great muscular pressure is necessary for movement; herniation and/or formation of sacs or diverticula result.

Metabolism of Carbohydrates—in General

The effect of low dietary intake of carbohydrates depends on whether the low intake is temporary or chronic. On a temporary basis, glycogenolysis, or breakdown of liver glycogen stores, will suffice. On a chronic basis, alternate supply mechanisms of lipolysis and proteolysis can be used singly or together. *Lipolysis* means conversion of storage energy to ready energy by breaking down triglycerides and using the glycerol portion to make glucose. This is the process used when people follow reducing diets, and will be discussed below. *Proteolysis* means conversion of a desperate energy source by breaking down tissue proteins, usually muscle proteins, and using the deaminated skeleton to make glucose. When the energy deficit has continued to a point where muscle wasting is evident, the system is desperate.

Metabolism Within Special Tissues

Brain, central nervous, and lung tissues require a glucose supply because they have only limited capacity to utilize lipids as an energy source. Their demand exceeds their capacity to produce glucose and there is some evidence that these tissues have a special, but undefined, demand for glucose *per se*. During a prolonged fast some adaptation occurs that enables these tissues to use ketone bodies derived from lipids.

In muscle tissues, the observed effects depend on whether the muscle tissue is resting or active and whether the deficit is temporary or chronic. IF the circulating glucose level is low AND muscle glycogen stores are adequate, THEN in the resting state there is no detrimental effect. IF the circulating level is low AND the muscle is exercised, THEN the glycogen stores are depleted AND fatigue results from a supply deficit. IF the circulating level is chronically low, THEN the system adapts with a decreased energy output and slow movement or resistance to movement. This is observed in the poor who show lassitude.

In the liver, the observed effects of a low circulating level of glucose are depletion of glycogen and fat stores. Use of the alternate pathways is evident as the circulating level of free fatty acids and ketone bodies rises.

In adipose tissues also, the effects can be observed. The stored triglycerides are degraded to glycerol and free fatty acids, both of which are transported to the liver for utilization.

CARBOHYDRATES: EXCESS SUPPLY

The results of excessive intake of carbohydrates have greater physiological effects in the short run than do those of deficient supply. These vary in importance between simple and complex carbohydrates.

Digestion/Absorption

The overall general effects of excess consumption of simple carbohydrates are irritation of the intestinal mucosa and development of an absorption/transport bottleneck. The transport rate is variable among the various simple sugars. For the rat, the known preference in decreasing order is galactose, glucose, fructose, mannose, xylose, arabinose. The order is assumed to hold for man, as well. Other effects are:

(a) sucrose—IF excess, THEN extra water is required for solution, THEREFORE thirst develops. Competition for carriers results in a slowdown of transport of glucose and fructose

(b) lactose—IF excess, THEN since galactose probably preempts transport, glucose uptake will be delayed.

(c) glucose—IF excess, and the circulating level is low, THEN passive diffusion will augment carrier facilitated transport and the circulating level will tend to peak rapidly and remain high.

The excess intake of starch has little observable effect, other than a slowdown of digestion due to a crowd syndrome. IF a large quantity of starch is consumed, the quantity of α-amylase secreted by the pancreas will be relatively short, THEN more will be produced and secreted. Also, IF the quantity of maltase and isomaltase is relatively short, THEN a bottleneck in degradation to glucose will occur, with the result that glucose uptake will be delayed and the lower peak will be sustained over a long time period. This action is similar to that of a time-release capsule.

The excess intake of fiber results in intestinal water retention, increased calibre of the mass, and consequent increase in the rate of passage. IF the frequency of elimination is increased, THEN diarrhea is the outcome. IF this occurs, then malabsorption of other nutrients, due to decreased digestion/absorption time, is the expected outcome.

Metabolism of Carbohydrates—in General

A temporarily excessive dietary intake of carbohydrate has a transient effect on the circulating blood sugar level. Because uptake of glucose by some specialized cells is uncontrolled, the circulating level must be controlled in order to prevent damage to those cells. Therefore, a rise in blood sugar elicits production and secretion of insulin which causes glucose to be stored in skeletal muscle cells (individual cell storage is low, but the cumulative and aggregate effect given the large muscle mass, is large), skin, and glandular tissues. This storage in peripheral tissues is necessary and sufficient to reduce the circulating level by two-thirds of its excess, if necessary.

Metabolism Within Specialized Cells

Insulin is not necessary for glucose entry into cells of the following tissues: brain, intestinal mucosa, kidneys, and liver. It is also unnecessary for uptake by RBC. Therefore, control by the adjustment of the circulating blood sugar level is necessary as a flood control mechanism. Metabolic effects of excess in these cells are outlined as follows:

(a) brain cells—These cells are super-sensitive to variation in the levels of nutrients in their environment. Fluctuations in circulating levels are so great that irreparable damage would occur. Therefore, as a protective measure, these cells are bathed in cerebrospinal fluid which is almost invariate in composition by comparison. Insulin appears to be unnecessary because historically the possibility of too little glucose was greater than the possibility of too much glucose. The control is on the limit of glucose in the cerebrospinal fluid.

(b) mucosal cells—The function of these cells is uptake. IF the circulating levels of insulin and glucose were low, THEN a requirement for insulin to facilitate uptake would obstruct function. This is the opposite of what is necessary to correct the problem.

(c) kidney cells—The function of these cells is to remove and prevent re-entry of excess nutrients. IF the circulating levels of insulin and glucose were low, THEN a requirement for insulin would obstruct function. This is the opposite of what is necessary to correct the problem. IF the circulating level of glucose is high, THEN glucose is removed from circulation by the kidney cells and is excreted in the urine (glycosuria). IF the circulating glucose level is chronically high, THEN kidney cells are damaged by dehydration because water must be excreted in order to keep the sugar in solution and dilute it (polyuria).

(d) liver or hepatic cells—The function of these cells is to control the circulating level. A requirement for insulin would obstruct function if insulin were insufficient to allow transport of excess glucose. This is the opposite of what would be necessary to correct the problem. Therefore, unlimited uptake facilitates the solution. IF a transient high circulating level occurs, THEN glycogenesis (synthesis of glycogen), lipogenesis (synthesis of fat), and/or synthesis of glucose derivatives occurs. IF a chronically high circulating level develops, THEN excessive fat formation results in a condition called fatty liver and failure to cope with the excess (diabetes) results in damage to other organ systems.

(e) red blood cells—The effect of excess glucose uptake has not been delineated.

The pancreas is the organ most affected by a chronic excess of glucose since it produces both insulin and glucagon. If the excess carbohydrate intake or excess circulating level of glucose persists for more than a week, the cells of the pancreas where insulin is produced will hypertrophy so as to increase insulin output. This correction in the circulating level of insulin promotes storage in peripheral tissues, so as to reduce the circulating level of glucose to normal. Prolonged elevation of the circulating glucose levels results in overstimulation of these pancreatic cells, which causes them to wear out. As a final outcome, little or no insulin is produced; diabetes mellitus is the result. From the above, the medical concern with high sugar intake becomes clear. IF the carbohydrate intake, especially of simple sugars which cause a peak in the circulating glucose level, is reduced and weight is returned to normal for the individual, THEN the quantity of insulin produced by undamaged cells may be sufficient to deal with a normal intake and may control the circulating glucose level within a normal range. From this, the medical concern with type of carbohydrate ingested, body weight, and control of diabetes becomes clear (this applies only to maturity onset diabetes).

Cardiovascular tissue is also damaged by a chronically high circulating blood sugar level. There is increasing evidence of the effect, but the identification of causes is incomplete at present. Partial speculative explanations relate to the effect (a) of the stress of the increased solids content of blood due to the solution of the glucose and its effects on osmotic pressure and (b) the continued production of lipids in order to remove the excess—when the concentration of lipids rises, less soluble varieties are produced and these precipitate in the arteries, forming the plaques of atherosclerosis.

CARBOHYDRATES: FOOD ECOLOGY AND LIFE EXPECTANCY

Man's relation to his food environment always has been important because it is critical to physiological survival and is related to safety-security and other basic needs. As discussed in Chapters 15 and 16, the same issues involved in eating with safety and security have confronted man since the beginning. These issues are edibility, perishability, control of defects, control of fraud, and public confidence in food quality. The contemporary twist to these problems confronts the current generation. Contemporary aspects, as related to the carbohydrate problem, are summarized below:

(a) edibility—Traditionally, the problem has been to make food edible. The carbohydrate problem is that it is too edible, enticing people into overconsumption. The sweetness of simple carbohydrates is a preferred and gratifying (or source of pleasure and satisfaction) attribute. So, consumption follows availability, displacing intake of complex carbohydrates and other nutrient sources. American carbohydrate production and processing technologies are the greatest man has ever known. With cereals, the bran and other portions can be removed from starchy seeds and the starch itself modified to produce sweetness. This not only increases the edibility of cereals but also tends to increase the quantity consumed. Consumption of such refined carbohydrates increases the caloric density of foods consumed, since the non-caloric indigestible portions are removed. The reported and usually accepted (known or postulated) effects of increased sugar consumption are:

-increased incidence of dental caries, due to overexposure of tooth surfaces to corrosive action of acids produced by bacteria

-increased incidence and prevalence of obesity, due to a habit-forming preference for sweets that contributes to overeating, especially of high caloric density foods

-increased incidence and prevalence of diseases of the colon, due to displacement of fiber by simple carbohydrates

-increased incidence and prevalence of diabetes mellitus (maturity onset type), due to elevated circulating blood sugar levels and/or obesity

-increased incidence and prevalence of cardiovascular disease, due to elevated circulating blood sugar levels and disposal of excess glucose by conversion to triglycerides and insoluble complex lipids

During the 1970s, Americans became aware of the problems associated with increased edibility and perceived a threat to life expectancy. There is no doubt that for some people the threat is real. It is an ecological problem, i.e., it results from a wrong relationship with the food environment. Some people want to eat as much simple carbohydrate as they like, irrespective of what their body can tolerate, and they do not want the consequences of immoderate consumption. So, they want the problem fractions removed, leaving the "healthful" and gratifying ones. Since the nature and extent of immoderate consumption have some unique aspects due to individual differences that create/maintain the wrong relationship, the real solution will have to come from within the individual. He/she must accept personal responsibility. Outside sources can provide only information and support.

(b) perishability—Perishability and unevenness of fresh fruit and vegetable supplies keep market cost high, which limits intake for many. Processing preserves, so fruits and vegetables are available in some form throughout the year. But, processing does reduce nutrient and fiber content. See Chapter 2.

Whole grain cereals are also perishable. The oil is subject to oxidative rancidity, a degrading process in which fragments that create off-flavors and off-odors are produced. Milling reduces the oil content to 3% or less, thus reducing the size of the problem. However, the bran coats are removed at the same time, creating another problem by elimination of the fiber. These can be separated from the oil and blended back in.

Bakery mixes and other products made from milled flour are also perishable. Shelf-life is insufficient for distribution and delayed sales. Fat added to aid incorporation of air for lightness, to provide shortness of crumb, and to impart flavor also becomes rancid; antioxidants are added to control this problem. Water content also must be stabilized; some products take up water and lump or become sticky, others dry out. Anti-caking agents and humectants are added to control these respective problems. Other technical problems related to perishability also have been encountered and solved by use of sophisticated processing techniques and/or food additives. Availability of these items in ready-to-eat form, since they are both sweet and rich, adds to the problems noted above.

(c) control of defects—Food sources of carbohydrates are plant materials. These are biological materials, and as such, are inherently highly variable in attributes. But, awareness of this fact has been obscured by lack of exposure to raw agricultural commodities, efficient sorting, and grading procedures that ensure relative uniformity within grades and reduce differences among grades, as well as increased consumer substitution of ready-to-eat items for ingredients to be used in food preparation. American processing technology has been deliberately designed for elimination or at least minimization of defined defects such as too short shelf-life or variability in attributes.

Planned shelf-life and uniformity in attributes are valued in industry. Absolute product quality may be sacrificed to these ends. To overcome defects, a number of food gums and/or modified starches are used in the formulation of fabricated foods that contain carbohydrate. (Fabricated foods are those items prepared commercially that formerly were prepared at home from a recipe, or that are created to fill a consumer need.) For example, food gums are added to chocolate milk and fruit drinks to suspend the solids, so that they will not settle out; frosting mixes, so that the frosting will not run off the bakery product; cake mixes, to form a film that traps gases, so that cakes will be light in spite of increased sugar and water content; bread doughs, to strengthen them so that extra gas can be incorporated, so the loaf will be large and light; and ice cream, to give body when melted and prevent formation of water and/or sugar crystals. The control of defects has increased the desirability of these products and results in increased consumption.

(d) control of fraud—The federal government has assigned program authority to the USDA and some other agencies to implement laws which protect consumers against specified kinds of fraud. The old idea of *caveat emptor* or let the buyer beware is no longer reasonable, above some basic level, because of the complexity of contemporary food technology. Few people have the technical expertise necessary to evaluate differences along what is often a fine line between technical necessity and fraud.

Three basic types of standards have been established to serve as a basis for control of fraud. Examples of applications to carbohydrate-containing foods are presented briefly:

-standard of quality—This requires that graded times, e.g., fruits and vegetables, meet established standards for tenderness, color, and freedom from defects.

-standard of identity—This defines what a food is, i.e., what ingredients and proportions can be used in preparing it. Standards have been established for items such as fruit cocktail, succotash, condensed milk, jams and jellies, and ice cream. Foods so defined do not need a label declaration of usual ingredients. Other foods must contain a label declaration of ingredients in decreasing order according to quantity.

Food additives can be used to achieve more than one purpose. For example, a money-saving decrease in carbohydrate content or an increase in air or water content can accompany the acknowledged functional role. Standards limit quantities allowed, the air or water content, etc.

-standard of fill—This requires that containers be properly filled with food, so that the purchaser is not deceived. Candy bars, cookies, and ready-to-eat breakfast cereals are fragile foods that require special packaging to reduce the probability of crumbling prior to purchase. Cardboard and/or plastic dividers are used to protect edges from impact and within-package movement. Ready-to-eat cereal packages are filled by volume; although the contents shake down in transit so that the package may not appear full, it is usually filled to the stated weight. Government inspectors purchase and check random package weights, which encourages control.

-nutrition labeling—For a number of reasons, some consumers need to know what nutrients are provided in the various foods in order to assess intake and/or control it. Label information on size of portions, number of portions, and carbohydrate content in grams are provided to meet this need. Federal control assures the validity of label statements; therefore, consumers can rely on them.

-advertising—Definitely false statements are prohibited; the problem lies with allusions and illusions which are difficult to control by legal means. Enticement is a major problem, given availability.

(e) public confidence in food quality—There are two aspects to this problem: one is related to food additives and the other to the value of carbohydrate-containing foods as a group. Both translate to "poisonous" and the question, "IF it is poisonous, THEN why eat it?"

The problem of acceptance of food additives *per se* is dealt with in Chapters 14 to 16. For those who can accept their use, an additional problem remains: What do we have, when we have what we have? Food gums and modified starches have distinctive flavor and texture effects that can be used to verify their presence. This clue can then be used in selecting the relevant food composition values, which is necessary for accurate assessment of carbohydrate intake.

In affluent America where excessive intake of simple carbohydrates and obesity have become problems, the value of carbohydrates has been undermined as part of the scare tactics used to deal with obesity. The resultant crisis in confidence has counter-productive effects. *Carbohydrate* has become a dirty word, with refined sugar and flour, potatoes, bread, and pasta the main targets. In some people's minds, refined sugar and flour have a negative food quality, i.e., they are poisonous, because they provide almost no nutrients other than carbohydrate, which is not valued. This is despite their purity which approximates perfect quality in a technological sense. Potatoes, bread, and pasta are perceived as having somewhat less negative food quality, i.e., they are marginal and best consumed in limited quantities. This situation is unfortunate. It is true that one serving does not provide a significant quantity of any nutrient other than carbohydrate. However, the traditional servings of some combination of items from this food group do provide significant quantities of the B vitamins (if they are made from whole grain or enriched cereals), and potatoes are a source of vitamin C as well.

Except for those foods made entirely from refined sugar and/or flour, this food group provides fiber. The newly acknowledged fiber requirement has created what is a forced choice situation, with two unacceptable alternatives. IF these foods are consumed for their contribution of B vitamins and fiber, THEN intake of other foods must be limited in order to control calories. IF this group of foods is avoided, THEN fiber intake will be too low. This dilemma has led to confusion accompanied by a lack of confidence in what to eat, resulting in alternating periods of consumption and rejection. The effects of this pattern have caused further degeneration in confidence. These, then, are the contemporary twists to the problem of eating carbohydrate foods with safety and security.

The 1970s was a period of cultural shock in relation to the ecological implications of the changes in carbohydrate intake that occurred in recent years. Although the changes were gradual and progressive, the nature and extent of the changes in the mean intakes of the various kinds of carbohydrates and carbohydrate-containing foods were documented.

The cumulative and aggregate effects on health have begun to surface. At least a first approximation of physiological environmental impacts has become available from epidemiological research. Questions of quality of life and various threats to life expectancy have emerged. These issues are being confronted in scientific circles and program authority has been mandated by Congress to seek alternate solutions and implement those that seem most promising.

Some segments of the general public have become aware of and alarmed by selected aspects of the problem. They have become emotionally involved, responding in a variety of counter-productive ways, e.g., with anxiety, fear, anger, hostility, and withdrawal. Credibility gaps, a crisis in confidence, and confrontations involving charges and counter-charges have resulted in a stand-off but not in resolution of the problems involved.

There are no easy solutions because the shape of the problem varies with the individual. There are some common elements that might be dealt with in a common way. But, comprehensive assessment is necessary prior to implementation in a specific case in order to avoid creating new problems. Certainly fads are to be avoided, e.g., misguided adherence to the low carbohydrate reducing diets can create a metabolic situation that threatens life expectancy by producing hypoglycemia and ketosis.

When all is said and done, people must consume an individually adjusted reasonable intake, i.e., one between ± 1. Otherwise, quality of life and life expectancy are threatened. This requires that the individual solve his ecological problem, i.e., become personally responsible and restore a correct relationship to his/her food environment.

BIBLIOGRAPHY

HUANG, C.T.L., GOPALAKRISHNA, G.S., and NICHOLS, B.L. 1978. Fiber, intestinal sterols, and colon cancer. Am. J. Clin. Nutr. *31*, 516-526.

KELSAY, J.L. 1978. A review of research on effects of fiber intake on man. Am. J. Clin. Nutr. *31*, 142-159.

VAN ITALIE, T.B., SMITH, N.S., and QUARTERMAIN, D. 1977. Short-term and long-term components in the regulation of food intake: evidence for a modulatory role of carbohydrate status. Am. J. Clin. Nutr. *30*, 742-757.

7

Energy

The American energy crisis involves dwindling supplies of fossil fuels and enlarging supplies in living depots. Only the latter aspect will be dealt with here.

The regulation of food intake, as related primarily to caloric value, has re-emerged as a major research interest in recent years. An oversimplified concept of the physiological demand for food and the mechanism for regulation of food intake sufficed for many years. Since human beings have the unique ability to impose mind over matter, research efforts were directed to psycho-social factors involved in food intake regulation. Then, in the 1950s, the number of adipose cells was identified as a critical variable in weight control. Since then, other breakthroughs have led to a new understanding of the mechanisms involved in regulation of food intake.

Obesity is the most common American form of malnutrition. It creates/contributes to the development of the most prevalent and life-threatening health problems experienced in contemporary society. An abnormal relationship between man and his food leads to obesity. Weight control involves manipulation of the food-related ecosystem. New definitions of what is food, modification of food ideology, retraining in meal/eating rituals, changes in food purchases, and food preparation practices can be used to restructure relations in the food-related ecosystem so as to control weight and improve life expectancy.

ENERGY: NORMALLY AVAILABLE FROM GLUCOSE AND FATTY ACIDS

The physiological regulation of food intake appears to involve several structures in the brain, neuro-muscular control of the rate of stomach emptying as discussed in Chapter 3, and body fat mass control mechanisms in adipose tissue. The role of each will be summarized briefly below:

119

(a) brain—The lateral hypothalamus or "feeding center" stimulates hunger at all times unless it is inhibited by the ventromedial nucleus or "satiety center." Only a partial explanation of the mechanism(s) whereby control is effected is available.

(b) small intestine—The presence of food, the pH of the chyme, and composition affect the level of *enterogastrone* secreted by cells of the duodenum. This hormone regulates the intensity of contractions in the stomach and thereby regulates the flow of chyme into the small intestine to a level that can be digested efficiently.

(c) adipose tissue—Both the number of adipose cells and their lipid content are involved. There are three periods when adipose cell number can be expanded, i.e., during the pre-natal period, during infancy, and finally during the growth phase of adolescence. The number of cells appears to be related somewhat to the ease of weight gain. IF the number of cells is greater than normal, i.e., hyperplasia, THEN the aggregate effect of a larger number taking up a little fat is a large total. However, recent findings show that surgical removal of fat storage tissue, i.e., lipectomy, results in hypertrophy of adipose tissue in other locations, tending to return the total adipose tissue mass to its presurgical mass in a matter of months. There are site differences in the degree of compensatory hypertrophy. Moreover, a high fat intake tends to promote greater adipocyte regeneration than does a moderate fat intake.

Body fat mass is probably regulated indirectly by control of adipocyte lipid content. The explanation at this time is that there appears to be a set-point for lipid content. This means that system control of feeding is regulated so as to maintain lipid stores at this level.

This is supported by the fact that the rate of release of glycerol and FFA from adipocytes is related to the cellular lipid content. The mechanism for control of lipolytic activity is unclear, but there is some evidence that insulin may be involved. Insulin resistance increases with increasing lipid content. So, although the circulating level of insulin is high, it is ineffective. Normally, insulin reduces the level of cAMP which results in a low level of lipolytic activity. However, when insulin resistance develops, a greater level of lipolytic activity creates a continuing mobilization of TG so that the set-point is not reached; in effect, the set-point is shifted upward.

The hypothetical explanation of the feeding compulsion is as follows: IF the set-point is shifted up, THEN the hypothalamus mediates a mandatory diversion of food calories to the adipocytes, which reduces the circulating level of glucose and/or fatty acids. This creates a signal to increase food intake.

The evidence for this comes from research that demonstrates that IF adipose tissue is removed and tissue regeneration is prevented, THEN food intake will not increase and weight will remain stable at the lower level. This finding implies that the critical lipid content is reached sooner in a smaller number of cells. As a result, intake is terminated before excess calories are consumed.

A feedback control mechanism also appears to be involved. When there are many cells, as long as the lipid content of adipocytes has not reached the set-point, the fatty acids available from absorption and conversion will be less than adipocyte uptake. Since there is a deficit, hunger pangs will result. So, more food will be ingested until the lipid content of the adipocytes reaches the set-point.

This is the long explanation for the operation of a vicious circle that determines the extent of the feeding compulsion. Thus far, the short-term stimulus has been considered. But, the long-term energy supply/demand situation is also involved. IF supply chronically exceeds demand, THEN the set-point shifts upward so that increased storage of lipid is possible. IF on the average, supply is equivalent to demand, THEN the set-point will remain fixed and weight will remain stable. IF supply is chronically less than demand, THEN a gap develops between demand and supply so withdrawal from storage results in an attempt to meet demand, lipid content drops below the set-point, and food intake signals are initiated. Thus, an obese person will have an elevated set-point and weight may be maintained on a long-term basis at the high level. To reduce weight and maintain it at the lower level will require a long-term effort that shifts the set-point down to the ideal level. This is why effective weight reduction is so difficult to achieve.

As a result of ingesting food and subsequent digestion/absorption processes, the body is supplied with four classes of molecules that yield energy from the degradative processes. These classes of molecules are:

(a) carbohydrate, as glucose and/or galactose—For quick energy or as a reserve stored as glycogen

(b) free fatty acids—For reserve energy, these are stored as TG

(c) amino acids—For desperate energy, these are stored as labile storage proteins and ultimately as structural proteins

(d) alcohol—For optional energy; this may be stored as TG

These kinds of molecules are low-energy sources, i.e., their physiologic fuel values are 4, 9, 4, and 7 kcal/g, respectively. A limited amount of glucose is stored as glucogen in liver and muscle tissues. The quantity of glycogen stored is small but sufficient for a quick response to demand. However, it is insufficient to sustain supply at a high level for more than a short time. Fatty acids are stored in highly variable quantities in adipose tissue and are degraded to meet sustained energy demands. A lead time is necessary to allow liberation, transport, and degradation; this lead time is provided by the immediate use of glycogen. When supplied in excess of needs or when energy from other sources is insufficient to meet demands, amino acids can be deaminated yielding keto acids which are degraded further, producing energy.

These low-energy molecules are degraded to intermediate energy sources that are called "common denominators" because the primary source no longer can be distinguished. Common denominators are pyruvic acid, acetyl CoA, and α-ketoglutaric acid.

These molecules are further degraded to CO_2, H_2O, and energy (chemical and thermal) via the common energy cycle (Krebs cycle). Degradation of the common denominators involves a series of steps that trap the energy given off. Instead of producing excess heat, the energy is transformed to chemical energy in the high energy phosphate bond of ATP.

Energy production is an on-going process in all cells. Since ATP is the necessary energy source in many other cell reactions, it is produced by this process on a continuous basis. In general, the process involves the following:

(a) activation of glucose by an endothermic reaction in which energy is shifted from the ATP to glucose by removal of one high-energy phosphate; glucose-6-phosphate and ADP are the end-products

(b) regeneration of ATP by an endothermic reaction in which energy is shifted to ADP from creatine phosphate (CP), by removing the high energy phosphate from CP and attaching it to ADP. CP is necessary as a phosphate energy storage compound because ATP is too reactive to serve as an energy repository

(c) oxidation of glucose-6-phosphate via the Krebs cycle (Fig. 7.1) occurs when intracellular supply of oxygen is adequate. Otherwise, glucose-6-phosphate is converted to pyruvic acid and then lactic acid and accumulates until oxygen supply is adequate for oxidation to proceed.

(d) oxidation of fatty acids involves removal of 2-carbon fragments which combine to form acetoacetic acid or β-hydroxybutyric acid. These are converted to acetyl CoA which enters the Krebs cycle by reacting with oxaloacetic acid to form citric acid.

(e) oxidation of amino acids involves removal of NH_2 with the formation of a keto acid. The keto acid formed from leucine forms acetyl CoA and is processed as described above. The keto acids formed by the other 21 amino acids form pyruvic acid, oxaloacetic acid, fumaric acid, succinic acid, or α-ketoglutaric acid, so enter the Krebs cycle as one of these reactants.

The process of converting food energy to physiological energy traps 55 to 60% of the energy in ATP, and 40 to 60% is lost as heat. Of the energy trapped in ATP, 20 to 40% is used to sustain metabolic functions, and 10 to 15% for cell maintenance. As a result, 0 to 20% of food energy may be used for muscular work when in caloric balance. Since consumption is

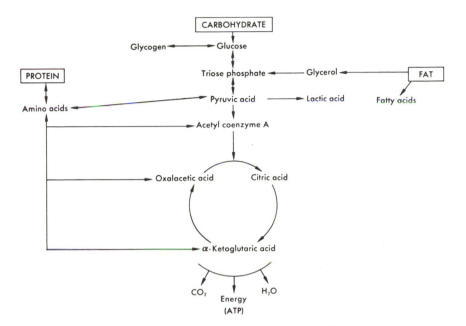

FIG. 7.1. CARBOHYDRATES, FATS, AND PROTEINS ARE INTERRELATED METABOL-
ICALLY BY THESE ANABOLIC AND CATABOLIC REACTION PATHWAYS

commonly greater than need, the low physiological efficiency in energy conversion is advantageous.

The bomb calorimeter is a device used to oxidize food samples in order to determine their caloric values. Because physiological efficiency is not as great as that obtained by the bomb calorimeter, physiologic fuel values are usually somewhat lower than those listed in tables of food composition.

For every individual, the demand for energy has two components. One is relatively fixed and the other is highly variable.

The fixed portion is called the Basal Metabolic Rate (BMR). BMR is defined as the physical demand for energy that is required to support life, i.e., the sum of the energy required for respiration, heart beat, maintenance of body temperature, and other essential functions. For purposes of comparison among individuals, BMR is measured under standardized conditions, i.e., when the individual is at rest, during the interdigestive period, and when relaxed. For an adult of average size, BMR is approximately 1800 kcal. BMR for adults of other sizes is shown in Table 7.1.

The variable portion is the physical demand for energy that is created by physical activity. Due to the increasingly sedentary life-style of most

Americans, this portion is a decreasing fraction of the total energy demand. Indeed, for many Americans, their total demand for energy is only slightly above that needed to keep them alive. Therefore, the problem of adjusting the supply of energy to the demand for it has become a major challenge.

TABLE 7.1. SUGGESTED ADULT WEIGHTS FOR HEIGHTS AND ASSOCIATED BMR[1]

Sex	Height		Median Weight[2]		BMR kcal/day
	in.	cm	lb	kg	
Male					
	64	163	133 ± 11	60 ± 5	1630
	66	168	142 ± 12	64 ± 5	1690
	68	173	151 ± 14	69 ± 6	1775
	70	178	159 ± 14	72 ± 6	1815
	72	183	167 ± 15	76 ± 7	1870
	74	188	175 ± 15	80 ± 7	1933
	76	193	182 ± 16	83 ± 7	1983
Female					
	60	152	109 ± 9	50 ± 4	1399
	62	158	115 ± 9	52 ± 4	1429
	64	163	122 ± 10	56 ± 5	1487
	66	168	129 ± 10	59 ± 5	1530
	68	173	136 ± 10	62 ± 5	1572
	70	178	144 ± 11	66 ± 5	1626
	72	183	152 ± 12	69 ± 5	1666

[1] Adapted from Food and Nutrition Board. 1974. Recommended Dietary Allowances, 8th rev. Natl. Acad. Sci. Washington, D.C.
[2] The "±" refers to the range from the 25th to 75th percentile of weight for height.

ENERGY: DEFICIENT SUPPLY OR INFLATED DEMAND— DEGRADATION OF PROTEINS

In normal healthy people, deficient caloric intake is not uncommon. It can be the result of deliberate action to effect a weight loss or it may be the result of excessive physical exercise, or due to inflated metabolic demands of pregnancy or growth. Lack of physical energy, nervous irritability, weight loss and/or muscle wasting are expected outcomes. The short-run and long-run metabolic conditions differ.

Persons who abruptly begin drastic weight reduction regimes may experience dizziness and/or muscular weakness at the outset. After the glycogen supply is exhausted, hypoglycemia results; fatty acids must be mobilized from adipose tissue and oxidized for energy. If the caloric intake is abruptly and markedly lower, the ability to mobilize fatty acids may be insufficient until adaptation occurs. This takes a week or more. In the interim, if the glucose supply to the brain and CNS tissue is reduced, dizziness and/or nervous irritability may occur. If the contractile proteins are mobilized for energy, muscular weakness will result.

If the reduction in caloric intake is severe, the degree of fatty acid mobilization and processing may result in ketoacidosis. This condition develops when the rate of mobilization exceeds the rate of degradation of acetoacetic acid, β-hydroxybutyric acid, and acetone. So, they accumulate. Since these would decrease blood pH, blood buffer base supplies must be expended to control pH. As buffer base is utilized toward the maximum, other metabolic abnormalities create additional imbalances and a systems crisis develops. It is to avoid this outcome that nutritionists recommend a maximum weight loss of two pounds per week. Even so, to lose two pounds, the daily deficit must be at least 1000 calories per day. Under these metabolic conditions, IF a person exercises heavily, THEN to meet the additional intermittent caloric demand muscle protein may be degraded. This accounts for the anguished cry of those dieters who quickly develop muscle fatigue when attempting to increase physical activity as part of their weight reduction program. In this case, muscle wasting is also accompanied by electrolyte and water loss. Between exercise periods, contractile protein replenishment may occur if intake or labile protein stores are adequate.

Excessive physical activity markedly inflates caloric demand so that even much greater than normal caloric intake is insufficient to prevent a relative deficit. IF this is the customary outcome, THEN lung capacity is increased in order to meet oxygen demand to enable rapid oxidation of glucose and fatty acids on a sustained basis. Under these metabolic conditions, ketoacidosis is unlikely to develop. The major negative outcome is that a gap between the adipose cell lipid content and the set-point results in habitually heavy food intake. IF the level of physical activity decreases for any reason, THEN problems in breaking the intake habits are experienced.

The inflated caloric demands of pregnancy and growth are not usually enough greater to present a problem to the normal, well nourished individual. However, those whose diet is only marginally adequate become high risk during these times. The implications and ramifications of the problem for pregnant women and their infants are discussed in Chapter 25. Similarly, discussions in Chapters 26 through 28 pertain to the effects on growth of infants, children, and adolescents.

ENERGY: EXCESS SUPPLY AND STORAGE PROBLEMS

Metabolic intermediates of energy metabolism create a leftover problem. Acetyl CoA, pyruvic acid, and α-ketoglutaric acid are unstable compounds that must NOT be allowed to convert to acetone, acetoacetic acid, β-hydroxybutyric acid, and lactic acid to any extent, since acidosis would result. Therefore, the preferred metabolic pathway is anabolic production of triglycerides. Since storage capacity in white adipose cells is essentially unlimited, the leftovers are recycled systematically and adiposity increases.

Control of the energy supply problem has become a major consideration for many Americans. The problem has many facets, e.g.,

(a) It is difficult to obtain all necessary nutrients on a customary intake of less than 1800 kcal/day. Recent research has documented the fact that trace minerals present an especially difficult problem.

(b) It is difficult to limit intake to 1800 kcal/day or less on a continuing basis. Three major reasons are that although a variety of foods can be consumed, whole categories of customary foods such as desserts or snack foods usually must be eliminated if nutritional balance is to be retained; the foods that are consumed lack richness and sweetness, so have low satiety value; and small quantities of food are all that are allowed, so oral gratification is less. Low-calorie foods do exist but they are neither nutritional nor taste-texture equivalents, and moreover, they are too expensive for use by an entire family for 60 years.

(c) The supply control problem is greater for women than for men and children. It turns out that in order to meet nutritional needs, women must consume a diet that is higher in nutrient density (ratio of nutrients to calories) than other family members. For many years, women have been taught that if they prepare nutritionally balanced meals for their husband and/or children, then if they consumed a somewhat smaller portion of everything they could meet nutritional needs within caloric allowances. New information has demonstrated that this is no longer true. As of now, it appears that a woman has only two nutritionally rational choices. Either she must eat smaller portions and supplement or she must eat differently from the other family members! Because many women will not do either, many have a supply problem that is creating a storage problem. The principles of diet management for weight control are discussed in Chapter 24.

8

Water and Electrolytes: Fluid Dynamics, Nerve Impulse Transmission, Muscular Contraction, and Acid–Base Balance

Ninety of the one hundred and three chemical elements known occur naturally. But, only 20 or so have nutriment roles, as far as is presently known. Of these, six are considered major minerals on a quantitative basis: calcium (Ca^{++}), phosphorus (as one of the phosphate radicals), potassium (K^+), sodium (Na^+), chlorine (Cl^-), and magnesium (Mg^{++}). Roles of these elements as electrolytes are discussed in this chapter. Other roles are discussed in succeeding chapters.

The food and people interactions in which water and the electrolytes involved in fluid dynamics are consumed have become critical to the health of many Americans. The recent drought in the western states has eliminated the traditional glass of ice water from the basic place setting. Water is provided only on request. Prices of coffee and tea have risen so high that these beverages are no longer consumed regularly by many people. One may well ask whether, under these circumstances, Americans continue to consume the five glasses of water that are recommended for health.

Consumption of processed foods, including convenience and snack foods, has increased. Most of these are salty, i.e., contain significant quantities of sodium and/or potassium salts, e.g., table salt (NaCl), monosodium glutamate (MSG), sodium citrate, potassium iodide, and potassium phosphate. Many phosphate compounds are common food additives.

The term *electrolyte* seems remote from foods. How is it relevant?

FOOD SOURCES OF WATER AND ELECTROLYTES

Water is commonly consumed as a beverage and as the major component of most beverages. Water in solid foods is present in free form embedded within plant and animal tissues. It also is present bound to various organic molecular constituents.

Calcium and magnesium exist in foods as the positively charged moiety of insoluble and soluble (a) inorganic salts, e.g., $CaCO_3$; (b) organic salts, e.g., calcium phytate or calcium lactate; and (c) protein complexes, e.g., calcium paracaseinate. In order for these minerals to be absorbed, they must be liberated to their free ionic form.

Phosphorus exists in foods in one of its oxygen-containing forms, i.e., as a part of the phosphate radical. At least 20 different phosphate compounds and their variants occur naturally and/or have been approved for food use. Five classes of these compounds are represented:

(a) orthophosphates (type formula X_3PO_4), e.g., anhydrous monocalcium phosphate (AMCP), which is used as the acid leavening agent in cake mixes, pancake and waffle mixes, and prepared biscuit mixes.

(b) pyrophosphates (type formula $X_4P_2O_7$), e.g., sodium acid pyrophate (SAPP), which is used as the acid leavening agent in refrigerated doughs, and as its iron salt as an iron enrichment compound.

(c) tripolyphosphates (type formula $X_5P_3O_{10}$), e.g., sodium tripolyphosphate (STP), which is used to retard development of rancid flavors in meat and to retain moisture in sausage products.

(d) straight-chain polyphosphates (type formula $((XPO_3)_n)$, e.g., sodium hexametaphosphate (SHMP), which is used as an emulsifier in processed cheeses, to increase gel strength in preserves, and to tenderize the skins of fruits canned whole.

(e) cyclic metaphosphates $((XPO_3)_4)$, e.g., sodium trimetaphosphate (STMP), which is used in preparation of modified starches.

Dietary potassium is an intracellular ionic constituent of muscle and tissues of meat, fruits, vegetables, and cereal grains (Table 8.1). It is liberated by digestion. It is also the positively charged moiety of many food additives.

Dietary sodium is commonly available from sodium chloride, monosodium glutamate, sodium nitrate and a number of other preservatives. Sodium chloride immediately dissolves in the water of chyme, dissociating into its constituent sodium and chloride ions. Sodium ions are liberated from other compounds by digestion.

Dietary chloride is commonly available from sodium and other chloride salts. When a sodium-restricted diet is consumed, a chloride supplement may be necessary.

TABLE 8.1. HOUSEHOLD MEASURES OF FOOD AS SOURCES OF POTASSIUM

	Potassium per Household Measure		
Food Group	300 mg and More	100-300 mg	Less than 100 mg
Dairy products and eggs	milk, whole, ½ pt milk, nonfat dry, ¼ cup	ice cream, 8 fl oz	egg, whole, one cottage cheese, ½ cup cheddar cheese, 1-in. cube butter, 1 tbsp
Meat, fish poultry (3 oz cooked, unless otherwise stated)	beef veal pork, fresh, roasted beef liver chicken, light meat salmon, pink, canned	frankfurter, one tuna, canned-in-oil chicken, dark meat ham, cured whitefish	
Vegetables and legumes (½ cup unless otherwise stated)	dry beans, cooked[1] soy flour, defatted[1] peanut butter, 3 tbsp potato, one, baked or boiled winter squash, cooked sweetpotato, one medium, cooked	lentils, cooked cauliflower, cooked broccoli, cooked brussels sprouts, cooked spinach, cooked kale, cooked carrots, cooked tomato, ½ raw	
Fruits and fruit juices (½ cup unless otherwise stated)	banana, one medium avocado, ½ medium[1] cantaloupe, ½ medium watermelon, wedge, 4 × 8 in. raisins, ¼ cup dried prunes, cooked or uncooked dried apricots, cooked or uncooked[1] dried peaches, cooked or uncooked[1] dried figs, 4 large dried dates prune juice	grapefruit, ½ medium apple, raw, one medium orange, navel, one medium peach, raw, one medium pear, raw, one medium strawberries, raw citrus juice, canned or frozen tomato juice, canned pineapple juice, canned or frozen	lemonade, limeade from frozen concentrate
Grain products (½ cup unless otherwise stated)		pie, apple, ⅐ of 9-in. pie	bread, one slice corn flakes, 2 oz oatmeal, cooked farina, cooked rice, white, cooked macaroni, spaghetti, or noodles, cooked grits, cooked pancakes, 2-3 doughnut, cake-type, one cupcake, plain, one cookies, plain, 5-6
Other foods	molasses, dark, 2 tbsp yeast, brewer's 2 tbsp	cocoa, 2 tbsp	sugar, 1 tbsp honey, 1 tbsp salad oil, 1 tbsp sherbet, 1 cup

Source: Murphy and Mangubat (1973).
[1] More than 500 mg potassium per common household measure.

FLUID DYNAMICS

Fluid dynamics refers to the pattern of changes in the movement of a fluid, such as water, that are related to the effects of various forces on its equilibrium under various circumstances. In this case, movement of water in and out of the cells, as well as within the circulatory system, is involved. Sodium and potassium ions and plasma proteins are the most important variables in the complex relationships which are described in terms of electrolyte balance, osmotic equilibria, and blood pressure. Fluid dynamics explains the mechanisms involved.

The term *ion* refers to an atom (e.g., sodium or potassium) or a radical (i.e., a fixed group of atoms such as sulfate or phosphate that remains unchanged during a series of reactions) that is positively or negatively charged as a result of having lost or gained one or more electrons, respectively. Ions involved in fluid dynamics include, but are not limited to, sodium (Na^+), potassium (K^+), calcium (Ca^{++}), magnesium (Mg^{++}), chloride (Cl^-), bicarbonate (HCO_3^-), phosphate (PO_4^{---}), sulfate (SO_4^{--}), and ammonium (NH_4^+) as well as ions of acetoacetic, lactic, pyruvic, and other organic acids. These electrolytes are involved in balancing charges within fluid media and across membranes. The relative combining power, based on charge, is expressed as milliequivalents (mEq).

The term *osmosis* refers to diffusion of water through a semi-permeable membrane of a cell or tissue (in the aggregate) to achieve an equilibrium concentration of solute or ions. Control of water balance is contingent on a balance of charges, which is computed in mEq Na^+ to K^+, the class representative extracellular and intracellular ions, respectively.

Water is the major constituent of the intracellular environment in which the life-sustaining reactions take place. The level of cellular hydration is critical to cellular survival. Both deficiency and excess pose a threat due to disruption of normal functions. Therefore, cellular hydration must be controlled, to the extent possible.

Water is the major constituent of the extracellular environment, especially of the circulatory system. The volume of plasma is critical to blood pressure and maintenance of nutrient supply. Both deficiency and excess pose a threat to survival due to disruption of normal functions. Therefore, blood volume must be controlled, to the extent possible.

Body Water: Normally Available

Water is the largest component of the human body. From a macro-view, this has implications in terms of the nutritional impact of variations in supply. From the macro-view, some important points are:

(a) The total amount of body water is highly variable within and among people, ranging from approximately 67 to 85% of body weight. Within people, there is variation due to variability in electrolyte intake; in women there is cyclic variation under control of estrogen level. Among people, body water varies as a percentage of weight due to variability in the proportion of lean muscle mass to adipose tissue mass (relatively anhydrous) and to heaviness of bone structure.

(b) Total body water is divided into 2 compartments, intracellular fluid (ICF) which makes up 55% of the total and extracellular fluid (ECF) which includes plasma, interstitial fluid, and integral bound water in solid tissues such as tendons, skin, collagen in elastin, and the skeleton.

(c) Water is a carrier, i.e., the continuous phase of the environment in the digestive juices, plasma, urine, and feces (Fig. 8.1). It is necessary for translocation of substrates and enzymes during digestion, of nutrients from point of liberation or storage to point of use in nourishment of a cell, and of indigestible food residues and metabolic end-products for disposal by excretion.

(d) Water pressure is a physical force to control migration of solids.

(e) Water is a heat regulator, i.e., it is involved in control of body temperature because of its capacity to absorb and disperse heat, as well as dispose of it by evaporation.

Digestion/Absorption.—Water is a major constituent of chyme. It is present as the major component of mucus, gastric juice, pancreatic juice, from consumption as a beverage, and as liberated from plant/animal tissues by mastication and digestion. Water is readily absorbed by dif-

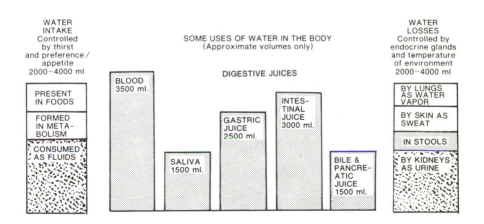

FIG. 8.1. BODY WATER—SOURCES OF SUPPLY AND DEMAND

fusion throughout the length of the GI tract.

Osmolality is a term that refers to the number of osmoles of solute in a kilogram of solvent—in this case the fluid portion of chyme. The osmolality of the chyme accounts for observed osmotic effects. The greater the number of dissolved particles, the higher the osmolality value assigned. At a given concentration, particle size is inversely related to osmolality. Thus, fats which are not dissolved have no effect and proteins which have a very large molecular weight have a small effect on osmotic pressure. As digestion progresses, osmolality of the chyme increases since amino acids are small molecular weight particles and become more numerous. A high molecular weight CHO, e.g., starch, has a lower osmolality than a low molecular weight CHO, e.g., a sugar. And, electrolytes, which are comparatively small molecular weight particles, have the highest values (Table 8.2).

TABLE 8.2. REPORTED OSMOLALITY OF FOODS USED ON LIQUID DIETS

Food	mOsm/kg
Whole milk	275
Gingerale	510
Gelatin dessert	535
Tomato juice	595
7-Up	640
Coca-Cola	680
Eggnog	695
Apple juice	870
Orange juice	935
Malted milk	940
Ice cream	1150
Grape juice	1170
Sherbet	1225

During digestion/absorption, gross adjustment of water balance is effected in the stomach by secretion of copious but variable quantities of mucus. Secretion results in localized dehydration of the mucus-secreting cells, which causes a sensation of thirst. Replenishment of cellular fluid as well as further dilution of the chyme results from water intake. Fine adjustment of the consistency of the chyme in the remainder of the GI tract is effected by continued secretion and absorption of a variable quantity of mucus.

Normal concentrations of sodium, potassium, and/or chloride salts contribute to the water-holding capacity of chyme because they draw water so as to dissolve and dissociate into ionic form. Active transport mechanisms have been identified for sodium and potassium; the mechanism for chloride transport is probably simple diffusion.

Water Balance, in General.—Water is technically a nutrient because it is utilized in a variety of roles that are necessary to keep tissues alive and able to grow or repair the effects of functional stress. Water has the following nutriment functions:

(a) constituent—For example, it is a basic component of cell sap and is adsorbed on the surface of crystals.

(b) diluent and dispersing medium—For example, it is the continuous phase of plasma and other fluids in which electrolytes, sugars, etc., are dissolved, proteins are colloidally dispersed, and lipids are emulsified.

(c) cofactor—For example, it is a catalyst in many reactions, especially those that are endothermic.

(d) reagent—For example, it is present in hydrolytic reactions where a substrate is split into two end-products with the addition of water.

Water is also an end-product, e.g., CO_2, water, and energy are produced by Krebs cycle reactions. The "metabolic water" produced is then available for nutriment functions. It is produced in the following proportions: 107 g water/100 g lipid, 55 g water/100 g carbohydrate, and 41 g water/100 g protein.

The state of cellular hydration is critical to survival of the cell, so water balance must be controlled. The cells are surrounded by a semi-permeable membrane which allows water, ions, and small molecules like sugars or amino acids to pass through in both directions. It is impermeable to large molecules like proteins. Control is effected at the cellular level by adjustment of the concentrations of sodium and potassium ions in ECF and ICF, which exert osmotic pressure.

Intracellular proteins remain within the cells and plasma proteins remain in circulation. They are amphoteric because they contain both an amino group (positively charged) and a carboxyl group (negatively charged). THEREFORE, they can react with anions (e.g., Cl^- and PO_4^{---}) and cations (e.g., Na^+ and K^+). For this reason, they function as buffers, stabilizing pH. Because of their dampening effect on fluctuation of electrolyte potential, they affect migration of ions and, hence, water balance. This function is important in fluid dynamics. The reader will recall that plasma proteins are in equilibrium with tissue proteins. Thus, any factor which increases tissue demand and results in a lower than normal plasma protein level, has an effect on water and electrolyte balance. Therefore, IF the circulating level of plasma proteins is low, THEN the effects of water loss, Na^+ excess, Na^+ loss, etc., are magnified. Indeed, low plasma protein level may decrease hydrodynamic pressure and result in edema.

Sodium is the main cation of ECF (Fig. 8.2) and potassium is the main cation of ICF. The potassium atom is larger than the sodium atom.

However, the hydrated sodium ion is larger than the hydrated potassium ion. Therefore, the inference is that cell membrane permeability to potassium in preference to sodium is related to size differences in solution. Normally, although there is continual translocation of Na^+ (K^+ to some extent) back and forth, the net effect is one of balance so that the cellular hydration level is relatively constant within the normal range.

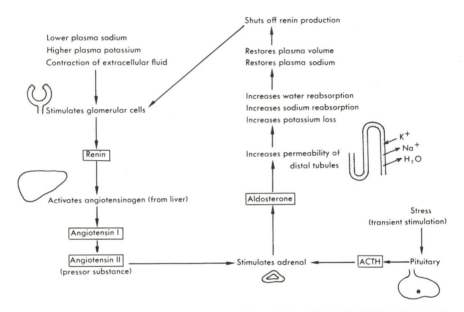

FIG. 8.2. THE REGULATION OF SODIUM CONCENTRATION IN EXTRACELLULAR FLUID

Control of water balance between plasma and interstitial fluid is effected by means of kidney excretion mediated by the hormone aldosterone (Figs. 8.3 and 8.4). This results in at least a minimum urine volume that, in adults, ranges from 200 to 900 ml in relation to the concentration of solutes to be excreted. Normally, urine volume exceeds this obligatory replacement level and approximates water intake.

Insensible water loss, i.e., that lost is respiration and by evaporation from the skin, is uncontrolled. In adults, this amounts to about 1200 ml/day. Replacement is obligatory.

Sweat losses are highly variable. All other things being equal, sweat losses increase with (a) physical activity (level of output and length of time), (b) environmental and/or body temperature, and (c) wind velocity. Sweat loss varies inversely with relative humidity, temperature and wind velocity remaining constant. Normally, sweat loss is low; replacement is obligatory.

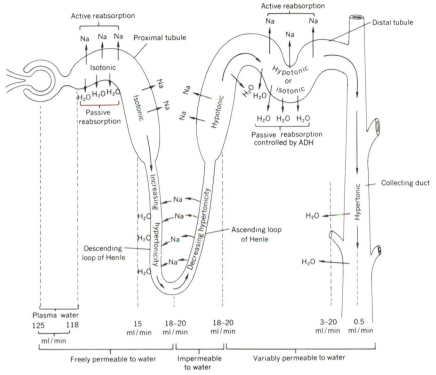

From Robinson (1978)

FIG. 8.3. FUNCTION OF THE NEPHRON IN ADJUSTING THE REABSORPTION OF SODIUM AND WATER, AND THE FORMATION OF URINE

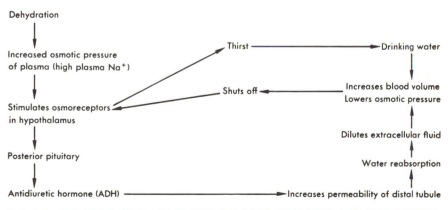

FIG. 8.4. THE REGULATION OF WATER BALANCE BY THIRST AND ANTIDIURETIC HORMONE MECHANISMS

Water: Deficient ICF Supply or Inflated Demand

Normally, thirst is related to the level of cellular hydration and a person will increase water intake with inflated demand. Heat exhaustion syndromes result from water and/or electrolyte (Na^+ and K^+) depletion. These syndromes can occur under conditions of strenuous exercise, especially at high ambient temperatures, encountered by those engaged in heavy physical labor as well as by athletes.

Digestion/Absorption.—The relative concentration of sodium ions is an additional factor determining the level of dilution of chyme. Sodium ions are readily absorbed and are actively transported in exchange for glucose molecules. IF the concentration of Na^+ ions in the chyme is higher than that in the mucosal cells, THEN water will be drawn from the mucosal cells into the intestinal lumen to disperse the Na^+ ions until the concentration is equivalent on both sides of the mucosal cell wall. Since the Na^+ ions are absorbed concurrently, the balance is continually shifting until at some point the rate of water absorption exceeds that of secretion and the chyme becomes progressively dehydrated. Whether water content will be normalized by the time the mass is evacuated depends on sodium intake and sodium need. IF intake is very excessive, THEN local dehydration of mucosal cells may be sufficient to cause cramps, nausea, vomiting, and loose stools.

To avoid salt depletion exhaustion, those engaged in strenuous physical activity must replace salts lost. Use of salt tablets may induce the symptoms just described. These can be avoided by ingesting liquid containing 1 tbsp table salt/gal.

Water Balance, in General.—The balance between K^+ of ICF and Na^+ of ECF determines the level of ICF hydration. IF the circulating level of Na^+ is high in relation to the ICF level of K^+, THEN water is drawn from the cell, which becomes dehydrated, and the volume of ECF is expanded, i.e., edema results. AND, IF water is removed by sweating or use of a diuretic, THEN because there is alway some loss of K^+ from the cells, cellular dehydration and edema occur at a lower equilibrium point. This situation is progressive and can result in symptoms such as cardiac arrythmias due to K^+ deficiency.

Water Balance, Effects on Specific Tissues.—Two tissues are severely stressed by the edema that results from withdrawal of water from ICF. The workload of the kidney is greatly increased. The increased volume of fluid to be circulated stresses the cardiovascular system.

Control of water balance between plasma and interstitial fluid is effected by means of kidney excretion, mediated by the circulating level of aldosterone. IF the circulating level of Na^+ is high (hypernatremia) AND the volume of interstitial fluid and plasma is high as a result, THEN the circulating level of aldosterone will be relatively low. THEREFORE, some plasma water and Na^+ will be excreted by the kidney, allowing a redistribution of both from interstitial fluid into the plasma until new equilibrium concentrations are reached. This action will be progressive in this direction as long as the concentration of extracellular electrolytes (measured as Na^+) exceeds that of the intracellular electrolytes (measured as K^+).

When the rate of kidney excretion of water is insufficient to control the volume of plasma within normal limits, cardiovascular effects of edema result. The increased plasma volume requires greater pumping action by the heart. The blood vessels have limited expansion capacity, so the push must be greater. So, blood pressure rises, and pressure damage causes weak spots to balloon and/or blow out. Because of the increase in volume, the plasma is relatively dilute in nutrients. Either normal circulating levels must be maintained or other tissues will be undersupplied. This is an unwanted but frequent outcome, resulting in increased pumping activity—from normally accommodating to urgent to frantic pumping as the gap between demand for oxygen and nutrients and supply levels increases. Congestive heart failure is the end-stage result.

Water: Excess ICF Supply

Salt depletion heat exhaustion is observed in summer but it is not as prevalent as edema. The observed symptoms depend to some degree on the amount of water imbibed in relation to the thirst created by sweat loss.

Sometimes availability of water is limited. IF plasma volume decreases below its normal circulating range, THEN blood pressure drops and weakness, etc., develop.

When water availability is unrestricted, too much water may be imbibed. IF the water lost by sweating is replaced but salt replacement is insufficient, THEN the ICF concentration of K^+ will be high in relation to the ECF concentration of Na^+. THEREFORE, water will migrate into the cells and aldosterone will be secreted by the adrenal glands. This causes the kidney to reabsorb Na^+ and Cl^-, and to excrete K^+ and water. As a result of this alteration in electrolyte balance, K^+ and water migrate from the cells to return to an equilibrium. This action is progressive in this direction until a stable equilibrium is reached. IF sweating continues beyond the heat exhaustion stage, THEN no equilibrium may be reached and water intoxication occurs. Also, loss of K^+ from ECF results in a low circulating level of K^+ (hypokalemia).

NERVE IMPULSE TRANSMISSION

Nerve impulse transmission is a complex process. It involves stimulation of one of the sensory end organs (vision, hearing, taste, smell, touch or pain) and communication of the resultant sensation to the central nervous system (brain and spinal cord). Communication is by means of a transduction process. This involves propagation of the electrical impulse, created by stimulation of the end organs, along the neuronal cell membrane and supply of chemical power at the cell terminal to neurotransmitter compounds, e.g., monoamines such as serotonin and norepinephrine; acetylcholine; amino acids such as glycine and glutamate; and peptides such as thyrotropin-releasing hormone. Recent research also has identified a number of peptides (e.g., angiotensin, cholecystokinen, endorphins, and enkephalins) in brain tissue that are involved. Whether their roles are as neurotransmitters, neuromodulators, or neurohormones is presently unresolved. The explanation of propagation of the electrical impulse is well developed and is outlined below. The mode of operation of the neurotransmitters is not well understood, so the explanation is tenuous and has not been integrated with the discussion. Even less is known about the peptides; limited information with respect to each group suggests what their functions may be and their possible mode(s) of action; explanation has not been attempted.

Sodium and potassium are the major ions involved in nerve impulse transmission, though chloride (Cl^-), calcium (Ca^{++}), and magnesium (Mg^{++}) ions are also involved. Normally, in the resting state between impulses, the following supply situation is observed:

(a) Na^+ concentration in ECF is greatly above that in nerve cell ICF, so only a few diffuse inside. K^+ concentration in ICF is greatly above that of ECF and although the K^+ ions migrate out freely, K^+ is returned to the cell by the potassium pump. Membrane potential is largely determined by the rate of outward migration of K^+ ions.

(b) The nerve cell ICF contains a large number of ions that are too large to diffuse through the cell membrane, e.g., organic phosphates, organic sulfates, and proteins.

(c) Cl^- ions distribute themselves in both ICF and ECF according to electrical potential, thus the majority are in ECF because the intracellular membrane potential is negative. Like charges repel, thus inhibiting inward migration.

(d) Ca^{++} and Mg^{++} ions distribute themselves in ICF and ECF in proportions similar to Na^+ and K^+ ions, respectively. Their overall effect on membrane potential is unimportant due to the small number of these ions involved.

Normally, in the excited state during transmission of an impulse, an action potential develops. A two-stage series of supply states results:

(a) depolarization—Since Na^+ is external and K^+ is internal, when a nerve cell is excited a local segment of the cell membrane is depolarized (membrane potential becomes positive), allowing a sudden influx of Na^+ ions.

(b) repolarization—Adjacent segments of the membrane are progressively depolarized, resulting in propagation of the action potential, i.e., a nerve impulse is transmitted. Each segment repolarizes immediately after the impulse moves on, because Na^+ is pumped back out against a gradient. Removal of the positively charged ions causes the intracellular membrane potential to repolarize to its resting negative charge in readiness for subsequent restimulation. Thus, Na^+ and K^+ balance is restored.

The explanation of the role of Ca^{++} ions in this process is that in the normal resting state, Ca^{++} ions which are bound to nerve cell wall proteins decrease permeability to Na^+ ions because their positive charge repels the positively charged sodium ion. When excitation occurs, some Ca^{++} ions become detached from their proteins. Removal of the Ca^{++} barrier to Na^+ ions enables the influx of Na^+ ions to surge inward, removing the remaining Ca^{++} ions from their protein sites. Once the impulse is past, the Ca^{++} ions progressively rebind to the membrane proteins. This progressively reduces permeability to Na^+ ions to its normally low level.

Clearly, the supply of Na^+, K^+, and Ca^{++} ions is critical to the level of nerve cell membrane excitability. Excitability is increased when the circulating level of Ca^{++} ions is low since lack of availability reduces the number of sites bound and the number of ions available to repel Na^+. So, the result is increased membrane permeability to Na^+ ions. Therefore, excitability is increased due to spontaneous impulses created by Na^+ migration. On the other hand, high circulating levels of Ca^{++} and/or low circulating levels of K^+ decrease the level of excitability.

MUSCULAR CONTRACTION

Muscle fiber contraction is controlled by electrolyte migration in a manner that is separate but similar to that described for nerve impulse transmission. The inotropic action, i.e., action affecting the force of muscle contraction, is mediated by an enzyme system is which (a) ATP is hydrolyzed and (b) Na^+ and K^+ are translocated across the cell membrane between ECF and ICF. Cardiac muscle, though it functions somewhat differently from skeletal muscle, will be used for illustration.

This is because inadequate supply of K^+ results in a life-threatening situation.

In cardiac muscle, the impulse to contract is spontaneous and immediately spreads throughout the muscle. Excitation results in depolarization of the membrane, a surging influx of Na^+ ions into the cell, and release of protein bound Ca^{++} ions. The Ca^{++} ions migrate into the myofibrils and catalyze the reactions that result in contraction. Contraction occurs by the interleaving of the proteins actin and myosin, forming actomyosin. The Na^+ ions are then pumped out, the membrane repolarizes, the Ca^{++} ions rebind, and the actomyosin relaxes to its resting state. The greater the Ca^{++} migration, the greater the contraction.

The supply of Na^+, K^+, and Ca^{++} ions affects the quality of cardiac muscle contraction. In theory, but not observed, excess Na^+ in ECF could prevent Ca^{++} ions from detaching from binding sites, thus preventing them from initiating contraction. An excess of K^+ ions in ECF (hyperkalemia) is known to result in blocking of the cardiac impulse and/or a decrease in the force of contraction. An excess of Ca^{++} ions in ECF results in spastic contractions, due to overexcitation. In theory, but not observed, a deficiency of Ca^{++} ions could result in decreased force of contraction.

Basomotor tone of arterial and venous smooth muscle appears to be regulated by Mg^{++}. The critical role of Mg^{++} appears to be to control the influx of Ca^{++} ion, which controls the level of contraction (Turlapaty and Altura 1980). In cases of hypomagnesemia, there is a marked increase in contractile response resulting in progressive basoconstriction that can lead to arterial spasms.

ACID–BASE BALANCE

Activation of many enzymes is pH dependent. Thus, the pH of ECF and ICF, which are in equilibrium, is critical to survival. Therefore, pH is maintained within narrowly controlled limits. This is accomplished by a system involving (a) buffers, (b) changes in the rate and volume of ventilation, and (c) adjustments in kidney excretion of acids and reabsorption of bicarbonate.

Body fluids are buffered by the bicarbonate-carbonic acid system, the phosphate system, the hemoglobin-oxyhemoglobin system, and plasma proteins, which are amphoteric. Of these, the bicarbonate-carbonic acid system has the greatest effect on circulating pH. It is described below.

A large number of metabolic reactions produce CO_2 as an end-product. Energy production via the Krebs cycle is one example. So, a number of mechanisms are necessary to trap it until disposal can be achieved. In body fluids, CO_2 exists in equilibrium with carbonic acid (H_2CO_3) as a result of a reversible reaction catalyzed by the enzyme *carbonic anhydrase*. The carbonic acid formed by this reaction immediately dissociates into H^+ and HCO_3^- ions. Disposal of CO_2 is achieved by a combination of two mechanisms. The first mechanism involves ventilation, which responds quickly to increased levels of CO_2 by increasing the rate and/or depth of respiration. Dissolved CO_2 is exhaled. Some carbonic acid is reconverted to CO_2 by the action of carbonic anhydrase; once liberated, this CO_2 is also exhaled. The second mechanism involves kidney excretion of ammonium phosphate and retention of sodium bicarbonate, according to the reactions given below:

$$H_2CO_3 + Na_2HPO_4 \rightarrow NaH_2PO_4 + NaHCO_3$$

$$2NH_3 + 2H_2CO_3 + Na_2HPO_4 \rightarrow (NH_4)_2HPO_4 + 2NaHCO_3$$

Metabolic acidosis results from a deficit of bicarbonate. This can occur under several metabolic circumstances which include, but are not limited to:

(a) Formation of excess keto acids when body protein and lipids are metabolized to produce energy, as in uncontrolled diabetes, starvation, or in severe dehydration.

(b) Retention of sulfates, phosphates, and hydrogen ions as in uremia. Respiration rate, kidney conservation of bicarbonate and excretion of H^+ ions, and liver conversion of lactate, citrate, and acetate ions to bicarbonate ions are part of the mechanisms for restoring bicarbonate base.

Metabolic alkalosis, i.e., a deficit of carbonic acid, occurs as a result of excess intake of sodium bicarbonate for GI distress, severe vomiting loss of HCl, and Na^+ and/or K^+ depletion resulting from sweating or use of diuretics. In the latter case, when excessive K^+ is excreted in the urine, K^+ migrates from the cells to maintain a normal circulating level of K^+. H^+ and Na^+ migrate into the cells to replace the K^+. The normal circulating level of H^+ ions is reduced, hence alkalosis occurs.

Extreme cases may show some shift in pH of the blood, but even so the shift is not great. Instead, the circulating levels of keto acids, sulfates, phosphates, and bicarbonates are used as an index to acid-base balance.

WATER AND ELECTROLYTES: FOOD ECOLOGY AND LIFE EXPECTANCY

In relation to customary intakes of sodium, potassium, and phosphate ions involved in fluid dynamics, etc., signs of disturbance of the normal intake-outgo balance are increasingly common. The customary intakes of the others are not yet out of line. Man's relation to his food was in balance with regard to intake of Na, K, and phosphates until recently. But, sodium chloride is abundant, inexpensive, and useful in stimulating consumption as well as in preserving food. Consumption of amino acid mixtures and formulated foods lacking K is a new alternative. And, phosphates are added to many foods for a variety of purposes. All of these changes have upset the balance in the food-related ecosystem. Individually all of these changes benefit man in one way or another; their cumulative and aggregate effect has not been studied. None are likely to be reversed, so some other solution must be sought. As of now, awareness and informed choice make mindful consumption the most feasible possibility in reducing the life-threatening hazard.

Hypertension has become a major problem for many Americans. Although sodium intake has not been proved to be the cause, reduction in sodium intake does result in reduced blood pressure. For this reason, a limited intake of 3 g sodium chloride has been recommended as a preventive measure.

Use of diuretics, which are potassium-wasting, and/or consumption of a liquid protein diet (a mixture of amino acids without potassium) has created an unnatural potassium supply deficit for some people. Use of a diuretic is effective but treats the symptom, not the cause. In most cases, fluid retention can be corrected by decreasing sodium chloride consumption. This has no unwanted physical effects, but it does create a need for change in man's relation to his food. Similarly, consumption of a liquid protein diet is effective in weight reduction in the short-run, but it treats the symptom not the cause. It is simply one of a number of fad diets that limits intake and is effective while followed but does not change poor habits. When the novelty wears off, one reverts to customary poor habits and weight gain resumes. Use of a weight reduction plan that is coupled with development of good eating habits is the best way to avoid the unwanted outcomes of this fad.

BIBLIOGRAPHY

MURPHY, E.W., and MANGUBAT, A.P. 1973. Potassium in common foods. Family Econ. Rev., Summer, p. 22-23. Consumer & Food Econ. Inst., Agric. Res. Serv., USDA. Washington, D.C.

ROBINSON, C.H. 1978. Fundamentals of Normal Nutrition. Macmillan, New York.

TURLAPATY, P.B.M.V., and ALTURA, B.M. 1980. Magnesium deficiency produces spasms of coronary arteries: relationship to etiology of sudden death is ischemic heart disease. Science 208 (4440) 198-200.

9

Major Minerals

The roles of the six major minerals in fluid balance, nerve impulse transmission, muscle contraction, and acid-base balance were discussed in the previous chapter. Other nutriment functions of these minerals are addressed in this chapter.

For centuries, milk has been considered to be food for young mammals and unnatural for adults. Use of milk in cooking and consumption of cheese and other dairy products have been highly variable within and among cultures. Dietary surveys usually have identified calcium as one of the nutrients supplied at marginal or deficient levels in segments of the American population.

In recent years, in some areas of the United States, milk drinking has become excessive. It displaces other foods from the diet because of its volume and/or calories. The long-term effects on mineralization of bone and other tissues are not well understood, so there is concern.

CALCIUM: NORMALLY AVAILABLE

The role of calcium in mineralizing bones and teeth has long been recognized. Calcium is also Factor IV in the blood clotting process.

Digestion/Absorption

Calcium salts are more soluble in acid medium. Absorption has been observed to occur primarily in the upper end of the small intestine close to the duodenum. The explanation for this site is based on solubility, i.e., at this location the chyme is still acid from gastric HCl, since it has not yet been neutralized by pancreatic secretions. THEREFORE, all other things being equal, a greater percentage of calcium will be available in the free ionic form so it can be absorbed.

A secondary site of absorption is the ileum. The hypothesis offered to explain absorption at this location is that lactate is converted to lactic acid by the normal bacterial flora. The lactic acid lowers the pH to the range at which the calcium salts are again soluble, so calcium is liberated and may be absorbed.

Another factor that facilitates absorption is the presence of selected amino acids. Lysine, arginine, and serine form soluble complexes with calcium, but calcium is easily liberated from these complexes.

Simultaneous ingestion of some other food substances may decrease the relative proportion of Ca^{++} that can be absorbed. The safety factor built into the RDA for Ca^{++} takes into account the normal effect of these, so that given normal ingestion levels, the effect is trivial. Substances known to form insoluble calcium salts include, but are not limited to:

(a) oxalic acid from vegetables such as spinach and rhubarb

(b) phytic acid from whole grain cereals

(c) free fatty acids

(d) free phosphate ion

Findings reported by Spencer *et al.* (1978) demonstrate that there is no significant difference in Ca^{++} absorption whether phosphate intake is high or low.

The rate of absorption is controlled by the circulating level. IF the circulating level is normal, THEN a normal percentage, approximately 30%, will be absorbed. Calcium is the alkaline constituent of intestinal juices. The quantity secreted is variable according to the amount of acid to be neutralized. The quantity of Ca^{++} is also variable.

Calcium absorption requires active transport. Absorption efficiency is mediated by the active form of vitamin D and two hormones. The accepted explanation for the process until 1974 was as follows:

(a) IF the circulating level of calcium is within its normal circulating range, THEN thyrocalcitonin will be secreted and will inhibit the parathyroid hormone mediated activation of the hydroxylating enzyme. In the liver, vitamin D is converted to 25-hydroxycholecalciferol (25-HCC) as the first step. Then, in the kidney 25-HCC is hydroxylated to its active form 1,25-dihydroxycholecalciferol (1,25-DHCC). By inhibiting the hydroxylating enzyme, this second step is blocked.

(b) Lack of the active form represses production of calcium-binding protein (CaBP). THEREFORE, permeability of the intestinal mucosa to, and transport of, calcium will be limited.

A study by another group (Anon. 1978) showed that CaBP is not obligatory in calcium transport across the mucosal wall. Ca^{++} transport occurs even when CaBP is absent. Moreover, there is some evidence that Ca^{++} transport is reduced when CaBP is present. However, there is no doubt that 1,25-DHCC does induce mRNA for synthesis of CaBP. And, while CaBP has a function in calcium transport, it may not be the only protein involved. Therefore, there has been speculation that the initial Ca^{++} transport is in response to vitamin D and that later, CaBP is involved. Other proteins in the brush border may be involved, e.g., alkaline phosphatase and a Ca-dependent ATPase.

Metabolism of Calcium—in General

The supply of Ca^{++} ions is normally adjusted to maintain a circulating level of 9 to 11 mg/100 ml. Of this, 50% is bound to plasma proteins and 5% is combined in unionizeable form. The remaining 45% is in the free ionic form for translocation throughout the body to meet needs for two of its nutriment functions:

(a) to increase permeability of cell walls to fluid, as described in the previous chapter

(b) to activate several enzymes

Recent evidence indicates a relationship between protein intake and the level of urinary calcium excretion. The findings suggest that when protein intake is high, the requirement for calcium may be inflated due to greater excretion. Because the mean protein intake in the United States is twice the recommended quantity, the RDA for calcium has been continued at a generous level, pending additional information.

Metabolism of Calcium—in Specific Tissues

Calcium has unique functions in blood and bone tissue. In blood, calcium is the catalyst for the conversion of prothrombin to thrombin. This conversion is a necessary step in the series of reactions that results in blood clotting.

In bone, crystals of apatite, which are composed of $Ca_{10}(PO_4)_6(OH)_2$ and $CaCO_3$, are deposited within a protein-based structure composed of collagen, hyaluronic acid, and chondroitin sulfates. The density of crystallization is related to calcium intake.

Some apatite crystals are hardened by formation of insoluble fluoride salts. For example, the hydroxyl group can be replaced by F^- or CaF_2 can be formed.

In addition, a readily exchangeable source of Ca is necessary for rapid adjustment of the circulating level. This calcium is adsorbed on the surface of bones.

Most bone tissue participates in the concurrent anabolism/catabolism process in which the circulating levels of Ca^{++}, PO_4^{---}, and Mg^{++} are adjusted, given variable dietary intake and withdrawal for cell use. The balance between anabolism and catabolism is controlled by the same mechanism involving circulating levels of parathyroid hormone (mobilizes Ca) and thyrocalcitonin (stores Ca) that control uptake by the intestinal mucosa. The currently accepted explanation is:

(a) IF the circulating level of calcium is within its normal circulating range, THEN thyrocalcitonin will be secreted and will inhibit the parathyroid hormone mediated activation of the hydroxylating enzyme that converts vitamin D to its active form.

(b) The presence of 1,25-DHCC will increase the action of the osteolytic cells somewhat; resorption will occur, liberating Ca^{++}, PO_4^{---}, and Mg^{++} ions into circulation.

(c) AND, the presence of 1,25-DHCC will increase the action of the osteoblasts, leading to deposition of the Ca^{++}, PO_4^{---}, and Mg^{++} ions when intestinal uptake corrects the temporary imbalance.

Kidney excretion of calcium is also used to adjust circulating levels. The normally low levels of parathyroid hormone and 1,25-DHCC do not permit active reabsorption of Ca.

CALCIUM: DEFICIENT SUPPLY OR INFLATED DEMAND

Rickets and osteoporosis are the deficiency diseases that result when dietary intake of calcium is chronically insufficient to meet tissue needs. Such chronic lack is rarely seen in children in this country, so rickets is rare. Prevalence of osteoporosis among the elderly is low, but of concern.

Digestion/Absorption

Absorption efficiency is determined partly by need and can be increased somewhat in order to compensate for (a) chronic ingestion of an insufficient quantity or (b) inflated demand, as during growth stages or pregnancy. When the circulating level of calcium falls below the normal range, the circulating level of 1,25-DHCC increases, which causes an increase in the calcium-binding protein in the mucosal wall. Therefore, absorption, or transport of calcium through the mucosal wall, is facilitated. However, even if the percentage is increased, the absolute quantity may still be insufficient since no amount of increase in transport capacity can overcome an absolute lack of calcium.

Many adults probably ingest marginally adequate quantities of calcium as a matter of food preference. In this case, the additive effect of a factor that decreases bioavailability would be to create a deficiency. For example, with a normal intake of calcium, formation of calcium phytate has a trivial effect since only about 30% of ingested calcium is absorbed anyway. However, when ingestion is marginal the percentage absorbed has to be much higher in order to obtain as much as possible, so the percentage unavailable as a result of formation of the insoluble salt may be a critical variable. Hence, there is concern for those on strict vegetarian diets unless non-dairy sources are conscientiously selected in generous amounts.

Another intervening variable that may result in inadequate calcium absorption is the condition achlorhydria, or lack of gastric HCl. This condition afflicts approximately one-third of the elderly. Since calcium salts are more soluble in acid medium, a lack of gastric acidity decreases their solubility. Therefore, absorption is impaired.

Metabolism of Calcium—in General

No general effect of low calcium intake has been observed. Well nourished bone contains approximately a 20-year supply of calcium. Therefore, the effect of low calcium intake would be manifest in bone long before the critical level was reached in other tissues.

Metabolism of Calcium—in Specific Tissues

When dietary intake of calcium is insufficient to maintain the circulating level within a normal range, even temporarily, the rate of resorption of bone is increased over the rate of mineralization. The calcium that is liberated is used to maintain the circulating level. Since urinary and fecal calcium loss occur continuously, progressive bone demineralization results.

In children, extension of the long bones is expected. IF less than normal mineralization occurs, THEN the bones will be soft and will bend as weight increases. Hence, the bow legs of rickets.

In adults, reduced bone density due to demineralization is called osteoporosis. A triangular shape provides the greatest load-bearing strength. So, the weight-bearing bones of the spine, etc., bend to approximate this shape and loss of stature occurs. Spontaneous fractures occur if the weight on a demineralized bone is too great for it to bear.

CALCIUM: EXCESS SUPPLY

The effects of chronic excess intake of calcium have not been defined. Hypercalcemia, hypercalcinuria, calcification of soft tissues, and renal stones (mostly calcium) are known but these effects are not related to calcium intake *per se*. However, a high calcium intake does exacerbate these conditions. What is known about effects of high intake is largely limited to digestion/absorption and excretion.

Digestion/Absorption

When the amount of calcium ingested greatly exceeds the amount needed, it exceeds the amount of calcium-binding protein available for transport of calcium through the intestinal wall. So, it remains in the chyme and is eliminated in the feces. Because absorption efficiency is low, fecal losses are high. Moreover, since calcium and magnesium compete for some of the carriers, and calcium is preferentially transported, development of a magnesium deficiency is a possibility, albeit infrequently observed.

Excretion of Ca is under control of parathyroid hormone and 1,25-DHCC. A minute increase in the circulating level of Ca results in a marked increase in urinary excretion. It is for this reason that high calcium intakes exacerbate kidney stone formation.

PHOSPHORUS AS THE PHOSPHATE ION: NORMALLY AVAILABLE

Phosphorus is a poisonous ion sometimes used for medicinal purposes. However, the phosphate ion is an essential nutrient, i.e., it must be provided by diet and/or supplements since it cannot be synthesized. While phosphates are known to sequester other nutrient minerals, i.e., calcium, copper, iron, magnesium, etc., the overall absorption of them is not inhibited by the presence of dietary phosphates, to any extent.

Digestion/Absorption

Each of the different phosphate forms appears to be absorbed somewhat differently, although the process involves active transport and is the same mechanism that controls calcium absorption. Nearly all ingested phosphate is absorbed. Some additional facts that pertain to each of the phosphate forms are listed below:

(a) orthophosphates are readily absorbed

(b) pyrophosphates are readily absorbed and are hydrolyzed to orthophosphate by an enzyme in the blood (alkaline phosphatase)

(c) tripolyphosphates, e.g., STP, are absorbed and are then hydrolyzed to orthophosphate in the blood

(d) straight-chain polyphosphates, e.g., SHMP, are complexed with calcium and are absorbed intact; they are then hydrolyzed to orthophosphate in the blood

(e) cyclic metaphosphates are hydrolyzed to tripolyphosphates and then to orthophosphate, prior to absorption

Metabolism of Phosphate—in General

The phosphate radical is required for nearly every function of respiration and biosynthesis. It is the major anion of ICF. Thus, supply must be controlled. The normal circulating level is 2.5 to 4.5 mg PO_4^{---}/100 ml. Both free inorganic HPO_4^{--} and $H_2PO_4^{-}$ and compounds such as phospholipids and phosphoproteins contribute to the circulating level. The level is controlled partly by the circulating levels of parathyroid hormone and calcitonin, in conjunction with the circulating level of calcium. A second mechanism, the phosphatase enzyme system, is also operative. Activation of this system is a function of the circulating level of magnesium as well as calcium. Phosphate is translocated throughout the body to supply target tissues for purposes which include, but are not limited to:

(a) constituent of ribose- and deoxyribose phosphate, the bases of nucleic acids

(b) phosphorylation of glucose to glucose-6-PO_4 to activate it for degradation via the Krebs cycle in energy production

(c) constituent of the active high energy compounds, e.g., creatine phosphate (CP) and adenosine triphosphate (ATP)

(d) activation of vitamin-containing coenzymes, e.g., nicotinamide adenine dinucleotide phosphate (NADP), pyridoxal phosphate (PLP), thiamin pyrophosphate (TPP), riboflavin monophosphate (FMN), and flavin adenine dinucleotide phosphate (FAD).

Although phosphate has many general functions, particular functions in specific tissues have not been identified. Phosphate is stored in considerable quantities in bone. When parathyroid hormone is secreted to mobilize Ca^{++} from bone, the circulating Ca:P ratio is adjusted by kidney excretion of phosphate and reabsorption of Ca.

PHOSPHATES: DEFICIENT SUPPLY OR INFLATED DEMAND

A deficient dietary intake of phosphate is unknown in man. A depletion syndrome has been observed as a result of chronically excessive use of non-absorbable antacids. Symptoms associated with the drug-induced nutritional deficiency are weakness, anorexia, malaise, and bone pain.

PHOSPHATES: EXCESS SUPPLY

The traditional dietary ratio of phosphate to calcium has been 1½ to 2:1. The new uses of phosphates as food additives have resulted in imbalances and reconsideration of toxicity probabilities. Orthophosphoric acid is classified as Generally Recognized as Safe (GRAS) according to the FDA, so it is approved for food use. Polyphosphoric acids as well as their calcium, potassium, sodium, and ammonium salts are also classified as GRAS substances, since all have been demonstrated to be converted to orthphosphoric acid. The Meat Inspection Division of the USDA also has approved of these compounds for use as additives to meat products, as regulated in the Code of Federal Regulations. Nonetheless, an excess intake from inherent and/or additives is acknowledged to be toxic. In consequence, the FAO has established Acceptable Daily Intake (ADI) levels for humans. These are expressed in mg/kg body weight:

(a) acceptable levels for all diets—less than 30

(b) acceptable levels for high calcium diets—30 to 70

Orthophosphates and short-chain polyphosphates are more toxic than sodium chloride when ingested orally. However, long-chain and cyclic polyphosphates are less toxic. The extent of toxicity is directly related to the extent of intestinal hydrolysis to ortho- and/or pyrophosphates, which is highly variable but not well defined.

Concern with the effects of high phosphate intake is not limited to ingestion of toxic doses. A recent study by Bell *et al.* (1977) reported that depending on the subset of foods selected, food additive-related phosphate might increase dietary phosphate by ½ to 1 g per day. These investigators also found that at the higher level of phosphate intake calcium absorption was reduced, hydroxyproline and cAMP were elevated, and urinary excretion of calcium was decreased. These findings suggested that an increased circulating level of parathyroid hormone (PTH) was the cause.

Many of the phosphate additives were sodium polyphosphate compounds. The foods were also high in sodium and/or added salt. Under these conditions of high sodium intake, antidiuretic hormone (ADH) and cAMP are commonly elevated. Therefore, the elevated cAMP may be due to PTH and/or ADH, reflecting both phosphate and sodium levels.

Abdominal distress is a common side-effect of high phosphate intakes. This may be due to the osmotic effect. A 4 g dose of phosphate is known to be cathartic. The dietary intake in this study was 5[+] g. Although this quantity was divided among three meals, the quantity may have been sufficient to cause distress in sensitive individuals. Moreover, since the sodium polyphosphates are more readily hydrolyzed in the GI tract than are other phosphate compounds, they may have contributed more than proportionally to the osmotic and other effects.

MAGNESIUM: NORMALLY AVAILABLE

Magnesium is the second most important cation in ICF. It is a catalyst involved in many enzyme systems.

Digestion/Absorption

Magnesium, like calcium, exists in foods as both inorganic and organic salts. It also must be liberated to the free ionic state in order to be absorbed. Normally, 40% of the ingested magnesium is absorbed.

Magnesium is more soluble in acid medium, so it is absorbed close to the duodenum. An active transport mechanism is involved, but at this point no vitamin or hormonal mediation seems to be necessary.

Metabolism of Magnesium—in General

The circulating level of magnesium normally ranges from 1.7 to 3.0 mg/100 ml. Magnesium circulates as the free Mg^{++} ion and in a non-diffusible form, bound to plasma proteins. It is translocated to the various cells, where uptake is paired with K^+ uptake.

In the mitochondria, Mg^{++} activates ATPase, coenzyme A, etc. Thus, it is involved as a co-factor in (a) transfer of energy from ATP, (b) synthesis and degradation of glycogen, and (c) energy production. It is a coenzyme with a role in DNA and RNA structure and, therefore, in ribosomal protein synthesis. Another function is with the mineral-ocorticoids in regulation of the circulating phosphate levels—an involvement in acid-base balance. A newly acknowledged critical function is in regulation of smooth muscle contraction.

Metabolism of Magnesium—in Specific Tissues

Magnesium is combined with calcium and phosphorus as one of the bone salts. About 70% of the body magnesium is utilized in this function.

MAGNESIUM: DEFICIENT SUPPLY

Magnesium deficiency in man is rare but not unknown. Symptoms involve increased neuromuscular excitability, resulting in tremor and convulsions, and finally in tetany.

Digestion/Absorption

Magnesium is widely distributed in foods. Deficiency is seen only occasionally in alcoholics or in starvation. However, in theory, reduced intake can result from presence of excessive amounts of fatty acids that result in formation of insoluble soaps, thus increasing fecal losses. As noted above, excessive calcium intake also may reduce absorption, due to competition for carriers.

MAGNESIUM: EXCESS SUPPLY

Depression of the CNS is the effect of a high circulating level of magnesium. This has been observed as a complication of kidney failure. Otherwise, the excess is deposited in bone or is excreted by the kidney.

CHLORINE: NORMALLY AVAILABLE

The chloride requirement is easily met by normal intake of sodium chloride. Therefore, although the essentiality of this nutrient is indisputable, it is often taken for granted and little information is available.

The chloride ion is readily and almost completely absorbed. The mechanism has not been described. As the main anion of ECF, it is involved in fluid balance and respiration, as discussed in the previous chapter.

Gastric HCl is formed in the parietal cells. The postulated mechanism for secretion of HCl is as follows:

(a) hydrogen ion—CO_2 combines with water, mediated by the enzyme carbonic anhydrase, to form carbonic acid which dissociates into the H^+ and bicarbonate ions. The bicarbonate ion is removed by out-migration. The H^+ ion remains in solution.

(b) chloride ion—It is actively transported into the cell by an unknown process. Inside, it associates with the H^+ ion forming HCl. When the parietal cells are stimulated, the HCl is secreted into the lumen of the stomach.

MAJOR MINERALS: FOOD ECOLOGY AND LIFE EXPECTANCY

Within the limits of current knowledge, neither deficit nor excess intake of calcium, magnesium, nor chlorine seems to be possible at a level that is life-threatening. Nonetheless, lesser effects are known and are to be avoided by monitoring intake.

Dental decay is a prevalent disease. The number of new caries and the extent of decay can be modified by use of one of the phosphate compounds as a food additive (Schiff 1977). Phosphates have a local effect in tooth enamel protection during maturation phases. Dental research has presented indicative evidence that IF one of the phosphates is present in fermentable carbohydrate-containing foods, e.g., candy, gums, THEN the phosphate remineralizes the demineralized areas, thus filling in the defects and resulting in a smooth surface (Nizel 1977). This smooth surface is probably less vulnerable to attack by plaque bacteria produced acids. One or more phosphates of each type have been tested; all are effective (Baron 1977; Nizel 1977; Schiff 1977). Effectiveness is variable in different foods, so the type of phosphate compound must be selected for the particular food application. Presence in an individual food item will not appreciably reduce overall decay since no one food is eaten with sufficient frequency. It is the cumulative and aggregate effect that is important. So, for maximum effectiveness, the phosphates would need to be present in many foods. Present usage of phosphates is extensive; whether it coincides with need for dental protection has not been determined. However, it is unlikely.

BIBLIOGRAPHY

ANON. 1978. Vitamin D, calcium binding protein and the intestinal transport of calcium. Nutr. Rev. *36*, 90-93.

BARON, H.J. 1977. Modifying the cariogenicity of foods with dicalcium phosphate. *In* Proc. Workshop in Cariogenicity of Food, Beverages, Confections and Chewing Gum, Sept. 15-17, 1977, Chicago. Res. Inst. Am. Dental Health Foundation.

BELL, R.R. *et al.* 1977. Physiologic responses of human adults to foods containing phosphate additives. J. Nutr. *107*, 42-50.

NIZEL, A.E. 1977. The anticaries effects of trimetaphosphates. *In* Proc. Workshop in Cariogenicity of Food, Beverages, Confections and Chewing Gum, Sept. 15-17, 1977, Chicago. Res. Inst. Am. Dental Health Foundation.

SCHIFF, T. 1977. Phosphate compounds used in caries research with some degree of success. *In* Proc. Workshop on Cariogenicity of Food, Beverages, Confections and Chewing Gum, Sept. 15-17, 1977, Chicago. Res. Inst. Am. Dental Health Foundation.

SPENCER, H., KRAMER, L., OSIO, D., and NORRIS, C. 1978. Effect of phosphorus on the absorption of calcium and on calcium balance in man. J. Nutr. *108*, 447-457.

Trace Minerals

Human need for iron and iodine is known to and acknowledged by most people. Moreover, the deficiency diseases associated with lack of these trace minerals have been so prevalent that people are generally aware of their major manifestations. The nutritional need for sulfur is not well known and it is not usually addressed *per se*, though need for the sulfur-containing amino acids and vitamins is acknowledged.

With the exception of these three elements, micronutrient needs pose a perplexing problem for the consumer because there are so many unanswered questions. Requirements, when known, are often expressed in quantities such as micrograms, inconceivably small amounts. Since only a trace is necessary, a deficiency seems unreasonable to expect, yet it occurs. Some of these elements are antagonists of others; if present, then absorption/utilization of others is impaired. More than a trace is toxic. There is almost no information available on food sources of micronutrients. Some have not been demonstrated to be necessary to humans; they are only presumed to be necessary, given animal data. Food processing is known to remove macronutrients; does it also remove trace minerals? There are new micronutrients announced at frequent intervals. Mineral supplements do not contain micronutrients—is that bad? Food labels do not indicate presence or absence. Even more of a problem is the fact that there are so many trace elements, and more are announced all the time. All of this complexity overwhelms the consumer.

Iron, iodine, and sulfur nutriture have been studied extensively. Nutriture with respect to each will be considered separately. Then, general points regarding trace mineral nutriture will precede a brief discussion of what is known concerning each of the remaining trace minerals.

IRON: NORMALLY AVAILABLE

Nutrition survey results suggest that about one-fourth of the American population is anemic, especially infants and women of child-bearing age. Hence, iron nutriture is a major contemporary nutritional concern. The salient nutriment function of iron is related to its oxygen-carrying capacity as a constituent of the hemoglobin molecule.

Digestion/Absorption

Bioavailability of food iron depends not only on the amount contained in a food but on the nature of the iron compound, the presence of absorption enhancing factors in the meal, the presence of absorption blocking factors in the meal, and the individual's need for iron (Monsen *et al.* 1978). Therefore, the total iron content of the diet is an unreliable index to the supply of iron.

Dietary iron is ingested in two forms. Heme iron is the iron porphyrin complex from muscle myoglobin and hemoglobin. According to Monsen *et al.* (1978), the heme ratio is 30 to 40% in pork, liver, and fish and 50 to 60% in beef, lamb, and chicken. Nonheme iron is bound to other proteins in dairy products, eggs, fruits, grains, vegetables, meat, poultry, and fish. It is also a component of the inorganic salts such as ferrous sulfate or one of the organic salts such as ferrous citrate or ferrous gluconate. The latter are used in food supplements or for enrichment.

Heme and nonheme iron are absorbed by separate mechanisms. Heme iron is absorbed with greater efficiency but the quantity present is small. Nonheme iron is absorbed with lower efficiency but the aggregate quantity is large, so in the aggregate it is the largest source of dietary iron.

Heme iron is absorbed as the intact iron porphyrin complex. This heme moiety is degraded within the intestinal mucosal cell, liberating free iron. IF a person has little or no iron stores, THEN he/she may absorb up to 35% of the heme iron ingested. IF a person has average iron stores, which are estimated to be 500 mg, THEN he/she may absorb up to 25% of the heme iron.

Nonheme iron must be reduced to its ferrous state and liberated to its free ionic form prior to formation of soluble complexes with gastric juice. Concomitant ingestion of some substances enhances nonheme iron absorption. These substances are ascorbic acid, which reduces ferric iron to ferrous iron; citric, lactic, pyruvic, and succinic acids; fructose and sorbitol; and many amino acids. There is a "meat factor" in meat, poultry, and fish that also enhances absorption four-fold. This factor is absent in other protein-rich foods such as milk, eggs, and cheese. So, these are associated with decreased iron absorption.

Many substances block iron absorption. These include, but are not limited to, calcium and phosphate salts—these may completely block iron absorption; EDTA; phosvitin of egg yolk; phytic acid from cereal grains; polyphenols from tea; and several trace elements that compete for binding sites, e.g., copper, zinc, cadmium, cobalt, and manganese. Zinc also interferes with iron incorporation into mucosal ferritin. IF a person has little or no iron stores AND many enhancers are present, THEN he/she may absorb up to 20% of the nonheme iron ingested. IF a person has average iron stores of 500 mg AND/OR iron enhancers are not present AND/OR iron blockers are present, THEN he/she may absorb only 2% of the nonheme iron present.

The quantity absorbed is also controlled in relation to need by other mechanisms, but the process(es) of regulation is/are not completely understood (Fig. 10.1). Recent evidence suggests that the iron is stored as ferritin within the mucosal cells and is bound to the plasma membrane. The explanatory hypothesis that has been generally accepted is that when the level of iron saturation of transferrin, the iron transport protein (Fe^{+++}), is below normal, an interaction at these membrane binding sites releases the iron from ferritin so that it can rebind to transferrin for translocation to the liver, spleen, and bone marrow. As a result, additional iron can be absorbed by the mucosal cell and bound to the free sites.

Mucosal cells are replaced every three days. Degradation of the cellular debris by intestinal enzymes liberates the iron from the ferritin. This iron is reabsorbed along with newly ingested iron.

Metabolism—in General

Transferrin provides the link for distribution of iron in its various metabolic cycles. In order to release iron from transferrin (40% saturation potential), ATP and ascorbic acid must be present in adequate quantity. Ascorbic acid reduces the iron from ferric to ferrous form so that it will dissociate from the globulin protein and be free to enter the cells. ATP supplies the energy for liberation. The iron cycles are:

(a) The hemoglobin cycle for oxygen transport—Plasma transferrin to bone marrow to red blood cell (RBC) to senescent RBC to plasma transferrin. The ferrous form is incorporated into the heme portion of the hemoglobin molecule of the RBC, which has a normal lifespan of 120 to 125 days. The senescent RBC are removed by the reticuloendothelial cells of the liver, spleen, and bone marrow. The heme moiety is removed and degraded. The iron is released and is recycled by incorporation into newly forming hemoglobin molecules. Approximately 21 to 24 mg are recycled daily.

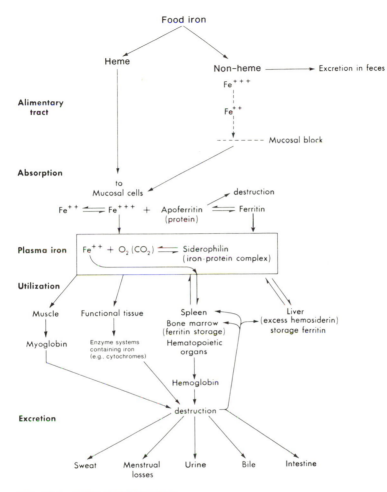

FIG. 10.1. IRON METABOLISM

The explanation of the mechanism by which the supply of iron for heme formation is adjusted to oxygen-carrying capacity is beginning to emerge. It appears that IF absorbed iron ferritin stores in the intestinal mucosa are short but liver ferritin/hemosiderin stores are normal, THEN when the oxygen-carrying capacity of the blood is decreased due to insufficient hemoglobin, a rising level of hypoxanthine in the liver cell activates xanthine dehydrogenase which interacts with ferritin, resulting in release of iron. The iron then becomes available for incorporation in transferrin, to be translocated to the bone marrow for incorporation in heme. When iron is incorporated into hemoglobin, the rising oxygen-carrying capacity results in conversion of hypoxanthine to xanthine, thus deactivating xanthine dehydrogenase. Thus, by this mechanism normal iron nutriture enables a normal level of heme formation and normal oxygen-carrying capacity.

(b) The ferritin/hemosiderin storage cycle—Plasma transferrin to liver, spleen and/or bone marrow ferritin (20% iron saturation) to hemosiderin (35% iron saturation potential) to plasma transferrin. Iron is stored in the ferric form. At low levels of iron storage, iron is distributed approximately equally in these two compounds and it is exchanged between them. However, it first must be incorporated into ferritin before it can be transferred to hemosiderin. At high levels of storage, the quantity of hemosiderin exceeds that of ferritin.

Release of stored iron from ferritin involves reduction to the ferrous form by riboflavin, which allows dissociation from the protein moiety prior to binding to apotransferrin for transport. Ceruloplasmin, a copper-containing enzyme, oxidizes ferrous to ferric form, creating a gradient that favors mobilization from storage.

(c) The oxygen exchange and electron transport cycle—Plasma transferrin to myoglobin (in skeletal muscle) or iron-containing enzymes, e.g., cytochrome oxidase, to plasma transferrin. Myoglobin is a protein molecule similar to hemoglobin and is the oxygen-storing compound of muscle. Although the concentration of iron in myoglobin is low, in the aggregate the quantity of iron stored approximates that in liver.

IRON: DEFICIENT SUPPLY OR INFLATED DEMAND (BLOOD LOSS)

Iron deficiency results in a hypochromic microcytic anemia. It occurs as a result of inadequate iron intake and/or inflated demand created/maintained by chronic blood loss. Chronic blood loss due to the following has been associated with a secondary anemia: excessive menstrual losses, repeated pregnancies, infections, malignancies, ulcers, frequent blood donation, and use of drugs such as aspirin (one tablet results in mean blood loss of 5 ml). Dietary intake is usually insufficient to correct a secondary anemia; it may be refractory.

The currently accepted explanation for the anemia that develops as a result of iron deficiency is acknowledged to be incomplete. It appears that IF the level of iron saturation of the circulating transferrin is low and cannot be increased by liver stores, THEN the quantity of iron available for incorporation in heme is decreased, oxygen-carrying capacity of the blood which depends on heme concentration is reduced (anemia), and a low cellular supply of oxygen results. Many reactions, especially those energy-producing reactions of the Krebs cycle, require oxygen. Lack of oxygen prevents the reactions and results in a systems slowdown, hence, the popular term "tired blood."

IRON: AVAILABLE IN EXCESS

The quantity of iron which, if ingested chronically, would result in toxicity is unknown. One study reports that a mean intake of 50 mg/day is safe, although ingestion of a greater quantity with no observable effects in known.

Both hemosiderosis, a non-damaging deposition of excess hemosiderin, and hemochromatosis, a damaging deposition of hemosiderin due to iron overload, are known. In some cases, the factors predisposing to one over the other are unknown. The explanation for the development of these conditions is as follows:

(a) Apoferritin in the mucosal cells combines with available ferrous up to its saturation point when all sites are engaged.

(b) When transferrin saturation falls, mucosal ferritin iron is released and combines with transferrin until it is resaturated to its normal level.

(c) Liver cells remove the iron from the transferrin and recombine it with liver ferritin. Then it is transferred to hemosiderin. The normal cycle, which is progressive, results in excessive deposition of hemosiderin. Until recently, the condition was considered irreversible. A chelating compound which can be used to reduce the excess iron stores is now available.

IODINE: NORMALLY AVAILABLE

The nutriment functions, as far as is known, are related solely to iodine's role as a constituent of the hormone thyroxine and its more active form triiodothyronine. Thyroxine is a high-use hormone. Its primary function is to stimulate energy metabolism at the cellular level, which is a major factor in the expression of the genetic potentialities of the human being. The mechanisms of this process are unknown. Subsidiary functions include, but are not limited to, neuromuscular functions especially of the CNS (mechanism unknown); cellular differentiation resulting in growth and development of tissues/organs (mechanism unknown); health of skin and hair, decreasing the circulating level of cholesterol, and conversion of β-carotene to vitamin A. Accordingly, the requirement for replenishment is such that the supply of thyroxine or its circulating level must be controlled.

Iodine is present in food in both organic and free (I_2) forms. During digestion, conversion to the inorganic ionic I^- form is necessary for absorption, except for iodated amino acids which are absorbed intact. In its ionic form, iodine absorption is rapid and complete. The salivary and gastric secretions contain organic iodides which are digested; the I^- is reabsorbed.

The mechanism for control of the circulating level of thyroxine functions as follows: IF the circulating level of thyroxine is low, THEN the hypothalamus releases thyrotropin releasing factor (TRF). TRF stimulates the adenohypophysis to release thyroid stimulating hormone (TSH). A high circulating level of TSH causes iodine to be removed from systemic circulation via active transport into the cells of the thyroid gland. The iodide ion is immediately incorporated into a storage protein, thyroglobulin. The quantity withdrawn from circulation is approximately one-third, given a normal intake. The remainder of the ingested iodide ion is excreted in the urine.

To form thyroxine, I^- is liberated from thyroglobulin to form I_2, then monoiodotyrosine, then diiodotyrosine (DIT), and finally, thyroxine. Thyroxine is a compound comprised of two molecules of DIT minus the amino acid alanine. Thyroxine is bound to plasma protein for translocation to the various sites for utilization.

IODINE: DEFICIENT SUPPLY

Deficiency has been recognized for centuries. IF the dietary intake is somewhat low on a continuing basis, THEN hypothyroidism results, i.e., the metabolic rate is decreased with the observed effect of loss of vigor AND the tissue of the thyroid gland hypertrophies to form a goiter, in an attempt to increase capacity to produce a necessary and sufficient quantity of thyroxine (Fig. 10.2). IF the dietary intake is very low on a continuing basis, THEN myxedema results, i.e., the metabolic rate is greatly reduced with the observed effects of a firm inelastic edema, dry skin and hair, loss of physical vigor, and mental retardation. IF the dietary intake of a pregnant woman has been so deficient that her stores are depleted, THEN fetal development will be modified producing a cretin with characteristic physical and mental retardation.

A deficient supply of thyroxine can result from ingestion of an interfering factor. Goitrogens, inherent in some foods, are substances that cause a goiter to develop. Since the circulating level of thyroxine is critical to survival, IF low, THEN the pituitary gland attempts to increase it by increasing its output of TSH. This induces compensatory proliferation of the thyroid tissue.

Goitrogens are of three types. *Goitrin* interferes with thyroxine synthesis. Its effects can be partially reversed by increased iodine intake. It is found in vegetables of the cabbage family. *Thioglycosides* are converted to thiocyanate which inhibits the selective concentration of iodine by inhibiting the iodination of tyrosine. Its effects can be reversed by increased iodine intake. This goitrogen is found in vegetables of the mustard family. A *sulfated unsaturated hydrocarbon* (undefined) is found in water (mode of action unknown).

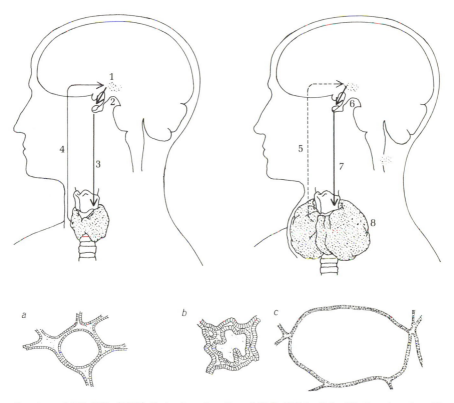

FIG. 10.2. NEGATIVE FEEDBACK SYSTEM

Negative feedback system controlling production of thyroid hormones begins with the neurosecretion from the hypothalamus (1) of thyrotropin–releasing factor (TRF), which goes directly to the pituitary (2) and causes it to release thyrotropin, or thyroid-stimulating hormone (TSH), into the bloodstream (3). In the thyroid gland TSH acts to bring about the synthesis and secretion into the circulation of the thyroid hormones thyroxine and tri-iodothyronine (4); the amount of thyroid hormones reaching the hypothalamus in turn controls the secretion of TSH, completing the negative-feedback loop. In the absence of iodine, an essential substrate for thyroid hormones, not enough hormone is produced (5) to "turn off" the system; excessive TRF (6) and TSH (7) are secreted, stimulating the iodine–depleted thyroid tissue to grow (8). A normal thyroid follicle, in which hormones are synthesized and stored, consists of an envelope of cells containing a colloid, thyroglobulin (a). In the absence of iodine TSH causes the cells to proliferate and become more columnar (b) and then to produce more colloid, so that the follicles become distended (c), forming a goiter.

Normally, the quantity of ingested foods containing goitrogens is insufficient to produce goiter. However, in exceptional cases, goitrogens have been known to induce goiter even when the iodine intake is normal. Cooking, a procedure that destroys the enzyme that liberates goitrin from its precursor, is recommended when large quantities of cabbage are consumed regularly.

IODINE: EXCESS SUPPLY

Persons consuming excessive quantities of iodine from kelp or other sources may develop a toxicity syndrome. IF intake is as much as ten times the RDA on a continuing basis, THEN thyrotoxicosis or hyper-thyroidism may develop in individuals with a defective iodine regulatory system. This condition is characterized by increased metabolic rate, rapid heart rate, and high blood pressure. Excessive intake of iodine results in progressive toxicity to the thyroid gland itself. Wolff (1969) has defined four levels of toxicity as follows:

(a) A small excess, leading to increased storage of thyroglobulin up to capacity. An increased percentage of iodine is excreted in the urine.

(b) A moderate excess inhibits release of iodine for incorporation into thyroxine.

(c) A larger excess decreases thyroxine production and results in development of a goiter.

(d) A very large excess saturates the active transport mechanism.

SULFUR: NORMALLY AVAILABLE

Sulfur is a nutrient and it is essential in the sense that it must be supplied by dietary intake. It is a necessary constituent of several amino acids and vitamins. Often the focus of discussion is on the need for the amino acids and vitamins rather than on the role of sulfur *per se*. However, as details of the sulfur cycle have emerged, the need to view sulfur metabolism in a larger frame has become clear.

Digestion/Absorption

Sulfur in foods is contained in both organic and inorganic compounds. In organic form, it is a constituent of (a) the essential amino acids methionine and cystine and the nonessential amino acid cysteine, (b) the B vitamins thiamin and biotin, and (c) the malodorous flavor/odor compounds of many vegetables, especially of the onion family (S-allyl-1-cysteine sulfoxide, diallyl thiosulfonate, diallyl disulfide, etc.) and the cabbage family (S-methyl-L-cysteine sulfoxide and isothiocyanates or mustard oils). Inorganic sulfur is present as sulfate (SO_4^{--}), sulfite (SO_3^{--}), elemental sulfur (S), and sulfide (S^{--}). Sulfites and sulfates often are used as preservatives. The amino acid and vitamin forms are absorbed intact. Otherwise, the compound must be degraded and the ionic form liberated. The mechanism of S^{--} absorption has not been delineated.

Sulfur Metabolism—in General

Sulfur in its sulfate form is very active metabolically. The known nutriment functions for which sulfur must be supplied are as follows:

(a) constituent of all proteins—It is the linking agent between chains which stabilize the tertiary structure; disulfide bonds form the link. When the disulfide bond is hydrolyzed, a sulfhydryl group results; the chains are no longer linked so they are considered "denatured" and they are usually no longer functional. Metabolism of the sulfur-containing amino acids yields H_2SO_4 (sulfuric acid). It is immediately neutralized by conversion to its ammonium salt for urinary excretion.

(b) constituent of mucopolysaccharides and chondroitin sulfates—It is part of the ground substance of the cells.

(c) constituent of sulfolipids (sphinganine + sulfate on galactose).

(d) constituent of insulin and heparin.

(e) constituent of sulfate esters—These include steroid and phenol sulfates, choline sulfate, etc.

(f) constituent of many enzymes—It is the active site that reacts with substrates.

(g) constituent of coenzyme A—SH is the high energy active form.

(h) participant in oxidation-reduction reactions—It is a constituent of glutathione.

(i) detoxification of poisonous compounds and drugs—Metabolism of phenols, cresols, and sex hormones produces toxic compounds. Conjugation with SO_4^{--} is the mechanism for formation of excretion compounds.

In order to function metabolically, sulfur must be activated. This is a two-step process. The first step, catalyzed by a *sulfurylase*, results in formation of adenosine-5'-phosphosulfate (APS). The second step, which requires ATP and involves mediation by an APS kinase, results in formation of adenosine-3'-phosphate-5'-phosphosulfate (PAPS). PAPS is the active sulfate donor that participates in sulfur metabolism. Subsequent metabolic pathways involving sulfate reduction, incorporation of H_2S into organic compounds, sulfate respiration, and release of sulfur from organic compounds have been partially defined in microorganisms and higher plants. These pathways may function in humans as well.

Mammals, including man, are unable to make cysteine from H_2S and SO_4^{--}. Instead, cysteine is synthesized from methionine, which is why it is essential and cysteine is not. First, methionine is demethylated to homocysteine. Next, *cystathionine synthase II* catalyzes the combination of homocysteine and serine to form cystathionine and H_2O. Lastly, cystathionine is hydrolyzed to α-ketobutyrate and cysteine in a reaction mediated by a cystathionase.

In its active form, methionine is a methyl donor and participates in numerous reactions. The active form is produced by a reaction of methionine with ATP in which a high-energy sulfonium derivative, S-adenosyl methionine, is formed.

SULFUR: DEFICIENT SUPPLY

The effects of deficiency are associated with the form of sulfur that is in deficient supply. For example, IF the essential sulfur-containing amino acids are not supplied, THEN protein metabolism is impaired due to lack of active methionine and cysteine. IF the B vitamins are not supplied, THEN their cofactor roles are not performed and many reactions are halted. Death may result from these deficiencies as discussed in the chapters on protein and B vitamins.

The essentiality of nonamino acid and nonvitamin sulfur has not been established for humans. Effects of deficiency or excess in these forms are unknown.

OTHER TRACE MINERALS

With the exceptions of iron, iodine, and sulfur, trace element needs have been recognized only recently. So, evaluation of needs is incomplete. Therefore, one is probably privileged to conclude that, with these exceptions, trace elements are normally supplied in sufficient quantity. Otherwise, effects of gross deficiency or excess would have been evident much earlier.

The limits of the class of essential micronutrients called trace elements are unclear, and a number of unique considerations apply. Currently, trace elements as a class include, but are not limited to, iron, iodine, sulfur, copper, fluorine, zinc, chromium, selenium, cobalt, manganese, and molybdenum. Other elements presumed to be essential in human nutrition include, but are not limited to, vanadium, tin, nickel, cadmium, and boron. A 1973 WHO report summarized considerations that apply to this class of micronutrients as follows:

(a) A quantitative size limit that will distinguish between a trace and a major mineral under all circumstances cannot be established. Arbitrarily, the boundary designated is 1 mcg. Those elements that occur or seem to be required in quantities less than this are considered to be trace elements.

(b) Classification based on essentiality versus toxicity is inaccurate and/or misleading, since all essential trace elements are toxic at some level of intake. Moreover, only a trace is required and only a trace more is toxic.

(c) Until about 1970, these elements were regarded as natural contaminants or nuisance variables in research rather than as micronutrients. Moreover, essentiality and requirement levels are difficult to establish for nutrients required in trace amounts. However, using sophisticated analytical techniques and purified diets, some were identified as essential to animals and then to human beings. Essentiality of some is still questionable.

(d) Since these elements are widely distributed in nature, they are normally available unless there is an intervening variable.

Essentiality has been redefined by Cotzias (1967): present in all healthy tissues of all living things, its concentration is relatively invariate among species, its withdrawal results in identical reproducible physiological and structural abnormalities in various species, addition prevents/reverses the abnormalities, the deficiency is always accompanied by the same set of biochemical effects, the biochemical effects are directly related to the deficiency, and prevention/cure of deficiency is accompanied by prevention/cure of the biochemical change.

Trace elements are micronutrients because of their role either as a constituent of an enzyme or hormone, or structure of a tissue/organ, or as a cofactor in a necessary metabolic reaction. What is known is summarized for each of the trace elements.

Copper (Cu)

There are six known nutriment functions. One is as a constituent of cytochrome oxidase and other oxidases. A second is as a constituent of erythrocuprein, an enzyme that catalyzes the combination of superoxides to form peroxides and/or oxygen scavengers. A third is as a constituent of the cofactor ceruloplasmin which is necessary for incorporation of ferric iron from mucosal ferritin, liver ferritin or recycled from the reticuloendothelial system into transferrin. Lack leads to reduced transport of iron and, therefore, decreased incorporation in hemoglobin and results in anemia. Other functions (not well defined) include roles in melanin formation, in phospholipid synthesis, particularly those in brain and CNS tissue, and in bone development. Serum copper levels are greatly increased by use of the estrogen type of OCA; the meaning of this fact is unclear.

Dietary copper is present in a variety of forms. Copper is absorbed in the stomach and all along the small intestine. Absorption efficiency is low and is related to age, amount available, and level of competing metal ions. The mechanism of absorption is unknown, but intake appears to be regulated according to need. Copper is absorbed as the free ion and is complexed with amino acids. Phytic acid forms an insoluble complex, decreasing absorption. High levels of ascorbic acid also depress absorption efficiency.

Absorbed copper is immediately bound to plasma albumin for transport to the liver. The liver is the main organ for metabolism of copper—production of ceruloplasmin, storage, and excretion via the bile.

Between one-half and three-fourths of the body stores of copper are dispersed in muscle tissue in the aggregate. Concentrated storage depots also exist in the liver, heart, kidneys, and CNS. The nutritional significance of these storage sites is unknown.

Deficiency was demonstrated about 20 years ago in children whose single source of nourishment was milk (this results because milk is processed in copper-free equipment in order to minimize development of copper-catalyzed off-flavors). IF copper intake is low on a continuing basis, THEN anemia and decreased rate of cellular oxidation in liver, muscles, and nervous tissue lead to lassitude. A very recent finding is that in adults, IF copper intake is marginal on a continuing basis, THEN the risk of coronary heart disease is increased.

Toxicity has been reported only in persons with an inherited degenerative disease, i.e., Wilson's disease, in which the quantity of ceruloplasmin is limited and results in excessive storage of copper in the liver and other organs.

Fluorine (F)

The nutriment function of fluorine is as a structural element in teeth and bones, to a limited extent. The rate of F uptake by bone depends on its growth rate. Therefore, uptake is higher in children since their bones are growing. It is incorporated in bone in two steps: it exchanges with OH or CO_3 ions on the surface of bone tissue and then is incorporated into hydroxyapatite, maybe by replacing CO_3 with F or as MgF_2.

A deficient intake results in risk of dental caries. IF intake is low on a continuing basis, THEN in children, all other things being equal, the incidence of (number of new) caries is greater than normal AND in adults the incidence of osteoporosis and other demineralizing diseases is greater than normal. Symptoms of bone pain, decreased bone density, and elevated circulating calcium level can be reduced by treatment with sodium fluoride. Some very recent evidence suggests that fluorine deficiency may be associated with reduced hematocrit levels, fertility, and growth rate.

Excessive intake of F causes fluorosis. The most noticeable symptom is unsightly mottled tooth enamel.

Zinc (Zn)

The nutriment functions of zinc are as a constituent of enzymes such as *thymidine kinase*, which is necessary for nucleic acid synthesis; *carbonic anhydrase*, which is involved in CO_2 transport; *lactic dehydrogenase*, which is involved in the interconversion of pyruvic to lactic acid; and *alkaline phosphatase*, which liberates inorganic phosphate. Another function is as a structural element in storage of insulin in the pancreas.

Zinc is absorbed in the small intestine, but efficiency is low and highly variable among its different forms. It forms insoluble salts with phytic acid, etc. The explanation of the absorption process is incomplete. The current hypothesis is that the pancreatic fluid contains a Zn-binding ligand that leads to transport across the mucosal wall. It is bound to the plasma membrane and then interacts with albumin for transport through and within plasma. Therefore, the efficiency of uptake is regulated by the amount bound to the plasma membrane. IF Zn is retained in the mucosal wall, THEN it will be lost when the senescent mucosal cell is sloughed off. Copper and other metals compete for transport sites.

Once absorbed, Zn is bound loosely to albumin and tightly to transferrin or to a globulin for transport. It is also bound to the amino acids cysteine and histidine, which results in loss by kidney excretion. Conditions which increase the rate of tissue protein catabolism liberate these amino acids, resulting in high Zn losses. Since the amino acids compete effectively with albumin for the Zn, progressive losses result in depletion.

Deficient intake of Zn results in observable effects: growth retardation or dwarfism and sexual infantilism result from decreased thymidine kinase activity which reduces DNA synthesis and cell division; decreased appetite, decreased sense of taste and smell; skeletal abnormalities; and poor healing of burns and other wounds where high Zn losses occur. Conditioning factors resulting in zinc deficiency include, but are not limited to, malabsorption syndromes, stress from surgery or burns, chronic fevers, cirrhosis, or renal dialysis. Sources of Zn are listed in Table 10.1.

Toxicity is known to occur. IF an excess is ingested all at one time, THEN vomiting, dehydration, electrolyte imbalance, nausea, lethargy, dizziness, and lack of muscular coordination result. A gross excess may be ingested from acidic foods that are stored in galvanized containers.

Chromium (Cr)

Only the trivalent ion has bioactivity. The nutriment function is as a cofactor with insulin, so this element is known as the Glucose Tolerance Factor. The accepted hypothesis explaining its mode of action is that it decreases peripheral resistance to insulin, thus facilitating transport and utilization. Other functions involve lipid, especially cholesterol, levels (unexplained) and protein metabolism.

Inorganic Cr is poorly absorbed (1 to 3%), but the organic forms are absorbed somewhat better. The hexavalent ions are more readily absorbed than the trivalent forms. The site and mechanism of absorption are unknown. Presence of zinc and vanadium decrease Cr absorption.

Transport of the hexavalent ion involves penetration of the RBC and binding to hemoglobin. The trivalent ion complexes with transferrin for transport. Cr is widely distributed among the tissues. The circulating level is not in equilibrium with tissue concentrations, which precludes use of a hematologic index to Cr status. Instead, hair samples are used.

Deficiency has been linked to growth retardation and decreased longevity. Since protein, fat, and carbohydrate metabolism are affected by insulin activity, these outcomes are not surprising. They are not clearly understood, either. Deficiency is associated with reduced glucose tolerance and has occasionally been observed in pregnant women with a history of frequent pregnancies, insulin-requiring diabetics who lose it in the urine, and in older people.

TABLE 10.1. ZINC IN HOUSEHOLD MEASURES OF FOOD

	Zinc per Household Measure			
Food Group	More Than 3 mg	1–3 mg	0.5–0.9 mg	Less Than 0.5 mg
Shellfish, meat, poultry, fish (3 oz cooked, unless otherwise stated)	oysters, raw[1] beef beef or calves liver poultry heart lamb turkey, dark meat crab gizzard veal pork	chicken, dark meat lobster turkey, light meat shrimp, 6 salmon, solids & liquid, ½ cup clams (4 or 5)	tunafish fish, white chicken breast sausage, cold cuts and luncheon meats, 1 slice	
Dairy products and eggs	milk, nonfat, dry, 1 cup	cheese, 1 oz	milk, whole, 1 cup ice cream, 1 cup egg, whole, 1	margarine, ½ cup butter, ½ cup
Grain products (1 cup unless otherwise stated)		flour, whole wheat cornmeal, degermed oatmeal, cooked rice, cooked, brown bread, whole wheat, 2 slices	cookies, 10 vanilla wafers rice, cooked, white wheat germ, toasted, 1 tbsp wheat cereals, ready-to-eat, 1 oz macaroni, cooked bread flour all purpose flour	corn chips, 1 oz bread, white, 2 slices cake or pastry flour cake, white 1 piece, 3 × 3 × 2 in. crackers, graham, 2 squares popcorn, popped crackers, saltines, 10 crackers corn flakes, 1 oz

TABLE 10.1 *(Continued)*

Food Group	Zinc per Household Measure			
	More Than 3 mg	1–3 mg	0.5–0.9 mg	Less Than 0.5 mg
Vegetables and legumes (½ cup unless otherwise stated)		beans, mature, dry cowpeas, cooked peas, mature chickpeas lentils	peas, immature, cooked spinach, cooked	beans, green, cooked corn, canned lettuce, ⅙ head potato, 1 med., cooked carrot, 1 med., raw cabbage, raw, shredded onions, mature or green tomato, ripe 2⅗ in. diam.
Fruits and fruit juices (½ cup unless otherwise stated)				applesauce banana, 1 med. orange, 1, raw orange juice, canned, unsweetened peach, 1, raw, peeled apple, 1, raw
Other foods		cocoa, approx. 5 tbsp		coffee, fluid beverage, 1 cup chocolate syrup, 2 tbsp beverages, carbonated, 12 fl. oz tea, fluid beverage, 1 cup

Source: Willis and Mangubat (1975).
[1] More than 5 mg zinc per common household unit.

Selenium (Se)

The nutriment function is as a constituent of glutathione peroxidase, which is involved in destruction of lipid peroxidases. This is the basis for its role as an antioxidant and in maintenance of membrane structure by preventing breakdown of the lipid components. Selenium is also known to substitute for sulfur, forming selenium analogs of the S-containing amino acids in some protein structures and in some reactions (some of these substitutions are unwanted effects), but sulfur cannot replace selenium in its nutritional role. Selenium is incorporated into myoglobin, cytochrome c, muscle enzymes—e.g., aldolase, myosin, and nucleoproteins.

Little is known about the absorption and transport of Se. It is absorbed in the duodenum and is carried in plasma after an intra-RBC transformation that enables it to be bound to plasma β-lipoprotein.

The human requirement for Se is unknown, but the value extrapolated from animal nutrition is 60 to 120 mcg/day. A range is given to indicate that the requirement is dependent on such factors as bioavailability and the supply/demand situation with regard to other nutrients. A deficiency syndrome has not been observed in human beings. At the present time, the estimated mean intake of Americans is above the requirement range. Soils are highly variable in Se content. However, human beings, unlike animals, do not consume food produced predominantly on local soils. Therefore, Se deficiency is unlikely and Se supplementation is not justified.

Selenosis, the human toxicity syndrome resulting from chronic intake of Se in excess quantities, has been observed. Reported clinical manifestations are loss of hair, brittle fingernails, garlic breath odor, and nonspecific complaint of fatigue and irritability.

Cobalt (Co)

The known human nutriment function is as a constituent of vitamin B_{12}. But, there are other forms of Co in other species, so it may be bioactive in other forms in humans as well.

Variable amounts of Co are absorbed from the intestine. Both Fe deficiency and Fe excess result in increased Co absorption. Hence, it has been postulated that Co may share a common mucosal transport mechanism. Co is excreted in the urine and to some extent via bile.

Cobalt as B_{12} is an essential nutrient. It will be discussed in Chapter 13.

Toxicity has been demonstrated. Symptoms include thyroid hyperplasia, myxedema, and congestive heart failure.

Manganese (Mn)

The nutriment functions of Mn are as a constituent of pyruvate carboxylase and superoxide dismutases and as a cofactor to activate hydrolases, kinases, decarboxylases, and transferases, including glycosyl transferases which are necessary for polysaccharide and glycoprotein synthesis. These nutriment functions of Mn can be met partially by other metal ions, especially Mg, Cu, Zn, and Fe.

Manganese is absorbed as the bivalent ion, is carried as the free or bound ion in portal blood to the liver, and is converted to the trivalent form in addition to being hooked to its specific transport protein, transmanganin. Nothing is known of food forms nor the percentages absorbed/retained.

Manganese deficiency, associated with a vitamin K deficiency, has been observed in man. Symptoms include impaired mucopolysaccharide synthesis, impaired growth, skeletal abnormalities, defects in carbohydrate metabolism (mechanism unknown) and in fat metabolism (linked to choline, fatty acid, and cholesterol synthesis blockages). Blood clotting is also impaired, since Mn is a cofactor for vitamin K in prothrombin synthesis. The mode of action probably is by activation of the glycosyl transferase that adds the last part of the carbohydrate chain to the immediate precursor of prothrombin (a glycoprotein).

Manganese is relatively non-toxic. A toxicity syndrome is known, but has not been produced from diet intake.

Molybdenum (Mo)

The nutriment functions of Mo are as a constituent of metalloenzymes and as a cofactor for several enzymes. Mo is a constituent of xanthine oxidase which is involved in purine degradation to uric acid, aldehyde oxidase which is involved in conversion of liver aldehydes to their carboxylic acids, sulfite oxidases, and probably of nitrogenases and nitrate reductases. It is a cofactor for FAD and other flavine enzymes as well as in the reaction of xanthine oxidase with cytochrome c and reduction of cytochrome c with aldehyde oxidase. It is also an anti-metabolite, i.e., it substitutes metabolically and interferes with the function of copper.

Both inorganic and organic forms of Mo are readily absorbed, especially the hexavalent water-soluble sodium and ammonium salts. The circulating level reflects intake when sulfur and sulfur-containing amino acid status is controlled. Sulfur increases Mo excretion but the mechanism is unknown; the postulated mechanism is a blockage in kidney reabsorption of Mo.

No deficiency has been observed in man but excess intake (10 to 15 mg/day) results in gout. Both an increased uric acid level and increased xanthine oxidase activity have been observed in cases of toxicity. Since Mo is an anti-metabolite of copper, an excess intake results in development of a copper deficiency syndrome.

Elements That May Be Nutrients

A number of other elements have postulated roles in human nutrition, i.e., they have been demonstrated to be essential to some species, so are expected to be essential to humans as well. These elements include, but are not limited to:

(a) vanadium (V)—In pharmacologic doses, it decreases plasma phospholipid levels and plasma cholesterol levels. It also decreases cholesterol synthesis. Recent evidence suggests effects on bone development and growth rate.

(b) tin (Sn)—It has chemical properties that suggest possibilities for bio-function, e.g., it forms coordination complexes with 4, 5, 6, and 8 ligands so it may have a constituent role in tertiary structures of proteins and it may be a cofactor since it has an oxidation-reduction potential near that for the flavine enzymes.

(c) nickel (Ni)—It may be involved as a constituent of liver cell structures and as a cofactor in liver cell functions involving oxidation and lipid levels. It is stored and released under stress of myocardial infarction, stroke, burns, and major sweating episodes.

(d) cadmium (Cd)—It may have a role in control of blood pressure. It is poorly absorbed (3 to 8%) but accumulates with age, concentrating in liver and kidney tissue. It is bound to metallothionein for storage or as a means of sequestering it in detoxification. There is no homeostatic control mechanism, so it just accumulates. It is toxic to all systems. An anemia develops due to the effect of Cd on absorption of iron and copper as well as on their utilization.

(e) silicon (Si)—It is a constituent of mucopolysaccharides with a structural role in linking portions of the mucopolysaccharides to themselves and/or to proteins—thus its role is as a biological cross-linking agent. Its concentration is high in skin and connective tissues where it performs these roles.

Food forms of Si are as monosilicic acid, as solid silica, and in organic form bound to pectins, mucopolysaccharides, etc. The extent and mechanism of absorption are unknown. The amount ingested is excreted in the urine, since the circulating level remains essentially the same.

Other elements also may be nutrients. Even less is known about them nutritionally. What is known is summarized in Table 10.2.

TRACE MINERALS: FOOD ECOLOGY AND LIFE EXPECTANCY

With the exception of iron, iodine, and sulfur, little detailed information is available about the distribution of trace elements in food, i.e., their sources, varietal and other inherent differences in content, processing and/or preparation losses, and bioavailability. Therefore, although common sense leads to the conclusion that some dietary changes probably would be detrimental to trace element nutriture, the exact nature and extent of the effects are not predictable, given current knowledge.

Man's relation to his food supply has changed radically in this century. Prior to this century and probably through the first half of it, when the diet consisted of a variety of foods prepared at home from basic commodities, neither a deficit nor an excess of trace elements (except iron, iodine, and sulfur) was likely. However, uninformed consumption of low calorie diets or those composed largely of refined and/or formulated foods raises the possibility of deficit. And, uninformed use of food supplements raises the possibility of excess and toxicity. For the first time, then, changes in food ecology introduce the possibility of a threat to life expectancy. Given limited information on trace mineral requirements, lack of a RDA for most trace minerals, and almost no information on distribution in foods, the traditional advice of nutritionists is still the best possible at this time: *Eat a variety of items prepared from basic commodities, in moderation.*

TABLE 10.2. TRACE ELEMENT STATUS SUMMARY, HUMAN NUTRITION, JUNE 1978

Aluminum, Al
Known human need?	cytochrome oxidase component
Known animal need?	no
Absorption facts known?	poor, F alters rate, efficiency
Metabolic fate known?	no
Effects of deficiency known?	no
Effects of excess known?	interferes with phosphorylating mechanism, phosphate absorption

Antimony, Sb
Known human need?	none?
Known animal need?	yes
Absorption facts known?	no
Metabolic fate known?	no
Effects of deficiency known?	no
Effects of excess known?	no

Arsenic, As
Known human need?	no
Known animal need?	yes
Absorption facts known?	high absorption rate
Metabolic fate known?	rapidly excreted in the urine
Effects of deficiency known?	no
Effects of excess known?	nausea, vomiting, burning mouth, burning throat, abdominal pain, weakness, muscle ache, inhibits S-enzymes

Barium, Ba
Known human need?	no
Known animal need?	no
Absorption facts known?	poorly absorbed
Metabolic fate known?	no
Effects of deficiency known?	no
Effects of excess known?	no

Boron, B
Known human need?	no
Known animal need?	no, but higher plants need
Absorption facts known?	rapidly absorbed
Metabolic fate known?	rapidly excreted
Effects of deficiency known?	no
Effects of excess known?	no

Bromine, Br
Known human need?	no, but can substitute for Cl
Known animal need?	no
Absorption facts known?	rapidly absorbed
Metabolic fate known?	rapidly excreted
Effects of deficiency known?	no
Effects of excess known?	no

TABLE 10.2 *(Continued)*

Germanium, Ge
  Known human need?   no
  Known animal need?   no
  Absorption facts known?   rapidly and completely absorbed
  Metabolic fate known?   excreted within a week
  Effects of deficiency known?   no
  Effects of excess known?   no

Lead, Pb
  Known human need?   suspected but unconfirmed
  Known animal need?   suspected but unconfirmed
  Absorption facts known?   rapidly absorbed; Cu, Fe, Co, and Zn reduce absorption
  Metabolic fate known?   excreted in bile and feces
  Effects of deficiency known?   no
  Effects of excess known?   toxicity: CNS damage causes encephalopathy and neuropathy; anemia due to interference with heme synthesis and increased RBC fragility; renal tubular dysfunction; depressed endocrine gland function

Lithium, Li
  Known human need?   no
  Known animal need?   no
  Absorption facts known?   no
  Effects of deficiency known?   no
  Effects of excess known?   possible side-effects: polyuria, ataxia, hypothyroidism, weight gain; mild to severe toxicity known when pharmacologic dose is continued

Rubidium, Rb
  Known human need?   no
  Known animal need?   lower animals use as a substitute for K
  Absorption facts known?   no
  Metabolic fate known?   slowly excreted in urine
  Effects of deficiency known?   no
  Effects of excess known?   no

Silver, Ag
  Known human need?   no
  Known animal need?   no
  Absorption facts known?   no
  Metabolic fate known?   no
  Effects of deficiency known?   no
  Effects of excess known?   copper and selenium antagonist

Strontium, Sr
  Known human need?   no
  Known animal need?   one report of need by rats and guinea pigs; unconfirmed
  Absorption facts known?   presence of food interferes with absorption; absorption inversely related to age and Ca intake; poorly absorbed
  Metabolic fate known?   preferentially deposited in bones and teeth
  Effects of deficiency known?   no
  Effects of excess known?   in animals only

Tin, Sn
  Known human need?   no
  Known animal need?   rats
  Absorption facts known?   poorly absorbed, poorly retained
  Metabolic fate known?   no
  Effects of deficiency known?   no
  Effects of excess known?   low toxicity

TABLE 10.2 *(Continued)*

Titanium, Ti	
Known human need?	no, not essential
Known animal need?	no, not essential
Absorption facts known?	poorly absorbed, poorly retained
Metabolic fate known?	no
Effects of deficiency known?	no
Effects of excess known?	no
Zirconium, Zr	
Known human need?	no, not essential
Known animal need?	no, not essential
Absorption facts known?	no
Metabolic fate known?	not excreted in urine, via intestine?
Effects of deficiency known?	no
Effects of excess known?	no

Since requirements for trace minerals are minute and the minerals appear to be widely distributed in nature, a deficient intake is unlikely unless one consistently consumes a diet of less than 1000 kcal or consisting largely of highly refined and/or synthetically formulated foods. When low calorie diets are consumed on a continuing basis, a high nutrient density is necessary to maintain adequacy of intake of nutrients other than calories.

Refining is known to reduce the mineral content somewhat, e.g., flour milling decreases zinc, manganese, copper, and molybdenum content by approximately 20%. Textured vegetable protein, which is formulated to be equivalent to meat in amino acid content (therefore, sulfur content), is not equivalent in mineral content since minerals are not included in the formula. Neither refined foods nor textured vegetable protein presents a nutritional problem when consumption frequency is low, but the cumulative or the aggregate effect of consumption of many items that are somewhat lacking is dietary inadequacy. Thus, it is the relative rather than the absolute lack that is of concern to scientists. So, an emotional overreaction is unwarranted; informed monitoring in a mindful way is the appropriate response to this concern.

Iron intake of many women and children appears to be marginal; iron intake of men is occasionally excessive. Fortification will benefit women but men consume more of the foods proposed for fortification. Fortification has been delayed because this dilemma has not been resolved. In the short run, the alternatives for improvement of intake are (a) conscious and conscientious selection of iron-rich foods, (b) increased cooking by long, slow moist-heat methods in iron pots so that leaching of iron from the pot is maximized, and/or (c) use of low-dose iron supplements. In the long run, either fortification or naturally high-iron foods may become available. One study has shown that the mean iron content of some wild plants is greater than the mean iron content of their domesticated counterparts and other members of the same families; plant and animal breeding for higher iron content would seem possible.

Iodine intake is low in some areas due to iodine-poor soil. Because Americans no longer consume a diet based largely on local produce and because of the availability of iodized salt, there is no reason for deficiency to develop.

Faddish consumption of kelp is both unnecessary and undesirable. While some people probably do not meet their iodine needs because of failure to recognize them, this is no sign that anyone needs a kelp supplement. Those whose diet intake is demonstrated to be suboptimal should increase their intake. One alternative is to use iodized salt, another is to increase consumption of sea foods (kelp is one kind of sea food). In any case, the quantity should be limited in order to control sodium intake.

BIBLIOGRAPHY

COTZIAS, G.C. 1967. Conference on Trace Substances and Environmental Health—Proc. 1st Annu. Conf., Univ. of Missouri, Columbia.

CULLEN, R.W., and OACE, S.M. 1976. Iodine: current status. J. Nutr. Educ. *8* (3) 101-102.

FISHER, K.D., and CARR, C.J. 1974. Iodine in Foods: Chemical Methodology and Sources of Iodine in the Human Diet. Federation of the American Society of Experimental Biology, Bethesda, Md.

FREELAND, J.H., and COUSINS, R.J. 1976. Zinc content of selected foods. J. Am. Dietet. Assoc. *68*, 526-529.

GILLIE, R.B. 1971. Endemic goiter. Sci. Am. *224*, 93-101.

HALSTED, J.A., SMITH, J.C., and IRWIN, M.I. 1974. A conspectus of research on zinc requirements of man. J. Nutr. *104*, 345-378.

HAMBRIDGE, K.M. 1974. Chromium nutrition in man. Am. J. Clin. Nutr. *27*, 505-514.

KIDD, P.S., TROWBRIDGE, F.L., GOLDSBY, J.B., and NICHAMAN, M.Z. 1974. Sources of dietary iodine. J. Am. Dietet. Assoc. *65*, 143-153.

LEVANDER, O.A. 1975. Selenium and chromium in human nutrition: a review. J. Am. Dietet. Assoc. *66*, 338-344.

MONSEN, E.R. *et al.* 1978. Estimation of available dietary iron. Am. J. Clin. Nutr. *31*, 134-141.

MURPHY, E.W., WILLIS, B.W., and WATT, B.K. 1975. Provisional tables on the zinc content of foods. J. Am. Dietet. Assoc. *66*, 345-355.

NATIONAL RESEARCH COUNC., DIV. BIOL. SCI., FOOD & NUTRITION BOARD. 1977. Commentary: Are selenium supplements needed (by the general public)? J. Am. Dietet. Assoc. *70*, 249-250.

NIELSEN, F.H.   1974.   "Newer" trace elements in human nutrition. Food Technol. *28* (1) 38-44.

NIELSEN, F.H., and SANDSTEAD, H.H.   1974.   Are nickel, vanadium, silicon, fluorine, and tin essential for man? A review. Am. J. Clin. Nutr. *27*, 515-520.

PENNINGTON, J.T., and CALLOWAY, D.H.   1973.   Copper content of foods. Factors affecting reported values. J. Am. Dietet. Assoc. *63*, 143-153.

SANDSTEAD, H.H.   1973.   Zinc nutrition in the United States. Am. J. Clin. Nutr. *26*, 1251-1260.

UNDERWOOD, E.J.   1977.   Trace Elements in Human and Animal Nutrition. 4th edition. Academic Press, New York.

WHO.   1973.   Trace elements in human nutrition. WHO Tech. Rept. Ser. *532*. Geneva.

WILLIS, B.W., and MANGUBAT, A.P.   1975.   Zinc in foods. Family Econ. Rev., Spring.

WOLFF, J.   1969.   Iodide goiter and the pharmacologic effects of excess iodide. Am. J. Med. *47*, 101-124.

11

The Fat–Soluble Vitamins: A, D, E, and K

Interest in the fat-soluble vitamins has flared sporadically. The need for vitamin A was the first to be announced. Since its distribution in foods is very uneven, dietary intake studies (unconfirmed by biochemical measures) usually report inadequate intakes for a portion of the group sampled. This fact is always remarkable and revives interest. Vitamin D nutriture is routinely monitored and for adults is adequate; fortification of dairy products assures adequacy for milk-drinking children. Recently, intense interest was elicited when researchers demonstrated that a unique bi-phase biotransformation is necessary to convert this vitamin to its active form. In the active form, it is a hormone. Interest in vitamin E has been kindled by the tantalizing but false hope that some of the functions demonstrated in animal nutrition might hold for human nutrition. The role of vitamin K in blood clotting is interesting but not of general concern.

Essentiality, i.e., need for an exogenous supply, is indisputable and their nutriment functions are well identified. And yet, only a portion of the nutritional picture is clear. Perhaps some aspects are unknowable.

THE FAT-SOLUBLE VITAMINS: NORMALLY AVAILABLE

These vitamins are found in conjunction with the lipid fractions in plant and/or animal tissues. Vitamin A is found in both plant and animal tissues, especially liver. Its provitamin form, carotene, is found only in plants. Food forms of vitamin A include the provitamin carotenes, preformed vitamin A esters of the various fatty acids, and free vitamin A. Vitamin D is found only in animal foods, particularly fish liver oils. There are ten known forms of vitamin D. Vitamin D_3 is most available and is most important nutritionally. There are eight known forms of vitamin E. α-Tocopherol is most available and is most important nutritionally, although availability of γ-tocopherol has increased with use of soybean oil. The richest sources of vitamin E are oils pressed from oilseeds, e.g., corn or safflower and those of legumes or nuts, e.g., soybeans or peanuts. There are two known forms of vitamin K. Good food sources are cabbage, cauliflower, spinach, and soybeans. Wheat and oats also contain some.

Digestion/Absorption/Biosynthesis

The process(es) of digestion/absorption of the fat-soluble vitamins has been assumed to be similar to and contingent upon absorption of lipids. Somewhat more detailed explanations of these processes are available for vitamins A and D than for the others. The extent to which the explanation for vitamin A is generalizeable to the other fat-soluble vitamins is unknown. The same or separate but similar processes may be involved.

The accepted explanation for digestion/absorption of vitamin A is:

(a) When food fat containing any of the forms of vitamin A mixes with bile, it is emulsified. This increases the surface available for penetration by pancreatic lipases.

(b) Vitamin A as retinol or dehydroretinol or the corresponding aldehyde or acid forms is liberated by the lipases and is reemulsified for transport to the mucosal wall where the emulsion is broken immediately prior to absorption. A low fat intake, use of mineral oil which is not absorbed, or use of a drug that binds fats thus precluding absorption— any of these will block this step and reduce vitamin A absorption. Vitamin A is easily oxidized; presence of a reducing agent such as ascorbic acid protects its potency.

(c) Like the various lipid fractions, vitamin A crosses the mucosal wall via the lipid portion of the cell membrane.

(d) Inside the mucosal cell, the various forms of vitamin A are pre-processed differently and are incorporated into the forming chylomicrons. Some of the carotene is split to form retinol. It is then esterified with palmitic acid (retinyl palmitate) for transport. The remainder of the carotene is esterified to the fatty acids. Preformed vitamin A esters are hydrolyzed to retinol and are re-esterified with palmitic acid.

(e) The chylomicra are released into the lymphatic system and then into systemic circulation for translocation to adipose and/or liver cells for use or storage. Vitamin A is stored as retinyl palmitate, stearate, and oleate. These are hydrolyzed to retinol and it is bound to retinol-binding protein for transport.

The processes of absorption for vitamins D, E, and K have not been delineated. However, steps "a" to "c" are believed to be applicable.

These fat-soluble vitamins are also available in aqueous or water-miscible preparations. These vitamins are absorbed more rapidly and efficiently from these water-miscible forms. Fat is not involved in the absorption process. So, greater care in controlling dosage is necessary in order to avoid unwanted effects.

Vitamin D is also synthesized cutaneously, by actinic conversion (utilizing ultraviolet light), from its common endogenous precursor 7-dehydrocholesterol. The amount available from this source is highly variable and probably indeterminate because it depends on climate, level of dust and smoke pollution, level of skin pigmentation, duration and area of skin exposed, and whether or not a topical sunscreen is applied to the skin. For the most part, current lifestyles do not favor actinic conversion. So, a dietary source is now considered necessary for adults as well as children. Once produced, the vitamin D diffuses into the lymphatic system where it is indistinguishable from that obtained exogenously. Via the lymphatic system it is transported to the liver for processing.

A second mechanism also exists for absorption of vitamin K. About 50% of the vitamin K absorbed is produced by colon bacteria for their own use. It is liberated when they die. Bile salts are used to emulsify lipids in the small intestine. These are liberated when the lipids are absorbed, and as they remain in the chyme, they are carried along to the colon where they emulsify the newly liberated vitamin K. They carry the vitamin K across the mucosal wall when they are reabsorbed.

Metabolism of Fat-soluble Vitamins—in General

At the liver, the chylomicrons are removed from circulation and are processed, starting with release of the fats and fat-soluble vitamins. The details of liver cell processing are not clearly understood. Vitamin A esters are hydrolyzed and recombined with a specific protein for transport. During vitamin A processing, some vitamin E is utilized as an oxygen scavenger (it preferentially combines with the oxygen) to prevent unwanted destructive oxidation. In any case, IF the circulating level of any one of the fat-soluble vitamins is low, THEN it is packaged as a low density (LDL), very low density (VLDL), or particularly as a high density (HDL) lipoprotein and is released for translocation to the point of use. IF the circulating level of any one of the fat-soluble vitamins is within normal range, THEN it is converted to a storage form (process unknown) and is stored locally.

Metabolism of Fat-soluble Vitamins—in Specific Organs/Tissues

Although the site for concentrated storage of the fat-soluble vitamins is the liver, storage in low concentration is distributed throughout the adipose cells of the body. In the aggregate, the dispersed storage potential is almost unlimited. Therefore, in adults supply is seldom a problem. Infants and children, however, are vulnerable to supply problems until liver and adipose reserves are developed. Usually, the circulating level is maintained within normal range and cells can withdraw on demand. Utilization of the vitamins by specific organs/tissues will be discussed in turn.

Vitamin A.—Recent research in animals, as yet unconfirmed in humans, suggests that Zn is essential in mobilization of vitamin A from liver stores. Smith *et al.* (1973) have reported the following:

(a) Circulating plasma vitamin A and Zn levels are significantly correlated.

(b) IF a deficient animal is given vitamin A, THEN it will be stored in the liver.

(c) IF an animal deficient in both vitamin A and Zn is given both, THEN liver stores will not develop but the circulating level of vitamin A will rise.

(d) IF an animal deficient in both vitamin A and Zn is given only vitamin A, THEN the circulating vitamin A level will remain low AND IF the vitamin A is discontinued and Zn is given, THEN liver vitamin A stores will decrease and the circulating level of vitamin A will increase.

Clearly, this relationship requires further investigation. The mechanism of Zn involvement in the mobilization of vitamin A is unknown. It may be involved in either the synthesis or function of retinol-binding protein; this is under investigation.

A recent review (Rodriquez and Irwin 1972) concluded that little information about vitamin A requirements at various stages of the life cycle is available. For example, various investigators have deduced infant requirements from their findings. The values are highly variable according to the criteria used. No studies of the needs of adolescents have been reported, and only a few studies of the needs of the elderly have been located.

The review did outline the factors affecting the amount of vitamin A to be ingested. These are:

(a) activity of the compound

(b) amount of dietary protein present

(c) frequency and duration of exercise—need increases with physical activity

(d) exposure to sunlight—conflicting reports on effect

(e) environmental temperature—there are seasonal differences in need according to need for dark adaptability of vision

(f) thyroid activity—there is a positive correlation between the circulating level of vitamin A and the circulating level of thyroxine

(g) infection—the relationship is unclear, but an infection seems to decrease the circulating level

The transmission of the visual impulse, especially in dim light, requires a continuous supply of vitamin A. Retinol is released from retinol-binding protein and is converted to retinaldehyde. Retinaldehyde, in the *cis* form, complexes with opsin to form rhodopsin, in which vitamin A exists as the alcohol retinol in the *trans* form. This *cis-trans* shift results in transmission of the impulse that causes the psycho-physical translation that we call vision. After the impulse has been transmitted, the *trans* form reverts to the *cis* form, but there is a short lag time. IF the supply of *cis* retinaldehyde is adequate, THEN every stimulus will generate an impulse and it will be transmitted.

The nutriment role of vitamin A in epithelial tissues is as a constituent of the mucopolysaccharides and mucoproteins of mucus. Although some details are unclear, when the supply of vitamin A is adequate, mucus-secreting cells are formed at the normal level and secretion of mucus is adequate to protect the tissues. Mucus forms a slick dense physical barrier that protects the tissue from invasion by bacteria. They cannot penetrate. It is in this sense that vitamin A protects against infection.

Vitamin A is necessary for normal development of bones and teeth. It is a necessary constituent of mucopolysaccharides of ground substances. And, it is necessary in the step where cartilage is degraded in preparation for development of the matrix base on which the calcium-phosphate-magnesium apatite salts are deposited. Without the normal base, the shape cannot be controlled.

The adrenal cortex withdraws vitamin A for production of the steroid hormones. Growth and reproduction depend on the circulating level of these hormones. Vitamin A is involved in the synthesis of corticosterone, deoxycorticosterone, and progesterone.

Spermatogenesis requires that retinol be converted to retinaldehyde. Alcohol dehydrogenase, the enzyme involved in this conversion, is the one necessary for metabolism of ethanol. Since ethanol is preferentially metabolized, this conversion is inhibited. Hence, some investigators have proposed that alcoholic impotence results from this interference with vitamin A metabolism.

Vitamin D.—Recent research has revealed that prior to utilization in its nutriment function, vitamin D undergoes a two-step transformation. The first step takes place in liver cells where it is converted to 25-hydroxycholecalciferol (25-HCC), which is its active form. Then, the second step takes place in the kidney where 25-HCC is converted to 1,25-dihydroxycholecalciferol (1,25-DHCC), which is its hormonal form. In these forms it is secreted into systemic circulation for translocation to its sites of use.

The new theoretical explanation offered by DeLuca (1976) for the interaction of vitamin D and calcium and phosphate is as follows:

(a) IF vitamin D is adequate, THEN the l-hydroxylase, i.e., the enzyme that adds OH at position 1, is sensitive to the circulating Ca^{++} and phosphate levels.

(b) IF vitamin D is adequate, AND the circulating Ca^{++} and/or phosphate level is normal, THEN production of 1,25-DHCC (in renal tissues) and 24,25-DHCC (in renal and other tissues) is stimulated.

(c) IF vitamin D is adequate AND dietary Ca^{++} and/or phosphate intake is low AND the circulating level of Ca^{++} and/or phosphate is low, THEN parathyroid hormone is secreted which stimulates production of 1,25-DHCC and suppresses production of 24,25-DHCC.

(d) IF vitamin D is adequate AND dietary intake and the circulating level of Ca^{++} are high, THEN the 1-hydroxylase is inhibited, so production of 1,25-DHCC is suppressed and 24,25-DHCC is produced.

Explanations for the action of vitamin D in controlling Ca^{++} absorption and mineralization of bone have been revised (Fig. 11.1). Partial explanations of the processes can be summarized as follows:

(a) In the intestinal mucosa, vitamin D facilitates absorption in the initial phase before calcium binding protein (CABP) becomes available. And, IF 1,25-DHCC is circulating, THEN additional Ca^{++} will be absorbed because the presence of this hormone induces production of CaBP (Anon. 1978). This protein is involved in the active transport of Ca^{++} and phosphate ions because it makes the mucosal wall permeable to them. Note: parathyroid hormone is not involved in intestinal transport of Ca^{++} and phosphate. Since 24,25-DHCC is inactive, IF it has been formed, THEN Ca^{++} and/or phosphate uptake will be reduced.

(b) In bones, IF 1,25-DHCC is present, THEN the action of the osteolytic cells is increased and resorption occurs. Ca^{++}, inorganic phosphate, etc., are liberated and released into systemic circulation. At the same time, IF 1,25-DHCC is present, THEN the action of the osteoblasts is stimulated. Ca^{++}, phosphate, etc., are deposited. The balance between these two processes allows adjustment of the circulating Ca^{++} and phosphate levels.

Vitamin E.—The nutriment role of vitamin E is as an oxygen scavenger, i.e., it preferentially combines with available oxygen, preventing destructive oxidations. This function has long been known in relation to plant tissue lipids. Recently, it has been observed in animal tissues, e.g., intestinal mucosa, adipose tissue, and skeletal muscle tissue. Vitamin E appears to work in conjunction with the selenium-glutathione (Se-GSH) peroxidase system in performing its role.

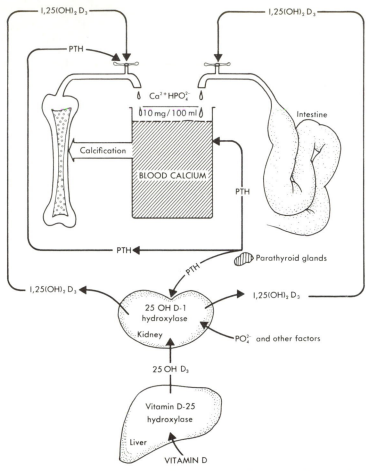

Courtesy of Dr. H.F. DeLuca and Federation Proceedings

FIG. 11.1. HORMONAL LOOP DERIVED FROM VITAMIN D

Diagram shows calcium homeostatic system. In the intestine 1,25–$(OH)_2D_3$ functions without the presence of parathyroid hormone; in bone the presence of parathyroid hormone is essential.

The human requirement for vitamin E largely depends on PUFA intake. A recent study by Lehmann *et al.* (1977) found that the natural vitamin E content of a mixed diet with 25% calories as fat was 0.17 to 1.18 mcg/g PUFA. The natural vitamin E content of a mixed diet with 35% calories as fat was 0.31 to 0.93 mcg/g PUFA. A level of 0.6 mcg/g PUFA is the recommended intake (1974). Using a circulating level of 0.5 mg/100 ml total tocopherol as the difference criterion, the vitamin E intake of those on a 25% fat-calories intake was borderline to deficient for one-third of the subjects; the 35% fat-calories intake was adequate. Sex differences in relationships between circulating levels of vitamin E and lipid fractions also were found. For women, there was a high correlation between total cholesterol level and α-tocopherol level. For men, there was a high correlation between TG level and α-tocopherol level. These sex differences need to be taken into account in assessment of vitamin E nutriture. As a result of these findings, i.e., that the 25% fat-calorie diets provided 12 IU and 15 IU of vitamin E to women and men, respectively, and that the 35% fat-calorie diets provided 21 IU and 26 IU of vitamin E to women and men, respectively, the adequacy of the current RDA of 8 to 10 mg has been questioned.

In the intestinal mucosa, free oxygen is occluded in the foods and has not yet diffused from the food across the mucosal wall to the systemic circulation. As a result, it can oxidize some nutrients, destroying their nutrient activity. Because vitamin E is an oxygen scavenger, it indirectly protects these nutrients. Vitamin A is particularly vulnerable on liberation from food fat esters. All other things being equal, vitamin A absorption is related to effectiveness of vitamin E protection. In the process, vitamin E is used up, so the amount absorbed is reduced.

In adipose cells, the role of vitamin E is similar but the process is more complex, involving stabilization of PUFA. IF a person consumes a diet high in PUFA, THEN stored TG in adipose cells will be partially composed of PUFA. PUFA are not very stable. The unsaturated bonds are easily broken, resulting in the formation of free radicals. We are continually subjected to radiation, which breaks the unsaturated bonds. The free radicals formed are of random size. They are rapidly moving fragments and they bombard the structures of the adipose cells (others as well), damaging them. When damage is great enough, cell function is interfered with to such an extent that cell death ensues. The cumulative and aggregate effect is tissue aging.

Vitamin E, as an oxygen scavenger, protects cell life by combining with available oxygen, making it unavailable for combination with PUFA. This breaks the chain reaction by which the free radicals are formed, and so prevents aging in this sense. THEREFORE, IF a diet high in PUFA is customarily consumed, THEN there is a need for vitamin E.

The role of vitamin E in muscles is to protect the integrity of the stored triglycerides, which are a reserve energy source. Normally, glycogen is stored for immediate energy. IF a person is well-nourished calorically, in addition to adipose tissue stores of lipid, THEN intramuscular deposits of lipids will develop, e.g., the meat of obese animals is well-marbled. IF the diet has been rich in PUFA, THEN the stored triacylglycerols will contain PUFA. Vitamin E protects these fatty acids from radiation-induced free radical formation by the same mechanism operative in adipose cells.

Vitamin K.—The nutriment role of vitamin K in formation of prothrombin for blood clotting involves four vitamin K-dependent factors: factor II (prothrombin), factor VII (proconvertin), factor IX (Christmas factor), and factor X (Stuart-Prower factor). These four factors are involved in the extrinsic (injury-activated) and intrinsic (platelet-activated) coagulation system by which clots are formed. Details of the system are not completely known; two alternate roles for vitamin K have been postulated, i.e., in regulation of the synthesis of these coagulation factors or in conversion of their precursors to active forms. Vitamin K is stored in the liver in at least two forms, one of which is an epoxide. IF the circulating level of prothrombin is low, THEN the following sequence of reactions occurs: the epoxide is activated, vitamin K is released and reduced to its active form, it modifies the four dependent factors which activates them and allows calcium binding of prothrombin to form thrombin, and thrombin interacts with fibrinogen to form fibrin, the base of the blood clot.

THE FAT-SOLUBLE VITAMINS: DEFICIENT SUPPLY

Clinical symptoms have been attributed to deficient intake of and/or block in utilization of vitamins A, D, and K. When the intake of these vitamins increases or when it is provided in its active form, remission of symptoms occurs. From these observations, nutritionists have inferred that intake from exogenous sources is essential. In the case of vitamin E, deficiency in premature infants has been demonstrated but not in adults. Discussion of the effects of deficient supply of each vitamin follows.

Vitamin A

Deficiency is progressive; three levels of severity of deficiency have been characterized.

IF intake is low for a long period of time AND liver stores are depleted, THEN mild clinical symptoms will develop. Vision is affected; nyctalopia or night blindness is the symptom. The accepted explanation for this manifestation is: since *cis* vitamin A aldehyde is not regenerated as rapidly as it is converted to *trans* retinol, it will be in short supply. *Trans* retinol accumulates and is translocated to the liver via systemic circulation. The liver reconverts it to the *cis* retinal form. Since the circulating level of *cis* retinal is low because of continuous withdrawal by the eye, *cis* retinal is released into circulation as rapidly as it is formed. But, since the eye tissue is rapidly metabolizing the *cis* form, its demand exceeds the supply. Because supply takes longer, some impulses are not transmitted, so one is night blind.

IF supply is very short, THEN moderate clinical symptoms develop and epithelial tissue becomes involved in addition to optical symptoms. IF the supply of vitamin A is very short, THEN squamous cells are formed in lieu of mucus cells. As a result, there is no mucus. So, the tissues become dry and hard. Thus, the barrier to bacteria is destroyed and they invade and infect.

IF almost no vitamin A is available, THEN severe clinical symptoms develop. Xerophthalmia progresses to blindness. The lacrimal glands cease production of tears, so the corneal tissue dries up and becomes hard. It then lacks resistance to attack by bacteria, so it becomes infected, When scar tissue develops, blindness results. Follicular hyperkeratosis develops in the skin. The ducts of the sweat glands and hair follicles are destroyed, so the skin is no longer moisturized. It becomes rough, dry, and scaly and covered with petechia, i.e., a roughness that looks like goose flesh. Bone growth also is affected. The cartilage is abnormal and the crystals of apatite are deposited irregularly so bones are misshapen. Bone and joint pain is excruciating.

Vitamin D

Rickets and osteomalacia are the common manifestations; both result because calcium metabolism is impaired. Recent evidence supports the position that rickets may result from the combination of vitamin D deficiency with a preexisting metabolic defect in phosphate transport (Bronner 1976).

In this deficiency state, the 25-HCC is not converted to 1,25-DHCC in response to low circulating levels of Ca^{++} and/or phosphate. IF the vitamin D supply is low, THEN CaBP is not produced in the intestinal mucosa, so both Ca^{++} and phosphate absorption are impaired. THEREFORE, the circulating level of Ca^{++} and phosphate falls AND they are mobilized from bone in order to maintain the circulating level for supply to muscles and nerves. Heart and lung action are critical to survival and take priority over bone mineralization.

Since demand is continuous and supply is low, withdrawal from bones results in progressive demineralization. In the case of a child, the effects are observed sooner and are more severe since growth needs inflate demand. Because the bone tissue cannot mineralize properly, the protein base that should extend is squashed into an irregular shape. Any long bones that are weight-bearing bend to approximate a triangle, the strongest shape. Hence, bow legs develop. In the case of an adult who is tall and heavy, when resorption reaches a critical point, the bones are so weakened that they cannot bear the weight. Spontaneous fractures result. These conditions are painful like arthritis because when the bones bend, they pull muscles, ligaments, etc., in an unnatural way. The stress causes the pain.

Vitamin E

IF vitamin E stores have not been developed in a premature infant via placental transfer, AND IF the child is fed a cow's milk formula, THEN a deficiency syndrome involving capillary fragility (bruising) may develop. IF an adult consumes a diet that is low in vitamin E for 6 years or so, THEN the mean survival time for RBC is reduced from 120^+ days to approximately 110 days, but the time of onset of this manifestation is unknown as it was unlooked for. Otherwise, there is no detectable mental or physical impairment even when the circulating level of vitamin E is reduced to 20% of normal.

Vitamin K

Because of intestinal production, dietary deficiency is rare. Deficiency is more likely to result from administration of too large a dose of dicoumerol, a drug that is structurally similar to vitamin K and acts as its antagonist. It is given to heart patients to decrease the probability of clotting. When too much is given, a medical problem, vitamin K is given to restore clotting time.

THE FAT-SOLUBLE VITAMINS: AVAILABLE IN EXCESS

Some Americans are taking megadoses of vitamins A and/or E, having accepted some of the popular myths that have resulted from misinterpretation of the facts. This is an unfortunate outcome, as the cumulative effect can be development of a toxicity syndrome. The fat-soluble vitamins are highly soluble in triacylglycerols, including those of adipose tissue and intramuscular deposits. Since fat deposits in many people are extensive and increasing, potential uptake is almost unlimited. Fat-soluble vitamin uptake is progressive. IF the circulating level increases, THEN uptake by adipose cells is facilitated. A slight drop in the circulating level then facilitates additional absorption. So, more is dissolved in adipose tissue. Since uptake potential is open-ended, and at some concentration it interferes with cellular functions, toxic side-effects are observed. The minimum toxic dose is unknown as is the cumulative level at which symptoms develop. People are highly variable in the amount of fat stored and, therefore, probably in the amount of excess vitamins that they can tolerate. The effects of toxicity of the fat-soluble vitamins are described below.

Vitamin A and the Carotenes

Not much is known. Acute cases are a public health problem. About 75% of these occur in infants 2 to 8 months of age. A dose of 300,000+ IU will cause symptoms in an adult in 1½ to 36 hours. The main manifestation in children is deformed bones. The syndrome in adults is more severe in women. For women, the symptoms are amenorrhea and consequent sterility, irritability, loss of hair, jaundice, and bone pain. In men, the symptoms are joint pain, thickening of the long bones, baldness, and jaundice. When the circulating level of carotenes is high (carotenemia), the skin of the palms of the hands and soles of the feet turn orange.

Vitamin D

The basic symptoms in children and adults are similar: weakness, lethargy, anorexia, and constipation. Also, the circulating level of calcium is reset to a high level (hypercalcemia, and may persist for months after intake is reduced to zero) so bones soften and soft tissues such as those of the kidney may calcify.

Vitamin E

No effects have been observed and no known excretion mechanism exists. Pharmacologic doses, i.e., 300 to 600 IU/day, lead to tissue saturation; since information is limited, an intake this high is not recommended, pending further information.

Vitamin K

The effects in infants and children differ from those in adults. Since the colon is sterile at birth and placental transfer may not have occurred, infants are routinely given a shot of vitamin K. The margin between too little and too much is narrow. IF an excess is given, THEN jaundice results because when the blood clots there is an increase in breakdown of RBC, resulting in production of the by-product bilirubin (a yellow pigment). In adults, IF an excess is taken, THEN it is excreted.

THE FAT–SOLUBLE VITAMINS: FOOD ECOLOGY AND LIFE EXPECTANCY

Exogenous supply of fat-soluble vitamins can result in toxicity, so warnings have been issued and a movement to limit availability has gained favor. An overdose (O.D.) from food alone, except for polar bear liver which contains toxic amounts of vitamin A, does not occur. Rather, in the case of infants and children, it is a result of a mistake in dose; a teaspoonful rather than a drop is given. In the case of adults, continued therapeutic doses of vitamin A for acne have resulted in toxicity. Some concern has also been raised about consumption of a cup or more of carrot juice per day (a fad utilizing a juicer gimmick) on a continuing basis. Usually, such fads wear out before harm can be done, but the possibility exists that a compulsive person might continue to use the juicer for a much greater than normal length of time.

BIBLIOGRAPHY

ANON. 1978. Vitamin D, calcium-binding protein and the intestinal transport of calcium. Nutr. Rev. *36*, 90-93.

BRONNER, F. 1976. Vitamin D deficiency and rickets. Am. J. Clin. Nutr. *29*, 1307-1314.

DELUCA, H.F. 1976. Metabolism of vitamin D: current status. Am. J. Clin. Nutr. *29*, 1258-1270.

HORWITT, M.K. 1976. Vitamin E: a reexamination. Am. J. Clin. Nutr. *29*, 569-578.

LEHMANN, J., MARSHALL, M.W., SLOVER, H.T., and IACONO, J.M. 1977. Influence of dietary fat level and dietary tocopherol on plasma tocopherols of human subjects. J. Nutr. *107*, 1006-1015.

RODRIQUEZ, M.S., and IRWIN, M.I. 1972. A conspectus of research on vitamin A requirements of man. J. Nutr. *102*, 909-968.

SMITH, J.C., MCDANIAL, E.G., FAN, F.F., and HALSTED, J.A. 1973. Zinc: A trace element essential in vitamin A metabolism. Science *181*, 954-955.

12

The Water–Soluble Vitamins: Ascorbic Acid

Since 1970, there has been much controversy among scientists regarding the need for ascorbic acid and the quantity necessary. The controversy is not resolved. Linus Pauling's book has created a furor, and some Americans have been induced to take pharmacologic doses of ascorbic acid on a regular basis. The position of the "Nutrition Establishment" is that such doses are both unnecessary and undesirable. It could be dangerous and there are many unknowns.

ASCORBIC ACID: NORMALLY AVAILABLE

Food sources of ascorbic acid are citrus fruits (oranges, lemons, limes, grapefruit, etc.), tomatoes which contain only one-third to one-half as much of the vitamin per serving, and strawberries and cantaloupe which are consumed only seasonally. Some tropical fruits are also good sources, but availability in the continental United States is limited. Ascorbic acid is easily destroyed by heat and/or oxidation. Therefore, careful handling is necessary to protect vitamin activity. Sodium ascorbate, the compound added to cereals, is stable. Rose hips is a good source, but the quantity available is limited.

Digestion/Absorption

Ascorbic acid is absorbed from the small intestine. Since no transport mechanism has been identified, absorption is presumably by passive diffusion. Given ingestion of a known quantity of ascorbic acid, the percentage absorbed is variable depending on its use as a reducing agent.

It is carried by the portal blood flow to the liver for use and/or distribution.

Metabolism of Ascorbic Acid—in General

The body pool of ascorbic acid is small and must be resupplied frequently. Since people tend to forget whether they have consumed a rich or a moderately good source the previous day or several days previously, nutritionists recommend a daily intake to be sure. There is no accepted storage site where a major concentration accumulates, although the adrenal cortex does accumulate some. All cells, especially leucocytes, retain a small quantity for local use. The circulating level is low and any excess is excreted. The urinary excretion point is 1.4 mg/100 ml.

The salient nutriment role of ascorbic acid is as the universal reducing agent in biological reactions. Unlike most other vitamins, ascorbic acid has no known coenzyme function. Other nutriment functions have been identified, but the mechanisms by which they are accomplished are delineated only partially. These known functions include roles as:

(a) a cofactor in the conversion of proline to hydroxyproline and lysine to hydroxylysine in collagen formation. This is the basis of involvement in wound healing, bone and tooth formation, and capillary wall strength/fragility.

(b) a cofactor in conversion of phenylalanine to tyrosine

(c) a cofactor in conversion of the B vitamin folic acid to its active form, folinic acid

(d) a cofactor in reduction of Fe^{+++} to Fe^{++} for absorption, for release from transferrin, and for release from ferritin

(e) a cofactor to phosphorylation and deamidation reactions

(f) an agent in response to stress—infection, injury, shock. All of these decrease the stores in the adrenal cortex and depress the circulating level, suggesting either increased need or increased destruction.

ASCORBIC ACID: DEFICIENT SUPPLY OR INFLATED DEMAND

For centuries, man has suffered and died from scurvy, the severe deficiency disease that results from continued lack of ascorbic acid. In this severe form, deficiency is rare among Americans.

The development of deficiency is progressive. Observation of persons with no exogenous source of ascorbic acid has defined the clinical picture. Development of symptoms, though continuous, has been divided into three stages.

In Stage I, symptoms are mild. IF deficient for some weeks, THEN the circulating level falls so response to stress is slow.

In Stage II, moderate symptoms develop. These involve several organs/tissues:

(a) skin—IF deficient 4 to 6 months, THEN the hair follicles become clogged and hairs ingrown, the texture becomes hard and horny (keratosis), and pinpoint bumps like goosebumps appear. As a result, a circulation problem develops, pressure builds up and small hemorrhages occur so that the skin looks like it has been bruised.

(b) gums—IF deficient 6 months, THEN the tissues become swollen, tiny hemorrhages appear, infection sets in, and the teeth become loose due to lack of intercellular cement. The mouth becomes very sore.

(c) CNS—IF deficient for at least 6 months, THEN the adrenal hormones are secreted in excess. The abnormal stimulation causes nerves to fatigue a little sooner, so irritability develops. Personality changes may develop from lack of control in reactions.

(d) any tissue—Rate of wound healing is decreased; surgical patients must be watched. IF supply has been deficient and/or is insufficient to meet the inflated demand, THEN the quantity and quality of intercellular cement is decreased. Both the rate of wound healing and the strength of the scar tissue are reduced. Skin, which should heal in five days, requires ten or more days to heal. Deep tissues show no healing in ten days (normal healing rate allows stitches to be removed in five days). When the tissues do heal, the scar is not strong and wounds will reopen with slight stress.

In Stage III, life is endangered. This is the stage traditionally associated with scurvy. Manifestations are as follows:

(a) heart-lung function is impaired—These are active muscles that need continuous renewal and repair. Since collagen formation is impaired and nerve impulse transmission is abnormal, function is impaired.

(b) bones are deformed and painful—Interference with normal collagen formation results in abnormal deposition of the mineral salts; the matrix is squashed so shape is deformed. In children, the long bones are stunted and buttons develop on the ends of ribs. Moreover, lack of collagen weakens ligaments and tendons, so failure to maintain normal bone alignment leads to pain.

(c) blood—A megaloblastic anemia develops. Iron absorption, transport, and release from storage are impaired, so the quantity of iron available for incorporation in hemoglobin is reduced. Moreover, since folic acid is not activated to folinic acid which is required for synthesis of some amino acids and purines used in DNA and RNA formation, RBC formation is reduced. Together, these two combine to cause the development of the megaloblastic anemia.

ASCORBIC ACID: AVAILABLE IN EXCESS

The general effects of chronic ingestion of a small excess (still at physiologic levels) have long been known and are trivial. IF a person chronically ingests a slight excess or intermittently a larger excess, THEN some is not absorbed, some is absorbed and excreted, and some is absorbed and retained.

The effects of chronic ingestion of pharmacologic doses (1 g or more per day) are different, and may be harmful. IF a megadose is ingested chronically so that a greater-than-normal quantity accumulates, THEN the set-point for the circulating level is reset at a higher level. IF the person reduces intake sharply (it may still be greatly above normal) or when the demand is sharply increased by stress, THEN the body will respond to the relative supply deficit with deficiency symptoms of Stage II or Stage III, depending on the magnitude of the supply deficit. Thus, chronic ingestion of a megadose results in addiction and can result in conditioned deficiency. The body will go through withdrawal symptoms. This state can be very dangerous.

Intermittent use of megadose ingestion of ascorbic acid in treatment of a "cold" may be appropriate; no preventive action has been observed. The explanation for the effect of a pharmacologic dose is incomplete but it appears that IF a megadose is ingested with aspirin at the onset of a "cold," THEN it increases membrane permeability to aspirin, thus increasing its effectiveness in decreasing the fever and in fighting the virus. As a result, there is some alleviation of symptoms. Ascorbic acid does not cure the "cold"; its role is that of a cofactor.

Chronic ingestion of ascorbic acid in megadose quantities is a recent phenomenon, so long-term effects are unknown. Some facts that have begun to emerge have created a cause for concern. Until more is known, megadose consumption is not recommended. The most recent findings are:

(a) hemosiderosis—IF ascorbic acid is chronically ingested in excess, THEN intestinal absorption of iron is augmented and the quantity stored may become excessive, especially in men.

(b) acidosis—A negligible problem because of buffer base reserves.

(c) oxaluria—50% of the quantity of urinary oxalate is normally derived from ingested ascorbic acid. If the person has normal kidney function, kidney stones are unlikely to develop.

(d) hypoglycemia—No relationship has been demonstrated. However, a false positive test results because ascorbate is a reducing agent. The physician should be notified of customary megadose intake so that an alternate lab method of testing is used.

(e) gastrointestinal disturbances—A sensitivity can develop that causes the symptoms of nausea, cramps, and diarrhea. In this case, the ascorbic acid should be taken with or following meals so that it is diluted.

(f) serum cholesterol levels—The circulating level may be elevated and atherosclerosis may be aggravated.

At the present time, the known effects of megadose consumption of ascorbic acid are trivial or rare except for the problems of systemic conditioning, and increasing the serum cholesterol level. However, these effects may be more important than currently recognized so they are under study. Destruction of vitamin B_{12} by ascorbic acid was reported as a hazard of megadose consumption. On further study, however, the point was refuted (Newmark *et al.* 1976) with evidence of a technical problem leading to erroneous findings. Clearly, the effects of megadose consumption of ascorbic acid are not fully understood. In the meantime, a moderate intake is recommended.

ASCORBIC ACID: FOOD ECOLOGY AND LIFE EXPECTANCY

Ascorbic acid intake from exogenous sources is required by man and a few other species that lack one of the enzymes necessary for its synthesis. Dietary surveys have repeatedly shown that ascorbic acid intake of Americans is highly variable; some take too little and some take too much and many are erratic in intake.

Although some dietary changes were evident, until the mid-1960s potatoes and cabbage were still major sources. Potatoes, though only half as rich a source as orange juice, were consumed daily by many Americans; more than two servings per day was not uncommon. Cabbage, which is approximately equal to orange juice in its ascorbic acid content, was consumed several times a week.

Consumption trend lines for potatoes and cabbage have shown a downturn for some years, so other foods have become major sources of ascorbic acid. Availability of and consumption of citrus fruits, especially oranges and grapefruit, have increased. In addition, fruit drinks have been fortified. Even more recently, ready-to-eat breakfast cereals have been fortified to provide about one-fourth of the amount needed.

Since the mid-1960s, questions of the comparative stability of natural and added synthetic ascorbic acid in fruit drinks and other foods have been investigated and partially resolved. Findings are:

(a) In order to make a label claim that fruit drinks contain 25 to 30 mg/serving, the quantity added by manufacturers must exceed this amount.

(b) Stability of synthetic ascorbic acid in fruit drinks is a function of pH and time; in acid fruit drinks it is stable for several days after opening.

(c) The bioavailability of synthetic ascorbic acid is slightly greater than that of natural ascorbic acid in orange juice.

Timing of ascorbic acid intake in relation to intake of iron, and perhaps other nutrients, is a critical variable related to its effectiveness as a reducing agent. In this regard, research has demonstrated that there is no carryover effect. Therefore, to potentiate iron uptake, both ascorbic acid and iron must be present in the chyme simultaneously. Therefore, IF this beneficial effect in potentiating iron uptake is desired, THEN food and/or supplement intake must be distributed among feedings or consciously paired with ingestion of sources of iron.

BIBLIOGRAPHY

BARNESS, L.A. 1975. Safety considerations with high ascorbic acid dosage. *In* Second Conference on Vitamin C. C.G. King and J.J. Burns (Editors). Ann. N.Y. Acad. Sci. *258*.

FOX, M.R.S. 1975. Protective effects of ascorbic acid against toxicity of heavy metals. *In* Second Conference on Vitamin C. C.G. King and J.J. Burns (Editors). Ann. N.Y. Acad. Sci. *258*.

GINTER, E. 1975. Ascorbic acid in cholesterol and bile acid metabolism. *In* Second Conference on Vitamin C. C.G. King and J.J. Burns (Editors). Ann. N.Y. Acad. Sci. *258*.

HARPER, A.E. 1975. The recommended dietary allowances for ascorbic acid. *In* Second Conference on Vitamin C. C.G. King and J.J. Burns (Editors). Ann. N.Y. Acad. Sci. *258*.

LEWIS, T.L. *et al.* 1975. A controlled clinical trial of ascorbic acid for the common cold. *In* Second Conference on Vitamin C. C.G. King and J.J. Burns (Editors). Ann. N.Y. Acad. Sci. *258*.

NEWMARK, H.L., SCHEINER, J., MARCUS, M., and PRABHUDESAI, M. 1976. Stability of vitamin B_{12} in the presence of ascorbic acid. Am. J. Clin. Nutr. *29*, 645-649.

SAUBERLICH, H.E. 1975. Vitamin C status: methods and findings. *In* Second Conference on Vitamin C. C.G. King and J.J. Burns (Editors). Ann. N.Y. Acad. Sci. *258*.

SCOTT, M.L. 1975. Environmental influences on ascorbic acid requirements in animals. *In* Second Conference on Vitamin C. C.G. King and J.J. Burns (Editors). Ann. N.Y. Acad. Sci. *258*.

STREET, J.C., and CHADWICK, R.W. 1975. Ascorbic acid requirements and metabolism is relation to organochlorine pesticides. *In* Second Conference on Vitamin C. C.G. King and J.J. Burns (Editors). Ann. N.Y. Acad. Sci. *258*.

SULKIN, N.M., and SULKIN, D.F. 1975. Tissue changes induced by marginal vitamin C deficiency. *In* Second Conference on Vitamin C. C.G. King and J.J. Burns (Editors). Ann. N.Y. Acad. Sci. *258*.

WILSON, C.W.M. 1975A. Ascorbic acid function and metabolism during colds. *In* Second Conference on Vitamin C. C.G. King and J.J. Burns (Editors). Ann. N.Y. Acad. Sci. *258*.

WILSON, C.W.M. 1975B. Clinical pharmacological aspects of ascorbic acid. *In* Second Conference on Vitamin C. C.G. King and J.J. Burns (Editors). Ann. N.Y. Acad. Sci. *258*.

YEW, M.L.S. 1975. Biological variation in ascorbic acid needs. *In* Second Conference on Vitamin C. C.G. King and J.J. Burns (Editors). Ann. N.Y. Acad. Sci. *258*.

13

The Water–Soluble Vitamins: The B Complex

Thiamin, riboflavin, niacin, B_6 (pyridoxine), pantothenic acid, folic acid, biotin, and B_{12} are the B vitamins. The essentiality of consumption of an exogenous source of these vitamins was demonstrated years ago. Nonetheless, according to the 1976 Report of the President's Biomedical Research Panel,

Large areas of ignorance exist concerning: (1) the interplay between nutrients; (2) the effects of vitamin undersupply or oversupply on the development and treatment of acute or subacute disease conditions; (3) the extent of variability in vitamin requirements (or vitamin toxicity at high levels) in different members of the population; and (4) the interrelationships of vitamins and drugs. . . Almost nothing is known about (1) the comparative rate of turnover of individual vitamin-dependent enzymes in intact organisms; (2) the relative rates of turnover of apoenzymes and their coenzymes; (3) the rates of coenzyme loss from individual enzymes during states of vitamin deficiency; (4) the efficiency of salvage pathways for individual vitamins; (5) the metabolic control devices that operate at high levels of vitamin feeding; (6) the schemes for metabolic degradation of vitamins in animals and man; and (7) the rates at which degradation or excretion occur at different levels of vitamin intake. Such studies are essential if the relationship of deficiency disease to vitamin level is to be understood.

From the above, it is clear that there are many unknowns. It is for this reason that nutritionists recommend moderate intakes.

THE WATER–SOLUBLE B VITAMINS: NORMALLY AVAILABLE

The B vitamins can be supplied from the plant and/or animal tissues consumed as food. But, a variety of foods is necessary since no one food is a concentrated source of any and may not be a good source of another,

198

e.g., pork is a good source of thiamin and milk is a good source of riboflavin. Whole grain breads and cereals are generally good sources, as are their enriched white flour versions (except for folic acid which was unknown at the time the enrichment legislation was enacted).

The supply of vitamin B_{12} is an exception. Omnivores and carnivores usually ingest a sufficient quantity of B_{12} to meet their metabolic needs. Vegetarians may not. This is because vitamin B_{12} is synthesized by bacteria and fungi but not by yeasts, plants, animals, or man. Grains, fruits, and vegetables may contain trace amounts absorbed from the soil. Since B_{12} is stored in glandular and muscle tissues, good sources are muscle meats, liver, fish and shellfish, eggs, and dairy products. Some of these sources may be proscribed, so the amount available to the vegetarian is limited. A concentrated source from bacterial production is a commercially available alternative.

Digestion/Absorption

With the exception of vitamin B_{12}, absorption of these vitamins takes place in the upper end of the small intestine. In general, they are destroyed by alkaline medium, so absorption must take place prior to infusion of the pancreatic fluids. Proteases liberate the vitamins from their protein bases. Some are then phosphorylated for rapid transport through the mucosal wall.

Vitamin B_{12} is absorbed in the ileum, after a long and complex sequence of steps. HCl in gastric juice splits B_{12} from its animal protein matrix. Then, the free B_{12} combines with intrinsic factor (IF) for transport along the alimentary canal to the ileum. In the ileum, it is liberated from IF and combines with calcium for transport across the mucosal wall. Within the ileal cells, it is converted to its coenzyme form 5'-deoxyadenosylcobalamin. Then it enters portal blood for transport to the liver and attaches to its transport protein Transcobalamin II, which also facilitates its uptake by cells of target tissues such as the liver and bone marrow.

New information on the processes of digestion and absorption of folic acid indicates some unique factors that affect bioavailability of this vitamin. Folic acid is pteroylglutamic acid (PGA), but it is not found in foods and is not biologically active in this form. In foods, it occurs as one of the polyglutamates. These are related to PGA by:

(a) containing additional glutamic acid residues

(b) being reduced by the addition of H^+ at positions 5, 6, 7, and 8, i.e., they are tetrahydrofolates

(c) having single carbon substituents at positions 5 or 10, e.g., methylfolates, formylfolates

The most common food form is 5-methyl tetrahydrofolate. In order to be absorbed, these pteroylpolyglutamates must be hydrolyzed to pteroylmonoglutamate. The enzyme γ-glutamyl hydrolase, also known as folate conjugase, catalyzes this reaction. Apparently, according to Reisenauer, Krumdieck, and Halsted (1977), conjugase activity occurs at two points. Membrane-bound conjugase in the brush border of the jejunum probably partially hydrolyzes the polyglutamates to the monoglutamate form so that it can enter the mucosal cell. An additional soluble conjugase inside the mucosal cell may complete the task. Beyond this, the sequence of steps in folate absorption and membrane transport is unclear.

The liver is the storage site for B vitamins. The quantity stored, with the exception of B_{12}, is only sufficient for two to three months. Therefore, consumption of an exogenous source must be frequent. Here again, to circumvent the memory problem of the timing and quantity of the previous dose, nutritionists recommend a daily intake. Vitamin B_{12} is stored in micro-quantities in the liver, kidneys, heart, muscles, pancreas, testes, brain, blood, spleen, and bone marrow. The liver alone can store 2,000 to 5,000 mcg, a 3- to 5-year supply.

Water–Soluble B Vitamin Metabolism—in General

The most frequent nutriment function of B vitamins is as a constituent of a coenzyme. In many series of reactions, the exact step where a specific vitamin-activated coenzyme is required as a cofactor for a specific enzyme has been identified. There may be additional steps that are presently unknown. Known nutriment functions for each of the B vitamins are listed below:

Thiamin.—As thiamin pyrophosphate (TPP), also called cocarboxylase, which is one of its metabolically active forms, it is involved as a coenzyme in reactions involving oxidative decarboxylation in carbohydrate metabolism, e.g., conversion of pyruvic acid to active acetate and carbon dioxide, which initiates the reactions of the Krebs cycle. As thiamin diphosphate (TDP), which is the other metabolically active form of thiamin, it is involved in the transketolation step in which glucose is converted to active glyceraldehyde as the first step in transformation of carbohydrate to fat.

Riboflavin.—As flavin mononucleotide (FMN, a riboflavin monophosphate compound), it is involved as a coenzyme in deamination of amino acids. As the coenzyme flavin adenine dinucleotide (FAD, a riboflavin diphosphate compound), it is involved as a cofactor in numerous reactions of amino acid, fatty acid, and glucose metabolism. It also is involved in the systems of H^+ transfer in cellular oxidation.

In this role riboflavin is a constituent of one of the metalloflavoprotein enzymes. These contain molybdenum and/or iron. The function of the flavin moiety is to accept or donate an electron in the oxidation-reduction process. Important enzymes of this type are the *ferredoxins* in which Fe is bonded to the S of cysteine, forming an iron-sulfur bridge as a part of the enzyme structure. In the oxidized form, both iron atoms are in the Fe^{+++} form. In the reduced form, one is Fe^{++} and the other is Fe^{+++}.

Niacin (Nicotinic Acid).—Its coenzyme form is a cofactor with thiamin and/or riboflavin in the anaerobic oxidation via the "respiratory chain" of reactions by which amino acids and fatty acids are oxidized as well as in several reactions in the Krebs cycle that transform glucose to energy, carbon dioxide, and water. For example, nicotinamide adenine dinucleotide (NAD, a niacin diphosphate compound) is involved with TPP in the Krebs cycle initiating step of conversion of pyruvic acid to active acetate. Nicotinamide adenine dinucleotide phosphate (NADP, a niacin triphosphate compound), as well as NAD, is involved in the Krebs cycle with FMN and FAD.

NADPH is produced primarily by the pentose phosphate pathway. The major function of this pathway is to produce NADPH, which must be supplied in sufficient quantities to meet demands for it as a reductant in numerous biosynthetic reactions involving NAD. These include, but may not be limited to:

(a) formation of long-chain fatty acids and steroids
(b) conversion of glucose to sorbitol
(c) conversion of dihydrofolic acid to tetrahydrofolic acid
(d) conversion of glucuronic acid to L-gulonic acid
(e) conversion of pyruvic acid to malic acid
(f) hydroxylation in forming PUFA and in the conversion of phenylalanine to tyrosine.

The utilization of NAD in these reactions does not require ATP or metabolites of the Krebs cycle so it provides an alternative. It may be regulated by need for NADPH.

Niacin is a nutrient because an exogenous source is necessary. However, unlike many other nutrients, its supply needs are partially met by an endogenous source. Tryptophan, an amino acid, is a precursor of niacin. Therefore, in assessment of niacin nutriture, the concept of niacin equivalents is used. This means that the expected amount of niacin available from endogenous sources should be added to that from exogenous (dietary and/or supplements) sources. Research has demonstrated that the mean tryptophan content of animal protein is 1.4% and of vegetable protein is 1%. For convenience, 1% is used in computing the quantity of niacin that may be produced by endogenous conversion. The mean quantity of niacin produced by the conversion is 1 mg/60 mg tryptophan ingested. A sample calculation follows:

(a) IF the protein intake is 125 g, the mean American intake, THEN 1250 mg tryptophan will be involved (125 g protein × 0.01 = 1.25 g or 1250 mg tryptophan).

(b) Since 1 mg niacin is produced/60 mg tryptophan, 21 mg niacin will be produced (1250 ÷ 60 = 21).

Pyridoxine (B$_6$).— This is the group designation for the three known forms, i.e., pyridoxine, pyridoxal, and pyridoxamine. In its active form of pyridoxal phosphate (PLP), its nutriment function is as a coenzyme in many reactions of protein, fat, and carbohydrate metabolism.

B_6 as a coenzyme in protein metabolism is involved in numerous types of reactions that include, but are not limited to:

(a) decarboxylation of amino acids, e.g., the conversion of tryptophan to serotonin which is a vasoconstrictor

(b) deamination, e.g., of serine and threonine

(c) transamination of the various amino acids to form nonessential amino acids or other non-protein nitrogen compounds

(d) transsulfuration, e.g., from methionine to serine

(e) conversion of tryptophan to niacin

(f) incorporation of glycine in heme

(g) active transport of amino acids across the mucosal wall and into cells

(h) biosynthesis of cysteine

B_6 has an indirect role in CHO metabolism because the end-products of the transformations listed above are finally degraded through the Krebs cycle. The role of PLP in fatty acid metabolism is related to its function in the conversion of linoleic acid to arachidonic acid.

B_6 exists in foods in the bound form. In some foods it is bound to proteins, but in others it is bound to an undefined substance (Nelson, Burgin, and Cerda 1977). Cooking has been demonstrated to enhance bioavailability. Otherwise, it is more available in the synthetic than in the natural food form.

Pantothenic Acid.—Its most widely recognized nutriment function is as a constituent of coenzyme A, which is converted to active acetate. This vitamin coenzyme role in acetylation reactions includes, but is not limited to, the following:

(a) Active acetate derived from amino acid, CHO and/or fatty acid metabolism combines with oxaloacetate derived from amino acid or CHO metabolism as the first reaction in the Krebs cycle.

(b) Active acetate activates fatty acids, which then form either TG or keto acids to be degraded via the Krebs cycle.

(c) Active acetate combines with amino acids, activating them, which enables their entry into the series of reactions that produce TG or glucose.

(d) Active acetate is one of the basic units from which cholesterol is synthesized; all of its carbon atoms are supplied by active acetate. In turn, cholesterol is a precursor of the steroid hormones.

(e) Active acetate is a precursor of active succinic acid, succinyl CoA, which combines with glycine in the initial reaction by which heme is synthesized.

A less widely recognized nutriment function of pantothenic acid is as a constituent of fatty acid synthetase (ACP). This enzyme is necessary in fatty acid synthesis after the initial step in which active acetate condenses with malonyl CoA to form a short-chain fatty acid. ACP combines with the short-chain fatty acid, which activates it and enables it to continue elongation by stepwise condensation with malonyl CoA. Whether pantothenic acid is a constituent of other enzymes or has unidentified nutriment functions is unknown.

Folic Acid or Folacin.— It is reduced to its active form, folinic acid, as the first step in preparation for subsequent interactions. The nutriment function of folinic acid relates primarily to its role in 1-carbon transfer in the synthesis of thymine, which is a pyrimidine base, and purines, both of which are constituents of DNA. Cell growth and reproduction are thus folic acid dependent; this is especially noticeable in relation to RBC formation. THFA also is involved in the conversions of glycine to serine and of phenylalanine to tyrosine. Methyl THFA provides the methyl group for synthesis of methionine, choline, and neurotransmitters such as serotonin. THFA also is involved in hydroxylation of proline, a step in collagen formation.

Para-aminobenzoic acid (PABA) is not a nutrient in human nutrition, although it is essential for some microorganisms. It is only a necessary constituent of folic acid.

Biotin.—Its major nutriment function is as a coenzyme in carboxylation reactions, in which carbon dioxide is transferred from one compound to another. For example, it is necessary in the reaction by which the chain length of fatty acids is increased, and in the reaction of pyruvic acid and oxaloacetic acid in the Krebs cycle, and two other reactions in the Krebs cycle. Its other functions are related to synthesis of purines and in activation of deaminases for threonine, serine, and aspartic acids—by which these are converted to keto acids.

B$_{12}$ (Cobalamin).—The cobalamide coenzymes are necessary for methyl group transfers in numerous reactions in amino acid, glucose, and fatty acid metabolism. B$_{12}$ is a coenzyme in the transfer of three methyl groups from methionine to serine in the synthesis of choline, which is a component of lecithin and the sphingomyelins. It is also necessary, in conjunction with ascorbic acid, for the conversion of folic acid to THFA, hence its roles in DNA synthesis and RBC formation.

Water–Soluble B Vitamin Metabolism—in Specific Tissues

The B vitamins are active primarily as cofactors in common metabolic reactions that occur in all cells. From the available evidence, there is no indication that particular tissues have specific needs.

THE WATER–SOLUBLE B VITAMINS: DEFICIENT SUPPLY OR INFLATED DEMAND

Although the exact steps where the various vitamins are required are known and well defined deficiency syndromes have been identified with classic cases of gross deficiency, a generalized deficiency syndrome is more typical. Usually, protein, calcium, and vitamins A and C are also deficient when intake of the B vitamins is deficient. The observed GI, CNS, and cardiovascular symptoms are a direct effect of decreased glucose supply and are only indirectly related to lack of the B vitamins. The effects of deficiency of each of the B vitamins are summarized below.

Thiamin

The classic syndrome beri-beri is characterized by polyneuritis, muscular weakness, and GI disturbance. The polyneuritis reflects a decreased supply of glucose, which is the predominant fuel of CNS tissue. When insufficient, motor control is impaired, alertness and reflex responses are decreased, and general symptoms of lethargy and lassitude are observed. Symptoms are progressive through nerve irritation to paralysis. Muscle weakness of heart and vascular tissue leads to edema and cardiac failure. GI distress is due to decreased mucosal supply of glucose which precludes normal function of the musculature, secretory glands, and absorption mechanisms. The results are anorexia, decreased HCl secretion, and constipation.

Riboflavin

The classic syndrome is a result of epithelial tissue inflammation and breakdown. It is characterized by the following symptoms: cheilosis, i.e., cracking and dry scaliness of the lips and corners of the mouth; cracks at the angles of the nose; glossitis, i.e., the tongue is swollen and typically red; corneal vascularization accompanied by burning and itching; and seborrheic dermatitis, i.e., a scaly, greasy skin eruption. The links between lack at the biochemical level and clinical manifestations are unknown.

Niacin

The classic syndrome pellagra is characterized by dermatitis in areas exposed to sunlight—the reddish rash later turns dark and the skin is very rough; diarrhea; dementia—irritability, anxiety, depression, confusion or delerium, etc.; and finally, death. Here again, the links between lack at the biochemical level and clinical manifestations are unknown.

B_6

The deficiency is associated with development of a hypochromic, microcytic anemia and/or by CNS disturbances as a result of impairment of the conversions resulting in the formation of γ-aminobutyric acid and serotonin, compounds important in the regulation of brain activity.

A majority of women using oral contraceptive agents (OCA) develop functional biochemical manifestations that suggest B_6 deficiency. This is a relative deficiency induced by inflated demand. Mean serum levels of PLP are significantly lower when OCA are first used, but in some women serum levels rise toward normal by the sixth month of use. An increased exogenous supply of B_6 is necessary in order for some to achieve normal circulating levels.

Pantothenic Acid.—This is unknown under natural conditions.

Folic Acid.—The macrocytic anemia of pregnancy and the megaloblastic anemia in premature infants have been attributed to folic acid deficiency. During the third trimester of pregnancy, the circulating levels of hemoglobin and folic acid fall below the normal standard for nonpregnant women. The prevalence of macrocytic anemia is small, and has been estimated as less than 2% of pregnant women. Apparently, despite the relative deficiency induced by the inflated demand to supply situation, there is enough to enable substantial nucleic acid synthesis for production of placental as well as fetal tissues. Among those whose customary folic acid intake is marginal, some will be deficient and the macrocytic anemia may be manifest. Infants born to these mothers present a megaloblastic anemia, i.e., the RBC are large and immature.

Folic acid deficiency is a deliberate iatrogenic deficiency that is intermittently induced in leukemia patients by the drug aminopterin, used to cause remission of the disease. It is a folic acid antagonist, i.e., it blocks nucleic acid synthesis and, hence, the rapid proliferation of leukemic cells. When remission occurs, the deficiency and the resultant anemia are corrected. This induced deficiency is greater in severity than that resulting from simple dietary lack. Glossitis, diarrhea, weight loss, decreased RBC levels, and urinary excretion of the metabolite FIGLU are manifest.

Biotin.—A deficiency syndrome has been produced in man, but it is not known to occur naturally. Avidin, a glycoprotein in egg white, combines with biotin in the intestine, preventing its absorption. To cause a deficiency, abnormally large quantities of raw eggwhite must be consumed—an unlikely event. So this effect is of theoretical interest only.

B_{12}.—The deficiency disease is pernicious anemia. The classic cause of this disease is the result of a rare metabolic disorder which causes a lack of intrinsic factor (IF); malabsorption results. Symptoms are severe. A more common, although infrequently observed, cause is inadequate dietary intake. Mild nervous symptoms but not anemia are seen.

In severe form, pernicious anemia is a highly injurious, destructive, and potentially deadly disease in which the lack of vitamin B_{12} undermines health by:

(a) creating a severe macrocytic hypochromic anemia which is marked by a progressive decrease in the number and increase in size of RBC, which results in physical symptoms of pallor and weakness.

(b) causing achlorhydria, which results in decreased efficiency of digestion and/or malabsorption of proteins and amino acids, B vitamins, Ca, PO_4, etc., and in generalized GI disturbances as a secondary effect.

(c) nervous disturbances that result in a typical gait.

This disease develops gradually by corrupting and undermining tissue processes. It is well established before it becomes apparent.

The accepted explanation for the macrocytic hypochromic anemia is that lack of cobalamides has an indirect effect which is produced by blocking the conversion of folic acid to folinic acid. This, in turn, prevents synthesis of the pyrimidines and purines that are constituents of DNA. Lack of DNA results in incomplete RBC division, so macrocytes develop. Lack of folinic acid also blocks heme formation, so the cells are hypochromic. Insufficient hemoglobin impairs oxygen transport, hence the typical symptoms of anemia. See Chapter 10.

The neurologic damage results from impaired formyl and methyl group transfer and consequent blocking of choline synthesis. Choline is a necessary constituent of acetylcholine, which is involved in nerve impulse transmission at the synapse, and of sphingomyelin, which is a nerve insulator. Hence, the impairment. Also, an observed, but not clearly understood effect is increased circulating levels of branched chain fatty acids such as methyl malonic acid and odd-numbered fatty acids.

Treatment of pernicious anemia depends on its cause. When lack of IF is the cause, B_{12} injections are necessary on a monthly basis. When dietary lack results from nonconsumption of animal products, then use of a commercially available bacterial production concentrate is recommended. One should note that the anemia can be corrected by administration of folinic acid, but it does not correct the more serious neurologic damage that is directly related to the B_{12} deficiency.

THE WATER-SOLUBLE B VITAMINS: EXCESS SUPPLY

Little is known about the effects of chronic excess supply of the B vitamins. An excess from dietary sources is unknown. With the exception of niacin, which is used medicinally, toxicity from megadoses is unknown.

The requirements for the various B vitamins are not accurately known in relation to nutriment function because quantitative analysis *in vivo* is impossible. Some, and perhaps most or all of the steps in various pathways where one or more of the B vitamins is necessary, have been identified. However, the information is qualitative rather than quantitative. That is, the quantity used up is unknown as are the number of reactions per cell per day and the number of cells in which the function is performed. Therefore, the value obtained from studies at low intake is only an approximation of the cumulative and aggregate quantity necessary. Such studies determine the intake level associated with development of clinical manifestations and the quantity per day that is necessary to relieve the symptoms. The quantity designated as excess is an arbitrary value. It is the quantity that spills into the urine.

Load dose studies have yielded some additional information which shows that the renal threshold for the various water-soluble vitamins is low. The accepted assumptions and inferences that are associated with load dose testing are:

(a) assumption—Plasma uptake will continue to its maximum. Withdrawal or redistribution to tissues is minimal since storage capacity is small.

(b) assumption—IF intake is increased greatly with a load dose, THEN one can obtain an indirect measure of uptake by computing the percentage of the dose that is excreted.

(c) inference—IF a person has had an adequate intake, THEN the percentage of the load dose that is excreted will be high or close to 100%.

(d) inference—IF the previous intake has been marginal to low, THEN the percentage retained will be high and the percentage excreted will be low.

(e) inference—Since kidney excretion occurs when even a small dose is ingested, there is no value in ingesting a greater quantity.

At the present time, the reason for kidney excretion is unknown. Two plausible, but unverified, explanations are that the kidney lacks the capacity to reabsorb these vitamins and that the circulating set-point is low, and the kidney is programmed to exclude any excess above the set-point. Undoubtedly, the fact that the urinary excretion point is low has been a factor in preventing development of a recognizable toxicity syndrome.

Niacin is used therapeutically in treatment of a number of medical conditions. The standard dose administered is 100 mg, which is approximately 10 times the RDA. Toxicity can be produced with doses 1000 times the standard dose.

Side-effects are common when even the standard therapeutic dose is ingested. Observation has led to the following conclusions:

(a) IF a therapeutic dose of 50 to 100 mg is given on an empty stomach, THEN a temporary speed-up of energy metabolism occurs which results in vasodilation accompanied by flushing of the ears, face, and neck.

(b) IF a greater dose is given, THEN the whole body may flush and the individual may experience burning, tingling, and/or itching sensations. These symptoms may last a few minutes or may persist an hour or longer. Body temperature also may rise and fever effects may result. Since enzymes can be inactivated at high temperatures, medical supervision is required in order to prevent extensive damage. A large dose also results in an increase in free and total HCl in gastric juice. Therefore, symptoms of nausea, vomiting, and diarrhea may result.

THE WATER–SOLUBLE B VITAMINS: FOOD ECOLOGY AND LIFE EXPECTANCY

Although unable to identify the names of the vitamins in the B-complex, the general public has accepted the need for supply. To many people this means the need to take vitamin pills every morning.

Discovery of most of the B vitamins resulted from studies of people with gross deficiencies created by consumption of an almost single-food refined cereal diet. Dietary surveys in the 1930s and 1940s revealed a marginal to low intake in many segments of the American population. As a result, legislation for enrichment of cereals and flour was enacted in the

1940s. Since then, until recently, there have been few cases of deficiency of any of the B vitamins.

Since the nutriment function of several of the B vitamins is as cofactors for various reactions in the Krebs cycle in the production of energy, the demand is linked to carbohydrate intake/metabolism. At the present time, some Americans are consuming quantities of unenriched flour-based junk foods and others eat no bread but sizeable quantities of simple sugars. Both groups may show symptoms of relative B vitamin deficiency. Others, with different food preferences, eat ready-to-eat cereals which are fortified with B vitamins and other nutrients; their intakes may be adequate to abundant. Since intakes have changed, the first step is to expand people's consciousness of this fact and its expected nutritional effects.

At the present time, life expectancy is not threatened by deficiency or excess intake of any of the B vitamins. However, quality of life may be suboptimal due to lethargy or lassitude or annoying skin conditions associated with chronic marginal intakes.

Vitamin pills are available over-the-counter (OTC) as an alternative to dietary intake. Careful label reading is required to determine whether all of the B vitamins are included in meaningful quantities. Moreover, a number of substances with vitamin or partial vitamin function, but not demonstrated to be essential from exogenous sources, may be included as a profit-making feature. These harmless, but unnecessary substances include, but are not limited to:

(a) lipoic acid—This is a sulfur-containing fatty acid with a coenzyme function in the initial decarboxylation step where pyruvate is reduced to active acetate on entry to the Krebs cycle.

(b) PABA—This is a fragment of folic acid, discussed above.

(c) inositol—It has no known role in human nutrition.

(d) choline—It is a lipotropic agent in the liver, i.e., it is involved in changing fat from its storage form to its transport form, which involves conversion from fatty acids to lipoproteins. The necessity of ingestion of an exogenous source has not been established, so it is not considered to be a nutrient in human nutrition.

(e) bioflavonoids, e.g., citrin and rutin—These have no known function in human nutrition.

The recently revised booklet listing Diabetic Exchanges includes a statement with respect to vegetable sources of folic acid. However, there is no implication that diabetics' need is any different from that of non-diabetics.

For the first time, the 1980 RDA for niacin is listed in niacin equivalents. Tables of food composition list preformed niacin. To determine the quantity of niacin equivalents, the amount available by conversion is computed and is added to the sum of the preformed values obtained from the food composition tables. Then, valid inferences about intake can be drawn.

BIBLIOGRAPHY

ANON. 1975. Report of the President's Biomedical Research Panel. DHEW Publ. (05)76-501. GPO, Washington, D.C.

NELSON, E.W., BURGIN, C.W., and CERDA, J.J. 1977. Characterization of food binding of vitamin B_6 in orange juice. J. Nutr. *107*, 2128-2134.

REISENAUER, A.M., KRUMDIECK, C.L., and HALSTED, C.H. 1977. Folate conjugase: two separate activities in human jejunum. Science *198* (4313) 196-197.

14

Food and People

Human food ecology and life expectancy—how are they related? Is longevity identical to life expectancy? Is there some subset of the contemporary array of food and people interactions that creates/maintains nutritional vulnerability? What is the relationship between an intake of nutrient X that is too low or high and life expectancy? What are the expected effects in terms of short-term and long-term quality of life? These are some of the relevant questions. They are eternally at issue and require a personal and continuing assessment and solution.

HUMAN FOOD ECOLOGY

The food environment of an American involves food and people interactions at three levels: (a) personal, (b) domestic, and (c) international. An observation at any given point in time can be evaluated to provide an index to the quality of the interactions at that time and implications for life expectancy. A dynamic interaction exists among the various factors operative at these three levels. Thus, the pattern of man's relation to his food environment, i.e., human food ecology, is complex and subject to continuous change.

Personal Component

A life-long series of problems associated with food and people interactions presents a continuing challenge and opportunity for growth/development to all personally responsible adults. Some problems are related to governing food intake and others to modification of food and people interactions for other purposes. Some problems are small and are a trivial challenge. Others are large and may test one's limit of adaptability. Success or failure in adaptation appears to derive from one's basic disposition rather than from one's motives, all other things being equal.

Initially, a motive, i.e., the need or desire, that operates on a person's will, causing an action to change food intake and/or other aspects of food and people interactions, is frequently supplied by a nutrition counselor or physician. But, to be effective, the individual must identify with the motive and internalize it as an integral part of his/her will. That is, the individual's mental powers must be manifested as wishing, choosing, desiring, and intending to act in a way that is controlled, directed, and/or strongly influenced by the motive. When the motive has been internalized, one becomes motivated to change pertinent aspects of food intake and/or food and people interactions.

Implementation involves thinking in four categories of thought with respect to the problem. These categories (Mahoney and Caggiula 1978) are:

(a) personal ability to deal with problems associated with food intake or customary food and people interactions

(b) personal goals to be achieved by problem-oriented modification of food intake and/or food and people interactions

(c) customary and/or preferred methods used in problem-oriented modification of food intake and/or food and people interactions

(d) nature and adequacy of progress

One's basic disposition may support (or undermine) one's will, which works for (or against) goal attainment. It conditions the nature and extent of one's thinking in each of the four thought categories and the tone of one's transactions in food and people interactions.

Disposition is the dominant quality, i.e., nature and distinguishing attribute, of customary moods and attitudes toward life and the normal transactions that are a part of living. Disposition is represented as a continuous variable with infinite gradations along a bi-polar continuum from positive to negative. It varies among people and for an individual over time according to the quality of experiences. Even so, a discrete point is used to characterize its quality at a particular place in time for the purposes of distinguishing differences in disposition among people. Thus, some are described as optimists and others as pessimists. These orientations result in very different thought and response patterns. Both are discussed below in some detail so that implications and ramifications in nutrition counseling will become clear.

Optimism is defined as an inclination to put the most favorable construction upon actions or happenings or to anticipate the best possible outcome. This sets up what has been called a "self-fulfilling prophecy." An optimistic orientation causes a person to approach situations/challenges with a hopeful, cheerful, encouraging, enthusiastic, confident, and assured manner. Thus, even when an action or happening is less positive than expected, the construction is facilitating toward acceptance or solution. The individual construes, i.e., understands or explains the sense or intention of the action or happening, in a positive way or with respect to having done the best possible, given the circumstances. The construction, i.e., the acts or results that follow from construing, interpreting, or explaining in a positive manner, sets up a situation in which the individual is open to suggestions for modification of the goals, methods, and other aspects related to the circumstances under which the less positive actions or happenings occurred. Thus, progress evaluation focuses on emerging aspects that can be changed.

The explanation of why an optimistic person eats/does not eat food X is related to the use of reason in implementation of methods of modifying food intake and/or food and people interactions. This focus suppresses emotional counter-productive thoughts and responses. Thus, actions tend to be rational, i.e., related to, based on, or agreeable to reason. So, reason is restored to consciousness, is held in the mind, and thereby exerts a positive influence or force in the modification of food intake and/or some aspect of the food and people interaction. Accordingly, the rationale for behavior modification, i.e., explanations of controlling principles of opinion, belief, practices, and phenomena associated with food intake and/or the food and people interactions tend to be rational. And, the optimist uses supportive rationalization, i.e., the attribution of one's actions to rational, credible, and creditable motives without analysis of true (especially unconscious) motives so as to provide plausible but untrue reasons for behavior. The individual may need additional information or new techniques but can independently work through a series of progressively closer approximations to what is wanted. Thus, use of reason reinforces other positive aspects.

Pessimism is defined as an inclination to emphasize adverse aspects, conditions, and possibilities or to expect the worst possible outcome. This also sets up what has been called a "self-fulfilling prophecy." A pessimistic orientation causes a person to deny the existence and/or effects of situations/challenges or at best to approach them in a hopeless, doubting, dispairing, anxious, and insecure manner. Thus, when an action or happening is less positive than expected, the construction is negative. Therefore, innumerable difficulties surface that appear to mitigate against attainment of a satisfactory solution. The person construes the action or happening in a defeatist way. As a result, the person becomes defensive and looks for excuses. Therefore, progress evaluation becomes reflexive unless redirected—it tends to focus on the person's failures, which are beside the point. If the action or happening is a small thing, the individual needs to be given assistance in refocusing on modification of the methods or other aspects of the circumstances that can be changed to bring action back on a positive course. IF the action or happening is a major thing, THEN the individual needs to be given assistance in finding a face-saving alternative goal. Note: Many pessimists view retargeting downward as totally unacceptable. As a result of efforts to get them to retarget, they become fatalistic and abandon the goal.

The explanation of why a pessimistic person eats/does not eat food X is related to the lack of reason in implementation of problem-oriented methods of modifying food intake and/or food and people interactions. The pessimistic focus allows emotional counter-productive thoughts and responses to overwhelm the will. The result is that the person loses any semblance of self-control. Actions tend to be irrational, i.e., not governed or guided by reason. Instead, some active power such as rebellion, vengeance, or fear becomes a compelling force. This force then creates resistance to positive modifications and/or sets in motion dysfunctional negative modifications of some aspect of the food and people interaction. The unwanted outcomes that result reinforce the pessimistic disposition. Moreover, rationalizations tend to be given in lieu of a rationale for behavior. As a result, the individual cannot work through a series of approximations toward goal attainment without extensive help.

A person with a generally optimistic disposition may have a pessimistic outlook with respect to any one of the four categories of thought as a result of previous negative experiences in that domain. IF one is insecure with respect to personal ability in dealing with problems, THEN supportive review of planned changes will decrease anxiety and the likelihood of panic-related impulsive actions. IF one is uncertain about goals, THEN supportive discussion of alternatives will decrease the likelihood of unfocused activity. IF one is uncertain about methods, THEN supportive review of appropriateness of applications of particular method(s) and steps in the process can minimize the likelihood of disappointing mistakes. IF one is impatient with limited progress, THEN supportive review of accomplishments can reveal whether the pace can be increased or one has to be content with small but continued improvement. Care must be taken to avoid development of a dependency.

In the context of the person's disposition as it conditions responses to the need for dietary change, other aspects of the personal component of the food environment begin to make sense. The personal component is based on the particulars of the near environment of the individual, i.e., physical, emotional/psychological, aesthetic, economic, social. To define the personal component, one must obtain information of the following types:

(a) who he/she eats with

(b) what plant or animal tissues are defined as food (or poison)

(c) when foods are consumed, i.e., time of day, season of the year for specific items

(d) where food is consumed, i.e., the boundaries of the eating territory, both at home and away from home

(e) why some foods are consumed at certain times, under certain conditions

(f) how food is consumed, e.g., state—raw or cooked, speed—fast or slow, utensils used, type of service involved, etc.

Resources of time, energy, money, skills, and food/nutrition information may be involved variously with different expectations for outcome at different points in time. This chapter and subsequent chapters in this section discuss many facets of these and other related aspects.

Time available for acquisition, preparation, and service of food determines, at least to some degree, what is consumed and its eating qualities. All other things being equal, when time and skill come together, the potential for a positive food and people interaction is increased. Otherwise, quality may have to be sacrificed to convenience.

Energy available (physical, mental, or petro-chemical) is also a factor in the ecological relationship between a person and his/her food. It is often a limiting factor, e.g., physical energy limits may determine shopping frequency, degree of convenience purchased, quantity of food prepared. Mental energy is one of the determinants of the go-no go decision on whether to plan menus, control nutrient intake, etc. Petro-chemical energy availability determines whether conservation and recycling measures predominate in food product design as well as the degree of convenience that can be purchased. This is because highly processed foods require more energy input at each step and also often in handling and/or storage than products prepared at home from "scratch." These energy relationships are just beginning to affect food ecology.

Money available for food and the accoutrements of food service is another aspect of food ecology. For an individual, the money available for food determines choices among alternate items in the array of foods available for purchase, the frequency with which some items can be served, what quality is purchased, the level of physical defects tolerated, the degree of convenience that can be afforded, portion size, and so on. Money also determines the size and type of eating territory and the quality of its furnishings, which includes everything from wallpaper to linens and flatware. In turn, all of these factors affect the perceived quality of the meal climate and eating experience and, hence, the affective component of man's relationship to his food environment.

Skills in food preparation, service, etc., determine the items selected, whether ready-to-eat or prepared according to an elaborate ritual, the aesthetic qualities of the items, and their elaborateness. This in turn is important to the quality of the eating experience and the value accorded it.

Knowledge of food attributes, food composition, menu planning methods, food purchasing principles, food storage principles, food preservation methods, food preparation techniques, and food service methods determine what can be done with what one has to work with. Knowledge gives the power to compensate for lack of time, energy, and/or money, to some degree. Thus, knowledge has a major impact on food ecology. The quality of food and nutrition information sources used is also important. Access to scientific rather than food faddist explanations leads to different conclusions and actions. Quality of information also determines the nature and extent of changes perceived as necessary to maintain health. Scientific information tends to take a conservative view that leads to moderate action, whereas food faddist sources tend to cause alarm and result in precipitate action. Any or all of these may be critical variables affecting the nutriture of an individual.

Domestic Component

The domestic component is composed of (a) those elements of the food supply/demand situation that control local food availability, (b) the culture-based food ideology and food practices, and (c) food/nutrition education and/or information sources. The overall relationships are sketched below and will be developed in subsequent chapters.

Food production technology and capacity are important as they largely determine the types of food available for consumption, given consumer acceptability and preferences. Fruits, vegetables, and cereals available commercially are only a limited subset of the wild edible plants that may be used for food locally and/or nationally. Technological considerations, e.g., ability to withstand the rigors of mechanical harvesting, limit the varieties selected. The number and kinds of animals that have been domesticated and used for or to produce food are also small. Technology has produced a controlled environment that enables a continuous supply of milk and eggs. The aggregate effect is a unique array of foods. The nature of items included and the supply of each determine the distribution of nutrients available from foods. Moreover, production efficiency has a major effect on price, which determines who can purchase what and how much. Thus, by adjusting food production technology and/or capacity, man can modify his relation to his food environment and his potential for adequate nutrient intake.

Food processing technology and capacity largely control the nature and extent of preservation methods and preservatives used. In theory, the nutritive content of fresh foods exceeds that of preserved foods. In practice, while a reduction in nutritional value that varies with the food, the preservation method, and the nutrient cannot be denied, fresh food cannot be supplied countrywide, year-round at a reasonable price. So, processing to preserve is necessary. The net effect of increased and continuous supply is an improved potential for adequate intake despite the fact that the nutrient contribution of individual items is somewhat less. The use of preservatives retards or prevents some common kinds of deteriorative reactions. In some cases, the effect is to retard or to prevent destruction of particular nutrients and, in any case, to maintain the food in a condition fit for consumption, making its nutrients available. Food processing capacity makes highly processed foods available at a relatively low price, which determines who can purchase what and how much. The result is that man can modify his food environment so as to reduce the variability in the supply of nutrients.

Food availability policies are manipulated to control food commodity prices. Policies limit, encourage, or channel food production. Policies of the following types are among the means used: subsidies for production of specific crops, intervention levels that allow production to a specified level, variable levies or charges, tariffs, import quotas, acreage quotas, price guarantees, export subsidies, land banks. Other policies limit, encourage, or channel consumer demand for food. Policies of the following types are used: purchase of surplus commodities; advice to the consumer on items that are plentiful; price controls; concessionary food programs for the young, pregnant, disabled, and elderly; rationing; public health legislation; quality controls; licensing laws; consumer protection laws; taxes on luxuries and duty on imports; foreign aid; and consumer subsidy to create new purchasing power. Thus, man can use food production and/or consumption policies to manipulate the supply and demand for food and, hence, food ecology.

Food distribution/marketing technology and capacity are also factors that determine local item availability, demand, and prices. Distribution technology allows refrigerated shipment of perishable fresh foods and transport of frozen foods. Marketing technology entices people into the stores and encourages impulse buying. Availability in relation to demand determines the mark-up. Thus, man can affect this aspect of the food environment.

Food control legislation encompasses food inspection, food additives, good manufacturing practices, food labeling, and food advertising. Food inspection procedures control the safety and wholesomeness of the food available. Food additives allow man to control color, texture, and flavor attributes, thus affecting quality and item choices made by the consumer. Good manufacturing practices followed within food processing plants assure nutrient conservation, wholesomeness, safety, and economy as well as control of air, heat, and water pollution. Controls on labeling are designed to aid the consumer in selecting appropriate foods to meet general and/or special dietary needs. Such legislation is designed to strengthen security while allowing for the level of choice that is necessary to self-esteem and self-actualization. Controls on food advertising are necessary to restrict claims while allowing product awareness to develop. All of these have important effects on food and people interactions.

Generally accepted food-related beliefs underlie personal decisions in food purchasing, storage, and preparation. Some are based on fact, others on myths. But, all are controlling factors, usually learned from others in an effort to deal with the food environment in the common way. As a result, a common pattern develops. It is carefully monitored by the food industry.

Usual food practices are the immediate and culminating factors in determining nutritional status, except in cases where nutrient supply and/or demand is altered by injury, infection, or malfunction. These include observable behaviors associated with food purchasing, food preparation, food service. These have a major impact on the food environment because they create/maintain/modify the aggregate demand for foods of various types, which in turn, results in marketing transactions, i.e., create a new product, discontinue a product, modify a product, increase production control on a specific aspect of a product, augment or decrease the supply of a product, etc.

Special food practices in relation to holidays, celebrations, and other social occasions reflect the status of man's relation to his food environment, at a given time. When food is scarce and limited to a few items, then samples with few physical defects are presented with elaborate ritual, and thus, status is maintained. When food is generally abundant, high quality items and elaborate ritual are understood to be basic and emphasis tends to shift to rarity, costliness, and/or prodigality as means of maintaining status. The aggregate effect is to create a demand for fancy quality and specialty items.

Paradoxically, in times of scarcity, the importance of these rituals increases and probably has a greater impact on man's relation to his food environment than when food is abundant. This effect probably results from the fact that when food is scarce, it receives more attention and its relative importance increases. Thus, behaviors of individuals, such as hoarding and selectivity, become important in maintaining status, which is under pressure for other reasons. The aggregate effect is to inflate demand for scarce items.

International Component

The international component began to have a marked effect on the food environment of Americans in 1972. At that time, the world food supply situation was transformed from one in which producer nations had surpluses and low food prices to one of relative scarcity and high prices. Prior to that time, American food giveaways of surplus foods had little effect on domestic availability and prices. However, when surpluses were reduced and other nations decided to purchase large quantities of American grains, although domestic supplies remained adequate, prices rose. On top of this, the world food crisis developed and resulted in a crisis in confidence, a credibility gap, and widespread insecurity regarding the American food supply. These events have altered the perceived relation to the American food environment. It is now regarded as threatened.

The food and people interaction is very complex. Its many components are under the control of world markets, national policies, commercial interests, and personal choice. Though these are operative at different levels, all are interdependent and the interaction among them shapes the nutritional outcomes for the American society and its individual members.

LIFE EXPECTANCY

Fundamentally, life expectancy or physiological survival depends on the supply of the right nutrients (assortment and quantity) on a continuous basis, all other things being equal. That is, consumption of a nutritionally adequate diet now and again or only some nutrients will not suffice. Nor can consumption of a nutritionally adequate diet overcome the lack of clothing or shelter nor the effects of mortal injury, infection, or organ malfunction.

Throughout history, a large proportion of mankind has lived with a marginal quality of life which was in part due to inadequate food intake. Life expectancy for this segment always has been low, although in this century improved sanitation and medical assistance have improved life expectancy. At the same time, in every society there have been some rich people who were obese, but their general health was better and their life expectancy was greater. These people often suffered from what are now called the degenerative diseases, namely heart disease, strokes, gout, and diabetes. Until lately, these diseases have been accepted as natural accompaniments of old age. Although these presented a threat, the threat was less immediate than the threat of starvation. Thus, people valued the good life, which was defined to include an abundance of food of ever-increasing quality and variety.

Since hunting/gathering times, the agricultural revolution and the industrial revolution have facilitated improvement in the lot of mankind. An ever-increasing proportion of people has consumed an adequate diet, and life expectancy has improved as has the prevalence of degenerative diseases.

In American society, in this century, the prevalence or number of cases of degenerative diseases has become a matter of increasing concern. Moreover, the incidence or number of new cases is growing as is the mortality rate, i.e., the proportion of deaths in the population. The forces at work in American society have increased life expectancy to about 70 years. While life expectancy has been stable at this point for some years, there is increasing evidence that acute manifestations of degenerative diseases are occurring at increasingly younger ages. Although the causes are unclear, there is some evidence to implicate food intake. Therefore, various preventive diets have been advocated in order to retard or prevent development of the degenerative diseases and their threat to life expectancy.

The opening paragraph raised some relevant questions. The answers are unknowable. Given current knowledge, some hypotheses and theories can be stated but in many cases we can only speculate, i.e., give a reasoned explanation, since the answer is problematic. Consensus is reached in each generation on the basis of understandings that result from the particular approximation to truth that emerges under the circumstances. Intervention programs to correct malnutrition must be implemented with care, since the implications and ramifications of such actions change man's relation to his food environment and may have an impact on almost every other aspect of his existence.

BIBLIOGRAPHY

MAHONEY, M.J., and CAGGIULA, A.W. 1978. Applying behavioral methods to nutritional counseling. J. Am. Dietet. Assoc. 72, 372-377.

15

Why Do People Eat or Not Eat X ?

At the personal level, food and people interactions in a society are related to (a) satisfaction of the basic human needs and (b) people's beliefs concerning the proper relation to their food, which may reduce to a definition of which foods are suitable to eat under certain circumstances.

This chapter examines generalizations that apply to the level(s) of satisfaction achieved by Americans as a people and/or its major subgroups. Discussion is organized according to the following topics:

(a) implications of the food and people interaction
(b) basic human needs and implications of satisfaction at various levels
(c) hunger, surfeit, nutritional status, and individual potential
(d) eating with safety and security—the issues
(e) eating or not eating and social acceptance
(f) religious functions of food
(g) foods and nutrition: "Doing your own thing"

The next chapter introduces concepts of individual intolerances and idiosyncrasies as related to food ideology. Then, the bases of subgroup beliefs are explored and the foodways of some of the major subgroups are described. These two chapters provide the foundation for understanding what you have when you have what you have, i.e., the data collected as a basis for nutritional assessment.

IMPLICATIONS OF THE FOOD AND PEOPLE INTERACTION

The three levels of food and people interactions were indicated briefly in the previous chapter. At all levels, there is an on-going concern with adequacy of the food supply. The food supply would be adequate to meet the needs of all people were it not for an anthropocentric view that creates defective and corrupt food and people interactions. The imposition of man's will (individual and collective) on the food ecosystem can have unlooked-for effects. Since man is not all-knowing, mindless mistakes can be made. Ultimately, man suffers the consequences. Man needs to be cognizant or mindful of this truth. Some effects at the personal and domestic levels have been discussed in previous chapters. Others pertaining to domestic and international levels are discussed in Chapter 32.

An assessment of an individual's true position would include a status evaluation of all aspects of all components and their expected effects. But, to evaluate all of these prior to working with a given individual would be prohibitive in terms of time, energy, and money. Therefore, some generalizations with respect to critical variables have been developed for people in various situations. These are revised from time to time, as the need is recognized. The use of generalizations releases professional time. Attention is then focused on the quality of choices made by an individual. Alternatives that can help the individual improve food choices in relation to his/her food environment are suggested so as to achieve/maintain the desired quality of life, all other things being equal.

Before discussing some of the elements of American food and people interactions, a number of terms need to be defined. Some of these are used with a meaning that differs from the popular one. Important terms are:

(a) Foodways—This is a genus term referring to internalized beliefs and customary patterns of activities associated with acquisition, preparation, serving, consumption, and storage of food. It includes all relevant factors in the food and people interaction—who, what, when, where, why, and how.

(b) Food habits—This is a species term referring to the practices associated with consumption of food, e.g., the usual or customary items preferred and selected, the rituals of eating under variable circumstances, eating territory, eating times and frequency, meal climate.

(c) Food ideology—This is a species term referring to the beliefs and attitudes people have that determine their personal definition of food and their activities in relation to food, e.g.,

-what people *think* about each of the different items that might be considered as food; the sorting factors

-what people *think* the effects of eating various "foods" might be on their health and well-being

-what kinds of "foods" people *think* are suitable for individuals and categories of people, e.g., old, infants, sick, pregnant, lactating

-what kinds of "foods" people *think* are suitable at certain times, e.g., one is not permitted to eat X from April to June; it is poisonous

-what kinds of "foods" people *think* are not suitable in certain conditions, e.g., pregnant women are not permitted to eat X or the baby will have symptoms Y, Z, and Q

The foodways of Americans are very diverse because the availability of foods is essentially unrestricted for most people; freedom of choice is not limited arbitrarily. We are a nation of peoples from everywhere who have introduced many new items and variations of existing items, and we have free communication of food ideas, practices, etc.

Nonetheless, the foodways of individuals and groups can be characterized at any given point in time according to similarities. Thus, anthropologists write long descriptions of beliefs, cooking pots and other utensils, the rituals of processing and preparation as well as service, food gifts, and the like. Statisticians prepare tables using descriptive statistics or measures of central tendency, i.e., mean, median, mode, and percentage. Tables are interpreted with statements such as "The mean number of people preferring food item X is . . . ," "Half the people of type X now eat dinner on TV trays in front of the television," "The most frequent (modal) cut of meat purchased is X, followed by Y," and "The percentage of people eating X on Friday is Y."

The foodways of individuals and groups can be compared at different points in time. The result is identification and documentation of variability or changes in foodways. Anthropologists and statisticians have techniques for characterizing the nature and extent of change. For this purpose they usually plot a trend. They may prepare a descriptive explanation, having identified the differences between two groups or among more than two groups. Another approach is to compare the effects of foodways to some standard, e.g., nutritional. In this case some are below standard, many are close to the standard, and a few exceed it. Many alternate patterns of nutriture can be observed, depending on the nutrient under study and the age or other basis used for segmenting the group.

American society has taken the position that professionals must intervene in the lives of those whose diet is not satisfactory nutritionally, whenever such cases come to their attention. A series of sorting factors for identifying the particular aspect(s) of the foodways of individuals and groups that will help one find the starting point for effective intervention has been developed. Three classes of variables are scrutinized routinely in making a dietary assessment. These are indicated here and are developed in Chapter 18. The classes of variables are:

(a) ingredient variables—The personal array of ingredients and/or ready-to-eat items consumed customarily and occasionally is identified and evaluated. Tables of food composition are used to compute the mean intake of various nutrients.

(b) environmental variables—The differences in personal food habits and food ideology (specific points) that make the difference in selection are identified and evaluated. Then a big matrix of variables is constructed with age, income, education, etc., as column headings and individual particulars in rows.

(c) Individual variables—The peculiarities of the foodways of an individual and/or known facts about particular biological needs that make the person vulnerable are identified and evaluated.

All of the factors that create the diversity of foodways are operative simultaneously and there are many interaction effects. In order to make the points clear, each aspect will be discussed as though it were the only variable. That is, with all other things being equal, the effect is X. Though in reality, the effect may be magnified or negated and masked by other coexisting and operative patterns.

BASIC HUMAN NEEDS AND IMPLICATIONS OF VARIOUS LEVELS OF SATISFACTION

Above all else, the foodways of an individual are determined by his status in relation to satisfaction of basic human needs. A person at or near the subsistence level assigns top priority to food acquisition activities. Above this point, the expected priorities are unpredictable as they change as a result of internal-external interactions. Observed foodways often reveal some pattern that has developed as a result of the interactions, in the same way that personality develops.

For the purposes of intervention foodways need to be reviewed and characterized. The first step is observation which should focus on obtaining a definition of where the person is at, at a specific point in time, in regard to satisfaction of the basic needs; the description should be recorded.

Then assessment of food ecology or the individual's relation to his particular food environment will provide meaningful detail. The elements of food ecology to be assessed and associated considerations and procedures will be described in Chapters 17 through 21.

Apparent inconsistency between observed food habits and expected food habits, given expressed food ideology, often can be explained by some problem in satisfying one or more of the basic human needs at some level. The problem may be one of frustration because of inability to satisfy. Or, the problem may be one of conflict between competing but equally important needs. In this case, the result is what Festinger (1962) called cognitive dissonance, which is internal war. Ultimately, a trade-off or compromise is reached. The conflicting points are rejected by a process called rationalization, and internal harmony is restored. Once this point is reached, seemingly inconsistent behavior disappears.

Basic Human Needs

In 1943, Maslow (1943) identified the basic human needs as phys-iological, safety-security, love or belongingness, esteem or status, and self-actualization. Maslow, in discussing the motivations of people in satisfying these needs, made a number of points that are fundamental to an understanding of the food and people interaction. In general, all human activity is organized to satisfy one or more of these needs, at some level. Generally, these needs can be arranged in a hierarchy at their lowest level of satisfaction; above the minimum, other considerations take priority.

What this means is that, when it comes right down to it, the highest priority of all is physiological survival. People will eat anything that they perceive might provide nourishment. A person is occupied with the prob-lem of the definition of *What is food?* And, the definition includes anything that the person perceives will supply nutrients to meet phys-iological demand.

But, as soon as enough "food" is supplied to meet the demand for nutrients and assure survival, man becomes concerned with safety-secur-ity considerations. A person is then occupied with the problem of the distinction between "food" and "poison" in relation to health. The result is that the definition of "food" is restricted to those items that are least associated with illness, i.e., those that appear to be least poisonous and reliably non-toxic. At the same time, man is occupied with problems of storing food for future use, i.e., to provide some security. Food clas-sification and beliefs begin to form.

When this distinction has been made and a person is secure with regard to the safety and stores of food, he then becomes concerned with love-belongingness considerations. A person is then occupied with the problem of defining what is OK/NOT OK to eat from a socio-cultural standpoint. The result is that the definition of what is food is restricted to those items accepted by the local peer group. The definition of what is "poison" is expanded to include unfamiliar or strange items and proscribed items. Observation will quickly identify who is in the "in" group and who is in the "out" group. The process of food classification and development of belief structures continues.

When these basic needs have been met, man becomes concerned with esteem or status. A person is then occupied with the problem of defining *What is food?* on an economic basis. This is an important consideration as it has a major impact on variety. The definition of what is "poison" is expanded to include inexpensive low quality items and items "given" in charity to those less fortunate.

When these needs have been met, man becomes concerned with self-actualization which is the process of establishing a personal identity. A person is then occupied with the problem of defining *What is food?* in terms of style that becomes a trademark. This is often an aesthetic definition. The result may be restriction of the definition of "food" to combinations that are harmonious in color, texture, and shape. The definition of "poison" may imply lack of harmony or it may connote monotony. A dinner of steamed chicken, mashed potatoes, and cauliflower on a white plate is deemed poisonous for this reason.

Implications

Above the minimum level of satisfaction, there is the potential of a continuous distribution of levels or gradations in satisfaction of each of these needs. The basic needs can never really be satisfied. This has both fortunate and unfortunate implications. It is fortunate as it allows flexibility in the food and people interaction and thereby permits healthy adjustment to changing circumstances. Elusiveness is also unfortunate as some individuals become compulsively obsessed with seeking continuous improvement in one aspect or another. There is more to life than this. IF one can get beyond obsession with pursuit of improvement, THEN satisfaction is not that important and is easily attained at a reasonable level.

For each individual, there is a characteristic band of expected levels of satisfaction for each of the needs. This is the result of self-concept and life-style. These motivate control of activity to assure expected satisfaction, to the extent possible. Within this characteristic band, there is some minor shifting up and down according to immediate considerations. A shift outside this band requires great adjustment. A shift down is traumatic and results in feelings of deprivation. For example, this occurs with every sharp price rise when some items are eliminated or served less frequently. A shift up implies that life is improving. It is accompanied by feelings of insecurity over appropriateness of choices at the new level, unless the shift was slight.

For every individual, the priorities for satisfaction of the basic needs are in a continuous state of change in response to internal and external forces. Any force which causes a shift in level of satisfaction of one need may result in a chain of responses involving any or all of the other needs.

From the above, it is clear that observable behaviors are a result of many interactions. Although the same food behaviors may be observed over time, they may result from different interactions and integrations. The change agent must be aware of this fact since strategies for change must be based on the causes, not the observable behaviors.

HUNGER, SURFEIT, NUTRITIONAL STATUS AND INDIVIDUAL POTENTIAL

The top priority need is to assure physiological survival. Too little or too much food can be life-threatening as will be discussed in this section. At the very least too much or too little food tends to modify individual potential. Before discussing the issues, a few terms will be defined.

(a) Hunger is a sensation occasioned by lack of food and results in a craving or urgent need for food or a specific nutrient.

(b) Surfeit refers to an overabundant supply of food, i.e., an excess or an intemperate/immoderate indulgence in food or drink, e.g., by a glutton.

(c) Nutritional status refers to the state of supply of an assortment of about 50 nutrients, in some known ratio and quantity, at a particular time in relation to expected metabolic demand.

(d) Good nutrition means that the supply of the right assortment (ratio and quantity) is adjusted continuously to meet expected metabolic demand.

(e) Malnutrition means inadequate or inappropriate supply in relation to expected demand, i.e., right nutrients in the wrong ratio, right nutrients but supply is erratic, wrong nutrients—miss one or more, or wrong nutrients—supply is so high that it poisons the system.

Nutritional status is related to health. Health has been defined in the preamble to the WHO constitution as "... a state of complete physical, mental, and social well-being and not merely the absence of disease or infirmity." Health is directly affected by injury, infection, and malfunction of organs and systems and indirectly by nutritional status. Nutritional status is an environmental factor that affects the body's ability to deal with injury, infection, and/or malfunction. If nutritional status is good, then effects can be reduced, i.e., a fast return to good health is possible or minimal problems result. If nutritional status is not good, then the effects are magnified and can slow or prevent a return to good health. Herein lies the importance of good nutrition.

As people always have known, a person who is chronically hungry is nearly always poorly nourished. A person who is surfeited traditionally has been considered to be well nourished. However, in the past 20 years, accumulated evidence supports the position that surfeit also results in malnutrition, but of a different kind. Thus, the problem of physiological survival is still a relevant issue.

Hunger

Hunger is not an all or none variable. Rather, it is continuous in degree from not very hungry to very hungry. Basically, hunger is related to physiologic need but the appetite response is unreliable. Everybody becomes hungry at intervals during the day, but responses vary among people (both in terms of quality and quantity of food consumed) along a continuum. Some people tune out the signals; they become hungrier and temporarily undernourished. Some people accept the signals but delay action; they often become hungrier to a point and then overreact. Some people accept the signals and eat appropriately. Some people accept the signals and overreact. Hence, the nutritional outcomes vary and the signals may cease, continue at a low level, or increase in intensity. A person also can override the physiological signals because of other needs. And, in some cases physiological need will take over at the subconscious level, resulting in uncontrollable cravings.

A pattern of behavior usually associated with simple starvation has been observed in milder form in persons who are temporarily hungry, such as dieters. If the pattern is present, then it must be dealt with before any progress can be made in dealing with other needs.

According to Maslow (1943), in the case of simple starvation,

. . . all other needs may become simply non-existent or be pushed into the background . . . For the man who is simply and dangerously hungry, no other interest exists but food. He dreams food, he remembers food, he emotes only about food, he perceives only food . . . Utopia can be defined very simply as a place where there is plenty of food. He tends to think that, if only he is guaranteed food for the rest of his life, he will be perfectly happy and will never want anything else.[1]

But, it turns out as soon as *some* food is obtained which partially satisfies hunger, then the person's scale of values changes—quality or variety becomes important or some other physiological or other need takes priority.

Hunger also is related to the safety-security need. In general, an emotional-psychological crisis resulting from a threat to safety-security results in a depressed appetite in the short-run. This occurs because the fright-fight-flight response is to release adrenalin in order to deal with the crisis. The effect is to shunt blood from the stomach and intestines to heart and muscles. If a person were to eat at this time, absorption would bottleneck since the blood flow for distribution of nutrients would be reduced. The result is anorexia, nausea, and cramps.

In general, in chronic cases of emotional-psychological crisis and after a discrete event, a person will experience hunger pangs and increased appetite. Originally, the fright-fight-flight response resulted in a major output of physical energy; it was then necessary to replenish energy stores. Emotional-psychological balance is necessary and people eat to symbolically replenish stores.

---

[1] From Maslow (1943). Quoted with permission of *Psychologic Reviews*.

Hunger also is related to the love-belongingness need. People who are lonely feel unwanted and ill at ease. They often do not eat except when invited out to dinner. Usually they subsist on tea and toast rather than meals.

Hunger or lack of hunger may result from frustration in obtaining status. People may be observed to eat to excess or to refuse food in order to gain attention, which increases status, in a sense.

Strength and integrity of food ideology may stimulate or suppress hunger pangs. Those who eat by the clock do so because they believe that they should eat regularly. The same type of person who does not eat enough at one time may suppress hunger pangs until "mealtime" as determined by the clock. Food beliefs are not that important to most Americans. So, if a person is very hungry, he/she probably will eat whatever is available, all other things being equal. If a person is not that hungry, then behavior is unpredictable.

Many people are hungry. The May 6, 1969 Message of the President to the Congress of the United States (Nixon 1970B) includes this passage:

. . . in the past few years we have awakened to the distressing fact that despite our material abundance and agricultural wealth, many Americans suffer from malnutrition. Precise factual descriptions of its extent are not presently available, but there can be no doubt that hunger and malnutrition exist in America, and that some millions may be affected.

Real hunger or food deprivation of sufficient extent and duration to result in medical cases of malnutrition usually are seen only in populations at marginal levels of subsistence. At least that was the consensus of opinion at the time. So, where did the President obtain information that caused him to make the above statement?

In 1969, the documentary film "Hunger in America" was shown in prime time on major TV networks. It showed hunger in Appalachia among coal mining families, hunger among Native Americans living on reservations, hunger of intermittently employed migrant workers, in rural areas and in city slums. It showed the hungry to be young, old, pregnant women, the employed as well as the unemployed. Documentation was comprehensive and unequivocal; the point was irrefutable and unavoidable—in affluent America, real hunger exists.

The resultant shock waves were of sufficient magnitude that they could not be ignored. A White House Conference was called, resulting in some corrective legislation.

In 1969, in appointing Jean Mayer to organize the White House Conference on Food, Nutrition and Health, the President said (Nixon 1970A)

In calling the White House Conference on Food, Nutrition, and Health, we are both reaffirming our commitment to a full and healthful diet for all Americans and exploring what we yet need to know and do to achieve that goal.

The White House Conference came and went. There was much talk and some immediate food aid. "Bread now" was the concept. But, man must eat every day, not just now and again. And the aggregate cost of feeding millions daily adds up quickly. Moreover, public opinion is fickle and shifts from one crisis to another. So, when budgets were juggled because of the next political exigency, feeding programs turned out to be approved but not funded. So, things have not changed. "The poor are with us always." And, poverty results in food deprivation and concomitant malnutrition.

Surfeit

Surfeit is not an all or none condition. It is a matter of degree and is the antithesis of hunger. Basically, surfeit is related to lack of physiological need for food. Here again, the appetite is an unreliable guide. Some people ignore the response and make themselves sick by overeating. Others accept the signal but delay action, continuing to eat mindlessly. These people have no will power and become obese. Some are easily satisfied and eat too little. In contemporary American society, availability of an abundant supply coupled with too little will power has led to development of the degenerative diseases. Prevalence is so high that a health crisis exists.

Nutritional Status

Nutritional science has established the fact that body stores of the various nutrients are highly variable. Since the reserve supply of some nutrients is small, they are critical to survival. The available evidence suggests that carbohydrate, potassium, sodium, and water are most critical, in that order. Normally, symptoms of deprivation of these have an acute onset and degeneration toward death is rapid. Consequently, man has learned to supply these and warning is passed among generations via folk tales and adages.

Fat and protein are the next most critical nutrients. Deprivation results in protein-energy malnutrition (PEM). This condition is seen among people of all ages, but most often among pre-school children.

Thiamin is the next most critical nutrient. It is a class representative, which means that it stands for all of the B vitamins except B_{12}. The expected effect of deprivation is similar for all since they all function as coenzymes. IF a low level of intake is maintained, THEN stores can be built to a limited extent that provides short-term reserve. IF intake is marginal, THEN deficiency results.

Stores of iron, vitamin A, and calcium are usually adequate for years. But, we hear of much anemia, and of deficiencies of vitamin A and calcium. Why? There are many causes of blood loss and iron intake is frequently low. Vitamin A is distributed unevenly in foods and not in the foods that are inexpensive and filling. So, people must select for it by conscious action and many do not. Deprivation of calcium in early childhood prevents normal storage so children have limited reserves and thereby become vulnerable. Development of a deficiency syndrome in an adult indicates real hunger of months' to years' duration, since stores are normally adequate.

Stores of ascorbic acid are diffuse. Nutritionists recommend a daily intake. Why? Ascorbic acid is not stored in any great quantity. Therefore, it must be supplied frequently. But, supply must not be left to chance. Since people forget or cannot get organized, it is more convenient to recommend a daily intake.

Other nutrients are not listed as being stored. They probably are, at least to some extent, but the quantities are small. In most cases, IF a variety of natural foods is consumed, THEN intake will be alright.

In summary, severe malnutrition is expected only when people are really hungry because of chronic food deprivation. IF it occurs during the period when brain tissue is developing, THEN development may be impaired. Otherwise, misery rather than great harm is the likeliest outcome. Suboptimal nutriture also can affect individual potential because performance is likely to be lower with consequent reduction in opportunities.

Individual Potential

Nutrition is a science and much is known about the general human physiological demand for a specific array of nutrients under certain conditions. But, we cannot know how much of a specific nutrient is needed by a specific individual at a specific time. This is unknowable. Some general concepts of what is wanted, given genetic and environmental factors, have emerged from extensive controlled investigations.

There is a basal metabolic demand that is determined by genetic potential. This is the amount needed to sustain vital functions of heart, lungs, etc., given individual bioefficiency. It varies among people with race, sex with respect to size-and-shape-related distributions, and age— older people have lower proportions of functioning cells so require less. In addition, there is a demand that is determined by growth and development status according to a biological time clock. Growth and/or development inflates the need for all nutrients, for some more than others depending on the nature and extent of growth and/or development in process. For example, infants have a small body size but their growth rate is steep so demands are relatively high. Teenagers have attained or are in the process of attaining maximum body size. Basal metabolic need is high and growth and/or development is rapid so the demand is inflated to a very high level. Adults have attained a large body size so basal metabolic need is high. But, since growth has stopped, overall demand is only moderate. In pregnancy body size is large and growing so the basal demand is high. Growth of maternal and fetal tissues is steep, so the overall demand is inflated to a super-high level.

Over and above these physiological needs for nutrients are needs created by various environmental factors. Physical activity is the first of these. Physical activity results in wear and tear on the tissues in addition to the need for fuel. For example, infants have relatively high needs because activity during waking hours is practically incessant. Adults, who in our society are practically sedentary, may have no need above their basal metabolic need.

Use of drugs, whether over-the-counter or prescription, inflates the need for some nutrients but not much is known about such effects. It is known that oral contraceptive agents (OCA) inflate the needs for B_6, nicotine inflates the need for ascorbic acid, and aspirin inflates the need for iron. If a person takes any drugs routinely, then serum levels of various nutrients should be monitored. However, the effects of many drugs on nutritional need are unknown.

In general, nutrient demand is correlated with stage in the life cycle. For this reason, statements of guidelines are related to the stages. In general, people should recheck needs at least at five-year intervals. To avoid mistakes, one automatically could review needs each time the new Recommended Dietary Allowances are published.

Individual potential for performing optimally, given genetic potential, is related to nutritional status. Deficiency in the supply of each of the nutrients is related to slowdown or cessation of some necessary metabolic activity. Marginal intake leads to minor stress and vague symptoms. Major deficiency results in a major stress, development of pathological conditions, and if prolonged, death. Excess in supply of each of the various nutrients is related to problems of flooding, resulting in storage and/ or poisoning problems. A chronic marginal excess causes a minor problem. A major chronic excess results in a major stress, pathological conditions, and/or death. Thus, it turns out that a person must determine his/her personal level of need, adjust intake to supply it, and continue that supply level in order to facilitate productivity according to potential.

EATING WITH SAFETY AND SECURITY: THE ISSUES

From time immemorial, problems of food safety and security have been a relevant major concern of society. Since the beginning of recorded history, the same issues have confronted mankind. In this sense, there is nothing new in this world, but there may be a new twist for the current generation to solve. The problems for the individual involve trust in others and personal food intolerance or allergies that create special individual problems. The problems for society are:

(a) What is naturally edible or can be processed so as to become edible?

(b) What is perishable and what can be stored as is or if processed to preserve?

(c) When food is obtained from others, what procedures can be used to control the nature and extent of defects that result from ignorance or negligence so as to be sure that the food is wholesome?

(d) When food is obtained from others, what procedures can be developed to prevent/protect it from adulteration or fraud?

(e) What procedures can be established to control the problem of poisoning out of malice for political reasons?

(f) What can be done to establish public confidence in the safety and wholesomeness of the food supply?

Between 1900 and the mid-1930s, the major issues were problems with standards, control of defects which until then had been accepted as natural, and adulteration. These problems were solved effectively for the time being.

The controls were so effective that people became secure and complacent. Businessmen knew their businesses and there seemed to be adequate laws to control and protect, for the level of problems that existed at that time. City people were not exposed to natural toxicants. The array of domesticated plants is small compared to natural variety, but people had access only to domesticated plants so the problem of natural toxicants was minimal. The pesticides and food additives used were few and easily detected because the technology was not that advanced.

But, since about 1970 Americans have been insecure with regard to the safety and supply of basic foodstuffs. Why? The true explanations are unknowable. A plausible explanation is offered for consideration. Edibility may have become an important issue because of the new labeling law which requires a more extensive listing of ingredients in their long, impossible-to-pronounce chemical names. This might be expected to evoke a response of fear of the unknown. It may be that the change was too abrupt. The general public previously had not been educated to regard foods as mixtures of chemicals. Understandably, many people may have rejected this concept as unacceptable. If so, an expected outcome would be that out of fear and/or ignorance they would reject the foods with the chemical names for common ingredients. In this case, label information may have been the only aspect that changed with respect to the food, but beliefs would cause rejection. So, questions of safety were raised and people became insecure.

Edibility also became an issue because new sophisticated processing techniques were introduced. People are no longer involved in processing their own food. And, they fear the unknown. Food processing is accomplished by the food processing industry, and an impersonal unknown "they" are not trusted by many people. So, again out of fear and/or ignorance people rejected processed foods. Thus, additional questions of safety were raised and another segment of the American population became insecure.

Perishability became an important issue because new intermediate moisture foods that are shelf-stable were introduced. From television and other sources, the consumer learned that perishability was not a problem. These items look and taste like their traditional counterparts, which is the cause of the problem that developed. Sometimes the traditional items were purchased and handled in the new way; these items spoiled. Confusion resulted, questions of safety were raised, and people became insecure.

The problem of too many defects became an important issue because foods are biological materials and are inherently highly variable. Many consumers did not know this since neither they nor any relatives were any longer involved in agriculture. So, consumers expected too much uniformity and perfection. When people became aware of food product recalls for reasons of defects they panicked (Fig. 15.1). And, when prices went up, they bought less expensive substitutes, found unaccustomed defects, and responded with "What are you trying to feed me?" They felt cheated, raised questions of safety, and became insecure.

The problems of adulteration and fraud became an issue because sophisticated technology, using a large array of food additives, evolved. The food processor has been confronted with an increasing demand for product control during processing, delivery, and home storage by the consumer. The solution was manipulation of product attributes by controlled use of food additives (Fig. 15.2). But, nearly all of these food additives, when listed by chemical name, resulted in fear of the unknown. Moreover, the average consumer is not technically competent to understand why each food additive is used. Plausible and acceptable explanations usually have not been made, so the consumer concluded that either adulteration or fraud was intended. So, questions of safety were raised again and people became even more insecure.

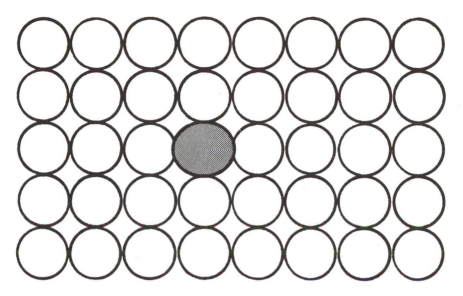

FIG. 15.1. PRODUCT RECALL—JUST ONE A LITTLE OFF RESULTS IN RECALL OF THE ENTIRE BATCH

The problem of poisoning out of malice or for political reasons has become an issue because sophisticated technology allows us to measure chemicals in parts per billion (p.p.b.). The question of natural contaminant versus deliberate low level poison, administered over time, has been raised. So people are anxious and insecure.

To top it all off, when crop short-falls abroad resulted in elimination of our surpluses from storage, the problem of possible death by starvation became an important issue. People became aware that greed and politics resulted in grain sales that depleted stores. At the same time, people became aware of the population explosion, and they became aware of waste on a grand scale. All in all, people became insecure regarding supply. In this country, which has the best agricultural productivity the world has ever known, some people have become afraid of death by starvation. See Chapters 32 and 33 for additional detail.

The wave of insecurity and lack of confidence in the safety of American foods was not confined to processed food. Techniques that enabled detection of substances in p.p.b. revealed the presence of pesticides, known poisons, in raw agricultural commodities. In the wake of this revelation, the "organic" foods movement was born.

Organic foods are purported to be raw agricultural commodities grown without benefit of chemical fertilizers or pesticides or such foodstuffs processed without the use of food chemicals or food additives. Thus, they are "pure" foods.

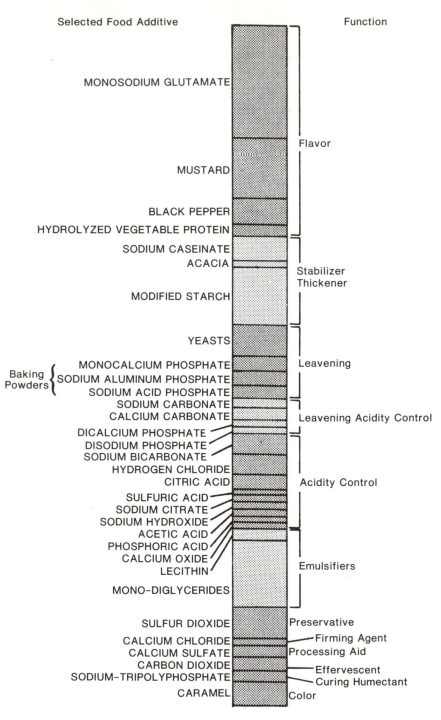

Selected Food Additive / Function

MONOSODIUM GLUTAMATE

MUSTARD

BLACK PEPPER
HYDROLYZED VEGETABLE PROTEIN

Flavor

SODIUM CASEINATE
ACACIA

MODIFIED STARCH

Stabilizer
Thickener

YEASTS

Leavening

Baking Powders {
MONOCALCIUM PHOSPHATE
SODIUM ALUMINUM PHOSPHATE
SODIUM ACID PHOSPHATE

SODIUM CARBONATE
CALCIUM CARBONATE

Leavening Acidity Control

DICALCIUM PHOSPHATE
DISODIUM PHOSPHATE
SODIUM BICARBONATE
HYDROGEN CHLORIDE
CITRIC ACID

Acidity Control

SULFURIC ACID
SODIUM CITRATE
SODIUM HYDROXIDE
ACETIC ACID
PHOSPHORIC ACID
CALCIUM OXIDE
LECITHIN

MONO-DIGLYCERIDES

Emulsifiers

SULFUR DIOXIDE

Preservative

CALCIUM CHLORIDE
CALCIUM SULFATE
CARBON DIOXIDE
SODIUM-TRIPOLYPHOSPHATE
CARAMEL

Firming Agent
Processing Aid
Effervescent
Curing Humectant
Color

FIG. 15.2. FOOD ADDITIVES IN COMMON USE

Average consumption total is 9 lb/year; proportionate usage shown.

Organic food stores opened throughout the land to cater to the needs of those who had to have organic foods. Some sell fancy grade produce or staples and assert that the superior quality is a direct outcome of the ecologically sound organic farming methods. Others sell substandard produce or staples. Natural defects such as apple scabs and worms, uneven color, or rancidity are accepted as evidence that the food is organically grown. Still others sell the same quality of items obtained from the same suppliers as the local supermarkets. In any case, organic food stores customarily charge "what the traffic will bear." Table 15.1 lists comparative prices. IF the assurance of safety and security derived from the label "organically grown" is sufficient to allay unreasonable fears, THEN such food and the peace of mind it creates is probably worth the price to the true believer.

TABLE 15.1. COST OF SELECTED FOODS ADVERTISED AS "ORGANIC" COMPARED WITH COST OF SIMILAR FOODS NOT LABELED "ORGANIC" (REGULAR), WASHINGTON, D.C., FEBRUARY 1976[1]

Foods	Unit	Regular Food Supermarket ($)	Organic as Percentage of Regular Food	
			Store No. 1[2]	Store No. 2[2]
			(%)	
Processed Foods				
Canned fruits and vegetables, juices and preserves				
Apple juice	qt	0.45	198	182
Apple sauce	lb	0.29	276	—
Peach preserves	lb	0.87	151	—
Pickles	qt	1.00	150	150
Tomatoes	lb	0.23	326	296
Dried fruits and vegetables				
Lentils, hulled	lb	0.37	338	100
Raisins	lb	0.78	—	89
Flour, cereals, pastas, and bread				
Cornmeal, yellow	lb	0.26	154	115
Granola	lb	0.69	—	132
Grits	lb	0.37	214	116
Oats, rolled (not quick-cooking)	lb	0.52	—	56
Wheat cereal	lb	0.49	82	61
Whole wheat bread	lb	0.55	—	144
Whole wheat flour	lb	0.22	205	177
Other				
Honey	lb	0.94	120	115
Peanut butter	lb	0.79	—	170
Vinegar, cider	qt	0.53	202	306
Unprocessed Foods				
Meat and poultry				
Ground beef, regular	lb	0.75	313	—
Chicken				
Fryer, whole	lb	0.65	254	—
Fryer, cut-up	lb	0.69	304	—
Breast with rib	lb	0.89	235	—
Leg	lb	0.79	265	—
Livers	lb	1.19	176	—
Eggs	doz	0.79	165	—

TABLE 15.1 *(Continued)*

Foods	Unit	Regular Food Supermarket ($)	Organic as Percentage of Regular Food	
			Store No. 1[2] (%)	Store No. 2[2]
Fresh fruits and vegetables				
Apples	lb	0.33	173	142
Grapefruit	lb	0.17	288	124
Oranges	lb	0.18	228	117
Tangerines	lb	0.21	186	143
Broccoli	lb	0.55	125	129
Brussels sprouts	lb	1.26	66	67
Cabbage, green	lb	0.10	550	430
Cabbage, red	lb	0.33	179	152
Carrots	lb	0.23	183	152
Celery, pascal	lb	0.44	148	109
Cucumbers	lb	0.53	160	160
Garlic	lb	2.45	90	65
Green beans	lb	0.59	151	180
Green pepper	lb	0.53	236	200
Greens (collards, kale)	lb	0.39	144	233
Lettuce, head	lb	0.39	164	144
Lettuce, romaine	lb	0.49	131	129
Mushrooms	lb	0.69	326	261
Onions	lb	0.23	343	343
Potatoes, white	lb	0.33	179	142
Spinach	lb	1.10	95	82
Squash, summer	lb	0.59	169	114
Tomatoes	lb	0.52	208	138

Source: Cromwell (1976).
[1] If a variety of brands or package sizes were available, the price of the best buy was chosen.
[2] Store No. 1 is a large natural food store that sells food, vitamins, cosmetics, and literature. Store No. 2 is a natural— almost completely organic—food store owned cooperatively by the workers. Many foods are purchased in bulk. Some are repackaged at the store in smaller containers; some are sold in the customer's own container.

EATING OR NOT EATING AND SOCIAL ACCEPTANCE

Wherever people meet, either informally or formally, food and drink are usually served. The offering, i.e., the sharing of food and/or drink, in the social situation serves as a unifying force with the functions of expressing love/friendship or belongingness/acceptance, status, hospitality, and celebration. Foodways are associated with each of these functions. In this context, foodways refer to the habits and beliefs of the group that reflect the way in which that culture standardizes behavior of the individual members of the group, in relation to food. As a group, Americans have developed certain foodways which form an identifiable pattern in terms of what is considered appropriate for picnics, pool parties, barbecues, teas, or brunches. Within American society, foodways of local social groups determine the who, what, when, where, why, and how of the food and people interaction. The connotations of eating or not eating, in regard to social acceptance, vary with the situation.

In the most common social eating situations, the functions of expressing love/friendship or belongingness/acceptance, status, and hospitality cannot be separated. The general situation will be outlined first, followed by some more specific functions.

A neighbor, a friend, a salesman admitted to the home—by tradition all of these are immediately offered some sweet and/or rich item and a beverage, even if the visit is unexpected. Appropriate items must be kept on hand against such an emergency; failure in this regard is embarrassing and decreases status. Failure to offer food and/or beverage usually implies flouting of custom and results in loss of status. To refuse an item offered is considered bad manners and implies rejection of friendship and results in loss of status. If for reasons of health, one cannot accept the item(s) offered, one feels obligated to apologize; nonetheless, the situation is awkward. If the timing of the visit is very close to a mealtime, non-acceptance of food and/or beverage may be alright but timing of the visit may be considered inappropriate and may be resented.

Food and/or drink is served as a planned but minor part of most meetings, except dinner meetings where it is more important. Usually, to refuse food is unacceptable. In some cases, arrangements are made for people to join a group after a meal just prior to the speaker. This alternative avoids the necessity for consumption of unwanted food, but is still not entirely acceptable socially.

Food and drink are a major part of social get-togethers such as teas, bridge parties, picnics, and ball games. If one anticipates that he/she will not be able to eat the type of food likely to be served, then the invitation usually is not accepted. To attend the function and refuse the food would be conspicuous and socially unacceptable behavior.

The type of food served on social occasions tends to be rich and/or sweet empty-calorie foods in keeping with the concept of generosity. Those individuals whose life-style involves frequent social eating become obese unless they compensate. One way to compensate is by selecting the best alternative item. Another is to eat slowly and leave a portion or at least to avoid additional portions. Another strategy is reduced eating at other times. The major difficulty is that the nutrient density of foods consumed socially is low. Supplementation may be the only feasible solution to control of nutrient intake.

Traditionally, American women have expressed love of family through careful selection, preparation, and service of meals. Accordingly, disparaging remarks about food are tabooed as bad manners. At the same time, a compliment expresses love in a socially acceptable way.

Love also is expressed through the system of rewards and punishments. In this sense, to publicly withhold food is equivalent to withdrawing love and social acceptance. This is a powerful means of applying social sanction.

Food gifts signify love/friendship and are universal symbols used for this purpose. A gift of wine is used to exchange for a meal. A gift of candy is expected at Valentines Day. Fudge, brownies, and special foods are prepared to strengthen relationships. A homemade food gift is offered as a "labor of love" and carries the message that "I care enough to use my time and talents to do this for you."

Belongingness/acceptance also is expressed by invitations to participate in social eating situations. Persons with reputations as gracious hostesses frequently invite old maids, bachelors, or the elderly to share Thanksgiving, Christmas, and other group dinners.

Status and social acceptance also are related. Newspaper gossip columns carry remarks about who was "seen" and therefore accepted as having sufficient status to belong to the "right" crowd. Invitations to "hundred-dollar-a-plate dinners" carry much status.

Serving of food and beverages has a central role in expressing hospitality with its implication of generosity. In this context, even the humblest of families shares their best food with guests. In fact, since other means are limited, food assumes greater importance. Indeed, it may be the social binder. More affluent families augment hospitality with a status-giving prodigal array of foods. Overeating and its sequelae are expected outcomes.

Food and drink play a well recognized role in celebration. Individuals celebrate special occasions of personal significance with culturally determined foods that have been assigned symbolic value by convention. For example, raises and promotions are celebrated with dinner out including wine and/or champagne, and birthdays are celebrated with cake and ice cream. American society celebrates most holidays with traditional foods. The women's magazines present new variations of traditional items and/or combinations each year. Thus, while turkey and cranberries are expected at Thanksgiving, the cranberries will be included in the different meal components from soup to nuts, e.g., one year a cranberry relish will be the rage and another a cranberry crunch.

Social acceptance limits freedom to choose. For example, consider the following situation. Three women enter a restaurant for lunch. As soon as the menu is presented, somebody mumbles her choice aloud. IF she selects a salad plate luncheon, THEN companions usually will select similarly light meals. In all probability, nobody will select the featured complete meal of entrée, vegetable, salad, and dessert. To do so would break an unwritten social rule.

FOOD AND ESTEEM: FREEDOM TO CHOOSE

Esteem was listed by Maslow (1943) as the fourth level need. To esteem means to have great regard for, to value highly, to respect. All of these imply status. High status is attributed to people, places, and things that are highly esteemed. American society teaches people to value freedom of choice. Consequently, self-esteem and the esteem of others are related to the number and kinds of alternatives available to an individual.

In American society money, rather than birth, is the basis for social position. Celebrations associated with the rites of passage always have been used to emphasize status differences. Also, conspicuous consumption has been the prerogative of those of high birth. But, in affluent America it is practiced by peoples of various levels. So, having money is not enough. It must be spent in socially acceptable ways. One of these is to purchase exotic expensive food and drink and/or serve it lavishly and conspicuously.

Operationally, status functions by accentuating the differences between the giver and the receiver. Suitable food gifts from high status people are extra quantities of deluxe items or strange and costly items.

The relationship between status and freedom of choice is that IF one has high status by means of being rich and/or famous, THEN one has a large array of alternatives from which to choose. IF one does not have high status, THEN one can make a showing and pretend, at least temporarily. The freedoms that status confers and that are emulated by others include:

(a) Freedom to choose rare and costly items with which to impress others. (When we go to C's house, she serves X! We accept invitations from C since they increase our status and we can impress others by relating the fact that we went to C's house and had X!)

(b) Freedom to select expensive restaurants, costly wines, and other luxury items for personal gratification. (When we switch from place A to place B or Brand A to Brand B, peers infer that we must be coming up in this world since these are more costly alternatives.)

(c) Freedom to prepare an especially difficult or time-consuming dish.

In addition to facilitating achievement of status in others' eyes, freedom to choose also provides the means for increasing self-esteem. For example:

(a) Freedom to choose luxury items. (I can afford X or I can afford X more often than anybody else in my group. Therefore, I feel good about myself.)

(b) Freedom to eat in restaurants, a more expensive alternative than eating a comparable meal at home. (I can afford to eat at place X or I can afford to eat at place X more often than previously. Therefore, I feel good about myself. I am coming up in this world.)

(c) Freedom to prepare X, which is difficult and time-consuming and which my neighbors or friends love but can not produce. (I can choose to make X for them because I have the skill. Then I can show off and feel good about myself.)

Lack of power to choose decreases self-esteem. The poverty problem is a case in point, whether people "feel poor" or are poor. IF people have less food purchasing power than usual or than others around them have, THEN they feel deprived. They become envious and the value of some items rises irrationally. They *must* have X. They spend scarce dollars to obtain X. Then, having obtained it, they may be able to endure the usual food for some time. When it is impossible to obtain X, the result is less variety by elimination of a coveted item. Sometimes the result is apathy and rejection of customary food, accompanied by an attitude of not caring whether any food is consumed.

The therapeutic diet problem is another case of deprivation. People feel restricted and their behavior reflects this. Some people accept or go along with the restriction. But, they fail to compensate in the food and people interaction so the total value of each meal is depreciated. After awhile, the diet is not followed. Some people cannot accept the lack of freedom, so reject the diet as impossible. These people regard physical discomfort as the lesser of two evils.

Institutions such as schools and hospitals often use a set or no-choice menu. Even when the food is acceptable, complaints arise due to lack of choice.

Another example is commonly observed in in-plant cafeterias. Everybody resents a situation which allows only a forced choice between two unacceptable alternatives such as lamb and liver. The problem arises because when such items are paired, they result in a no-choice situation for many people. Even when two equally popular items are paired, there may be resentment due to the problem of choice and the fact that the next pair is unlikely to be as good a choice.

RELIGIOUS FUNCTIONS OF FOOD (RELATED TO RELIGIOUS BELIEFS AND OBSERVANCES)

Freedom of religion is a constitutional right in the United States. More than 500 sects have taken advantage of this freedom and have become established. These have been grouped as follows:

(a) The Liturgical Family (Western or Roman Catholic and Episcopal)

(b) The Liturgical Family (Eastern Orthodox and Non-Chalcedonian Orthodox)

(c) The Lutheran Family

(d) The Reformed Presbyterian Family (Presbyterian and Congregational)

(e) The Liberal Family (Unitarian)

(f) The Pietist-Methodist Family (e.g., Moravian, Methodist)

(g) The Holiness Family (e.g., Church of God, Church of the Nazarene)

(h) The Pentecostal Family (e.g., Church of God, Pentecostal)

(i) The European Free-Church Family (e.g., Mennonite, Amish, Brethren, Quaker)

(j) The Baptist Family (Baptist and Church of Christ)

(k) The Independent-Fundamentalist Family (Plymouth Brethren, Grace Gospel Fellowship)

(l) The Adventist Family (Seventh Day Adventist, Church of God, sacred name churches, Jehovah's Witnesses)

(m) The Latter-Day Saints Family

(n) The Communal Family (e.g., Amana, Shakers)

(o) The Metaphysical Family (e.g., Christian Science)

(p) The Psychic and New Age Family (e.g., spiritualist churches, theosophy societies, the "I Am" movement, Rosicrucians, cosmic wisdom groups, Church of Scientology, ECKANKAR)

(q) The Magic Family (witchcraft, neo-paganism, satanism)

(r) The Eastern and Middle Eastern Family (Judaism, Islam, Hinduism, Sikhism, Jainism, Buddhism)

(s) The New Unaffiliated Religious Bodies (Jesus People)

Because many of these require strict adherence to dietary laws, awareness is essential so as to avoid giving offense. A simple case in point is when one party believes that to refuse food is to deny friendship when no such thing is intended by the other party, who may have no inkling of this belief. Moreover, when some refuse to eat there may be good reason for it. Adherents of many smaller religious groups have been taught that others do not understand and that they should not take offense when their religious scruples are ignored. Their coping mechanism is to withdraw and not eat rather than create a scene by requesting special food.

At this time in the United States, life is very secularized, and many people are only nominal Jews, Christians, Buddhists, etc. Even among adherents to the various religions, strength of belief and observance in practice is highly variable. Contemporary city territories and styles are informal and do not support religious observances.

A religion that is viable grows and evolves. As long as adherents give credence to the beliefs that underlie a rite, it will be performed in the right spirit. When they are disillusioned, it loses meaning and observance degenerates through erosion to detachment (*pro forma* observance) to separation (non-observance). In general, new converts are likely to be more zealous in observance than those who are raised in the faith. Thus, strength of belief and importance of adherence must be ascertained before implementing a diet or feeding program.

Spontaneous interpretations and revelations introduce new precepts that wax and wane. Over the centuries, splinter groups retaining the old or following the new break away from the main group. Thus, many versions coexist under the umbrella of a particular family of religions. No attempt has been made to identify all of the versions, since more than 500 are practiced in the United States.

A common religious belief is that people are capable of perfection and are responsible for choosing between right and wrong. Food is of fundamental importance in sustaining the physical body and is consumed several times a day, so it is a suitable vehicle for nourishing the soul by (a) communication with God by saying grace; (b) demonstrating faith through acceptance and observance of scriptural directions with respect to what may be consumed as food, what might otherwise be consumed as food but is detrimental to health, and the spirit with which food is to be consumed; and (c) developing discipline via fasting.

Observable behaviors with respect to choice of kind, quality, and amount of food consumed as well as food and people interactions also reflect obedience to and application of particular church dogmas. The subsequent discussion identifies similarities and differences among various religions, to the extent possible, given variability in the comprehensiveness of materials provided by the various churches.

All religions appear to have originally incorporated a belief that the provision of food involves some relation with the divine. However, in some of the older religions, only vestiges of the belief and means of observance remain. Christians have been provided with a scriptural admonition (1 Cor. 10:31):

Whether therefore ye eat, or drink, or whatsoever ye do, do all to the glory of God. (KJV)

This is the basic rule. All others are subsumed and provide specific guidance for dealing with particular positions which people always have taken that place an undesirable strain on food and people interactions.

Some Christian sects recognize and promote the ideal of religious liberty in a sense that precludes an official position or guidance with respect to social habits, diet, and domestic customs. Practices and avoidances involving food and people interactions are an individual matter. Churches with this persuasion include, but are not limited to, Baptist, Congregational, and Methodist.

Communication with God

A blessing is a short prayer said before a meal to ask God to bestow his favor on those assembled in order that the food might nourish the participant's body. A grace is a short prayer said at the close of a meal to express thankfulness or to acknowledge God's hand in what has been provided as a source of nourishment. Judaism, Islam, and Christianity have a precedent in a song of praise (Psalm 145:15):

The eyes of all wait upon thee; and thou givest them their meat in due season. (KJV)[1]

Both a blessing and a grace create a meal climate that affects the tone of the food and people interactions. When a sacrilegious grace such as "Rub-a-dub-dub, thanks God for the grub," is said, the tone of the meal tends to be light and joking; barbed, critical remarks about the food and/or cook are not uncommon. When a heartfelt grace is said, those who partake of the meal usually are more restrained and will refrain from disparaging remarks about the food and/or cook. Other aspects of table conversation are similarly constrained. Moreover, there is incentive to avoid misuse of the food provided. Thus, overindulgence, waste by taking more than can be consumed, and "pickiness" are less likely. The practice of asking a blessing or saying grace is practiced alone and in public by Jews, Protestants of all sects, Roman Catholics, Eastern Orthodox, Mormons, and Muslims.

The custom of offering a blessing by Jews and Christians is documented in scripture: Those seeking a seer were instructed that they might find him in a certain place on the day of sacrifice. (1 Sam. 9:13)

. . . for the people will not eat until he comes, because he doth bless the sacrifice; *and* afterwards they eat that be bidden. (KJV)

The model for behavior of Christians is contained in Acts 27:35:

And when he had thus spoken, he took bread, and gave thanks to God in presence of them all; and when he had broken *it*, he began to eat. (KJV)

Demonstration of Faith

Sharing of food to indicate a bond of friendship is an old Judeo-Christian tradition, as recorded in scripture (11 Sam. 9:7, 10, 11, 13). Similarly, to refuse food was an indication of anger (1 Sam. 20:34). Both aspects are recognized today. Churches in which fellowship and the interpersonal bond of love is strong emphasize this aspect. This is characteristic of Islam, Jehovah's Witnesses, Judaism, the Lutheran Family, Mormons, and Pentecostals.

Hospitality is encouraged by many religions; general scriptural references are numerous. For Christians, the specific scriptural references specify that hospitality is to be extended only to fellow Christians (1 Pet. 4:9 and 11 John 9−11).

---

[1] KJV = King James Version.

The custom of giving food gifts to gain or ensure the goodwill of another is an old Judaic custom. It puts the receiver under obligation to observe peaceful relations. Scriptural examples are 1 Sam. 25:18, 19, and 1 Ki. 14:1−3.

Gathering of relatives to partake of a common meal is one function recognized by many religious sects, including Catholic, Protestant, Mormon, Seventh Day Adventist, and Jewish. Some Oriental and African religions, especially polytheistic ones, do not; meals are consumed by members of the sexes separately and small children eat with the women.

A common Christian view with a scriptural basis (St. John 6:63) is:

It is the spirit that quickeneth; the flesh profiteth nothing...

This is true in all domains. Thus, the spirit with which food is consumed is the critical variable in obtaining maximum nourishment from food. Moreover, in this domain, the Christian view builds on the scriptural precedents of Judaism. (Prov. 15:17):

Better *is* a dinner of herbs where love is, than a stalled ox and hatred therewith. (KJV)

When people get along in harmony, food and people interactions are friendly, hearty, and pleasant. In this case, the meal is satisfying even if the actual food is limited to vegetables, i.e., the food of the poor. When people do not get along because of mutual envy and strife, malice causes hating and being hated. In this case, a prime cut from the best feedlot steer (the "stalled ox") cannot normalize the food and people interactions, so the meal is not satisfying. Hence, of the two alternatives, less desirable food is preferable to undesirable food and people interactions.

Another associated scriptural point (Eccl. 2:24) is:

There is nothing better for man, *than* that he should eat and drink and *that* he should make his soul enjoy good in his labor. This also I saw, that it *was* from the hand of God. (KJV)

One of the meanings of *enjoy* is "to have for one's use or benefit." Thus, in this context, it means that wages from labor should be used to provide food and drink for the body and the spirit. It is easily seen that this basic provision is from the hand of God.

Rest from work and cares on the Sabbath was enjoined on the Jews by Mosaic Law. This is a traditional convention observed to a variable degree by some Christian sects. The exception is the Mormons, on whom it was enjoined by prophetic revelation. Thus, Orthodox Jews do no food preparation on the Sabbath. One-dish meals requiring long, slow cooking overnight have been devised for Sabbath meals and are customary, as are cold food items. Similarly, since the Lord's Day is observed as a day of rest by the Mormons, basic preparation is completed the preceding day; this minimizes exertion. Finish food preparation designed to produce a meal that will evoke joy, thanksgiving, and cheerfulness is allowed by Mormon doctrine (D&C 59:13).[1]

In Judaism, the definition of what is food is delimited as a means to self-mastery. Hence, the stated position: "The dietary laws train us in the mastery over our principles, not to consider the pleasure of eating and drinking as the end of man's existence." (Maimonides)

The definition of what is food is also delimited by concepts of sanctity of life. Reverence for life is shown by different means in Eastern and Western religions. Vegetarianism, a feature of several Oriental religions (Buddhism, Hinduism), is the overt manifestation of a reverence for life. In some cases, meat is proscribed because of an associated belief that the souls of those who did not do well during their human existence devolve to lower forms in the subsequent incarnation, so reside in animals. To consume the flesh of animals so regarded would be tantamount to cannibalism.

In Western religions, proscription of blood as food is the overt manifestation of reverence for life. Consumption of blood was first forbidden to Noah (Gen. 9:4) and then was detailed in the Mosaic Law (Lev. 17:10–14):

And whatsoever man *there be* of the house of Israel, or of the strangers that sojourn among you, that eateth any manner of blood; I will even set my face against that soul that eateth blood, and will cut him off from among his people.

For the life of the flesh *is* in the blood. . .

Therefore, I said unto the children of Israel, No soul of you shall eat blood, neither shall any stranger that sojourneth among you eat blood.

And whatsoever man *there be* of the children of Israel, or of the strangers that sojourn among you, which hunteth and catcheth any beast or fowl that may be eaten; he shall even pour out the blood thereof, and cover it with dust.

For *it is* the life of all flesh; the blood of it *is* for life thereof; therefore I said unto the children of Israel, Ye shall eat the blood of no manner of flesh: for the life of all flesh *is* the blood thereof: whosoever eateth it shall be cut off. (KJV)

These scriptures are the basis for the koshering process (see discussion of Jewish foodways).

In New Testament times, the apostles and elders decreed that Christians should abstain from blood (Acts 15:20, 29; 21:25). Hence, consumption of blood puddings and blood sausages, etc., is forbidden.

In some of the other religions, the sanctity of life is expressed via strictures regarding the foods to eat for "health" and proscriptions to be observed to prevent bodily harm. Three major religions assert the im-

---

[1] D & C = Doctrine and Covenants of the Church of Jesus Christ of Latter-Day Saints.

portance of consuming a well balanced diet in order to nourish the body as the temple in which the soul resides. These are Seventh Day Adventists, Mormons, and Muslims.

For Seventh Day Adventists, the scriptural basis for their health emphasis is 1 Cor. 3:16—17:

> Know ye not that ye are the temple of God and *that* the spirit of God dwelleth within you?
> If any man defile the temple of God, him shall God destroy; for the temple of God is holy, which *temple* ye are. (KJV)

Ellen White (née Harmon), inspired by divine visions, called members' attention to their duty to maintain health by temperance in eating, drinking, and drugging. A corollary belief is that the body will function best on a diet of simple foods, i.e., grains, fruits, vegetables, and nuts. However, most members are lacto-ovo vegetarians. The rejection of flesh foods has three bases: (a) avoidance of scripturally unclean foods such as pork, (b) the suggestion that meat consumption causes diseases, and (c) the suggestion that meat consumption makes people more animalistic and less humanly sympathetic. Stimulants such as coffee, tea, alcohol, and tobacco are proscribed and use of strong spices and condiments that might harm the digestive tract is discouraged. Between-meal eating also is discouraged in order to rest the digestive organs.

For Mormons, the scriptural basis for their health emphasis has several scriptural bases including that of 1 Cor. 3:16—17 (quoted above) and D&C 89:18, 20:

> And all saints who remember to keep and do these sayings, walking in obedience to the commandments, shall receive health in their navel and marrow to their bones; ...
> And shall run and not be weary, and shall walk and not faint.

Prophetic revelation incapsulated as what is called the Word of Wisdom provides details in keeping the scripture of 1 Cor. 3:16—17. The basic point is stated as follows (D&C 89:10—12):

> And again, verily I say unto you, all wholesome herbs God hath ordained for the constitution, nature, and use of man—
> Every herb in the season thereof, and every fruit in the season thereof; all these to be used with prudence and thanksgiving.
> Yea, flesh also of beasts and of the fowls of the air, I the Lord, have ordained for the use of man with thanksgiving, nevertheless they are to be used sparingly;—

Other strictures recommend abstinence from alcohol (D&C 89:7), tobacco (D&C 89:8), and hot drinks such as coffee and tea (D&C 89:9).

Subsequent interpretation has extended the meaning of the latter to include cola drinks and other caffeine-containing foods. These doctrinal strictures were revealed in modern times. Hence, they supersede the scriptural injunctions. Furthermore, Mormons are expected to get enough physical exercise to maintain a healthy physique; obesity is not condoned. And, individual intolerances to particular foods are acknowledged and respected.

Other Christian sects, including Jehovah's Witnesses, take the position that individual Christians are personally responsible for ascertaining unhealthy sensitivities related to consumption of particular foods, i.e., alcoholic beverages, caffeine-containing beverages, sugar and/or honey, and salt. Individual sensitivities are regarded as dictating individual abstinence. These sects affirm the position that scripture does not categorically condemn consumption *per se*, but rather unwise selection or quantity. Additional scriptural wisdom (Prov. 25:16, 27) is also cited:

Hast thou found honey? eat so much as is sufficient for thee, lest thou be filled therewith, and vomit it.
It is not good to eat much honey; so *for men* to search their own glory *is not* glory. (KJV)

For Muslims, prophetic revelation documented in the Koran forbids consumption of the flesh of animals that die of disease or strangulation, blood, pork, or wine or other alcoholic beverages. Muslims are exhorted to eat foods necessary for development of strong bodies. To this end, a number of foods are stipulated: honey, milk, dates, meat, seafood, sweets, and vegetable oil. Fasting is used as a periodic means of restricting food intake for reasons of health.

The basic scriptural definition of food that is accepted by Jews and Christians alike is Gen. 1:29:

. . . I have given you every herb bearing seed, which *is* upon the face of all the earth, and every tree, in which *is* the fruit of a tree yielding seed; to you it shall be for meat. (KJV)

Thus, until the Flood, man was vegetarian. The distinction between clean and unclean animals apparently referred only to fitness for sacrificial purposes. After the Flood, Noah was instructed (Gen. 9:3, 4):

Every moving thing that liveth shall be meat for you; even as the green herb have I given you all things.
But the flesh with the life thereof, *which* is the blood thereof, shall ye not eat. (KJV)

Although God had decreed that man could eat all flesh, Mosaic law as interpreted by the Jewish rabbis prevented practicing Jews from consuming pork, shellfish, etc. (see discussion of Jewish foodways). In contrast, Christians were specifically warned by the Holy Spirit against such prohibitions as doctrines of the devil (1 Tim. 4:1, 3):

> . . . *and commanding* to abstain from meats, which God hath created to be received with thanksgiving of them which believe and know the truth. (KJV)

Thus, for many Christians, a religious regulation prohibiting consumption of meat is viewed as evidence that a religion is degenerate and has accepted doctrines of the devil. Jehovah's Witnesses and Mormons are warned against this problem.

Continuing, scripture indicates that any food can be eaten (1 Tim. 4:4—5):

> For every creature of God *is* good, and nothing to be refused, if it be received with thanksgiving;
> For it is sanctified by the word of God and prayer. (KJV)

Jews, Christians, and Muslims have long been informed of the proper way of dealing with drunkards and gluttons. Scriptural counsel is as follows (Deut. 21:20—21):

> And they shall say unto the elders of his city, This our son *is* stubborn and rebellious, he will not obey our voice; *he is* a glutton, and a drunkard.
> And all the men of his city shall stone him with stones, that he die: so shalt thou put away evil from among you; and all Israel shall hear, and fear. (KJV)

Warnings with respect to the consequences of intemperate eating and drinking have scriptural bases in many religions; in others, alcohol is proscribed, as noted. Scripture accepted by Jews, Muslims, and Christians (Prov. 20:1) says:

> Wine is a mocker, strong drink *is* raging; and whosoever is deceived thereby is not wise. (KJV)

Old Testament scripture provides further guidance for Jews, most Christians, including Pentecostal, and Muslims (Prov. 23:20, 21):

> Be not among winebibbers; among riotous eaters of flesh.
> For the drunkard and the glutton shall come to poverty: and drowsiness shall clothe a man in rags. (KJV)

This rather graphically depicts the effects. Excesses of wine and meat lead to drowsiness. As a result, men are stupified so that they cannot pay attention to their business by which they provide for themselves and their families. Then, their excesses become costly and they are impoverished. Clearly, this is a food and people interaction in which "the food and drink get even with the person." Thus, believers are warned against greediness leading to intemperance.

Use of alcohol in moderation is not forbidden. In fact, scripture acknowledges that wine is associated with joy and pleasure (Eccl. 9:7; John 2:2−10) and can be used to calm people in distress (Prov. 31:6, 7):

> Give strong drink unto him that is ready to perish, and wine unto these that be of heavy hearts.
> Let him drink, and forget his poverty, and remember his misery no more. (KJV)

Eating/not eating proscribed foods as a matter of conscience is another function circumscribed by religious strictures. For each dispensation (period in time involving a system of revealed commands and promises regulating human affairs), there has been a somewhat different set of particulars, apparently according to the needs of time and place. Thus, even for the sake of courtesy, practicing Jews, Hindus, Muslims, and members of some Christian sects do not consume proscribed foods. Following New Testament scriptures, Catholic and most Protestant sects do not make an issue of eating/not eating particular foods (Col. 2:16, 17; 1 Cor. 10:25-27, 31-32):

> Let no man therefore judge you in meat, or in drink . . . which are a shadow of things to come . . . (KJV)
> You may eat anything sold in the meat-market without raising questions of conscience; for the earth is the Lord's and everything *in* it.
> If an unbeliever invited you to a meal and you care to go, eat whatever is put before you, without raising questions of conscience.
> Well, whether you eat or drink, or whatever you are doing, do all for the honour of God; give no offence to Jews, or Greeks, or to the church of God. For my part I always try to meet everybody half-way, regarding not my own good but the good of the many . . . (NE)[1]

The point that Christians should not offend by eating/not eating particular foods is outlined in detail (Rom. 14: 1-23) and is reiterated (1 Cor. 8:1-13). This is coupled with the concept that one should not superimpose his food beliefs/practices on others. The reasons given are that (a) eating/not eating food X does not make or break a Christian, so it is not important enough to justify grieving others or becoming a model to lead another away from his/her beliefs (no matter how misguided they may

---

[1] NE = New English Version.

be), (b) out of respect for others one must not despise those with a more restricted definition of what is food, and in turn, the latter must not judge the former to be loose, (c) when in doubt about whether a food should be eaten/not eaten, then one should abstain, unless to do so would create a problem for others.

Some Protestant sects emphasize one aspect of the rules (Rom. 14:21):

It is a fine thing to abstain from eating meat or drinking wine, or doing anything which causes your brother's downfall (NE)

Thus, some groups, e.g., Southern Baptists, proscribe alcohol under any circumstances but otherwise consume whatever is offered, so as not to offend.

Mormonism is an exception among Christian sects in that proscriptions are observed as a matter of conscience. The underlying belief is that in these trying latter days, additional prophetic revelation known as the Word of Wisdom was given as a guide. Expedience and the possibility of giving offense to a fellow man are not accepted as relevant considerations for these times.

Fasting

Fasting is another common practice. Although exotic Oriental philosophical/religious styles of fasting recently have been applied in bizarre ways by Western atheists and agnostics, our Judeo-Christian heritage is not without precedents for fasting.

Jews have fasted since early times. The New Testament refers to Jewish observance of public fasts but nowhere does it contain a command enjoining Christian fasts. But, there is scriptural precedent for Christian fasting (Acts 13:2-3, 14-23). Catholics, some Protestant sects, and Mormons have long practiced fasting. In general, Christians are enjoined to give no outward sign of fasting; there is no merit, if one is praised for it (Matt. 6:17-18).

The World Food Problem developed in 1974. The World Council of Churches responded by recommending that one day per month be set apart as a fast day to save food for those in need. The various sects have used the released funds for various charitable purposes, including support of foreign disaster feeding programs.

Muslims observe three kinds of fasts (see discussion of Muslim foodways).

Jewish Fasting.—Fasts originally were observed by all of the people and their animals. Rabbinical exemptions for children under the age of 12, the ill, pregnant and lactating women, the very elderly, and animals have been granted since. On ordinary fast days, no food or drink is consumed during daylight hours. On special fast days, the fast is for the full 24 hours and extends to abstinence from other stipulated sources of sensual gratification. Fasts are one, three, or seven days in length; they usually do not include the Sabbath or festival periods. Public fast days are Mondays and Thursdays. Partial fasts limited to abstension from meat, wine, and pleasure also are observed, sometimes only for a few hours.

In common with other Near Eastern religions, fasting is viewed by Jews as the means of getting requests filled by God. God is expected to note that the pious afflict themselves as a symbol of humility and, therefore, compassion is called for. Exigencies for which fasting has a scriptural precedent are:

(a) To show Godly sorrow and repentence (1 Sam. 7:60, Joel 2:12-15, Jonah 3:5)

(b) In the face of great danger to avert or terminate a great calamity (11 Chron. 20:3, Esther 4:3)

(c) When in great need of divine guidance, especially when going on a journey (Ezra 8:21)

(d) When enduring tests and meeting temptations (Joel 2:12-15)

(e) When studying, meditating, or concentrating on understanding God's purposes

In modern times, only 2 fasts are widely observed: Yom Kippur (Day of Atonement), a complete 24-hour fast (Lev. 16:29-31, 23:27-32) and the Ninth of Av.

Jewish fasts are classified into 3 groups:

(a) Fasts decreed by God or referred to in scripture: Day of Atonement, Ninth of Av, 17th of Tammuz, 3rd of Tishri, and Fast of Esther

(b) Fasts decreed by the rabbis (selected): Ten Days of Penitence (between Rosh Hashanah and the Day of Atonement), the first Monday and Thursday following Passover and Sukkoth, 8 Thursdays in winter, the Three Weeks of Mourning between the 17th of Tammuz and the Ninth of Av, Seventh of Adar, Eve of Passover (firstborn males)

(c) Private fasts: anniversaries of parents' deaths or that of an esteemed teacher, the wedding day until the ceremony, as appropriate to avert the evil effects of nightmares.

Catholic Fasting.—Jesus affirmed the principle of fasting but left no rules. As a result, beliefs and practices have evolved over time; these differ among the various branches of the Catholic Church:

(a) Roman Catholic. Abstinence and fast have different meanings. Abstinence means that no meat is consumed, but the quantity of other foods is not restricted. Fast means that the total quantity of food is limited. Fast days are not observed by the ill. Current fasts include:

-40 days of Lent; each individual (children only?) gives up one favorite item which may be a food

-Ember Days—instituted in the 11th Century and discontinued as fast days in 1966. These are a relic of the old stations (weekly fast days), observed on Wednesdays, Fridays, and Saturdays in winter (the week after the third Sunday in Advent), in spring (the week after the first Sunday in Lent), in summer (the eight-day period beginning with Pentecost), and in autumn (the week after September 14, the Feast of Holy Cross).

-Rogation Days (gang days)—the three days before Holy Thursday. April 25 is the date of a pagan ceremony called the Robigalia, which was celebrated to protect sprouting crops from blight by rust or *robigo* by offering the entrails of a dog and a sheep to the god Robigus. Rogation Days supplant this ceremony and utilize processions or gangs.

-All Fridays, except Christmas Day if it falls on Friday

-Vigils before certain festivals

(b) Eastern Orthodox. *Fast* means abstinence from meat and other animal products including milk, cheese, eggs, and butter; fish (except clams, shrimp, and oysters); and some groups proscribe olive oil but not olives. Fast days are not observed by the ill.

Current fasts include:

-40 days of Lent (obligatory)—pre-Lenten preparation involves Meat Fare Sunday two weeks before Lent on which all remaining meat or fish is consumed. Cheese, eggs, milk, and butter are permitted during the ensuing week through Cheese Fare Sunday on which all remaining is consumed. Thereafter, that is, during Lent, none of these items are consumed except fish, which is consumed on Palm Sunday and on the Annunciation Day of the Virgin Mary.

-Fast of the Apostles for the octave of Pentecost to June 29th, St. Peter and St. Paul's Day

-Fast of the Mother of God—August 1 through 14

-Fast of the Nativity of Our Lord (Advent)—the 40 days between November 15 and December 25

-Decollation of John Baptist—August 29

-Holy Cross Day—September 14

-Wednesdays and Fridays throughout the year (obligatory), except on the day before Ascension Day (40 days after Easter) on which oil, wine, and fish are allowed

Protestant Fasting.—Although there is Biblical precedent for fasting, many Protestant churches do not encourage fasting. Those that do, including Pentecostal, regard fasting as a personal spontaneous act. Modes of fasting vary; fasts may be partial or complete, from brief periods of one meal to extended periods of several days.

Mormon Fasting.—Fasts are to be observed only by saints (members) in sound physical and mental health, so that there will be no adverse effects. Prophetic revelation of the Lord's command to continue in fasting and prayer (D&C 88:76) is partially implemented by organized fasting one day per month (instituted in 1855 as the first Thursday; changed in 1896 to the first Sunday (Rich 1972)). This is a 24-hour fast, from Saturday evening to Sunday evening, and includes abstinence from food, drink, and other forms of bodily gratification and indulgence. One of the chief purposes of fasting is the contribution of the food saved, or its equivalent in money, for the welfare of the poor. To be of value, fasting must be observed in the right spirit; true and hypocritical observances are contrasted (Isa. 58:3–8) and provide scriptural guidance. Additional discretionary fast days are observed as spiritual preparation for a variety of church rituals and purposes by participating individuals.

Buddhist Fasting.—Buddha was opposed to asceticism because in his view it was excessive, and anything excessive was anathema. Fasting was discredited in the *Dhammapada*. Several passages state that fasting is not useful to a person who has failed to overcome desire; fasts cannot purify the passions. Nonetheless, fasting was enjoined by monastic regulations; all males are expected to serve as monks for some period of time in their lives. The different monastic orders developed distinctive fasting regulations. In general, fasting is to be done for the sake of joy, frugality, purity, and contentedness. Hence, fasts are to be restrained rather than complete and prolonged. Fasting is practiced by monks and the laity as meritorious discipline. Ordinarily, they eat only at noon, only what is contained in the alms-bowl; second helpings are declined, and no food is consumed between meals. Water is permitted *ad libitum*. Complete fasts are observed four times per month, including the days of the new and full moon.

Muslim Fasting.—Mohammed, the prophet of Islam, was opposed to asceticism and did not advocate fasting. Nonetheless, prestigious followers instituted the practice of fasting as a time of reaffirmation of faith and for the remission of sins. Fasting is from sunrise to sunset; no food or drink is taken (requiring much discipline in lands where daytime temperatures may reach 140°F). Young children, the aged, the ill, travelers, and pregnant or lactating mothers are exempt from fasting. However, days missed for reasons of travel, pregnancy or lactation must be made up. (See discussion of Muslim foodways for particulars.)

Feasting associated with religious holidays is a common feature of many religions. Observance varies from vestiges of traditional rituals to a vital component of contemporary celebration. Feasting is a prominent feature of the Oriental religions. It is much less important to Christianity; indeed, it is not observed by some sects. Thus, important holy days are celebrated by Buddhists, Hindus, Jews, and Muslims with a feast. Holy days are joyous occasions to be celebrated with good food;

special foods are prepared and served on each. Involved ritual preparation is customary. For the Christian, plenty of somewhat dressed-up foods and a few traditional items are more typical. However, Pentecostals do not observe special feast days. In contrast, Lutherans feast by having pot-luck dinners to welcome new members, as socials, when the congregation gathers to vote and on secular and religious holidays as well. Even Sunday service is an occasion for coffee and sweets in most congregations.

Clearly the foodways and food and people interactions are greatly affected by religion, though each group has its own variation. To relate to peoples with differing beliefs one must expand one's consciousness and then proceed with sensitivity.

FOODS AND NUTRITION: "DOING YOUR OWN THING"

One of the answers to the question "Why do people eat or not eat X?" results from an attitude that values (or does not value) the use of foods and nutrition as a medium for self-actualization. Self-actualization or the power to express oneself is the lowest level of basic need. It is emphasized when higher level needs have been satisfied to some degree.

The food and people interaction provides many opportunities for self-expression that can be rewarding. The traditional role of a woman included home food production and service. But, over time the necessity for the woman to perform these functions diminished. So, now any family member can use this domain for self-expression. Increasingly, men have become weekend chefs, teenagers have made divinity or brownies, and even pre-school children have learned to prepare simple foods.

The problem in using food and people interactions for self-expression reduces to one of selecting which food(s) and which social food-serving situation(s) can be developed as a personal trademark for purposes of identity. The item(s) so selected then becomes a part of the array of foods consumed. The explanation for inclusion in the diet is that the item(s) is served because Person A enjoys preparing it.

Self-actualization can mean a number of things, for example: preparing tasty nutritious meals; developing skill in home gardening, home canning or home freezing, or home baking of breads, cakes, pies, or cookies; preparing ethnic meals; or preparing buffet and bridge luncheons that are perfect. On the other hand, it may mean development of a limited skill such as the ability to char-broil steaks, to make fudge or divinity, or to bake brownies. The range of possibilities is almost endless. In recent years, the domestic arts associated with food and people interactions have been revived for the specific purpose of self-expression.

The American culture traditionally has valued skill in the domestic arts. In part this stems from the early need to help family members deal with a hard existence in a hostile untamed land. The kitchen was the center of the home. And, a woman was valued if she could provide tasty meals and serve them in such a way as to affirm the strength and serenity of the family as a support unit.

But times and attitudes change. By 1938, the role of the food and people interaction in family support had diminished and had been devalued. The standard food and nutrition text of the day, *Feeding the Family* by Mary Swartz Rose, made the following point:

"I shouldn't mind housekeeping if it were not for planning meals"—how often have we heard this? There is a sort of inevitableness about meals which makes then seem truly awful at times. A hungry family and nothing on the table is terrible to contemplate. But routine (drudgery if you will) loses much of its depressing power when work gains significance. To see the children rosy, the family accounts free from doctor's bills, and an atmosphere of serenity in the home are surely compensations for the time and thought given to family meals[1]

The tradition-directed person can relate to this quotation. A person of this nature will begin to value the development of necessary skills and will find many opportunities for self-expression through food. But, before he/she can fully use this mechanism for self-actualization, the individual first has to value consumption of a nutritionally adequate diet. A person growing up in a home where tasty nutritious meals are valued may take them for granted. This depends on the amount and kind of dialogue in the home. Some homemakers are good providers out of duty. Others do it for the love and joy of it. Duty tends to generate neutral to negative feelings resulting in taking it for granted. Whereas, love and joy communicate a positive value.

In the 1970s Americans rejected the value of providing good meals. In part, this probably was because so few women had or would take the necessary time. Also, reasonably high quality convenience foods of many types became available. And, another set of factors may have been operative. Compared with previous times, children were healthy, people were relatively affluent and did not bother to calculate small differences in costs, and home serenity became only a dream, given the number of factors beyond immediate control. So, for many the value of attempting to provide good meals degenerated. For some, these points were less important so devaluation did not occur.

Because many devalued the traditional role of a woman in providing

---

[1] From Rose (1938). Copyrighted by and quoted with permission of the Macmillan Publishing Co., Inc.

tasty nutritious meals, the inner-directed person may have opted to use some aspect of the food and people interaction for self-actualization. Mastery, or "I can do X," is a power-giving self-concept. IF home-grown, home canned, home frozen, or home baked goods are valued, THEN a person is usually motivated to develop skills for producing them. Today, when skills of these types are unnecessary, pride in mastery becomes a value. So, new methods and new recipes have been introduced. These frequently use spices, seeds, honey, and other uncommon ingredients for reasons of distinctiveness. In this way, because these specialty items are produced they are consumed.

The other-directed person will utilize the food and people interaction or some aspect of it, for self-actualization if it is the current fad. Thus, in recent years, because there has been a wave of interest in foods and nutrition, those with skills in this area have reaped the rewards and have acquired status.

Food quality and other aspects of usual food and people interactions are symbols of high quality of life. Sharply rising food prices have threatened, if not reduced, customary levels of consumption. This is viewed as undermining and inconsistent with concepts of appropriate quality of life. Hence, resentment, resistance, and hostility have become manifest.

Some skills in food purchasing, money management, and the like have been revalued upward to meet the crisis. To maintain a normal facade and avoid embarrassment with respect to the question "Why do you eat or not eat X?," many have begun to employ these skills quietly and privately. To maintain quality of life in the face of rising food costs is not easy. According to Rose (1938), ". . . the satisfaction of ceasing to grope blindly (which is drudgery) and acquiring a conscious power over one's environment. . . makes even the difficult task interesting and joyous."[1] Thus, one way to fulfill one's self is to join the skill to work with the will to work in maintaining life-style. The food and people interactions provide many opportunities to do this.

BIBLIOGRAPHY

CROMWELL, C. 1976. Organic foods—an update. Fam. Econ. Rev., Consumer & Food Econ. Inst., Agric. Res. Serv., USDA, Washington, D.C.

FESTINGER, L. 1962. Cognitive dissonance. Sci. Am. *207* (10) 93-102.

MASLOW, A.H. 1943. A theory of human motivation. Psychol. Rev. *50*, 370-396.

NIXON, R.M. 1970A. Message of the President on appointing Jean Mayer to organize the Conference. *In* White House Conference on Food, Nutrition and Health, Final Report. GPO, Washington, D.C.

---

[1] From Rose (1938). Copyrighted by and quoted with permission of the Macmillan Publishing Co., Inc.

NIXON, R.M. 1970B. Message of the President to the Congress of the United States. *In* White House Conference on Food, Nutrition and Health. GPO, Washington, D.C.

RICH, R.R. 1972. Ensign to the Nation. BYU Publications, Provo, Utah.

ROSE, M.S. 1938. Feeding the Family. Macmillan, New York.

16

What Is Food? What Is Poison?

In man's near environment, there always have been many items that man perceived might be used for food. At the same time, some peoples have avoided eating available plant or animal tissues (specific items or classes of items) that could be used for food, as demonstrated by the fact that other peoples used them for food. That is, by convention, particular peoples had decreed that selected food items are inedible or poisons, i.e., something that would cause illness or death. Early on, man also learned that what appeared to be food might turn out to be poison and that some means to distinguish between the two classes of items was necessary in order to prevent illness and/or death. As man learned to sort items into "food" and "poison," some definitions and generalizations regarding the basis for sorting emerged.

This chapter reviews alternative definitions of food and poison from a variety of perspectives that account for the decision to eat/not eat an item. Topics include:

(a) Food rejection: food avoidances and food proscriptions
(b) Physiological definitions of food and poison
(c) Emotional/psychological definitions of food and poison
(d) Socio-cultural definitions of food and poison
(e) Health-related definitions of food and poison
(f) Economic definitions of food and poison
(g) Aesthetic definitions of food and poison
(h) Subgroup definitions of food and poison

An understanding of the various definitions of food and poison is a necessary prerequisite for the professional who is involved in assessment of an individual's relation to his/her food environment. Food avoidances restrict the array of foods consumed. The probability of an adequate nutrient intake is reduced and may vanish.

Since for a particular individual or group any food may be regarded as either food or poison, one must ascertain how it is classified. Using a standardized list of items with provision for write-ins, one may observe and/or question individuals or groups. Preferred items evoke an active response. Preferred foods are consumed by choice and will continue to be classified as food except under unusual circumstances. Items that are proscribed will be classed as poisons as long as the supporting beliefs continue.

IF one pursues the matter beyond the first response, THEN one usually finds that some items may be classified as either food or poison, depending on the circumstances. Items that are barely accepted evoke a passive response. They are consumed for lack of an alternative. Given an alternative, acceptance turns to rejection. Under special circumstances, some items that normally are avoided might be consumed. Without an understanding of the reasons for the distinction, one cannot predict the classification of these items.

FOOD REJECTION: FOOD AVOIDANCES AND PROSCRIPTIONS

Rejection of any food item or class of items is an overt individual action that may result from beliefs, attitudes, and/or intentions. Reasons for the action generally may be classed as personal avoidances or collective conventions and proscriptions. However, collective reasons must be internalized to be implemented. So, in the final analysis, all reasons are personal reflecting individual will.

Personal Avoidances

The degree of preference for or avoidance of an item is determined partly by exposure to and experience with it. For example, if a preferred food is served with a high frequency, one may become tired of it. Then one may rebel and avoid it, perhaps permanently. Or, a food that is usually enjoyed may have no appeal and may be avoided during illness. Or, a food that is preferred may not look quite right and may be temporarily avoided. This is especially likely to occur if previous experience with variable quality resulted in a negative association between appearance and presence of a defect that was unpleasant or harmful.

The array of reasons based on beliefs and attitudes is extensive. Many intentions are logical outgrowths. These include, but are not limited to, the following types:

(a) health-related—"I ate X and got a stomachache; I will never eat X again."

(b) association—"I had a pet duck (rabbit, goat, or whatever); I could never eat duck (or whatever)."

(c) surfeit—"I once had to eat turkey (or whatever) every day for period X; I can not tolerate the smell of it cooking much less eating it."

(d) snobbery—"Lesser beings of type X eat X; how could you suggest that a person of my class eat X!"

(e) preference—"I dislike X (no particular reason that I can (or will) state); I will never eat X."

(f) indifference—"I don't care that much about X; I just don't think of it."

Some people have an attitude that they have been eating food X all of their lives, so they will not stop for any reason. Others have the attitude that they have never eaten item X and will not start. In these cases, preferences or avoidances are based on permanent intentions.

Collective Conventions

Items that are defined as "food" may be avoided in a specific instance because they are perceived to be inappropriate under the circumstances. These are collective conventions; several examples follow:

(a) instant orange juice—It would be selected by those who prefer it, usually at breakfast or between meals. It would be avoided at lunch and dinner as unsuitable.

(b) butterscotch sauce—This item usually is served in conjunction with a dessert, which is served at lunch, dinner or p.m. snack. It would be avoided as inappropriate at breakfast as it would not complement the items served.

(c) mixed sweet pickles—This item usually is served with a sandwich. It is not appropriate at breakfast. Formerly, they were a daily accompaniment at both lunch and dinner meals. They were homemade and available. But, for whatever reasons, at the present time they are not valued enough to warrant purchase in a quantity sufficient for daily service. The result is that now it is considered inappropriate to serve them routinely at both lunch and dinner.

This type of avoidance is passive and simply results in failure to select. It is in contrast to other types of avoidance which are more active in that an emotional/psychological response is added to the avoidance behavior.

Because what we eat is limited largely to what items are commercially available, most people are only vaguely aware that they would avoid certain other foods. IF a person were to inquire whether an individual would eat dog or snake, THEN the individual would say no. But, IF the individual were asked to list items not eaten, THEN such items probably would not be recalled. They just are not considered as a possible source of food. For this reason, this emotional/psychological response is probably less than in an individual who has been trained to avoid such items. So, they are not recalled because by convention they are ignored.

Collective Proscriptions

Since the Year One, in almost every society, collective proscriptions have been used as a powerful means for social control. Society has used a number of measures to ensure that members were conscious of tabooed foods and would overreact if they ate a forbidden food, no matter how inadvertently. To this end, a response of fear and horror of the magnitude elicited by a callous murder was carefully cultivated.

Before proceeding with discussion, a number of terms need to be defined. Some of these are used with a meaning that differs from the popular one. Terms called to reader attention are:

(a) food—A solid or liquid that is consumed by members of a group. Context must be specified, because the definition applies only given a definition of the group's culture at a stated place and time.

(b) food aversion—An intense or definite dislike accompanied by feelings of repugnance, loathing, and/or revulsion. It is an avoidance based on an ingrained feeling against an item that is perceived to be disagreeable and offensive.

-repugnance—An emotional opposition to items incompatible with one's ideas and tastes; e.g., snake or lizard meat would evoke this response.

-loathing—An expression of extreme disgust.

-revulsion—A drawing away from the item in horror, e.g., the physical and mental response to the idea of eating pet dog.

(c) proscribe—To condemn or forbid as harmful; prohibit. Proscriptions are disseminated by formal decree.

(d) proscription—This is an imposed restraint or restriction.

(e) defiled—A person, place, or thing that is inherently or (corrupted so as to become) dirty or unclean, hence unfit.

-unclean—It is prohibited for use or contact (by ritual law). The implication is that the item is infected with harmful supernatural contagion.

-unfit—Not suitable.

-ceremonially defiled—Contact with X makes one unclean, according to church rules.

(f) religious observance—A customary practice or ceremony or an instance of following a religious custom, rule, or law.

The theoretical explanation for and mode of enforcement of collective food avoidances and aversions now must be considered. The leaders of a social group/religious group define what is food, i.e., which plant and/or animal items are OK/NOT OK for its members to eat. Then they explain the basis for the accept/reject decision.

The primary motivation behind the need to define what is food is group survival. Food is important to people, so it can be used as a lever in social pressure. Food is power. Food can be used as a factor in group cohesion and identification. People who have something in common tend to unite, then the common factor serves as a basis for identification. For example, people who do not eat X acquire a label and everybody knows that they do not eat X. Once branded with the label, people fight for survival of their group. It is worse to be beyond the pale.

On the other hand, leaders of an established group may wish to accentuate differences from other groups in their territory. To this end they study what nearby groups eat/do not eat and select some item(s) to create a difference. Then they set up rules to guide social pressure, in order to ensure group cohesion. In essence, group members must develop the designated kind of food discipline in order to demonstrate group loyalty. Once this goal is achieved, one can easily distinguish between members of the "in" group, i.e., those who have the food avoidance or aversion, and outsiders who do not.

It also turns out that over time the foods accepted by members of the "in" group increase in familiarity and the foods avoided become strange. Astute leaders magnify these differences with supportive myths to create fear and anxiety as a consequence of consumption of strange items. This sets up a conditioned response of tension and fear of the unknown. The result is that people become reluctant to try strange foods. So, these strange items become "not food," and not tried is equivalent to dislike. Thus, the array of potential foods is restricted by food avoidances.

From the above, one might conclude that the array of foods is continually shrinking. Fortunately, there is a counter-balancing process that occurs simultaneously. There is a continuous struggle by would-be leaders who introduce "out" group food(s) and attempt to induce people to accept it. If the item(s) is/are accepted, this is perceived as a vote of confidence for the would-be leader and the definition of what is food is expanded. Since there is frequent testing and acceptance by some, the food array is constantly changing.

In contemporary society, the subgroup where this pattern is most evident is that of Orthodox Jews. Originally, Jews and Moslems lived in the same territory and food taboos were one means of identification. Since the diaspora, Jewish leaders have found it necessary to inflate and strengthen differences from others in order to prevent integration and assimilation (which are equivalent to group dispersion, the opposite of what is wanted by group leaders since dispersion extinguishes power). So, in this group, food is power, and it must be controlled.

In contemporary society, collective food behavior has become very important to Black leaders—hence, Soul Food. Until the 1960s, Blacks were becoming integrated into the Caucasian society, so the Black leaders created an identity crisis as a means of reasserting their position. The outcome was the "Black is Beautiful" strategy, one outgrowth of which was Black studies. Since food is power, Soul Food surfaced and Blacks learned to prefer it for cultural reasons.

Since this strategy was successful for the Blacks, leaders of other ethnic groups tried it. They "discovered" that members of their groups had become assimilated and that they were losing/had lost power. So, they "discovered" the power of the food and people interaction. And, American society has witnessed a succession of ethnic food fads.

In the long run, it is apparent that the use of the food and people interaction in social power games cycles back and forth according to temporal importance of need for power. Success depends on timing. And, this depends on the aggregate need of individuals to belong to American or ethnic subgroups for reasons of identity. In any case, in contemporary American society, the overwhelming response to breaking a food taboo has been attenuated. Collective food proscriptions are not that powerful because of the diversity of backgrounds, mobility, and anonymity.

All individuals reject some foods. The professional who is trying to change food selections as part of a nutrition intervention program needs to distinguish between avoidances with personal and collective origins. Different strategies/actions may be required to deal with them successfully. For example, one may opt to ignore an avoidance based on a strong collective belief structure; any other course would be likely to terminate the relationship. Moreover, the method of presenting the need to change a weak belief differs according to whether the individual is tradition-, inner-, or other-directed. For example, one might appeal to the inner-directed person with a logical argument and to the other-directed individual with the argument that "everybody is doing it." When a food avoidance results from an individual intolerance, the appropriate response is to suggest a nutritional equivalent. When it is due to negative experiences, if important enough, one might attempt to overcome the aversion with a series of positive experiences.

PHYSIOLOGICAL DEFINITIONS

Some foods are forbidden and some foods are rejected, but what foods can man tolerate? Consideration of the physiological definitions of food and poison answers this question. IF *food* is a liquid or solid substance that is consumed and nourishes the body and *poison* is a substance that causes illness or death when eaten, drunk, or absorbed, THEN can one predict whether a substance is a food or a poison? Is quantity a factor in ability to tolerate?

The Case of Pure Foods

Pure foods are popularly believed to be non-toxic. Otherwise people would be afraid to eat most things. Nonetheless, Boyd and Boyd (1973) reported their research which shows that while the lethal dose of some pure foods is so high as to be unlikely to be consumed by human beings (½ ton/day), consumption of a lethal dose of other foods is a possibility. Moreover, the researchers present evidence that animals who grow and appear normal on diets containing very large amounts of pure foods become susceptible to effects of other stresses. Thus, the importance of the question of quantity begins to emerge. These authors state:

> The basic concept. . . is that there is probably a toxic dose or amount of everything. This dose is an amount that overwhelms the body mechanisms for dealing with the substance in question.[1]

This quantity is large for foods and small for poisons.

The operational definitions of food and poison are determined by careful research, using an index that defines relative toxicity as a criterion. LD_{50} is defined as a lethal dose for 50% of the sample. Subjects are given a series of graduated quantities and are observed. IF less than 50% die, THEN the quantity is manipulated until 50% die. This quantity is the dividing line between food and poison; greater quantities are poisonous. In this way, the physiological definitions of food and poisons are obtained for various substances. The Nuremburg Code prevents giving lethal doses to man; so animal studies are used and the quantities are extrapolated.

It turns out, that for pure foods, animals die when given a lethal dose of food all at once because (a) the substance irritates and inflames the mucosal lining of the GI tract which causes pain and malabsorption and (b) the osmolar load is so high that it draws water into the intestines, causing diarrhea and at the same time dehydrating blood and tissues. The stress is too great. It also turns out, that IF an animal survives the initial lethal dose, THEN it adapts. The effects disappear and the animal can continue to ingest the lethal doses with no observable effects. It also turns out, that IF the total lethal dose is divided into portions and given at intervals, THEN a much greater quantity is needed to have a lethal effect.

---

[1] Reprinted with permission from E.M. Boyd and C.E. Boyd (1973). Toxicity of Pure Foods. Copyright, The Chemical Rubber Co., CRC Press, Inc.

While large quantities of a particular food can be ingested, tolerated, and adapted to, the effects are unpleasant and some risk is involved. The evidence is limited and a particular person's LD is unknown. For this reason, some of the single-food fad diets are possibly hazardous.

Physiological Demand for Nutrients

All of the working cells of the body require variable quantities of a number of nutrients as raw materials used in cellular processes. Normally, the majority of nutrients are obtained by dietary intake. A few can be synthesized and some can be withdrawn from body stores, if available, to meet temporary needs. A nutrient supply/demand monitoring system is presented as a model that can be used in nutrition education to aid in conceptualization of the processes involved.

Normally, when intracellular supply of a nutrient is low, it is replenished from the blood, whose main function is translocation of nutrients throughout the body. A normal circulating level of each nutrient is maintained continuously, to the extent possible, at a level that will supply all cells' needs under normal circumstances. When the circulating level cannot be maintained, life is threatened.

Since the beginning, man's intake of the various nutrients has been highly variable, often taking wide swings. So, to deal with this situation, the body has evolved some mechanisms that provide flexibility for dealing with a range of intakes:

(a) flood extreme—The body can eliminate some of most nutrients in the urine, it can store some, or if levels are still too high nutrients can be detoxified.

(b) famine extreme—The body can draw some from reserve stores or it can recycle more effectively, or it can shift to low gear which reduces usage.

The brain functions as a monitoring screen with a translator/recorder unit attached. Feedback mechanisms are auto-correcting at the local level under normal circumstances. On a continuous basis, the cells send what amounts to a "state of the cell" message. Since the supply/demand situation is critical to survival, these messages are sent out "Special Delivery" as a strong signal that will register. However, under some circumstances it may not register or the appropriate action may not be made because of the following:

(a) busy signals—Human beings have the capacity for mind over matter. They can focus on something else and tune out the hunger/satiety signals.

(b) noise as a distractor—Worry, fear, etc., keep the mind occupied so that it cannot focus on other messages.

In response to various signals, various responses and messages are remitted. Some examples follow:

(a) IF the signals result in reception of a pattern that is within normal range and not highly variable, THEN the "message received" signal is remitted.

(b) IF the mean level registers high, THEN some organs are coping with flood conditions so the signal to GI tissue is "not necessary" so that the response to food translates "that's nice."

(c) IF the mean level registers low and this is a new message (temporary), THEN the translation is "that's OK" AND a message is sent that translates "draw from stores."

(d) IF the mean level registers low and the stores are low, THEN the message sent is "not OK, get food." The result is that hunger pangs are generated and conservation mechanisms are implemented. At the same time, a portion of the alarm system registers and keeps checking to see if status is transient or if more and stronger measures must be taken to ensure survival.

(e) IF the mean level registers low and stores are out AND no food intake continues, THEN the translator sends the message "NOT OK. Desperate, help, starving!" Since the gut and general conservation measures have failed, a rationing system is implemented in which brain, heart, circulation, liver, and kidneys function as best they can, as long as they can, and supply to other tissues an amount that is just sufficient to keep them marginally alive. After this point, the only remaining message is "Can't cope, sorry about that."

The situation described pertains to any nutrient, even those that are required only in trace quantities. By definition, IF a substance is a nutrient, THEN it is required in some quantity. One nutrient cannot be substituted for another. In a few cases, one nutrient can perform some, but not all, of the functions of another. So, the requirement is absolute. Therefore, a diet that is inadequate in even one nutrient is not OK. Some effect can be expected.

But, ability to observe effects is limited; small differences cannot be detected at the present time. In most cases only cumulative and aggregate effects resulting in major malfunctions, which are described as the classic deficiency diseases, are detected. In a few cases, effects of lesser levels of deficiency are known. But, the effects of marginal intake are unknown; these are under intensive investigation at the present time. Moreover, while the effects of absolute deficiency of one nutrient are known, with few exceptions the combined effects of multiple deficiencies are unknown. This is to be expected since (a) there are about 50 nutrients, (b) the number of combinations of multiple deficiencies is a very large number, and (c) the number of levels of deficiency is continuous from zero deficiency to total deficiency. Pre-selected combinations and levels of interest are under investigation. Because the task is infinite, the true definition of physiological demand for nutrients always will remain an unknown that challenges every generation. Man can have only the current approximation to truth; some inkling of past approximations also may be known. Details of the monitoring system were described in Chapter 3.

The appostat or appetite mechanism converts signals of cellular need for nutrients to conscious awareness of hunger and, unless there is an interfering factor, to food-getting behavior. A plausible explanation for variability in size of appetite is related to cellular demand for nutrients in the following way. For an individual, the aggregate demand of the *active* or processing cells is determined genetically by the basic architecture of the tissues and environmentally by physical exercise, which affects muscle development. Thus, a person with a large body developed for physical strength and endurance will have a different need for nutrients than one with a small and poorly developed body. The aggregate demand of adipose *storage* cells is determined by the number of storage cells required at three early periods in growth and development, i.e., prenatal, infancy, and during the teenage growth spurt. IF the need to store excess fat exists during these three periods, THEN the number of adipose cells is increased and maintained at the new number. The cumulative effect is a greatly inflated number of cells. This is important to appetite control because a greater number of cells can take up a greater quantity of nutrients, causing the circulating levels to fall. IF there are many cells, THEN the signal of need is greater, THEREFORE a person is programmed to "feel" hungry. IF there are few cells, THEN the signal of need is smaller, THEREFORE a person is programmed to "feel" not hungry, which programs for thin to normal weight.

Physiological Definition of Food

Until recently, the available information led to the conclusion that only a "hungry/not hungry" signal could be sent. A corollary idea was that if the signal was to fill the stomach, a mixture probably would provide some of the nutrient needed; if not, the signal could be continued. Newer evidence supports the position that the message may be somewhat more specific, at least for some nutrients like sodium.

Suppose nutrient X is deficient and has caused the signal to be sent. It is reasonable to suppose that IF the circulating level is low, THEN receptors in the intestinal wall will be unsaturated. Therefore, uptake from ingested food is facilitated. Since the circulating level is low, nutrient X will move from the receptors into venous circulation. Thus, removal will be continuous until the circulating level is approximately normal, at which equilibrium dynamics would slow uptake.

Foods are digested and absorbed at variable rates depending on their liquid-to-solid ratio and proportions of fat, carbohydrate, and/or protein since these require different processing in digestion. IF a food is rapidly digested and absorbed AND IF it contains some of nutrient X, THEN the signal of need shuts off. IF a food that is slowly digested contains nutrient X, THEN the signal of need shuts off and stays off because absorption continues over a long period of time, i.e., several hours. So unless a person eats by the clock or some other cue, no impulse to eat will occur. Thus, consumption of coffee, tea, and other clear liquids scarcely shuts off the signal since they are absorbed as is. In contrast, fat takes a long time to digest; so the signal will be shut off and a person will not desire food. Thus, fat has great satiety value. Simple sugars, e.g., sucrose, are easily degraded and absorbed; so they also have little satiety value. Starches require more extensive breakdown because of the long chain lengths; they have moderate satiety value. Protein itself is slowly degraded and in food it is usually associated with fat; therefore, it has almost as much satiety value. The satiety value of a meal containing a variety of foods is highly variable and depends on the proportions of fat, carbohydrate, and protein. Thus, it turns out that the physiological definition of food is determined by the nutrient needed and whether the substances ingested contain it in a quantity that shuts off the signal of need.

EMOTIONAL/PSYCHOLOGICAL DEFINITIONS

Contact with food or poison, or the thought of either, usually evokes an emotional/psychological response of some sort. The psychic and physical reaction to food and poison are experienced (a) subjectively as a strong feeling and (b) physiologically as a result of changes that prepare the body for immediate vigorous action, e.g., release of adrenalin in the fright, fight, flight sequence. Both aspects are involved in man's relation to his food as well as life expectancy.

Feelings are partly mental and partly physical responses characterized by pleasure, pain, attraction, and/or repulsion. The whole range of feelings can be evoked in response to the presence of or thought of food or poison. The feeling responses are variable in magnitude, intensity, and duration depending on the stimulus and experience with stimuli of the same kind.

People are highly variable in the degree to which they are aware of their feelings in relation to food and poison stimuli. Awareness or consciousness denotes: (a) realizing that the psychophysical response has occurred,

(b) perceiving or understanding what aspect of the stimulus or some association with it evoked the response, and (c) knowing or apprehending, i.e., grasping, the meaning of the response for oneself and outside observers.

In former times in America, people probably were more conscious of their feelings regarding food and poison. This is because of their religious mentality and the impression made by weekly sermons designed to raise their consciousness of (a) the temptations of pleasure, (b) the evils of being covetous, jealous, greedy etc., (c) the virtue of disciplining oneself to endure monotony, and (d) the need to be thankful. Feelings were accepted as natural but to be controlled; advice was given for dealing with them. Various sayings embodying the ideas, often as metaphors, were used to remind people of what they knew. In recent years the lack of meaning attributed to degenerating food and people interactions may reflect lack of understanding of emotional/psychological responses to food and poison and the definitions of food and poison that result.

The array of feelings is universal. However, how a people "feels" about food varies among groups. The observable behaviors used to denote or express the various emotions also vary. Little is known about this aspect as it has not been studied to any extent.

Prior to contact, one is *indifferent*[1] to a food. Contact is a prerequisite to the development of feelings regarding food, the eating experience, and the eating territory. Contact can be physical causing a *sensation*, or mental causing a *perception*. People are sentient beings, i.e., they are responsive to or conscious of sense impressions (Tables 16.1 and 16.2), so the attributes of the food itself may attract or repel. Moreover, people are perceptive and can pick up both verbal and non-verbal cues to other people's responses. From these experiences, people form beliefs and attitudes that reinforce the strength of emotions.

After initial contact, other feelings can be generated (Table 16.3). A basic attraction can become a *desire*. The desire may take the form of a *wish*. Or, it may become a *want* that initiates food getting behavior. A food that is desirable and can be enjoyed, i.e., it is available for one's use and benefit and can give pleasure (delight and joy), and satisfaction (fulfillment of a need or want) is considered *delicious* and *delectable* and may be consumed with *gusto*. The desire for a particular food may become stronger and compelling, so that the person responds when *enticed, lured, tempted,* or *tantalized—craving* and *greedy* consumption may result. Or, desire may be coupled with *envy* and *jealousy* and result in *covetousness*. So, ultimately some foods become so desirable that they

---

[1]Most of the italicized words in this chapter are defined in Tables 16.1−16.3. Definitions integrated with the text are also adapted from Webster's Seventh New Collegiate Dictionary, 1969, G. & C. Merriam Co., Publishers, Springfield, Mass.

cannot be served except to selected people because they have an *invidious* effect. Thus, a few favored items become "super-foods" with high status—a special definition.

TABLE 16.1.   TERMS[1] RELATED TO EMOTIONAL/PSYCHOLOGICAL RESPONSES

Term	Page(s)	Definition
EMOTION	271, 306	1. the subjective aspect of consciousness that results from the action of a stimulus strong enough to produce a noticeable response or reaction 2. a psychophysical response, i.e., a psychic and physical reaction subjectively experienced as strong feeling and physiologically involving changes that prepare the body for immediate vigorous action; excitement or agitation are implied reactions
FEELING	306	1. the undifferentiated background of one's awareness considered apart from any identifiable sensation, perception, or thought 2. denotes any partly mental, partly physical response characterized by pleasure, pain, attraction and/or repulsion; it may suggest the mere existence of a response without implying anything concerning the nature or intensity of it
EXCITE	289, 687	1. to rouse to feeling 2. to arouse as if by pricking and implies a stirring up or moving profoundly
Agitation	18	1. to move with an irregular, rapid, or violent action—used metaphorically to imply this 2. to excite the mind or feelings of; disturb
Irritate	449	1. to excite impatience, anger, or displeasure in; annoy 2. to induce irritability in or of 3. implies an often gradual arousing of angry feelings that may range from impatience to rage
Provoke	449, 687	1. to arouse or stir 2. to incite to anger 3. to call forth or evoke 4. to stir up purposely; induce 5. to provide the needed stimulus for 6. to arouse by pricking; directs attention to the response called forth and most often applies to an angry or vexed reaction 7. implies often gradual arousing of angry feelings that may range from impatience to rage that incites to action
Stimulate	687, 861	1. to excite to activity or arouse as if by a goad or stylus 2. to function as a physiological stimulus to 3. to arouse as if by pricking and suggests a rousing out of lethargy, quiescence, or indifference

[1] Adapted from Webster's Seventh New Collegiate Dictionary, 1969. G. & C. Merriam Co., Publishers, Springfield, Massachusetts.

TABLE 16.2. TERMS[1] THAT DENOTE AWARENESS

Term	Page(s)	Definition
AWARE	61	1. having or showing realization, perception or knowledge 2. implies vigilance in observing or alertness in drawing inferences from what one sees or hears or learns
Apprehend	43	1. perceive 2. to grasp with understanding: recognize the meaning of
Conscious	177	1. perceiving, apprehending, or noticing with a degree of controlled thought or observation 2. may suggest a dominating realization or even preoccupation
Consciousness	177	1. awareness 2. the state of being characterized by sensation, emotion, volition, and thought: mind
Perceive	625	1. to attain awareness or understanding of 2. to become aware of through the senses: observe
Sensation	789	1. a mental process (as seeing, hearing or smelling) due to immediate bodily stimulation often as distinguished from awareness of the process 2. awareness due to stimulation of a sense organ 3. a state of consciousness due to internal changes 4. a state of excited interest or feeling
Sense	789	1. to perceive by the senses 2. to become aware of or detect
Sentient	790	1. responsive to or conscious of sense impressions 2. aware

[1] Adapted from Webster's Seventh New Collegiate Dictionary, 1969. G. & C. Merriam Co., Publishers, Springfield Massachusetts.

Satisfaction of needs and desires can be achieved by everybody at a number of levels. One progresses from feeling *full* or *satiated* to *gorged* or *replete*. A *glut* or too much good food changes the food and people interaction from a positive experience to a negative one. Interest in the particular food or in any food *palls* and the person becomes indifferent; food has no interest for the person. *Surfeit* becomes *cloying* and even the thought of food is *wearisome. Monotony* and *boredom* undermine *tolerance* for the food(s) until finally the food is rejected as poisonous. Each of these emotional states is ecologically different and the implications of the resultant food and people interactions for life expectancy also differ.

Man has a tendency to think that if only he/she could have X, the desired food, then he/she would never want anything else. IF one has a mental set that predisposes one to *gratitude, appreciation,* and/or *con-*

TABLE 16.3. TERMS[1] THAT DESCRIBE EMOTIONAL /PSYCHOLOGICAL RESPONSES TO FOOD AND /OR THE FOOD AND PEOPLE INTERACTION

Term	Page(s)	Definition
PLEASURE	650	1. state of gratification or enjoyment 2. a sensual gratification 3. a source of delight or joy 4. an agreeable emotion accompanying the possession or expectation of what is good or greatly desired; stresses satisfaction or gratification rather than visible happiness
Appreciate	43	1. to evaluate the worth, quality or significance of 2. to admire greatly 3. to judge with heightened perception or understanding; to be fully aware of 4. to recognize with gratitude
Content(ment)	180, 765	1. appeases the desire of 2. to limit (oneself) in requirements, desires, or actions 3. manifests satisfaction with one's possessions (the kind of food and the appointments in the eating territory), status (who, what, when, where, and how one eats), or situation (able to sit up and take nourishment every day) 4. quality or state of being contented 5. implies gratification to the point where one is not disturbed or disquieted even though every wish is not fully realized
Delectable	218	1. highly pleasing—delightful or delicious food
Delectation	218, 650	1. reaction to a pleasurable eating experience that is consciously sought or provided
Delicacy	218	1. something pleasing to eat that is considered rare or luxurious
Delicious	218	1. a food that affords great pleasure 2. a food that is appealing to taste or smell
Delight	218	1. a high degree of gratification 2. extreme satisfaction 3. a food that gives great pleasure 4. to give keen enjoyment 5. gives visible happiness, not just satisfaction or gratification
Desirable	224	1. a food or food and people interaction having pleasing qualities or attractive properties
Desire	224	1. to long for or hope for 2. a strong feeling and often implies a strong intention to obtain 3. a conscious impulse toward a food or eating experience that promises enjoyment or satisfaction in its attainment
Enjoy(ment)	275	1. to have a food for one's use, benefit, or lot 2. to take pleasure or satisfaction in
Epicure	278	1. one with sensitive and discriminating tastes in food or wine

TABLE 16.3 *(Continued)*

Term	Page(s)	Definition
		2. one who takes pleasure in eating and drinking; implies fastidiousness (overly difficult to please, showing or demanding excessive delicacy or care) and voluptuousness (full of delight or pleasure to the senses, given to or spent in enjoyments of luxury, pleasure, or sensual gratification) of taste
Fruition	336	1. pleasurable use or possession 2. pleasure in possession or enjoyment in attainment
Gourmand	278, 361	1. one who is excessively fond of eating and drinking 2. a luxurious eater 3. one who takes pleasure in eating and drinking; a hearty interest in good food is suggested
Gourmet	278, 361	1. a connoisseur in eating and drinking 2. one who takes pleasure in eating and drinking with discriminating enjoyment of food and drink
Gratification	365, 650	1. to give or be a source of pleasure or satisfaction
Gratitude	365	1. the state of being gratified or thankful 2. showing gratitude or appreciation for the benefits received 3. expression of pleasure or contentment 4. showing that one is grateful (grateful commonly applies to a proper sense of favors received from one's fellow men whereas thankful may apply to a more generalized acknowledgement of what is vaguely felt to be providential) for food or a food and people interaction
Gust	371	1. inclination or liking for 2. enjoyment or appreciation
Gusto	371	1. taste, liking 2. enthusiastic and vigorous enjoyment or appreciation of food
Humor	430	1. yielding to a person's moods or whims by providing desired food, eating climate, or eating territory
Indulge	430	1. to give free reign to the appetite for a particular food or food in general 2. to take unrestrained pleasure in food 3. to treat leniently or generously in allowing to eat 4. to show undue favor to a person's desires and feelings for and about food; implies an excessive compliance and weakness in gratifying another's or one's own desires for food
Joy	459	1. the emotion evoked by well-being, success, or good fortune or by the prospect of possessing what one desires 2. expression of such, usually rapturous

TABLE 16.3 *(Continued)*

Term	Page(s)	Definition
Luxury	504	1. a food/appointment in the eating territory that gives unrestrained gratification to the senses; that is ostentatiously rich or magnificent 2. a food/appointment that is choice, costly, hard to get, and suggests gratification of the senses and desire for comfort
Satisfaction	765	1. a fulfillment of a need or want 2. a cause or means of enjoyment 3. full appeasement of a need or requirement
Spoil	430	1. to show undue favor to one's desires and feelings in a way that causes injurious effects on character by indulging or pampering (implies inordinate gratification of desire for luxury and comfort with consequent enervating effect)
Tickle	923	1. to have a tingling or prickling sensation 2. to excite the surface nerves to prickle 3. to excite or stir up agreeably
PAIN	605	1. an unpleasant or distressing sensation 2. acute mental or emotional distress or suffering (associated with sorrow, loss, and/or deprivation; results in not eating)
Anguish	35	1. extreme pain or distress of either body or mind caused by consumption of a forbidden food or an unpleasant food and people interaction 2. a torturing dread of eating a particular food
Apprehensive	43	1. discerning or cognizant—the knowledge of a connoisseur of food and drink makes the person apprehensive in this sense 2. viewing the future consumption of food(s) and/or food and people interactions with anxiety or alarm
Dread	253, 305	1. to fear greatly 2. great fear in the face of impending evil 3. painful agitation in the presence of or anticipation of danger and intense reluctance to face or meet it and suggests aversion as well as anxiety; the emotion of the obese facing a diet, for example
Fear	305	1. an unpleasant often strong emotion, including painful agitation, caused by anticipation or awareness of danger 2. to be afraid to eat a food or to be apprehensive about the outcome 3. to fear a food and people interaction or to be apprehensive about the outcome
Fearful	305	1. causing fear 2. extremely bad, intense or large 3. a food or food and people interaction that causes fear, agitation, or loss of courage (a dreadful eating experience has the power to make one shudder with mingled fear and aversion; fright-

TABLE 16.3 *(Continued)*

Term	Page(s)	Definition
		ful implies a startling or outrageous quality to the eating experience; a terrible eating experience is one that is so painful that it is beyond endurance; a terrific eating experience has the power to stimulate or strike terror by the release or display or imposition of great or explosive force, e.g., an allergic response might cause swelling of the mouth, nose, throat, and result in choking; an appalling eating experience terrifies and also dismays or dumbfounds)
		4. disturbed by fear and implies a timorous, worrying or imaginative temperament more often than a real cause for fear, which causes the person to overreact to a food or eating experience
Fright	305, 335	1. fear excited by sudden danger, as when a person with food allergies perceives that he/she has eaten a food that produces a response
		2. a food that is strange, ugly or shocking to consume
		3. painful agitation in the presence of or anticipation of danger from eating X; it may imply the shock of sudden, startling fear
Horror	401	1. painful and intense fear, dread, or dismay
		2. intense aversion or repugnance even at the thought of eating a food such as dog meat
Panic	304, 608	1. a sudden overpowering fright, especially a sudden unreasoning terror often accompanied by mass flight
		2. painful agitation in the presence of or anticipation of danger, as for example when one perceives that a food causing a severe allergic reaction has been eaten; it implies unreasoning and overmastering fear causing hysterical activity
Shock	802	1. a sudden or violent disturbance in the mental or emotional faculties
		2. to strike with surprise, terror, horror or disgust
Terror	305, 911	1. a state of intense fear
		2. a frightening aspect or cause of worry
		3. painful agitation in the presence of or anticipation of danger—the most extreme level of fear
ATTRACT	57	1. to cause to approach or to draw by appeal to natural or excited interest, emotion or aesthetic sense
		2. having the power to draw toward
Acquire	8, 351	1. to get or gain possession of a food; may not imply effort
		2. to come into possession of food by some uncertain or unspecified means; implies in addition to the quantity on hand
Cloy	157, 764	1. to surfeit with an excess, usually of a food that was originally attractive and pleasing
		2. results in disgust or boredom which detracts

TABLE 16.3 *(Continued)*

Term	Page(s)	Definition
Covet	192, 224	1. to wish for a food or a special food and people interaction in an envious way 2. to desire the food, food experiences, and/or eating climate that belongs to another inordinately (exceeding reasonable limits) or culpably (could be condemned for it) 3. implies a strong eager desire often inordinate and envious and often for what belongs to another
Crave	195	1. to have a strong inward desire 2. suggests the force of physical or emotional need
Entice	277, 504	1. to draw on by arousing hope or desire for an attractive food or eating experience; tempt 2. drawing by artful or adroit means
Envy	278	1. painful or resentful awareness of an advantage in food experience or eating situation enjoyed by another joined with a desire to possess the advantage 2. to begrudge the pleasure or enjoyment of an attractive food or eating experience
Full	377	1. containing as much as possible or normal to be held or contained 2. satisfied, especially with food or drink
Gorge	360, 764	1. to eat an attractive food greedily or to repletion 2. to stuff to capacity 3. suggests glutting to the point of bursting or choking on food
Glut	357, 764	1. to fill, especially with food, to satiety 2. to flood with food so that supply exceeds demand 3. implies an excess in feeding or supplying
Glutton	357	1. one who finds food so attractive that he/she eats too much, i.e., to excess
Greedy	192, 366	1. having a strong desire for food or drink 2. stresses lack of restraint and often of discrimination regarding attractiveness of the food or drink when satisfying the desire
Inclination	423	1. a propensity or bent or liking for 2. tending toward or will attempt, i.e., is inclined to try a new food
Jealous	455	1. intolerant of rivalry in the eating situation based on the definition of food 2. hostile toward a rival or one believed to enjoy an advantage in the eating situation
Lure	504	1. an inducement to pleasure in the eating situation 2. a food that is attractive or that has appeal 3. implies a drawing into danger, evil or difficulty through attracting and deceiving; snack foods lure people with weight problems into consuming unwanted calories

TABLE 16.3 *(Continued)*

Term	Page(s)	Definition
Obtain	583, 679	1. attainment of a food or eating experience sought for by the expenditure of time and effort 2. procure by putting out the effort
Prize	678	1. a food that is exceptionally desirable 2. to value a food or eating experience highly or with esteem
Replete	327, 727	1. abundantly fed; gorged 2. implies being filled to the brim or satiety
Satiate	764	1. to satisfy fully, may imply repletion that has destroyed interest or desire for food
Surfeit	764, 885	1. an overabundant supply or excess of food 2. an intemperate or immoderate indulgence in food or drink 3. disgust caused by excess food; implies a nauseating repletion
Tantalize	901	1. to tease or torment by or as if by presenting a desirable food to the view but continually keeping it out of reach
Tempt	504, 908	1. to entice to do wrong by promise of pleasure or gain 2. implies the presenting of an attraction so strong that it overcomes the restraints of conscience or better judgment
Value	980	1. to rate or scale a food or food experience in usefulness, importance or general worth 2. to consider or rate highly on the basis of its attractions
Want	224, 1003	1. to desire an attractive food earnestly 2. to be inclined to a food or food experience 3. to have or feel a need for a food or food experience; to long for—a felt need
Wish	224, 1025	1. to have a desire for a food or food experience 2. a vague or passing longing for an attractive food or food experience that is unattainable
REPULSION	729	1. the action of driving or beating back 2. the action of repelling by discourtesy, coldness, or denial 3. a feeling of aversion; repugnance
Abhorrent	2, 381, 729	1. regarded with extreme repugnance 2. to be turned aside from or kept away from, especially in scorn; to be rejected as unfit for food 3. not agreeable with 4. detestable 5. repugnant and implies a food or food and people interaction that causes active antagonism 6. a food experience that causes an emotional aversion with deep shuddering repugnance
Abomination	3, 381	1. a food worthy of or causing loathing or hatred; detestable

TABLE 16.3 *(Continued)*

Term	Page(s)	Definition
		2. a food that is quite disagreeable or unpleasant
		3. a food experience that causes disgust and hatred; loathing
		4. implies an emotional aversion and suggests strong detestation and often moral condemnation
Antipathy	39, 276	1. settled aversion or dislike 2. positive hatred which may be open or concealed and implies a natural or logical basis for one's hatred or dislike and suggests repugnance and a desire to avoid the eating experience or reject the food
Aversion	61	1. a feeling of repugnance toward a food or food and people interaction with a desire to avoid or turn from it
Bad	65	1. below standard: a poor food experience or an unfavorable food and people interaction or decayed or spoiled food 2. inadequate 3. disagreeable or unpleasant 4. injurious or harmful
Bore	97	1. to weary with ennui or tedium
Condemn	173	1. to declare to be wrong; censure 2. to adjudge a food unfit for use or consumption
Contempt	180	1. the act of despising a food or a food and people interaction, or the state of mind of one who despises 2. a lack of respect for something
Criticize	197	1. to consider the merits and demerits of and judge accordingly: evaluate 2. implies finding fault with a food and people interaction, especially with methods or policies or intentions
Despise	225	1. to look down on a food, a food experience or a food and people interaction with contempt or aversion 2. to regard as negligible, worthless or distasteful; may imply any emotional attitude ranging from indifferent disdain to loathing
Detest	226, 381	1. to dislike a food, a food experience, or food and people interaction intensely: loathe, abhor 2. an emotional aversion suggesting violent antipathy
Disapprove	236	1. to pass unfavorable judgment on 2. to reject 3. to feel or express an objection; implies dislike or distaste but not necessarily condemnation
Disdain	238	1. a feeling of contempt and aversion 2. to look with scorn on
Disfavor	239	1. disapproval, dislike 2. to withhold or withdraw favor from

TABLE 16.3 *(Continued)*

Term	Page(s)	Definition
Disgust	239	1. marked aversion excited by exposure to a food, food experience, or food and people interaction that is highly distasteful or loathsome 2. to provoke to loathing, repugnance, or aversion: to be offensive to 3. to cause (one) to lose an interest in a food, food experience or food and people interaction through exciting distaste
Dislike	240	1. disapprove 2. a feeling of distaste or disapproval
Displease	241	1. to incur the disapproval of, especially as accompanied by annoyance or dislike 2. to be offensive to
Disrepute	241	1. low esteem: discredit
Distaste	242	1. dislike of food or drink 2. unpleasant to the taste 3. offensive or disagreeable
Distasteful	242, 729	1. disinclination, aversion 2. offensive, displeasing food experience or food and people interaction 3. repugnant, implies a contrariness to one's taste or inclinations that causes shrinking or reluctance to accept or agree
Hate	381	1. intense hostility and aversion usually deriving from fear, anger, or sense of injury 2. a habitual emotional attitude of distaste coupled with sustained ill will for people involved in the particular type of food and people interaction 3. a very strong dislike or antipathy 4. to have a strong aversion to 5. to find distasteful
Indifferent	427	1. that does not matter one way or the other 2. marked by no special liking for or dislike of something 3. not showing or feeling interest 4. implies neutrality of attitude from lack of inclination, preference, or prejudice
Invidious	446	1. tending to cause discontent, animosity, or envy 2. repugnant, applies to a food that cannot be used without creating ill will, odium, or envy
Loathe	381, 496	1. to dislike greatly 2. extreme disgust 3. implies an emotional aversion including utter disgust and intolerance
Monotonous	549	1. tediously uniform or unvarying 2. tedious sameness in the food, eating experience
Nausea	564	1. a stomach distress with loathing for food and an urge to vomit 2. extreme disgust that is sickening

TABLE 16.3 (Continued)

Term	Page(s)	Definition
Objectionable	581	1. arousing a feeling of disapproval 2. offensive
Obnoxious	729	1. offensive 2. repugnant and suggests an objectionableness too great to tolerate
Odium, odious	585	1. the state or fact of being subjected to hatred and contempt as a result of a despicable act or blameworthy eating situation 2. hatred and condemnation marked by loathing or contempt 3. a mark of disgrace or reproach: stigma 4. disrepute or infamy attached to a food and people interaction 5. exciting or deserving hatred or repugnance
Offend	586	1. to cause dislike, anger, or vexation 2. to cause hurt feelings or deep resentment, may not imply intent; may suggest a violation of the victim's sense of what is proper or fitting
Offense	586	1. a food that offends the physical senses beyond endurance and calls forth extreme feelings 2. an emotional response to a slight or indignity in a food and people interaction
Offensive	586	1. giving painful or unpleasant sensations: nauseous and obnoxious
Pall	606, 764	1. to lose interest or attraction 2. to become tired of a food or food and people interaction 3. to cause a food to become insipid, i.e., to be lacking in taste or savor, or the qualities that interest, stimulate or challenge; emphasizes the loss of power to stimulate interest or appetite
Repellent	727, 729	1. a food or food and people interaction serving or tending to drive away 2. arousing aversion or disgust: repulsive 3. repugnant, implies a generally forbidding or unlovely quality of a food that causes one to back away
Repugnant	729	1. something reciprocally opposed 2. a food, food experience, or food and people interaction that excites distaste or aversion 3. a food and people interaction that is alien to one's ideas, principles, or tastes that arouses resistance or loathing
Revolt	737	1. to experience disgust or shock 2. to turn away with disgust 3. to cause to turn away or shrink with disgust or abhorrence: nauseate
Revulsion	737	1. a strong pulling or drawing away: withdrawal 2. a sense of utter repugnance
Scorn	773	1. an emotion involving both anger and disgust: vigorous contempt

TABLE 16.3 *(Continued)*

Term	Page(s)	Definition
		2. to reject with vigorous or angry contempt
Tedium	906	1. the quality or state of being tiresome because of length or dullness 2. to become disgusted with a food or food and people interaction because it is wearisome
Tolerance	930	1. relative capacity to endure an unfavorable environmental factor 2. sympathy or indulgence for beliefs or food practices differing from or conflicting with one's own
Weary	1010	1. having one's patience, tolerance or pleasure exhausted by a food or food and people interaction
Vex	989	1. to bring trouble, distress, or agitation 2. to annoy
UNCERTAINTY	964–965	1. lack of sureness about someone related to a food and people interaction or the food itself 2. a food and people interaction that is not reliable or cannot be trusted 3. not known beyond doubt 4. not having certain knowledge: doubtful, as wholesomeness or safety 5. not clearly identified or defined 6. indeterminate 7. may imply a falling short of certainty or almost complete lack of definite knowledge, especially about the outcome or result
Distrust	243	1. to have no confidence in
Doubt	250, 964	1. uncertainty of belief or opinion 2. lack of confidence or trust 3. an inclination not to believe or accept 4. lack of sureness about somebody or something which suggests both uncertainty and inability to make a decision
Dubiety	256, 964	1. a matter of doubt 2. lack of sureness about somebody or something in a food and people interaction that stresses a wavering between conclusions
Dubiosity	964	1. lack of sureness about someone or something in a food and people interaction; suggests vagueness or mental confusion
Mistrust	542, 965	1. a lack of confidence: distrust 2. to have no trust or confidence in; suspect 3. to doubt the truth, validity, or effectiveness of 4. lack of sureness about somebody or something in a food and people interaction; implies a genuine doubt based on suspicion
Skepticism	815, 964	1. an attitude of disposition toward doubt 2. lack of sureness about someone or something associated with a food and people interaction that implies unwillingness to believe without conclusive evidence

TABLE 16.3 (Continued)

Term	Page(s)	Definition
Suspicion	886, 964	1. the act or an instance of suspecting something wrong without truth or on slight evidence 2. lack of sureness about somebody or something in a food and people interaction; stresses the lack of faith in the truth, reality, fairness, or reliability of someone or something
Wary	1005	1. marked by keen caution, cunning, and watchful prudence in detecting and escaping danger
DISCIPLINE	237	1. training that corrects, molds or perfects the mental faculties or moral character 2. control gained by enforcing obedience and/or order 3. to train or develop by instruction and exercise, especially in self-control 4. to impose order upon
Addict	10	1. to devote or surrender (oneself) to something habitually or obsessively: antithesis of discipline
Compel	169, 326	1. to drive or urge with force 2. requires a personal object and suggests the working of an irresistible force that overcomes discipline
Compulsive	171	1. having power to compel 2. of, relating to, caused by or suggestive of psychological compulsion or obsession, e.g., compulsive eating is caused by a psychologically compelling force
Evil	288	1. not good morally: wicked 2. arising from actual or imputed bad character or conduct 3. causing discomfort or repulsion
Force	326	1. to compel by physical, moral or intellectual means: coerce 2. a general term that implies the overcoming of resistance or discipline by the exertion of strength, power, weight, stress, or duress
Obedient	581	1. submissive to the restraint or command of authority 2. implies compliance with the demands or requests of one in authority
Obsession	583	1. a persistent disturbing preoccupation with an often unreasonable idea or feeling
Rebel	713	1. to oppose or disobey one in authority or control 2. to act in or show disobedience 3. to feel or exhibit anger or revulsion
Resentment	730	1. a feeling of indignant displeasure at something regarded as a wrong, insult, or injury 2. offense

[1] Adapted from Webster's Seventh New Collegiate Dictionary, 1969. G. & C. Merriam Co., Publishers, Springfield, Massachusetts.

tentment, THEN this may be so. IF in pursuit of gustatory pleasure one acts to *indulge, humor,* or *spoil,* THEN one has become involved with a "more" spiral. All of these have negative connotations because they imply that one goes too far in satisfying desire. Temporarily, the definition of what is food is restricted to the few favored items. IF such a practice of restriction becomes customary, THEN an abnormal food and people interaction has been established—it may threaten life expectancy.

Hedonism is a life-style based on the doctrine that pleasure or happiness is the sole or chief good in life. IF enjoyment of food and drink becomes a predominant way for an individual to obtain pleasure, THEN the relationship may take on added emotional significance due to the concurrent satisfaction of status and self-actualization needs. Progressive levels of pleasure and satisfaction are involved, and different kinds of food and people interactions result. The definition of what is food is progressively restricted since the person becomes more discriminating; at the same time the concept of poison expands. At one level, one is a *gourmand;* at another, a *gourmet;* at the ultimate level, one is an *epicure.*

Normally, definition of what is food is not so narrow because people are generally less discriminating. However, within a group what food is good is defined. This enables people to *evaluate* food by comparison with a standard, which is often a mental construct. Given the standard, *objectionable* attributes are identified and serve as a basis for *criticism* or *condemnation* of the particular specimen(s). These are labeled as poisonous or *bad* and *disapproval* results. *Distaste* or *dislike* for an item may degenerate to *repugnance* and *avoidance.* IF too many people find that samples of a food are unsatisfactory, THEN the item falls into *disrepute* and people are *offended* if the item is served to them. After this point, *antipathy* develops and the food is regarded as an *abomination.* Such food is *repellent* and evokes *repulsion. Aversion* increases, resulting in *disgust.* Then even the thought of the food is *revolting.* Finally, the food becomes *abhorrent* and *detestable* and *loathsome;* it is *invidious* and *odious.* Thus, some foods that are usually acceptable are temporarily defined as poison and are rejected in the particular instance. Others lose favor and are permanently defined as poisonous and unfit for consumption. Such outcomes have an important effect on man's relation to his food.

The experience of physical pain as a result of consuming a food evokes a range of responses. A trivial amount of pain, by definition, *stimulates* or *excites.* Black pepper and mustard are added for their appetite stimulating effect that derives from their bite. At low levels the sensation is pleasant. At higher levels it is unpleasant because more *irritates* and may cause *agitation.*

The *shock* of unexpected and sharp pain as a result of injury or allergic response causes a person to be *apprehensive* about consuming more of the same lot of food and/or trying a sample from other lots. The effect is that the food is avoided as a result of fear. If the food was previously a favorite or it is forced on a person, considerable *anguish* may result. Thus, physical pain can result in restrictions on the definition of what is food.

Like physical pain, mental pain also can evoke a range of responses that result in the redefinition of what is food. In this case, it is not usually an inherent quality of the food that evokes the response, but an association with a painful food and people interaction. Nonetheless, IF a special food was served on the painful occasion, THEN whenever the food is served, the painful situation may be recalled. IF so, THEN the food is regarded as poisonous and may be rejected. Agitation and/or hurt feelings lead to irritation. Then a person becomes *offended* and later *disgusted*. Repetition creates repugnance. What is distasteful and repellent becomes abhorrent and loathsome and finally invidious and odious. Thus, what is food is redefined and a carryover effect that influences similar food and people interactions may result.

Emotional/psychological responses also are associated with status-seeking. Thus, nourishing foods consumed by low status persons are redefined as poisonous, are held in disrepute, and are *despised. Disgust, scorn,* and *disdain* may be shown whenever such foods are mentioned or contempt may be shown for persons who serve them. Thus, for high status people, the definition of what is food is restricted to exclude these items.

Uncertainty about food quality or the honesty/integrity of those who produce/process foods causes some people to redefine what is food so as to exclude items that they are unsure of. *Wariness* leads to *dubiosity* and *doubt*. These produce low level emotional/psychological responses and have only a minor effect on the definition of items to be included in the food array. *Distrust* and *suspicion* lead to *mistrust* and *skepticism*—emotional/psychological involvement is greater and more items become questionable. *Dubiety* and *agitation* characterize final stages where many items are suspect and therefore avoided. Moreover, the person at this stage selects information that reinforces his/her doubt in order to maintain the integrity of his/her beliefs.

Eating to excess on a continuing basis leads to obesity. Obesity is repulsive to many. So, eating to excess has long been considered *evil* because obesity arises from the actual or imputed bad conduct of eating to excess on a continuing basis.

Discipline is a means of perfecting moral character, in this case by imposing order on what is eaten and by training the person in self-control. So, a person is trained to redefine what is food to a smaller number of less satisfying items. Diets fail because *resentment* results, *obedience* gives way, and one *rebels*. As a result of rebelling, the restricted definition of what is food is rejected and many desirable "poisons" are redefined as food.

What is food is also determined in part by whether one eats alone or with companions. Emotional/psychological responses relating to social aspects of eating will be discussed in a later section.

Development of Emotional/Psychological Definitions

Each adult responds to items regarded as food in his/her culture according to the feeling evoked as a result of his/her original and/or continuous exposure to the item. The one exception is when the person is imitating the behavior of others. The observable behavior may or may not reflect the real response. Some people are overt. Others are covert and control themselves to project whatever response they plan to.

The definition of what is food in general is learned as is the unique overlay of personal restrictions. Little children will taste/eat anything within reach until they learn not to. Thus, they will "eat" cigarettes, dust balls, blocks, hair, a rattle, etc. Somebody says NO and projects an emotional/psychological vibration that gives the child the message. This child soon learns to label the item "not food." This is the first level of learning. Children also learn what is "not food" from other experiences, for example:

(a) imitation—A father gives a non-verbal negative reaction such as a grimace when food X is served. Thereafter, the child defines the item "not food" and resists the mother's efforts to coax the child into trying it.

(b) sensitivity to pain—Hot, sour, and biting are painful and a child is more sensitive than an adult due to a greater number of taste buds. After a painful experience, the child defines the item as "not food" and will not eat it.

(c) muscular fatigue—Children become tired of chewing. Tough meat or any meat may be defined as "not food" and rejected.

(d) ridicule—Little children lack refined muscular coordination so have difficulty handling slippery foods. If ridiculed or reprimanded for difficulties or an accident, they will define the item as "not food."

(e) television exposure—What is food and what is good are learned from commercials, i.e., sweet, chocolatey, crispy, crunchy are good and other flavors/textures are suspect so the items are rejected as "not food" when introduced.

(f) tiresome—Food jags are common. Children get turned on to an item and eat it to the exclusion of other foods, then suddenly they become tired of it and thereafter it is redefined as "not food."

It is clear that by the time a person becomes an adult, his/her food experience has personalized the definition of what is food. In order that a child develop accepting attitudes toward food, experiences that evoke positive emotional/psychological responses are necessary. The number one objective in establishing the food and child relationship is to create a positive feeling, i.e., a positive but undifferentiated background of awareness that is apart from any identifiable sensation, perception, or thought regarding food. Then, the objective shifts to providing eating experiences which evoke the range of feelings toward and away from foods, so that the child learns to distinguish and respond appropriately within the cultural context. These experiences form the basis for social competency in food and people interactions.

Although a child's initial response to a food may be negative, the response can be modified if the right strategy is employed. IF the food is available because it is served frequently AND others around the child consume it with enjoyment, THEN the child will be inclined to try it unless pressured to do so. IF plates are served and everybody is given some of everything (the child is given a "no thank you" portion) AND everybody eats what is given, THEN the child may manage to eat the small amount and over time come to accept the food unless pressured to eat more, in which case a mild dislike may be increased by an element of defiance. Firmness but avoidance of force is the key.

As teenagers or young adults, many people learn to use food to restore emotional/psychological balance after a crisis or on a chronic basis. Food provides transitory gratification. And, both food and food and people interactions are normally associated with deep feelings of security. So, food consumption is used symbolically to compensate. IF chronic anxiety or depression develops, THEN a person may become *obsessed* with the problem(s) and eat certain foods *compulsively*. These are defined as good because they provide immediate gratification.

In order to serve this function, the eating experience must evoke a positive emotional/psychological response. This response may be evoked by a sensory attribute, e.g., sweet and chocolatey in which case a person becomes a "chocoholic." Or, the response may be evoked by an association, for example:

(a) "I am cheating on my diet and getting away with it."—Fattening foods, i.e., those that are sweet and/or rich are "good" for this purpose.

(b) "I have been good. Therefore, I owe myself a treat."—Something sweet or expensive is "good" for this "lollipop mentality," which is a holdover from childhood when an authority figure gave the child a lollipop for being good at the doctor's office.

(c) "I am eating this because everybody else does; I know it is not good for *me*, but I want to be like everybody else."—All kinds of rich and salty snack foods are "good" for this purpose.

(d) "My feelings are hurt and nobody loves me. It doesn't matter what I look like."—A large bowl of a snack food or a box of chocolates is so "good" that it disappears.

(e) "I am just as good, strong, and brave as 'they' are."—IF I eat heart, kidneys, and liver, THEN I will be strong like a lion.

(f) "I almost starved to death during period X."—People who have been deprived of food on a continuing basis often will eat whatever they can obtain in order to become fat for the security of having calories to go on.

(g) "I am really up tight."—People who are anxious with a feeling that makes them aware of an undifferentiated background stimulation that is unrelated to an identifiable sensation, perception, or thought also eat to compensate. They are "driven" to eat mindlessly, i.e., they will eat whatever they can get and whenever they can get it.

(h) "That was a real put-down."—Persons who have been degraded or feel unwanted often will eat steak or lobster or some other status food to "even the score."

(i) "I shouldn't have said (done) that; it was not right. I feel guilty about that but I can not bring myself to admit it to X."—Because they are later uncomfortable with what they have said or done, they may symbolically do penance by bringing a food gift from their garden or a homemade cake, pie, or cookies. They have to exert themselves to provide the food gift and have to go out of their way to present it, so they have made an effort without having to rectify, recompense, or reconcile.

A number of other typical examples of compensatory eating and/or food and people interactions could be cited. However, these should be sufficient as "food for thought."

The attributes of a food may cause it to be regarded as poisonous, i.e., something harmful or an object of *aversion* and *abhorrence*. Allergy or intolerance causes people to regard some foods as poisons. Associations put other people off. Within a culture, people define what is food according to a common concept of what is "good" or what is an appropriate color, texture, flavor, temperature, etc. A deviation from a standard evokes the response "What are you trying to feed me? It is poisonous." Blue mashed potatoes, slimy sour smelling hamburger, unfamiliar spices, and tepid coffee are examples of inappropriate attributes that evoke this response.

Centuries ago, a sage stated, "It's not what is that is, but what people think is that is." Thus, it is not always undesirable attributes of a food that cause rejection but an association that evokes an emotional/psychological response causing a redefinition as poison. In this sense, "One man's meat is another man's poison." And, a person will "lose his/her appetite" and/or "feel sick" (nauseated—"It turns the stomach") when presented with a "food" that is regarded as poison. The non-verbal response to even the thought of baked potato with sour cream and a hair, or dog, squid, rat, or snake meat, illustrates this point. A number of other typical examples of poisons could be given. However, other bases for redefinition need to be considered.

One of these relates to changes in the eating environment, as for example when a student goes away to college or when a person is hospitalized. These are major changes that disrupt many personal routines and challenge personal definitions of what is good in every aspect of life. A major emotional/psychological adjustment is required. A person is likely to be so busy dealing with the major stress that he/she is indifferent to food.

Or, in the case of the college student, he/she may not be accustomed to planning for or procuring food; he/she may lack the necessary skills and have to be content with whatever he/she can obtain. Or, he/she may not accept the difference in food quality in the food that is provided so may avoid some items or classes of food; he/she may not be aware of diet quality deterioration as long as hunger is assuaged. When confronted with the reality of nutritional deficiency, he/she sees clearly that the definition of what is food has changed and can begin to adapt toward a balanced intake.

In the case of a hospitalized patient, a stress related to the attributes of, or the choices of items available in, the eating experience when food quality is different, or the food and people interaction when eating in bed alone or with only a random acquaintance rather than family may evoke a range of emotional/psychological responses including suspicion, embarrassment, fear, anger, hostility, and rejection. At a time when nutrient intake is important to recovery or control or mitigation of a medical condition, emotional/psychological responses may intervene and interfere with acceptance of an appropriate definition of what is food.

SOCIO-CULTURAL DEFINITION

The socio-cultural definition of what is food encompasses the various aspects of the ecology of man's social eating within the local cultural context. The terms *social* and *cultural* have a number of meanings with important implications that pertain to food and people interactions. Social means:

(a) Marked by or passed in pleasant companionship with one's friends and associates; engaged in for sociability. This aspect necessitates inclusion of the concepts of host, guest, hospitality, conviviality, comfortability, and congeniality as well as alone, lonely, lonesome, forlorn, and desolate.

(b) Tending to form cooperative and interdependent relationships with one's fellows; gregarious. This aspect necessitates inclusion of the traditional group activities, e.g., corn husking, canning and jam making, candy making, and pot luck suppers as well as contemporary ones, e.g., progressive parties and food cooperatives.

(c) Of or relating to human society, the interaction of the individual and the group, or the welfare of human beings as members of society. This aspect necessitates inclusion of the concepts of courtesy and table manners; acceptable, appropriate, and inoffensive behavior.

(d) Of, relating to, or based on rank or status in a particular society. This aspect necessitates inclusion of the concepts of appropriateness, competition, and rivalry. These are discussed in the section pertaining to cultural definitions.

Culture means:

(a) Enlightenment and excellence of taste acquired by intellectual and aesthetic training. This aspect necessitates inclusion of aesthetic definitions of what is food. This is to be discussed in a subsequent section.

(b) A particular stage of advancement in civilization, the characteristic features of such a stage or state. This aspect necessitates inclusion of concepts of traditions in food for different occasions.

(c) Behavior typical of a group or class. This aspect necessitates inclusion of concepts of sanctions applied in cases of mistakes and defiance and of barbarians.

In the United States, we serve food at or in relation to essentially every kind of gathering of people. The definition of what is food is determined as a socio-cultural, often local, definition of what is appropriate. Generalizable considerations are that items will (a) create/maintain a pleasant, relaxed atmosphere, (b) not offend, and (c) be customary for the kind of occasion. These considerations are all related to the objective of evoking a positive emotional/psychological response in the collective food and people interactions. The means to this end are socio-cultural imperatives in terms of who, what, when, where, and how food will be served and eaten. These are transmitted among members of a cultural group by the same type of strategies and means used in teaching behavior patterns related to other aspects of life.

Underlying Social Reasons

Amicable, friendly, and *genial* are terms that describe relations that are expected to characterize social eating situations. The *convivial* host provides the hospitality, i.e., receives and welcomes guests in a cordial manner and creates a pleasant or sustaining environment. The role of the host requires that one plan for the guest's(s') comfort.

A large heterogeneous group introduces many unknowns, as people differ in what they define as food. Because of the uncertainty in this situation, the definition of what is food is customarily restricted to commonly accepted items in order to minimize the risk of giving offense. Food offered must not offend by being strange, shocking or horrifying, or causing pain (physical or mental). In short, it must be innocuous and appropriate. It also may be interesting and mildly stimulating, perhaps a conversation piece to be used as an "ice breaker."

On the other hand, a large homogeneous group is more manageable in the sense that there are fewer unknowns. But, a mistake in item selection is more noticeable because the food will remain uneaten and people will remark on that fact.

A small heterogeneous group is also more manageable in the sense that there are fewer unknowns. But, IF a mistake is made in item selection, THEN it is likely to be noticeable when some individual(s) avoids the item(s). The response of the host/hostess is reflexive; an apology for the discomfort incurred is proffered immediately.

A small homogeneous group is the most manageable, as there are few unknowns to deal with. The probability of a mistake in selection of foods offered is expected to be low. When it does occur, discomfort is correspondingly greater.

Congeniality is managed by selection of persons for the guest list. When tastes are similar, the definition of what is good food is more likely to be similar. Thus, item quality must be acceptable and appropriate. IF strange, shocking, or a source of mental pain (distaste), THEN comfort has been compromised and the eating experience fails socially. This is because one or more people become alone as a result of the difference between their definition of what is food and the quality that is presented.

By nature, man is gregarious. IF a person is alone, i.e., separated from others for any reason, especially on a continuing basis, THEN normal food and people interactions occur with a low frequency. The result is that the definition of what is food shrinks for reasons that include, but are not limited to:

(a) The kinds of items prepared for one person and a group differ, e.g., casseroles, quick breads, cakes, pies, and cobblers are prepared from recipes that make six or more portions and roast meats serve a dozen or so. These items drop out and are replaced by eggs, sandwiches, salads, ice cream, and cookies, which are more easily managed.

(b) The items that would have been prepared as a "labor of love" to please somebody else are avoided because they call forth painful memories.

(c) The special foods that would be prepared/eaten in celebration of holidays, promotions, or other special occasions drop out unless the person is invited to join a group.

(d) The quality of the eating experience is low, creating a degenerative spiral in which interest in eating decreases progressively and many an item drops out because the person does not think of it or can not bring himself/herself to make the effort to prepare it; quick-fix and/or ready-to-eat items remain.

Loneliness and *lonesomeness* may restrict the food experience of people of any age; the *forlorn* and *desolate* are usually elderly. IF a person is lonely, i.e., apart from others with the implication that there are no others of the same kind around and the person longs for companionship so is sad and has feelings of bleakness or desolation, THEN in addition to the above, the person may not remember to eat, may eat whatever is available, or may be unaware of what he/she is eating. IF a person is lonely, i.e., sad and dejected as a result of a lack of companionship or separation from others and perceives existence to be dreary, THEN in addition to "a−d" above, the person may compensate by eating sweet and/or rich items almost continuously. IF the person is forlorn, i.e., apart from others and suffers miserably from a great sense of loss, or is desolate, i.e., apart from others with a sharp and poignant sense of loneliness that results in behavior showing the effects of abandonment and neglect, THEN the person may refuse to eat. The cause rather than the effect of a restricted food array must be dealt with.

Cooperative and interdependent food and people relationships are used to manage bigness and complexity, using a "divide and conquer" strategy. Many foods and many people can be served successively at a progressive party. A unique definition of what is food (kinds, amounts, quality, and perhaps brands) is created through discussion for the particular occasion, perhaps around a theme. The list of items is divided among participating hosts. A food co-op enables a group to purchase common items in bulk. These are cooperatively divided, packaged, and sold to members at a lower price. On "workdays" the members socialize while they work for the common good.

Courtesy, or behavior marked by respect for and consideration of others, dictates that an alternate item be provided unobtrusively when a person cannot eat one of the items served. In this way, the definition of what is food on the particular occasion is expanded to include special diet items, non-alcoholic beverages, etc.

Table manners are one means to control the quality of interaction among members of a group for their general welfare as individuals. In a formal social situation, the concept of good table manners precludes noisy chewing or picking up food with the fingers. So, the definition of what is food is redefined to exclude relishes, e.g., carrot and celery sticks, fried chicken, corn-on-the-cob, fresh cherries, lest fingerlicking and other inelegant habits offend someone. On the other hand, in an informal social eating situation such as a picnic, such items are customary. Indeed, the definition of what is food is expanded to include as many items that can be eaten without the use of utensils as is possible.

Variability in rank and status of the people, places, and things involved as well as in the occasion causes several kinds of redefinition of what is food in social eating situations such as dinner parties. For example,

(a) *Who* the honored guest is may be the major factor in deciding what to serve, e.g., when entertaining the boss, one serves food "fit for a king" whereas one may simply add another plate for a grandchild, nephew, or other relative. Moreover, some foods commonly served to the family would never be served to guests.

(b) *What* the occasion is is another factor, e.g., the usual items are served every day whereas familiar, acceptable but dressed up or special items are required when dinner becomes a dinner party or social gathering for dinner.

(c) *When* a person shares a meal with another of differing rank or status, both must subordinate or suspend their personal definitions of what is food in order to preserve the relationship that brought them together. Otherwise, differences may come between the parties.

(d) *Where* the particular dinner party is held may determine the definition of what is food. This is especially so when the meal is consumed in a commercial establishment. The rank and status of the restaurant are associated with its type, i.e., fast-food versus exotic table service or some type in-between. Menu offerings delimit the definition of what is food; these vary with the type of establishment. Therefore, when a steak tough as shoe leather and cold coffee are served in a high class French restaurant, the patrons react with shock and horror at the affront because such are not defined as food in these circumstances.

(e) *Why* people give dinner parties, e.g., to introduce a new person to the social group, to impress others, or to repay a social obligation may determine what is defined as food. When introducing a new person, some informality, certainly no stiffness or awkwardness, is desired. So, a buffet with spaghetti or other easy acceptable casserole is a common choice. To impress, the foods may require long painstaking preparation or be costly or rare or exotic. To repay a social obligation, the food is usually limited to items similar to those served previously by those being entertained as guests—type, cost, and elaborateness should be similar in deference to feelings.

Underlying Cultural Reasons

The culturally defined definition of what is food for different occasions provides a basic list of items that are expected to be served. Occasions for which the definitions of what is food can be obtained include, but are not limited to, birthday party; card party; koffee klatch; picnic; wake; dinner party, e.g., Chinese, German, Hawaiian, Italian, Japanese, Mexican; holiday dinner, e.g., Christmas, Easter, Thanksgiving.

In addition, in many local areas a competition develops in relation to food decoration, use of special optional ingredients in a creative way that adds interest. This aspect must be considered in the definition of what is food. Variation of this sort is approved and expected. Friendly rivalry of this sort is a social game used to introduce new status. Deviation, whether an unwitting mistake or in defiance, is not approved. To the newcomer, the distinction between variation and deviation may be unclear and result in the degrading designation of barbarian. Within a culture, people learn the boundaries of the definition of what is not food for every common circumstance, i.e., what is poison because of some off-note that turns people off in such a way that they respond with "The very idea of eating X!"

In the United States, what is meat, i.e., animal tissue used for food, is largely limited to muscular tissue. It is clearly defined and is known. There are also a number of "inedible" flesh foods that have been eaten and relied on by some other cultures as a source of high quality animal protein. These are consumed by some subcultures that accept the items as meats. However, all of these items generally evoke a learned emotional/psychological response that has a socio-cultural basis. The items and presumed reasons for non-consumption are:

(a) pig (pork)—A gross animal that will eat whatever it can obtain; in former times, it often ate garbage, which led to the idea that it is unclean.

(b) dog, cat, horsemeat—These have been domesticated as pets, which are friends. To eat a friend would be cannibalistic, so one withdraws in horror instinctively at the very idea of eating their flesh as meat.

(c) wolf or coyote meat—These are "bad animals" that kill sheep and other domestic animals; ranchers loathe these animals. Also, these animals have been vilified in folk tales so they are rejected as a source of meat.

(d) snakes, lizards, rodents, and insects—Contact has created fear in many people; the fear has generalized and people overreact with revulsion at the idea of eating such as meat.

(e) game, e.g., moose, elk, duck, rabbit, pheasant, deer, bear, squirrel—People do not think of these as food; unless one has access, and since the supply is seasonal, these are strange and therefore suspect.

(f) organ meats, e.g., tongue, heart, liver, kidneys, brains, tripe—Muscles but not organs are accepted as food. Organs are basically repugnant because of texture, and we have undercut the beliefs that gave magical qualities and overcame natural aversion.

(g) blood—The thought of drinking warm blood, which is a highly nutritious beverage, causes one to withdraw in horror.

(h) milk—It is produced by all mammals but only cows', humans', and possibly goats' milk are accepted. Others are strange and are considered suspect. Milk is the natural food for young mammals but it is rejected by many adults as "baby" food.

(i) eggs (hens' and possibly ducks')—These are accepted as food although the eggs of other birds are nutritional equivalents.

In addition to these reasons, some meats are not considered food because a person does not know how to cook them or does not think of them. And, flesh foods are avoided by vegetarians, as discussed elsewhere. Thus, flesh avoidances result from a variety of responses and derived rationale.

Historically, there have been few taboos against eating plants other than those containing natural toxicants, which are avoided for health reasons. Some plants are comparatively rich in iron and/or protein but are not regarded as food. For whatever reason(s), they are not grown commercially, so most people are not aware of their existence. Many of these were used by Native Americans and the settlers and now grow wild. Some that are used and could be used more extensively are nasturtium leaves, chrysanthemum leaves and buds, geranium leaves, dandelion leaves, poke, purslane, lamb's quarters, and horsetail ferns.

Legumes or pulses are in disfavor because they cause flatulence, which is socially embarrassing. Therefore, consumption by most Americans is limited to outside occasions.

Other items are not defined as food by some people under defined circumstances. These are avoided because of degrading associations. These foods are avoided because they are for (a) low class people, (b) children, (c) sick people, or (d) old people. Clearly, there are many factors that may determine the definition of what is food.

Learning Definitions of Food and Poison

The definitions of food and poison are part of our general cultural heritage of foodways. They are transmitted to succeeding generations by mothers and other parent figures by means of the same types of strategies and actions used in teaching behavior patterns related to other aspects of life. A system of rewards and punishment is used to encourage desired behavior. The following aspects are commonly taught:

(a) What is food, when to eat what, where to eat what, why eat, how to eat what (how much, how fast, manners, etc.)

(b) How much variety to expect within and among meals, by the example of what is provided. IF the food array is restricted by prejudice or economics, THEN children will have a restricted definition of what is food. The expected outcome is that children then will refuse to eat unfamiliar items, or at least they will be reluctant to try them.

(c) What is nutritious—items and what cluster of foods make up a balanced diet. IF one is knowledgeable about the nutrient contributions of various foods AND values consumption of a nutritious diet, THEN the nutrition information, attitudes, and associated behaviors he/she teaches will program a child for good nutrition later. Otherwise, the child will learn adages, attitudes, and behaviors that belittle the value of a nutritious diet.

In our mobile society, children have other learning experiences that program them nutritionally. IF a family is mobile and has to adjust to a difference in ingredient availability, price, or differences in regional food preparation methods and in the definition of what is food, THEN the child learns to be adaptable and somewhat more catholic (universal) in tastes. At least four expected outcomes have been identified:

(a) IF the change is sudden or drastic, THEN the family may not make a perfect adaptation so maladaptation results in less optimal nutritional status than previously.

(b) IF the change is slow and gradual, THEN nutritional status is likely to be stable at the normal level for the family.

(c) IF frequent changes are required, THEN the requirement for adaptations may exceed the capacity to cope and nutritional status may degenerate rapidly.

(d) IF the family regards changes as an opportunity for an eating adventure and recognizes the need to study the effects of item changes on nutrient intake, THEN necessary changes will be accepted more easily and unwanted effects will be minimized.

Children in a mobile family are more vulnerable nutritionally than their peers. They cannot evaluate the effects of so many complex factors. Lack of continuity in diet and inability to understand and deal with differences in nutrient intake lead to incomplete and/or incorrect concepts and habits. So, the child is less likely to redefine what is food in such a way that he/she chooses a balanced diet. The child needs both support and assistance in balancing the diet during the transitional phase while new habits are being formed. Lacking this, the child is likely to develop habits of food choice that are nutritionally unwise.

The adult who has grown up in a mobile family or who has moved from one region to another and has not given thought to changes in food intake may be nutritionally vulnerable. This is because of the cumulative and aggregate effects of failure to unlearn, or of incomplete and/or incorrect past learning. For example, people who live on a farm are accustomed to eating a variety of home-grown fruits and vegetables. These are eaten because they are available, customary, and enjoyed. When farm people move to urban areas, fresh fruits and vegetables are often no longer defined as food because of quality and availability differences. Moreover, purchase price is a deterrent to those who have not previously considered their cost. Commercially preserved forms are not substituted, so fruits and vegetables drop out of the diet of many. Of course, the nutritional quality of the diet suffers. But, often people do not recognize that such important changes have occurred in their diet, nor could they explain why. Expected effects are completely beyond them. Thus, people who have moved from one area to another need help in redefining what is food so as to retain the nutritional quality of their diet.

HEALTH–RELATED DEFINITIONS

"Good health!"—in every culture, one of the most common traditional rituals at a social gathering—is the proposing of this toast, first to the host and then to all gathered. Everybody can drink to this toast, which unites all with good wishes.

The concept of good health has three aspects: (a) the person gives the appearance of and is free from signs of disease, weakness, or malfunction; (b) the person behaves in a way that demonstrates full strength and vigor in performance of tasks; and (c) the person has a sense of physical and mental well-being.

From earliest times, man has perceived that food intake was related to health, i.e., consumption of the right food might remedy a disease whereas consumption of a poison might cause a disease. Man also learned that the possibility of demonstrating full strength and vigor was influenced by something inherent in the food itself, i.e., by nutrient intake, rather than food intake *per se* since consumption of different diets has different effects on health. And, sense of well-being was linked to man's perception of the relationship between food ecology and life expectancy.

The question has been asked, "Who eats for health?" The answer is, those who

(a) Have a chronic disease and must modify and/or control food consumption in order to remedy the condition or mitigate symptoms. (This group also includes the incurable who are seeking a miracle.)

(b) Opt to prevent or delay onset of symptoms by modifying food consumption to balanced moderation.

(c) Highly value physical prowess and actively pursue any means that promises improvement.

(d) Are losing or have lost a sense of well-being, e.g., the elderly who seek to recapture the strength of youth or members of the counterculture who seek health.

Everybody eats or avoids certain foods on a temporary basis during an acute illness. Thus, at some time or other, everybody eats for health.

It turns out that many persons in the first two groups have a rational basis in eating for health. The challenge in improving the nutriture of persons in these categories is to reach them with accurate information, assistance, and support so that they can accept personal responsibility for monitoring and control of their food intake. An appropriately modified definition of what is nutritious food, given physical limitations, is the basis for health maintenance.

Many persons in the latter categories eat for health on the basis of affective or emotional criteria. Food fads and cults are common among people in these categories. The challenge in this case is to improve diet intake without giving offense, which would alienate them. An appropriately modified definition of what is nutritious food, given beliefs, is the basis for health maintenance.

The mentality of a people determines the level at which they perceive and attempt to deal with health-related aspects of their life-style. Food ecology is closely related to the mentality and life-style of a person. For some, health is a blessing that they pray for because they fear that poor health will prevent happiness. People with this mentality often do not take the necessary actions in redefining what is food to assure a basis for health. Others feel that they are at the mercy of disease, which is a disaster that strikes randomly with appalling devastation. People with this mentality often adopt an attitude of utter hopelessness which precludes implementation of an assertive health maintenance program that includes diet control. Some people respond to any decrease in physical strength with a sharp decrease in sense of well-being; they feel abandoned. They will grasp at anything that appears to have promise in regaining vigor. So, unwittingly they may redefine what is food in a way that leads to nutritional disaster. For still others, the concept of health is inextricably bound to a cult of the body.

The quality of the observed food intake is determined by the quality of sources of food and nutrition information used. Use of a nutritionist is likely to lead to a nutritionally valid definition of what is food, which may improve physical capacity. Use of a quack is likely to lead to a nutritionally invalid definition of what is food, which may create a physical stress and/or waste money.

In recent years, there has been increasing evidence that the American people perceive unmet needs in relation to the way to eat for health. The number of courses, lectures, books, and articles on one aspect or another is phenomenal. Still, the demand is insatiable and people do not feel secure in their knowledge.

The "Establishments" have not dealt effectively with the need to eat for health. They provide some limited kinds of information in a fragmented way, for example:

(a) The "Nutrition Establishment" provides information on normal nutritional needs and how to use basic food guides. People learn about these in order to have some intellectual understanding of nutrition.

(b) The "Food Processing Establishment" provides some information on the nutritional value of foods, food processing methods, and the role of food additives.

(c) The "Health Care Establishment" provides some information on preventive and curative diets, and special foods to be used. Still, these inputs are not sufficient and are not used systematically in making daily food choices for health and people are uncomfortable.

So, many have turned to the person employed in health food stores for help. The lure of profit from the gullible encourages the glib to present their irresistible sales pitches. Thus, in good faith, many are enticed into spending large sums on innocuous and/or worthless foods that have been redefined as possessing some special value.

Therapeutic Diet Definitions

Diet therapy is used in prevention and/or control/cure of disease. It results in need for modification of food and people interactions, food experiences, food attributes, and food consumption behavior. A therapeutic diet is designed to treat a disease or disorder by application of a remedy. Terms with related connotations and implications are:

(a) remedy—A diet that relieves or corrects for effects of a disease (within an involved tissue) or disorder (some effect, e.g., high blood pressure, glucosuria, hyperlipidemia)

(b) relieve—Lift a burden to make it tolerable

(c) alleviate—Temporary or partial lessening of distress

(d) mitigate—Moderate or counteract the effect of something painful

(e) cure—To restore to health, soundness, and normality (implies permanence)

There are different types of modified diets for different conditions and levels of restriction that vary with the severity of the condition. The concept of modify includes, but is not limited to, the following aspects:

(a) to make less extreme—As when a person who habitually consumes a high fat diet must reduce fat intake to a moderate level

(b) to limit or restrict the meaning of and suggests a difference that limits, restricts, or adapts to a new purpose—As when one who has habitually consumed a salty rich diet must follow a low fat-low calorie diet until sufficient weight is lost that the gall bladder can be removed

(c) to make a minor change in—As when an ulcer patient is instructed to eat mid-morning, mid-afternoon, and bedtime snacks

(d) to make a basic or important change in—As in diabetes where the simple CHO content must be greatly restricted and the complex CHO content must be adjusted

Use of a modified diet requires changes. In this context, *change* means to make different in some particular(s) and may imply whatever level of variation, whether affecting some aspect of the food domain essentially or superficially. An *essential* difference amounts to a loss of original identity in one or more aspects of the food domain, i.e., that aspect is transformed or has a new direction. The magnitude of the change depends on the magnitude of the aspect changed. A *superficial* difference leads to substitution or replacement of one food/interaction by another, e.g., to exchange one food for an equivalent or comparable item. Between these two extremes are a number of levels of change. These include, but are not limited to:

(a) permutation—Transposition within a group of otherwise unchanged items, as in preventive modifications that are not followed rigorously.

(b) mutation—An inevitable change that lacks permanence and stability. This change is observed when people have distress from foods X, Y, Z, and Q. These may drop in and out of the diet or be replaced by other foods. The observed diet is usually very close to the customary since the effects of a few items are not far-reaching.

(c) major change—Either a transformation or a new direction. This is difficult and requires strong nutritional counseling. Many aspects of the food and people interactions may have to be changed in diseases such as ulcers, diabetes (maturity onset), and kidney failure.

(d) radical change—Either a transformation or a new direction of a magnitude great enough to constitute a reversal of what had been, as when one must change from high fat to low fat, high salt to low sodium, etc. This is very difficult and requires effective and continued nutritional counseling.

Both major and radical changes require extensive redefinition of what is food and what is poison and involve adjustment to changes in food attributes (color, texture, flavor, etc.), eating frequency and spacing of meals, size of meals, eating territory, and satisfactions resulting from food and people interactions. Counseling is needed to salvage as much positive reward as possible, given the new reality. It is used to assist the individual in returning to former health state and normal food and people interactions, to the extent possible. It provides suggestions for ways to lift the burdens of the dietary constraints via individualization of the diet, to the extent possible. Counseling seeks to assist individuals in compliance so as to reduce the probability of a recurrent episode and/or increase the probability of a return to a normal diet. It also provides guidance to assist individuals in returning to social eating in public, which involves instruction on selecting from restaurant menus.

Most people grow up with a vague awareness that adults and/or some children have some "condition" which requires that they may be served special foods or not served other foods. The "condition" for which such definitions are generally available include obesity, ulcers, diabetes, "heart trouble," and indigestion. Gradually, everybody acquires a definition of what is food and what is poison for each of these "conditions." These definitions are acquired piecemeal and out-of-context distortions occur. Unfortunately, the definitions are known and accepted and interfere with instruction by qualified professionals.

Some "conditions" require continuous adherence to a reasonably restricted definition of what is food in order to remain symptom-free or to avoid a catastrophe. Acceptance of personal responsibility is a necessity, but requires self-discipline.

Some subcultures have not accepted the concept of delayed gratification. Members from these subcultures will have two alternate definitions of what is food, which will be used alternately according to level of pain. These are: (a) the restricted definition, which is followed without deviation, when in acute pain, and (b) the usual subculture definition of what is food, which is indulged in during relatively asymptomatic periods. Continuing instruction is necessary to help individuals make a more appropriate adjustment for health.

When a diet has been prescribed, initial instruction provides definition of what is food and poison for most people. Because of individual differences in food ecology, additional and perhaps continuing instruction is necessary to individualize the definition of food and poison, to retain the quality of the eating experience, and to minimize disruption of food and people interactions. This is necessary in order to maintain long-term adherence and well-being; professional assistance should be sought.

Preventive Diet Definitions

The concept of a preventive diet to reduce the risk of heart attacks and strokes was introduced to the general public in the late 1960s. Whether an individual is at risk and whether diet modification will prevent one of these catastrophic events is unknowable for an individual. For the population-as-a-whole, the fact that risk is reduced has been established.

So, many people have been induced to redefine what is food. In this case, only a few foods are excluded. The emphasis is on making choices on a continuing basis so that the total intake of cholesterol, saturated fatty acids, and/or salt is below a defined daily limit. Particulars of a simplified pattern called "The Prudent Diet," discussed in Chapter 24, are quite restrictive but if one is willing to take the time, the definition need not be so narrow.

Body-Building Definitions

The masculine ideal of a strong, healthy, well developed body has been sought by teenage boys and men of every generation since the Golden Age of Greece when perfection of physical prowess was an obsession. Physical fitness programs have been revalued and revitalized since the 1960s finding that Americans were physically unfit due to a sedentary life-style. Men were encouraged to improve physical fitness in order to decrease risk of heart disease and physical exercise was advocated as a means to weight control. And, increasingly, women began to seek a healthy physique.

Control of food intake and a restricted definition of what is food have been a part of the body-building regimen since early times. The definition of what is food seemingly always has been an important issue, with many differing opinions among coaches and athletes. The decrees of the local coach(es) usually redefine what is food for the athlete in training. The idiosyncrasies of some nationally or internationally famous athlete(s) may result in a transitory redefinition of what is food as aspiring athletes imitate their idol in a faddish way.

From the scientific standpoint, the definition of what is food for body-building must be determined by the nutritional requirements of the individual as established by a biochemical evaluation of circulating levels of nutrients. Then lists of rich sources of needed nutrient(s) can be used as a basis for food choice. In this way, the definition of what is food can be modified to provide needed nutrients. No particular food is essential or possesses special virtue. It is only a better or poorer source of a needed nutrient(s), given the quantity consumed.

During training, protein (amino acid) needs are increased in the early stages while muscles are being developed. So, the need for high quality protein (any red meat, fish, poultry, or carefully chosen mixture of plant proteins can be used) is greater. After that, a normal maintenance quantity (RDA) suffices.

Strenuous exercise inflates the need for fluids and salts that are lost in sweat. These must be supplied for replacement. Many items may be defined as food for this purpose.

Public awareness of "body-building" foods is maintained by advertising slogans such as "Wonder Bread Builds Strong Bodies 12 Ways" or

"Every Body Needs Milk." Advocates of foods from each food group develop catch-phrases for this purpose.

Youth-Seeking Definitions

Approximately 15% of the American population lives to age 65 or older. Aging is accompanied by a decreased sense of well-being. As one becomes infirm, i.e., no longer strong enough to endure strain, pressure, or strenuous effort, and then feeble, i.e., almost totally lacking in strength, a panic may evolve. These natural outcomes are repugnant in a society that glorifies youth. So many, being unable to accept this problem, will grasp at anything that promises the "Fountain of Youth."

There is some evidence that some of the elderly have special difficulty in facing the normal fears, anxieties, and insecurities of old age and death. A crisis evolves since some ideologies do not deal with these aspects and to resort to religion would require an about-face that would be shattering to beliefs and self-concept. The solution to these problems that has been adopted by many has been the use of megadoses of selected vitamins. These are believed to postpone the effects of the aging process and ward off disease. For the elderly of this persuasion, the definition of what is food has been expanded to include large quantities of vitamin supplements. Other items such as bone meal, tiger's milk, kelp, carrot and kraut juices, and bran capsules also have been added to the definition of what is food.

Moreover, within memory of the elderly, many old people routinely took tonics and drank tisanes for health and comfort. When all else fails, many revive these customs and include these items in the definition of what is food. Indeed, such items may be infused with and invested with magical properties in restoring health and vigor. So, these are reinstated with a primary role. Thus, a tonic of sulfur and molasses (contemporary equivalent is Geritol) and various herbal teas are expected to have value and are consumed in hope. The observed euphoria, i.e., an often unaccountable feeling of well-being or elation, becomes understandable. When the elderly have established this link between their past, in dealing with present infirmities and in warding off future disease, they can experience a good feeling of accomplishment. Thus, a redefinition of what is food and drink can rekindle a sense of well-being.

Counterculture Health-Seeking Definitions

A health food diet works, i.e., it leads to improved health of those who follow it. How can this be? The answer is simple:

(a) A health food diet is based on foods of known nutritional quality, i.e., fresh meat, dairy products, fruits and vegetables, and minimally processed cereal products.

(b) It uses a combination of these in a simpler diet. The increased bulk causes people to feel full on a smaller quantity of food that also contains fewer calories. Such a diet avoids the common excesses that result from consumption of unsatisfying but enticing foods made from refined cereals and sugar.

(c) Greater interest in and knowledge of nutrition combined with religious, i.e., scrupulously and conscientiously faithful, control of intake. Together, these factors create and maintain a definition of what is food that leads to good health. Success in improving physical health naturally leads to a more positive mental outlook, even euphoria.

The need for internal balance and harmony has long been recognized as essential to good health. Since ancient times, man has believed that food has medicinal value, i.e., it can be used in treating disease—to alleviate or cure it and to relieve pain—and to improve one's sense of well-being. Bark, leaves, seeds, and roots are known to contain some substances that have healing power. Some plant materials have been processed since ancient times, albeit crudely, to remove the active principle and make them more convenient to use. So, some plant materials are dried and powdered and others are extracted. An infusion has been made from others and the liquid is drunk as tea. Still others, being used mainly for food, also have an effect; these traditionally have been classified as "hot" or "cold." This classification redefined usage or what is food for (a) certain people, e.g., old, sick, or weak and (b) certain circumstances, e.g., pregnancy, confinement, and lactation and a whole array of temporary minor illnesses such as flu, stomachache, and evil eye. The effects of "hot" diseases were believed to be alleviated by taking "cold" foods and vice versa, since these were believed to reestablish internal balance.

Acute Illness Definitions

Most people grow up with some vague memories that when they were sick with X (a common acute minor illness), they were served Y but not J. Y and J turn out to be variable among people; the common list of items has evolved from common experience. The items differ from place to place due to historical differences in availability. A few examples are listed below for illustration:

(a) nausea, vomiting, or stomachache—Y = dry toast, tea, plain carbonated beverage, gelatin dessert

(b) diarrhea— Y = tea and toast, carrot soup, chipped ice, boiled skim milk

(c) flu or common cold (starve a cold and feed a fever)—Y = chicken soup, milk toast, orange juice, fluids, whiskey and honey, honey hore-hound drops

(d) mumps—Y = chicken soup, ice cream; J = pickles, other sour foods

Learning Definitions of What Is Food for Health

Like other culturally defined aspects of the definitions of food and poison, the health-related portion is in part absorbed and in part careful-ly taught by means of the common system of rewards and punishment. The process begins early.

Everybody values a healthy baby, so most mothers try to create a situation in which the children will eat what they consider to be a healthful diet. A number of common phrases are used to impress upon the child the importance of eating X (an unwanted food), so one hears:

(a) "Eat your meat so you will be strong."

(b) "Eat your spinach; it's good for you."

(c) "Drink your milk so you will have strong bones and teeth."

(d) "You need your vitamins every day. Come on, chew it up. That's a good boy."

(e) "Eat your liver so you will be strong like a lion."

Even mothers who pay little or no attention to their own food intake are careful to buy baby meat, strained fruits and vegetables, and egg yolks for their babies. And, so it goes.

In a well meaning effort to be sure that the baby is well fed, some parents poison their babies with too much food. They give the baby a lot of juice, which is dilute. It fills the stomach but does not provide enough nourishment for the volume, so the baby is unsatisfied and continues to cry with hunger. It expands capacity and keeps food in the mouth; dental caries in erupting teeth result. When too much solid food is given, the baby becomes fat, which programs it for later problems. What is needed is balance. See Chapter 26.

School children become "junk-food junkies" as a result of an abundant supply of and free access to candy, soft drinks, and cookies. Peanuts, chips, ice cream, and other items also are staples of the diet. This definition of what is food is sweet, rich, and high in calories and little else. But, ten years of experience on this diet teaches the child many things. See Chapter 27.

The teenager learns more about food and health since physical de-mands for growth greatly inflate needs and appetite, concern with shape leads to body-building and/or weight control regimens, and belonging-ness needs require conformity to the current food fad. All of these aspects expand the teenager's consciousness of the health-related definitions of food and poison, as he/she attempts to conform to a defined diet rather than simply eating whatever is prepared and served in the home or is generally available. Typically, the teenager tries a variety of diets, so experience with redefinition of what is food for health can be considerable. Peers and popular literature are main sources of information about what is food for health under a variety of circumstances. See Chapter 28.

Normally, the primary health-related definitions of what are food and poison to be learned by young adults pertain to pregnancy and feeding of infants and children. Everybody, e.g., relatives, friends, and neighbors, frequently share opinions and repeat experiences as object lessons. Popular literature is also studied. From the process of sifting through this often conflicting information, a personalized definition of what is food emerges. See Chapter 29.

During the middle and later years, the personalization of the health-related definition of food and poison continues as one develops intolerances, opts to follow a preventive diet, and/or requires a therapeutic diet. A general accretion of common knowledge of the definition of food and poison for common acute illnesses also occurs. Normally, bit by bit the basic definitions formed at earlier periods are refined to meet new needs. See Chapters 30 and 31.

From early teenage years on, popular literature can have an important effect in redefining what is food and poison in relation to health. The half-truths that are presented and accepted are likely to be those portions of truth that are closest to what is already believed. The other half is beyond what one can understand; it may be there, but it is not revealed. It is in this way that people selectively learn or reinforce what they know.

Research has shown that people are more likely to select what they pay attention to because of the beliefs they have rather than base their belief systems and behavior on what they have just heard or read—nobody can change that fast and that consistently. IF this is so, THEN what is the explanation for the fact that many people have become health faddists? Consider the following: (a) most adults remember that they were healthy as children and (b) when most adults or their parents were young, food technology was not so advanced so food was processed less and did not contain the food additives that are commonly added today. In contemporary society, people are confronted with symptoms of poor health and/or reason to question food quality from the standpoint of health and safety. Since many people's beliefs about what is food were formed before food technology was so advanced or in a home where preparation from "scratch" was highly valued, it is reasonable to suppose that given uncertainty about health, some people will be receptive to the health food literature because it fits with long-held beliefs. Moreover, the fact that the beliefs were formed at a time when the person was healthy seems to confirm the suspicion that the simpler diet was healthier. This, then, is the basis on which a seemingly abrupt change can be made.

The revival of the cult of food as medicine can be explained similarly. Many adults from the various subcultures have grown up with some awareness that an older relative recommended X for "condition" Y and it worked. X is only half-remembered; but what is remembered is the resulting satisfaction. The impersonality of today's medical practice does not meet people's affective needs in times of stress in a society where many are anonymous and alone. Therefore, it is reasonable to suppose that given symptoms of poor health, some people will be receptive to a return to the use of food as medicine.

ECONOMIC DEFINITIONS

Seemingly food always has been considered to be costly; some foods such as salt were even precious in times past. And, food prices have been a major topic of discussion for centuries. Almost everybody has a mental idea of what the price of food X "should" be compared with what it is and what he/she "will" afford to pay for food X, irrespective of what he/she "can" pay. Therefore, IF the price of food X rises above what a person will afford, THEN it usually will not be purchased. The effects may be a temporary excluding from the definition of what is food, as in the case of foods with seasonally fluctuating prices. For example, meat, fruit, and vegetable prices are highly variable but the foods can be obtained year-round, e.g., strawberries may have to be flown in at $3.50 a quart in December. Or, the effects may be permanent, e.g., Salmon Loaf was served frequently when canned salmon was 59¢ per can but since the price has been beyond $1.25, it has been considered prohibitive.

In affluent America, most people can afford to purchase sufficient quantities of a reasonable variety of foods of good quality. Still, economic definitions affect everybody's food choices. In general, younger and older people differ in their expectations of and experiences with food prices and these factors affect their definition of what is food. Differing priorities at different stages of the life cycle also affect the definition of what is food. Some people cannot afford to purchase enough good food; a severely restricted definition of what is food is a common concomitant effect. Clearly, cost may be either a primary (critical variable) in the definition of what is food and the food choice decision-making process, or it may be one of a cluster of factors that together determine the decision outcome.

People appear to evaluate the cost of food simultaneously on two different scales. On the *normative* scale, the cost of an item is judged in comparison with the costs of other items in the same food class, e.g., the cost of hamburger is compared with that of chicken or T-bone steak. On the *ipsative* scale, the cost of an item is judged against itself at several points in time, starting with its cost at a base period, e.g., the cost of hamburger when one was a bride is compared with its current cost. Relative positions on both scales enter the decision-making process. However, the weights used depend on the age of the purchaser and food budget priorities. Thus, when somebody says, "The price of food X is outrageous—I just can't afford it anymore," the interpretation hinges on knowledge of the relative cost of alternate items as well as other demands of the person's food budget.

Economic Definitions When One Has Comfortable Means

Differing expectations concerning the cost of various foods is one independent factor that probably accounts for part of the differences between a younger and an older person's economic definition of what is food. It seems likely that because today's young people have generally grown up during a relatively affluent period, they can accept current prices of many foods as reasonable. And, they are more willing to purchase what they want, at what it costs. Since they have enough money, they can budget what is required. On the other hand, older persons generally grew up in a poverty or war-restricted period when both money and food were scarce, and prices were considerably lower. They feel virtuous when they feel that they can resist the impulse to purchase high-cost foods. Their hesitation is ingrained; they are not comfortable with the idea that they can expect to buy whatever they want, whatever it costs. Although they often have enough money and can budget what is required, they are reluctant to do so. And, they expect lower prices and are generally outraged with the price of many foods. Prices have not risen uniformly. So, those foods whose prices have risen most are targets for the outrage and are removed from the definition of what is food.

Differing experience with food prices is another independent factor that probably accounts for part of the differences in younger and older persons' definition of what is food. It appears that older people may be less willing to accept the continually rising price spiral as a normal outcome. They can remember when the price of food X was a nickel a pound; in their experience, this price is reasonable. No amount of explanation can reconcile them to the fact that the current high price is an outrage. They know that their income has risen and they read that personal disposable income has increased. But, these facts do not matter to them. What matters is that on the ipsative scale, the price of food X is "too much." So, this means that food X must be regarded as too expensive to be afforded. Younger women do not respond to current prices in the same way. This is because their experience is different. The purchase price at the time they started purchasing food X already was elevated, so the observed price rise is not yet too much. But, unless prices stabilize, the price of food X will reach a level that evokes the same response.

Except for the affluent, in order to meet expenses, people must set different spending priorities at the different periods of the life cycle. As a result, in some periods, the amount budgeted for food may be absolutely and/or relatively low in relation to other aspects of life-style. The resulting constraints on the definition of what is food may produce feelings of frustration, guilt, and anger. Thus, the incongruity creates a major conflict when it comes together with economic realities and results in feelings of deprivation in relation to an acquired need.

During the launching period, young people must (a) initiate purchase of basic household goods, (b) acquire a business wardrobe, and (c) start a family—on an income that is probably at its lifetime lowest. Life-style determines the level or quality of demands and thus associated costs. A higher income may not mean that more money is available for food. Sufficient money must be allocated for lunches and entertaining to maintain a socially acceptable food and people interaction front. But, behind this one may see that the amount budgeted for food is shockingly little—whatever is left. So, food is "gold" and the definition of what is food may be restricted to the less expensive cuts of meat which are extended when served, nuts and dairy products, and carbohydrate fillers. Fruits and vegetables may be too expensive to be used other than as treats.

During the coasting period, adults in the middle years must (a) complete purchase of original household goods and initiate replacement, (b) upgrade and update business apparel, and often (c) meet growing expenses of children's developmental education and experiences with an income that is climbing toward its lifetime maximum point. Here again, life-style determines the level or quality of demands and so the associated costs. Increasingly, during this stage the amount of money available for food rises. Sufficient money is available for and is allocated for lunches and entertainment that fit with life-style. Usually, the amount budgeted for food is relatively much greater. Food is still "gold"; however, the definition of what is food has been expanded to reinclude steaks, roasts, chops, fruits, vegetables, and other items formerly consumed during childhood and teenage years in the family home. As income expands, the less expensive items progressively drop out of the diet and are replaced by more highly valued and higher cost items since increasingly it is economically feasible to define them as food. Feelings of deprivation become only a memory. Luxuries that formerly were only dimly perceived on a distant horizon now become almost within reach and are tantalizing.

During the arrival period, spending priorities are rearranged to optimize satisfaction, given values and life-style. It seems that IF food is not an important source of satisfaction, THEN whatever definition of food applied in the preceding period is likely to continue. IF food becomes a major source of satisfaction, THEN its priority rises to its lifetime maximum and the definition of what is food will expand to include whatever is desired. So, food is "gold" and one enjoys its richness.

During the has-been period, which is highly variable in length from a few years to several decades, a sharply reduced income forces people to again redefine what is food within newly imposed economic limits. IF sufficient money is available, THEN a socially acceptable food and people interaction front may be maintained. But, often the amount of money available for food is shockingly little. So, food is "gold" and the definition of what is food is often sharply and painfully restricted to cheap and somewhat filling items. Loss in the economic sphere adds feelings of deprivation, bleakness, and desolation to the problems of aloneness of the elderly.

Another factor having an independent effect on the economic definition of what is food is advertising. Advertising is deliberately designed to create/maintain wants as well as to entice and tantalize. Carefully designed messages with multiple meanings that appeal differently to different segments of a reader/listener audience are disseminated via radio, TV, and magazines. These messages expand consciousness of alternate definitions of what is food to include similar items. This progressively expands the size of the food array and the want list. Unfortunately, when wants are created ahead of economic capability/access, then frustration and anger result.

The mentality of those with comfortable means and the mentality of the poor differ. As a result, there are different expectations/experiences in regard to food, eating, and the food and people interaction. These differences must be understood in order to respond appropriately to behavior of persons in both groups.

Economic Definition of the Poor

The level of uncertainty the poor have to live with makes a future orientation ridiculous. They cannot plan for the future as there are too many intervening variables that are beyond their control. In the resulting ecosystem, the definition of what is food reflects the "now" orientation, which is part of an appropriate adjustment mechanism that makes the deprived food and people interaction tolerable. Until now, attempts to change this situation have failed.

When the poor get a little money, they buy food and have a feast; between times, they may almost starve. So, efforts have been made to persuade the poor to allocate money received intermittently in such a way that a slightly better diet will be consumed on a continuing basis. The poor refuse to cooperate because a feast provides hope, relief from the monotony of a limited variety of foods, and the satisfactions of achievement. On the other hand, they perceive that a more uniform allocation might result in a somewhat better diet nutritionally, but that it would not be significantly different in terms of the items defined as food so it would still be monotonous and unsatisfying. Moreover, they would no longer be able to look forward to the occasional feast. And, this system would be impractical because other demands would take the money away from food anyway. So, it is not worth the effort.

It is for this reason that all enlightened contemporary proposals to help the poor obtain a better diet require that they be given enough money to obtain a basic level of other goods and services. The definition of what is food cannot rise above its minimum subsistence level to something with a potential of meeting nutritional needs when the level of other goods and services is similarly low. The money is simply spent on the other items.

When people consume a subsistence diet in the midst of a society where the majority have comfortable means, the poor are more aware of their deprivations than they would be in a society where nearly everybody shares the common lot. So, the poor covet the foods they cannot afford. And, their desires, which are fanned by advertising, become an obsession until they just must have food X, no matter what.

So, one observes that the poor purchase steak, lobster, and other luxuries with their Food Stamps. Public awareness results in expressions of outrage and demands for punitive action. Still, the "abuse" continues and it probably always will.

When people have a fixed low income, they accept the restricted definition of what is food as something they have to live with since they have no hope of obtaining luxuries. They do this by reducing awareness.

However, when people are given hope in the form of expanded food purchasing power, acceptance gives way to desire which frustrates them until they purchase the item(s). Under these changed circumstances, the accepted definition of what is food is rejected. A new definition emerges to take advantage of the expanded purchasing power in gratifying repressed desires. So, initially, a person on Food Stamps may feast. But, the reality of the continuation of the expanded food purchasing power is soon realized. Then, the wide swings of the feast or famine mode tend to even out toward the planned outcome of a nutritionally better diet.

Another behavior that at first glance appears to be an "abuse" of Food Stamps also can be observed: mothers use precious Food Stamps to obtain candy and soft drinks for the children. Here again, the explanation is simple and reasonable—on an occasional basis. At the subsistence level, a mother has difficulty in supplying rewards for desired behavior. Since food is scarce and is served monotonously, any variation takes on added significance. Everybody in the family, including very small children, know this. So, IF precious food money has been spent for candy or soft drinks, THEN the sense of satisfaction generated is all out of proportion to the monetary cost and thereby enables the food to serve as an important reward.

The poor long have had reduced purchasing power which has had a long-term effect on their definition of what is food. It is essentially limited to staples. Some rich sources of nutrients are not included in the definition of what is food because their absolute cost is too high. Many other foods that are good sources also are not regarded as food. Therefore, it should not be surprising that the nutritional quality of their diet is low. To improve nutritional quality, some of these foods must be consumed regularly. But, for most people an unknown food is rejected as readily as a disliked one. Therefore, unless steps are taken to correct the definition of what is food, increased purchasing power will not necessarily result in improved nutriture. It is for this reason that nutrition education, including the introduction of new foods, is a mandatory component of federal food programs. But, the solution to this problem creates another: IF one expands a person's consciousness of alternate foods in order to expand the definition of what is food, THEN one has changed the eating experience and has created an acquired need for the food(s) introduced. Unless access is provided simultaneously and on a continuing basis, dissatisfaction results and provides the seeds for rebellion. For this reason, control of the definition of the food of a people has political as well as economic importance; food is power.

Unlooked-for Gain

The notion of "getting something for nothing" is appealing and evokes gleeful exclamations. Everybody exults when food is obtained by give-aways or bargains. A windfall makes one jubilant. Whenever food is available free or at a cost below the going prices, especially when below the real value of it, the definition of what is food is adjusted to utilize the new item(s) to best advantage. A new item (introductory offer) or version (different brand) of a familiar item may be introduced into the food array by this means. Or, because of supply, frequency of consumption may be increased markedly. As long as supply lasts, which ordinarily is not that long, advantage overcomes the tendency to become tired of a perishable item that must be consumed intensely before it spoils. During the harvest season, this effect of the economic definition of what food is has a heavy impact on the diet.

AESTHETIC DEFINITIONS

The assessment of aesthetic quality is based on a psychological evaluation of the physical properties of foods, i.e., it is a psychophysical evaluation of appropriateness and composition. Color, texture, flavor, and odor are the attributes of foods that are evaluated for appropriateness. Composition of the plate and meal are evaluated on the bases of topography, neatness, quantity of food, harmony of attributes, and emphasis. Ornamentation is evaluated with respect to taste.

In the United States, we value artistic ability in a cook, i.e., showing taste in arrangement or execution, from the point of view of the cook who thinks in terms of creating beauty or form. But, most Americans are resigned to the fact that the majority of cooks make only a token effort to be artistic, e.g., they add something green, usually parsley, to the plate. On the other hand, as consumers we are highly variable in terms of the importance we place on aesthetic quality, i.e., assessment of beauty, from the point of view of one who analyzes and reflects upon the effect a work of art has upon him. Unless the cook is superb and evokes a response to his/her art, most of us focus on utilitarian aspects unless the food has some obvious defects.

The aesthetic definition of what is food and what is good is culturally determined. Each culture has its own scale of values for each quality; both scale factors and values are known. In some cultures, especially Japanese, perfection can be obtained only by a few—freshness and top color, texture, and flavor are prized. In the United States, we value what has been derisively called "uniform mediocrity"—a standard that is less than perfection but attainable almost everywhere, most of the time. Aesthetic values change with technological capabilities. The American standard for fruits and vegetables requires uniformity in size and color, which has been made possible by sizing and grading. Artificial colors and flavors are commonly added to foods to adjust color and flavor to a standardized level. Deviation from standard is a recognized defect that detracts from aesthetic quality. The accept/reject decision is based on attributes and composition.

Attributes

Foods are the source of nutrition. . . Since their nutritive properties are taken for granted, food items are not bought primarily on the basis of nutrition but rather on the basis of how well they are liked. While price and ease of use are interwoven in the fabric of food purchase, the inherent sensory properties of the food item *are* the primary determinants of its acceptance. How does it look? How does it smell? How does it taste? If the response to these questions is "O.K." or "all right," then acceptance will result. For acceptance implies neutrality: there is nothing particularly wrong with a product. Better yet, if the response to the question of looks, smell, and taste is "good" or "I like it" or "my family likes it," then preference is on the horizon. Preference implies the existence of plus factors over and above neutrality or acceptance.

In other words, people use their senses to determine if a food is edible and secondly if it pleases them. The first is a judgment, the second is a reaction.

People prejudge a food by its appearance. From its colour they can tell if a tomato is ripe; they can tell if a roast of meat will be juicy and succulent, if toasted bread will taste bitter, if coffee is weak. Its odour will tell them if a fish is fresh, if a fat is rancid, if milk is sour. Through previous experience they will frequently be able to predict the flavour and texture of the food from its appearance and aroma, and on the basis of this flash prediction they decide to accept or reject.

But the prime test of a food occurs when it is eaten. Its in-the-mouth or flavour properties are by far its most important sensory properties.[1]

As Sjostrom (1959) has pointed out, the decision to accept/reject a food item is based on the definition of what is good food, which involves a psychophysical multi-factor evaluation. A few examples of the role of food attributes in this evaluation follow.

Color as an Index to Eating Quality.—(a) appropriateness—The food has no off-color, usually it is uniform in color or has typical variegation, and has no color defects. It is not considered to be food if it is out of the ordinary, e.g., red French fries, green tinged meat. By convention, inappropriate food colors are blue and psychedelic hues such as electric pink and chartreuse.

(b) index to process control—The food is of the appropriate color, reflects light appropriately. A cooked food that is too brown is expected to have a flavor defect; color indicates overcooking. Juices that are expected to be clear but are turbid reflect overextraction in which the pulp has been extruded into the liquid; turbidity is expected in "natural" juices.

(c) index to flavor based on stage of maturity—This concept applies to fresh fruits and vegetables. IF the skin is green, THEN they are expected to be underripe. IF the skin is brown, THEN they are expected to be overripe or rotten.

(d) index to purity—This concept applies to sugar and cereals. IF white, THEN they have been refined or milled to a state of pure carbohydrate.

Texture as an Index to Eating Quality.—(a) appropriateness—The food has no abnormal texture and is uniform with no defects. IF a hard

---

[1]From Caul and Sjostrom (1959). Quoted with permission of Arthur D. Little, Inc.

spot is encountered, THEN it evokes a sense of fear of injury and the mouthful is ejected. IF an unusually soft spot is encountered unexpectedly, THEN the same response follows.

(b) index to deterioration—Prior experience creates an association, e.g., mushy (fruit or vegetable) is rotten, flexible (carrot, celery, potato, or the like) is wilted, hard (bread or other bakery product) is old and stale.

(c) index to cookery quality—Prior experience creates an association that serves as the basis for inference, e.g., lumpiness in a gravy or sauce indicates poor dispersion and smoothness indicates good mixing; stringiness (cheese) indicates too high and/or too long heat exposure; and smooth fluid texture indicates appropriate exposure.

Flavor and Odor as Indexes to Eating Quality.—Flavor and odor are expected to be typical for the item, with no off-flavor or off-odor. In the mouth, the action of chewing ruptures cellular structures and coatings, water-soluble compounds are dissolved, and heat volatilizes odorous fragments and molecules. Thus, a variety of stimuli are active, provoking an individual and/or collective response.

An individual is not always able to characterize and describe the specific aspects that create the "right" or "wrong" flavor/odor impression. Frequently a person can respond only in general, e.g., "It tastes good" or "I like it" or the contrary.

A "wrong" flavor or odor evokes a negative response. And, IF any stimulus is wrong, THEN the overall flavor and/or odor will be perceived as unpleasant. Also, the eater will be disappointed. In fact, the degree of unpleasantness appears to reflect the degree of wrongness. Wrongness includes, but is not limited to, sourness, bitterness, greasiness, bite, lack of salt, or strength of characteristic bouquet. Too much or too little implies existence of a range that cannot be exceeded without evoking a perception of wrongness.

(a) appropriateness—No off-flavor or off-odor, and usually it must be uniform with no defects. We accept differences in flavor of chicken and turkey that are reminiscent of nuts but not fish. Vegetables that taste like dirt or fertilizer also are rejected.

(b) index to deterioration—We smell a fish for ammonia, a fruit for alcohol, milk for sourness, fats and oils for rancidity or fishiness. Such defects cause instant rejection.

(c) index to cookery quality—Mellow flavors indicate a quality not achieved by a hurried sprinkle of a powdered spice or herb. The flavor of butter is distinctive and not replicated by butter-flavor. The tantalizing aroma of soups, stews, casseroles, and steaks attracts consumers. The pungent odor of over-heated oil advertises a "greasy spoon" restaurant.

The sulfurous odor of over-cooked cabbage precedes the item to the table. What is good has four aspects: an early impact of an appropriate flavor and/or odor, pleasant mouth sensations, absence of unpleasant sensations and/or character, and no bad lingering aftertaste. Cookery must avoid or mask salty, burned, or excessive sharpness in flavor and sweaty, goaty, or putrid odors.

IF any one of the above attributes is prominent, for whatever good or bad reason, THEN the eat/not eat decision is heavily affected by that attribute and conscious awareness is achieved. Otherwise, a cluster of attributes must create an effect in order for the impact to register at the conscious level. When the qualities balance out, one is unconscious of the individual attributes.

Perfection is sought. A perfect food is one that satisfies all of the requirements when judged against an ideal standard of soundness of every part and excellence in every quality. A blemish or surface defect or even a flaw such as a crack can be removed and the remainder diced, sliced, etc. But, if the fruit or vegetable is served intact, i.e., it is perfect in its natural or original state so that no part has been removed or destroyed, one perceives that it is of high quality and is suitably impressed. It is for this reason that whole fruits and vegetables are highly prized and give aesthetic satisfaction.

Composition

A mixed dish, a plate lunch, and a meal itself present the cook with opportunities for artistic expression that affects the aesthetic aspects of the eating experience. Topography, neatness, quantity, harmony of attributes, and emphasis are evaluated as separate aspects of composition. In achieving artistic composition, the cook uses several alternatives:

(a) food mixture—A dish prepared by combining two or more ingredients; a *mixture* is distinguished from a compound in that the ingredients are not present in absolutely fixed proportions, do not lose their individual characteristics, and can be separated by physical means.

(b) food combination—Foods commonly served together; an association links them because the sensory attributes are compatible.

(c) food flavor blend—The ingredients are mixed thoroughly so that the flavors of the individual ingredients merge and are no longer distinct.

(d) food carrier—A mild food used as a base to dilute the highly flavored food which may be costly, hard to handle, or need a frame to set it off.

(e) food mask—An optional ingredient added to disguise or interfere with perception so that off-color, off-flavor, or off-odor becomes indistinct or imperceptible.

For aesthetic reasons, a high quality mixed dish has the following attributes:

(a) topography—Some large and small pieces so that when it is served it forms a pile.

(b) neatness—Pieces are cut uniformly and any sauce is not runny; no part extends beyond the edge of the dish.

(c) quantity—Reasonable in proportion to the dish; neither skimpy or too much.

(d) harmony of attributes—A pleasing integration and arrangement of items—colors, textures, shapes, flavors, and odors are compatible.

(e) emphasis—Pleasing contrasts of color, texture, shape, flavor, and/or odor.

This standard is not often met, so when the definition of what is food is associated with this standard, anything less may be rejected; at least it is less satisfying.

The quality of a plate lunch also may be judged on the same bases. For example:

(a) topography—Some large and small pieces should be piled so as to create variation from high to low.

(b) neatness—Pieces of the same item should be uniform, any sauce should flow but not run, and no part should extend beyond the edge of the dish.

(c) quantity—The portions of the various items should be related to their nutritional density and satiety value as well as the size of the plate; neither a skimpy nor an excess amount should be served.

(d) harmony of attributes—A pleasing arrangement of items is essential; garnishing is customary but should be in harmony. Colors, textures, shapes, flavors, and odors should be integrated and/or compatible.

(e) emphasis—Pleasing contrasts of color, texture, shape, flavor, and/or odor are necessary for interest. A garnish may be used for accent.

The same bases are used for evaluating the aesthetic quality of a meal. However, select and/or superior items, rare and/or costly items also may be a major basis for aesthetic satisfaction. When the common bases are used, the focus is different.

(a) topography—The various foods should not all be the same height nor distinct pieces; one that is amorphous on the main plate integrates.

(b) neatness—The items served together on the plate should not run together nor extend beyond its edge.

(c) quantity—Same as above.

(d) harmony—Same as above.

(e) emphasis—Same as above and there should be variation in the temperature of the various courses. A meal that has too much sameness of any attribute lacks interest. Richness can be cloying or pleasing. Variation in all aspects of richness can be used for interest; i.e., among the various foods some can have high value or quality, some can be magnificently impressive, some can be vivid or deep in color, some can be full and mellow in tone and quality, some can have a pungent odor, some can be highly seasoned, fatty, or sweet. Any of these variations can give richness by means of a quantity greater than that necessary to gratify normal needs or desires.

High quality ingredients may be skillfully prepared to produce aesthetically pleasing meals that need no adornment, i.e., enhancement by addition of something beautiful in itself. But, many times, some addition is necessary and/or desirable. There are six concepts with respect to adornment that are applied in meeting different needs:

(a) decorate, i.e., to relieve plainness or monotony by adding color or design to the food to give it beauty

(b) ornament, i.e., to heighten or set off the original food's beauty by adding something

(c) embellish, i.e., to add something to the surface of the food as a decoration; often it is superfluous and/or adventitious, e.g., an inedible toy on a birthday cake

(d) beautify, i.e., to add an embellishment of a type that counterbalances inherent plainness or ugliness, e.g., swirling chocolate icing on a cake

(e) deck, i.e., to add something that contributes gaiety, splendor, or showiness, e.g, ice cookies with faces, add exotic fruits to a platter, heap a platter for a group or a plate for an individual and then embellish it lavishly

(f) garnish, i.e., to decorate with a small final touch of something at serving time

In any case, success in adornment is usually contingent on demonstration of good taste. Good taste means that the manner of adornment creates an aesthetic quality indicative of discernment and appreciation for what is artistically pleasing. IF one lacks discernment, THEN adornment fails by being (a) gaudy, i.e., by ostentatious or tasteless use of overly bright colors or lavish ornamentation; (b) tawdry, i.e., by gaudiness and cheapness of quality; or (c) garish, i.e., unpleasantly bright. Definitions of what is good are a matter of convention.

Aesthetically pleasing food is the basis for a pleasurable eating experience. It also adds to the quality of normal food and people interactions. It reaches its ultimate in importance to the gourmet.

DEFINITIONS OF FOOD/POISON, FOOD ECOLOGY AND LIFE EXPECTANCY

Clearly, the various definitions of what is food have individual effects on man's relation to his food. These definitions determine the accept/reject decision in regard to each possible food. What is food and what is poison are major factors in life expectancy. This point will become clear from subsequent discussion.

Subgroup Definitions of Food and Poison[1]

Most members of the various ethnic, religious, and/or socioeconomic subgroups that comprise the American population are familiar with and follow common American foodways to some extent. In addition, they have a set of foodways that are unique to their subgroup. Thus, they have two coexisting sets of foodways with which to respond in food and people interactions.

Usually one set of foodways is dominant and the other is recessive. For practical reasons, the American set is usually observed in public. But, they may follow their subgroup foodways at home, especially with respect to the main meal and on special occasions. Or, they may follow only subgroup foodways on ceremonial occasions or in times of emotional/psychological stress when the traditions are a source of comfort. However, some individuals in each subgroup consistently follow the subgroup foodways in their entirety, for example, new immigrants who may be unfamiliar with the common American foodways, or, new converts who are zealous in observance in their initial fervor.

The foodways of subgroups differ from the common American foodways because of differences in beliefs, attitudes, intentions, and/or codified behavior patterns related to any aspect in the food domain, including food and people interactions. Some overlap between the common and subgroup foodways is usual. However, disparate beliefs and differences in specification of important details of particular practices are inherent sources of conflict. The nature and extent of resolution of such conflicts vary within and among subgroups. Frequently, a particular point of view simply must be accepted. In some cases individuals are ambivalent and practice both ways, depending on the situation. And, inconsistencies between belief and intentions or behavior may be apparent to others but the member(s) of the subgroup may be oblivious to them. For these

---

[1]Some members of each of the various subgroups may perceive important similarities and differences between the foodways of their subgroup and the common American foodways, but they may be unable to communicate the spirit of such intimate matters. As a result, descriptions are apt to be sterile compilations of documented facts. This constraint imposes a barrier that can only be surmounted by those who have an open and non-judgmental approach that gains acceptance by members of the group.

A student may study descriptions and explanations of the foodways of a particular subgroup and thereby acquire a limited intellectual understanding and appreciation. But, to develop an intimate awareness of the symbolic meanings associated with the various aspects, extensive experience as a participant-observer in a variety of customary food and people interactions is necessary.

reasons, delineation of foodways may be a very complex and challenging undertaking.

Characteristically distinctive responses to particular items are due to differences in conditioning. Different beliefs and/or attitudes toward a particular plant or animal tissue that might be used for food make a different response appropriate. Differences in perception of an occasion, food and people interactions, etc., also evoke different responses. And, the definition of what is "good" in terms of color, texture, and/or flavor in general or in reference to particular foods also may differ; thus, different responses will result. So, composition of the arrays of items accepted as food and items avoided as poison differs from the norm.

The foodways of the various subgroups are not static. In the original form, they were relevant—they met human needs, given the constraints imposed by circumstances—and reliable in that they provided a structure that encouraged consumption of a nutritious diet. Since they first evolved, changes in some of the foodways or in the circumstances of the subgroup may have modified their basic validity. For example, scarcity or costliness of traditional ingredients may have caused some food to be eliminated or modified by substitutions with the result that nutrient intake is decreased significantly. Or, new life-styles may have precluded family gathering for meals at traditional times and places so the resultant lack of informed food choice caused nutritional quality of intake to fall. Exposure to alternative beliefs, attitudes, and/or practices may result in acceptance and incorporation into the contemporary foodways, i.e., they are assimilated. Thus, foodways evolve, becoming less divergent. On the other hand, an influx of new immigrants or converts tends to renew vigor of some traditions, causing them to wax stronger for a time. New ways also may be introduced as variations. Thus, the contemporary transitional version of a subgroup's foodways evolves. And, the historical cultural plurality of the United States continues, sustained in part by maintenance of traditions in the food domain.

Folk beliefs and practices related to the use of dietary adjustment and/or herbal remedies to create/maintain inner humoral harmony during periods of physical and/or emotional stress continue in many areas. These evolved from ancient Egyptian and Babylonian medicine and were introduced into Latin America at the close of the Middle Ages. Folk medicine quickly spread throughout the world. Modern medical care has long been available in major cities but has not been widespread in the rural areas. For this reason, folk medicine has continued. At present, it is used instead of and in addition to standard medical care.

The general system of folk medicine has the following features that are important in restoration of health and well-being. With respect to each specified medical condition, there is a definition of what is food—which items, modifications in preparation that are necessary; a definition of which standard foods are poisons to be avoided; an explanation of why the remedy is necessary and why its qualities are efficacious; and usually there is a ritual for cleansing and acknowledgment of the cure.

Examination of the foods in each classification reveals a general pattern. The dietary staples are usually classified as irrelevant to the remedy, so they can continue to be consumed *ad libitum*. The foods that must be eaten are scarce or costly, so consumption requires a sacrifice which can be justified by the forthcoming benefit. The foods to be avoided are usually desired for their sensory gratification, so a sacrifice is justified by the forthcoming benefit.

These practices and beliefs are very controlling. IF not followed correctly, THEN some overwhelming evil is predicted.

Having discussed some of the more prominent universal differences, particulars can now be addressed. The traditional and/or contemporary foodways of the following subgroups are outlined: Blacks, Latin Americans, Eastern Mediterranean peoples, Jews, Orientals, and vegetarians.

Black Definitions of Food and Poison.—The Blacks of the rural South have customarily followed simple foodways that developed during the antebellum era. The Black descendents of those that migrated from the rural South to the North Central and Northeast industrial cities of the United States have adapted the traditional foodways; the contemporary pattern is frequently a reflection of low socioeconomic status and may not include much of a residue of the traditional foodways of the rural South. Those on the West Coast consume a diet that is essentially the same as that of WASPs of the same economic level; they are unlikely to be familiar with the traditional foodways of the rural South.

The Rural Southern Traditions.—A residual set of folk beliefs with respect to what is appropriate for certain persons to consume under certain conditions may affect diet intake to some extent. The nature and extent of these folk beliefs that continue to be followed is a local matter. Some relate to cravings or avoidances for pregnancy and lactation, others pertain to the weaning diet for infants, others define consumption/avoidance of specific foods in relation to particular illnesses, and still others pertain to diets for the elderly. Pica, the eating of clay, soot, or other non-nutritious non-food items in a compulsive way, is one manifestation. Avoidance of a specific food to avoid a birthmark on the fetus is another.

The food and people interactions link beliefs, attitudes, intentions, and behavior in a positive way to make life more bearable. A basic belief is that food is a blessing to be used for reward and satisfaction. A pervasive attitude in the family-centered culture where togetherness and hospitality are a tradition is that food is provided, prepared, and served as a gift of love. The intent is to imply and reinforce the point that situational limitations can be overcome in such a way that love, security, happiness, enjoyment, and a sense of well-being are possible. Therefore, the behaviors that sustain the mealtime atmosphere radiate thankfulness and enjoyment, even when resources are limited.

Food preparation methods have been used ingeniously as a means of making use of less desirable but free or inexpensive ingredients into palatable and filling meals. For example, long slow cooking of fibrous plant and animal tissues was feasible since these items could be started prior to and simmered during the hours in the fields. Leftover mush, potatoes, grits, etc., could be fried quickly, either prior to leaving for the fields or upon return when one was too weary to engage in elaborate meal preparation. Over-mature peas, corn, and squash could be improved by routine addition of sugar to compensate. Quick breads such as biscuits and cornbread were practical since self-rising flour and meal were available.

The traditional diet prepared by a "labor of love" has been romanticized and stereotyped as Soul Food. Typical ingredients include, but are not limited to, fat meat (salt pork), tripe and other variety meats from the pig, pigs' feet, pigs' ears, pigs' tails, neckbones, and ham hocks; chicken; squirrel and other small game; starchy carbohydrates such as cornmeal used for breading, cornbread, and muffins and grits, rice, and wheat flour; legumes such as black-eyed peas and lima beans; greens such as mustard, collard, dandelion, turnip tops, and kale; and vegetables such as okra, squashes, onions, tomatoes, corn, sweet potatoes, and turnips; sweeteners such as molasses and cane syrup. Fresh garden vegetables and melons were eaten in season. Along the East and Gulf Coasts and in areas close to rivers, local fish and shellfish were consumed in quantity. Fish were conventionally coated in a cornmeal batter and fried; these were accompanied by hush puppies. Shellfish usually were simmered in a highly spiced mixture such as Creole Sauce or gumbo. Use of dairy products normally was limited to buttermilk and, later, evaporated milk. Candies, cakes, and pastries were very rich and very sweet. Iced tea was the omnipresent beverage; it was brewed by steeping tea in hot simple syrup.

Fieldwork requires hard physical labor, so large high-caloric meals were necessary to provide energy. A traditional breakfast included assorted fried meats and/or eggs with rice, grits, and fried potatoes and gravy. Biscuits and syrup accompanied the main course. Strong coffee extended with chicory was served with sugar and milk. A traditional dinner served at noon was a boiled dinner. It consisted of boiled vegetables and legumes seasoned with fat meat and onions, boiled sweet or white potatoes, cornbread, iced tea, and possibly a dessert or fruit. The evening meal consisted of fried meat or fish, fried leftover grits or rice with gravy, and cold biscuits or cornbread.

The Contemporary Southern Diet.—The increasing industrialization of the South since the 1940s has provided Blacks with the economic means to purchase standard American foods. Moreover, Blacks generally have accepted the values of the common middle-class WASP culture. However, many do not have sufficient money to purchase the full array of foods that symbolize these values on a regular basis. As a result, the contemporary Black diet continues to feature traditional items and methods of preparation more frequently than does the diet of WASPs in the same community. Otherwise, it is the same.

The Northern Black Diet.—Migration from the rural South to the industrial urban North necessitated some changes. These were described by Jerome (1968, 1969) for one group in the late 1960s as follows:

(a) An effort was made to retain as many features of the traditional meal pattern as possible. All items were retained, although some were served less frequently and/or at a different meal.

(b) The traditional breakfast was lightened to eggs with or without a meat such as bacon or sausage, hot biscuits or bread, and coffee.

(c) A lunch meal of soup, sandwich, fruit, and fruit drink replaced the boiled dinner.

(d) A heavier evening dinner replaced the warmed-over supper. The week was divided between boiling and frying days. The traditional noon boiled dinner was served on boiling days and the traditional fried breakfast on frying days.

There also is some indication that northern-born Blacks consume a diet that is essentially the same as that of their socioeconomic peers, with three exceptions:

(a) They purchase somewhat less frozen juices and frozen desserts.

(b) They purchase more pork, chicken, greens, baking supplies, and other foods associated with southern cookery.

(c) They purchase more soft drinks, candy, and other snack items which are status symbols used as rewards.

Those who have become Black Muslims follow the traditional proscriptions of Muslims. For a description, see chapter references.

The Western Black Diet.—The ingredients necessary for preparation of traditional southern fare are not readily available in western supermarkets, although some can be obtained in small neighborhood markets that cater to Blacks. However, prices are sharply higher. Moreover, life-styles and working hours do not favor continuance of traditional food preparation and meal patterns. So, they have been abandoned and have been replaced by the common western eating patterns.

Latin American Definitions of Food and Poison.—A common blend of foodways dominates from Mexico to Tierra del Fuego, including the Caribbean. The originally distinct foodways of many Native Americans, Spanish and Portuguese Roman Catholics, and various groups of African Blacks have been assimilated as a result of centuries of intermingling. In general, the same basic beliefs, attitudes, intentions, and behaviors are shared despite differences in dietary staple and economic level. Recent in-migration of sizeable groups of peoples from eastern Europe and the Orient has had a major impact on the foodways in some local areas. In the major urban areas, especially among the more affluent, cosmopolitan foodways are observed.

The Traditional Foodways Base.—The major factors determining the regional foodways are: basic foodstuffs available, food preparation methods, the social structure, influence of religion, and folk medicine. The contributions of each are outlined below:

(a) The indigenous foods of the Native Americans plus selected imported foods define what is food. The indigenous foods include, but are not limited to, corn, various starchy root vegetables, tubers such as white and sweet potatoes, various kinds of beans, tomatoes, chilis and sweet peppers, onions, squashes and melons, avocados, chocolate, vanilla, oregano, and coffee. Rice, wheat, pork, chicken, beef, mutton, salt codfish, olives, Mediterranean herbs, Oriental spices, and some fruits were contributed by the Spanish and Portuguese. Peanuts, okra, cowpeas, and sesame were introduced by the Blacks.

(b) Methods of preparation of common dishes and of preservation of the basic foodstuffs are largely Native American in origin. For example, in the northern areas where corn was the staple, it was parched, dried, and ground into meal. The meal was made into a gruel and consumed as a beverage. It also was blended with a small amount of water, forming a pour batter, and was baked on a hot rock—this unleavened water bread is called a *tortilla*. Another item, the *tamale*, is a steamed cornmeal mush envelope enclosing a piquant to pungent meat-tomato-chili paste. In other areas, starchy root vegetables were steamed and/or baked in fire pits. Large quantities of rice were steamed with fat, particularly lard, in some areas. The ration required about 7 oz raw rice. Pit barbecues, spit roasting, and stewing are indigenous methods of meat preparation.

Mixtures[1], combinations[2], and blends[3] are distinctive and ubiquitous. Bean and tomato mixtures, cactus and pumpkin or squash mixtures, and avocado, tomato, and chili mixtures are basic. Combinations of soup or stew with tortillas, bean mixtures with tortillas, and/or rice, mashed avocado and tortillas are typical. Blends of cumin, chilis, green peppers, onions, and tomato with and without oregano are the base of a sauce used for seasoning most entrées.

Spanish sauces, salt codfish stews, and baked custards with and without bread or rice, tortes, wheat flour breads, and pastas are the contributions of the Spanish and Portuguese. Hot, spicy, tomato-okra-onion dishes were contributed by the Blacks. Both groups also contributed some adjustments in spicing and refinements in tools and methods of food preparation. Other distinctive influences are:

(a) The male-oriented social structure dictates that food be served by the female to the male(s) present. The main mixture is ladled from a common serving bowl to an individual dish. Accompanying side dishes are offered or passed. Children and women then may be served, or they may be fed separately.

(b) The influence of the Roman Catholic church is pervasive. Grace is a part of the mealtime ritual and the traditional Roman Catholic feast and fast days are publicly observed. In each locale, special dishes are associated with each of the major religious festivals. Composition and preparation are a matter of local convention rather than standardized ritual. No meat is served on specified fast days or during Lent.

(c) Folk medicine is practiced widely. The "hot" and "cold" system is the one that has been retained. Physical and emotional conditions are classified as "hot" or "cold" according to some local convention which may have an empirical basis. The basic underlying belief is that the condition creates or results from a lack of harmony of the basic humors. This can be remedied by consumption of a food of the opposite character. Thus, a "hot" condition is treated by consumption of a "cold" food; all "hot" foods must be avoided. Within a particular locality, there is some consensus concerning which conditions are "hot" and which are "cold." There is usually much less agreement with respect to which foods are "hot" and "cold."

---

[1]Food mixture—A dish prepared by combining two or more ingredients; a *mixture* is distinguished from a *compound* in that the ingredients are not present in absolutely fixed proportions, do not lose their individual characteristics, and can be separated by physical means.
[2]Food combination—Foods commonly served together; an association links them because sensory qualities are compatible and the contrast provides interest.
[3]Food flavor blend—The ingredients are mixed thoroughly so that the flavors of the individual ingredients merge and are no longer distinct.

These beliefs and practices associated with folk medicine are determining factors with respect to the diets during pregnancy and lactation, weaning diets, and diets for the elderly. An infant with a birth defect is especially likely to be treated by dietary means. For specifics, see chapter references.

The Contemporary Chicano Foodways.—Most Chicanos in the United States reside in California, Arizona, New Mexico, or Texas; in some of these states they are the major population group, in others they are the largest minority. Others reside in surrounding western states, Michigan, or New York. Area of origin in Mexico, socioeconomic status, and length of time in the United States are major factors affecting their degree of acculturation.

The majority who have immigrated to the United States as unskilled labor are from the rural northern states of Mexico. Their foodways are traditional and change is relatively slow due to economic and educational limitations. Migrant workers are part of this group. Their meal pattern has been reported as: breakfast (consumed at 9:00 a.m. during a morning break)—eggs, tortillas, fried beans, cereal, and beverage; lunch (eaten between 12:00 and 2:00 p.m. in the field)—beans and/or tortillas, meat or stew, beverage; and supper (consumed at about 6:00 p.m.)—beans and/or meat, rice or potatoes, tortillas, and sometimes a vegetable, beverage. Cookies, doughnuts, and standard American snack foods are eaten at breaktime in the fields.

The foodways of American-born Chicanos from lower class families may be traditional due to limited exposure to the common American diet. However, when they do Americanize their meals, breakfast, lunch and/or snack foods are changed first. Often they repress traditional beliefs and attitudes learned at home for social reasons. They may follow American foodways mechanically, not having understood nor accepted the underlying beliefs. Preferences for traditional entrées, seasonings, and methods of preparation are usually retained.

The foodways of American-born Chicanos from middle and upper class homes are similar to those of their peers. In their homes they may continue to prepare and serve traditional foods more frequently than others in the same community. However, common exposure by the mass media is likely to result in loss of traditional beliefs, attitudes, and intentions rather than assimilation.

The Contemporary Puerto Rican Foodways.—Puerto Ricans have settled in groups in Florida, New York City, and Chicago. Many make intermittent extended trips back to Puerto Rico. This encourages retention of the traditional foodways as does concentration in neighborhoods of their own kind. However, lack of availability of familiar tropical fruits and high cost do modify the quantity and frequency of consumption of fruits and other items. The basic staples of the traditional diet are starchy root vegetables (plantains, sweet potatoes and yams, and cassava), rice, and beans. *Sofrito*, a variety of Spanish sauce, is used for seasoning the staples. Salt codfish, pork, eggs, avocados, and many other optional ingredients are used in small quantity to provide endless variety.

Eastern Mediterranean Definitions of Food and Poison.—The foodways of the peoples of Greece, Turkey, and the Arab lands of Lebanon, Syria, Iran, Iraq, Jordan, Egypt, Libya, etc., have many common features. Food is regarded as important both as a source of nourishment and as a medium of socio-religious ceremonial functions, e.g., families gather for meals, food is a central feature of hospitality, it is blessed before consumption, and it is eaten with enjoyment.

Ingredients, spicing, and preparation methods are distinctive. Food mixtures are used extensively. The lunch entrée is usually a stew. Pilaf is frequently a component of the evening meal.

Bread is the staple starchy food; in Greece it is a French-type often baked in a ring; in the other countries it is like a large chewy pancake. In any case it is eaten plain and is used to sop up juices from the entrée. Pasta is used to some extent. Rice is seasoned and stir-fried and then steamed with optional ingredients such as nuts and/or raisins to make a pilaf.

Lamb is the preferred meat but chicken and pork also are commonly consumed, as is fish. Meats and vegetables are frequently simmered together, seasoned with garlic, cinnamon, mint, lemon juice, and tomatoes. A similar lamb-rice mixture is rolled in cabbage or grape vine leaves and simmered in a tomato sauce. Legumes of many varieties are eaten in lieu of meat at many meals.

Vegetables are eaten raw in salads dressed with lemon juice and olive oil or sour cream and sesame seed. They are cooked by simmering pieces in broth, stuffed and baked, or are fried and served with a tomato-based sauce. Some are stored in brine or are pickled.

Desserts are very rich and very sweet; portions are small. They are usually spiced with lemon and cinnamon, contain ground or finely chopped nuts, and may contain raisins. Several kinds are typical, but are reserved primarily for holidays and special occasions. One is made by building a stack of layers of very thin pastry sprinkled lavishly with finely chopped nuts, sugar, and spices. This is baked, cut in diamonds, and is drenched in simple syrup prior to service. A second is a plain rounded fritter served in honey or simple syrup. A third is a congealed farina mush, cut in various shapes, and served with a simple syrup flavored with almond, orange, or rose water. A fourth is a coffee cake similar to that of the Slavs.

Common beverages are coffee, tea, and fruit juice mixtures. All are very sweet. Coffee is very strong. Tea is frequently flavored with mint. Wine, plain and flavored with resin, is consumed in quantity except by Muslims. Arak is a typical hard liquor.

Three major religions are practiced in this region: Jewish, Muslim, and various Christian sects including Eastern Orthodox. Jewish foodways are described in a subsequent section.

Muslim Dietary Practices.—Food proscriptions and fasting are distinguishing features. Building of strong bodies by consumption of a good diet is a sacred obligation.

There are two main types of proscription. Pork is forbidden in any form as is meat that has been slaughtered without mentioning God's name or by an athiest. Alcoholic beverages and food containing a flavoring with an alcoholic diluent or wine in a marinade are also forbidden.

Fasting is a religious obligation and is practiced for the purposes of earning God's favor testing and reconfirming the quality of one's self-discipline with respect to control of food intake, and to improve health by periodic restriction of intake. Salient differences in concept of fasting are:

(a) fasting is limited—The fast is from dawn to sunset, but neither food nor drink is taken during this time. On fast days, two meals are consumed. Well before dawn, a light meal of foods from the following classes is consumed: dairy products, fruits, vegetables, and breads. To break the fast, immediately after sunset a beverage such as water, milk, or juice is consumed with some dates. Later, a light festive dinner of customary foods is consumed.

(b) fasts of different types are observed—The differences in type result from variability in length of the fast and in the kind of obligation. The rules and practices are the same, irrespective of type.

The first type is a mandatory fast. All adult Muslims, i.e., those beyond puberty or age 15, fast for the entire month of Ramadan, which occurs at variable times of the year as determined by the Islamic lunar calendar.

The second type is a supererogatory fast. This is observed or practiced by an individual without the need to do so—the concept implies a level of observance that is not needed or wanted. There are 4 elective fast periods that may be used for this purpose: *Shawwal*, a six-day fast period which begins on the 4th day of this month; *Muharram*, the 10th day of this month is designated; *Sha'ban*, the 15th day of this month is designated; and in *Zul Hijjah*, the 9th day is designated.

The third type is optional fasts. A Muslim may fast on any unspecified day up to three days a month or twice a week (Mondays and

Thursdays are preferred). Fasting on consecutive days is not recommended except during the two months that precede Ramadan.

Eastern Orthodox Dietary Practices.—Numerous feast and fast days are observed. Easter is the main festival. The date is variable; it is always celebrated on the first Sunday after the full moon following the spring equinox according to the solar calendar. Moreover, it is never on the same day as Jewish Passover; it is always later. Many special foods are prepared. Twelve other feast days are also observed (Table 16.4). Major fast days and periods are listed in Table 16.5. On fast days, only animal products are proscribed. This includes milk, cheese, butter, and eggs.

TABLE 16.4. MAJOR FEAST DAYS OF THE EASTERN ORTHODOX CHURCH[1]

Gregorian Calendar Date (New Style)	Julian Calendar Date (Old Style)	Feast Day	Food
Dec. 25	Jan. 7	Christmas Eve (Nativity of Our Lord)	12 different dishes; e.g., dry mushroom soup, bread, sauerkraut and peas, beans, potatoes, fish (stuffed, baked, or fish balls), pickled herrings, stuffed cabbage, dried fruit compote or sweetened cereal desserts "Kutya," a fasting food served; made of boiled wheat, honey, nuts, poppy seeds, and fruit
		Christmas Day	for Russians: roast pork and turkey for Greeks, Serbians, and Syrians: roast lamb and various sweet yeast dough desserts
Jan. 6	Jan. 19	Theophany (12 days after Christmas)	
Feb. 2	Feb. 15	Presentation of Our Lord into the Temple	
Mar. 25	Apr. 7	The Annunciation	
Sunday before Easter		Palm Sunday	(a fast day)
40 days after Easter		The Ascension	
50 days after Easter		Pentecost (Trinity) Sunday	Kulich, saved from Easter
Aug. 6	Aug. 19	The Transfiguration	(blessing of fruit)
Aug. 15	Aug. 28	The Dormition of the Holy Theotokos	
Sept. 8	Sept. 21	The Nativity of the Holy Theotokos	
Sept. 14	Sept. 27	Elevation of the Holy Cross	(a strict fast day)
Nov. 21	Dec. 4	The Presentation of the Holy Theotokos	

[1] Note: Russians and most other Slavic Orthodox still follow the Julian calendar, which in the 20th Century is 13 days behind the Gregorian calendar. Thus, dates of the stationary feasts differ according to the calendar used. Frequently, a feast day is celebrated by a heavy meal that includes meat, milk, butter and/or cheese for the first time in days or weeks.

TABLE 16.5. FAST DAYS[1] OF THE EASTERN ORTHODOX CHURCH

Fast Days[2]

Wednesdays and Fridays of the year except for fast-free weeks:
  Week following Christmas to Eve of Theophany
  Bright Week, week following Easter
  Trinity Week, week following Trinity Sunday
Eve of Theophany (Jan. 6 or Jan. 18)
Beheading of John the Baptist (Aug. 29 or Sept. 11)
The Elevation of the Holy Cross (Sept. 14 or 27)

Fasting Periods[2]

Nativity Fast (Advent) (Nov. 15 or Nov. 28 to Dec. 24 or Jan. 6)
Great Lent and Holy Week (seven weeks prior to Easter)
  The week before Lent is Carnival Week or Cheese-Fare Week where no meat is eaten but
  only dairy products. Among the Russians it is the time when *blini* are eaten (pancakes
  made with a yeast batter and served with melted sweet butter, smoked salmon or caviar,
  and sour cream).
Fast of the Apostles (St. Peter and St. Paul)
  (May 23 or June 5 to June 16 or June 29)
Fast of the Dormition of the Holy Theotokos
  (Aug. 1 or Aug. 14 to Aug. 15 or Aug. 28)

[1] Exact dates depend upon whether the Julian or the Gregorian calendar is followed.
[2] No meat or animal products, such as milk, butter or cheese, or fish can be eaten. Some Greeks also abstain from olive oil.

Jewish Definitions of Food and Poison.—The foodways of Jews are complex and sophisticated because of strong religious and secular factors in their development. The religious aspect varies in importance as a determining factor, i.e., ritual laws dominate the foodways of the Orthodox Jews, and it is an unimportant factor in the foodways of Reform Jews so observance is nominal. The secular aspect derives from the historical dispersion of Jews throughout the world and the necessity of adapting their foodways to local conditions. As a result of assimilation, the foodways are cosmopolitan, i.e., they include selected ingredients, recipes for prepared foods, methods of preparation, and other practices common to most nations of the world. The definitions of food and poison are a function of the religious and/or secular traditions. These include, but are not limited to, those delineated below.

Religious.—The observance of the foodways is a sacred activity that controls the drive for food by means of a system of discipline that leads to self-purification, service to God, as well as moral and spiritual freedom in this domain. Beliefs and behaviors with respect to food selection, preparation, and consumption are specified in the dietary laws recorded in the Old Testament books of Leviticus and Deuteronomy. The dietary laws (Kashruth) define what is "right" and "fit" for consumption as food (Kosher) and what is poison. Explanations of traditional attitudes and intentions have been collected and interpreted in the text of the Talmud.

The Biblical stipulations pertain to the means by which pure, i.e., undefiled, food could be selected and prepared by the temple priests as sacrificial offerings to God. Animal sacrifices have greater value; muscle and fat tissues gain favor as thank offerings and blood is used for cleansing of sin. So, the requirements for selection, slaughter, preparation, and service are stipulated in greater detail. This model served as the basis for the ritual laws that specify practices to ensure consumption of acceptable food. In general, foods are classified into three groups:

(a) permitted or kosher—Fruits, vegetables, grains, tea, and coffee. These may be consumed with either dairy products or meats.

(b) permitted or kosher *if*, and only if, selected from a healthy live animal, slaughtered according to a ritual that provides a painless quick kill, and processed to eliminate all traces of blood from the meat—The koshering process involves draining of arterial and venous blood; soaking, rinsing, salting, further draining, and three final washes to remove any residual blood. The kosher process is used with meats from the forequarters of cloven-hoofed quadrupeds that chew a cud, i.e., cattle, sheep, goats, and deer; poultry, i.e., chickens, turkeys, geese, pheasants, and ducks; fish with fins and scales.

(c) not permitted or proscribed—Pork products, shellfish, birds of prey, insects except locusts, reptiles, amphibians, and cartilaginous fishes such as eels.

Other proscriptions and practices also are followed. For example:

(a) Foods that contain non-kosher additives or ingredients that are considered by rabbinical authorities to be waste products are proscribed.

(b) Dairy products and meat products may not be cooked together.

(c) Foods containing a mixture of dairy products and meat may not be consumed.

(d) The same utensils, dishes, and cutlery may not be used for preparation or service of meat and dairy products.

(e) After consuming meat, milk products may not be consumed within one, three, or six hours (the length of time varies with the interpretation of the particular sect).

(f) Two vegetables of the same botanical family are not served at the same meal.

(g) Chicken fat or vegetable oil is used in food preparation, not lard or tallow.

(h) Leftovers are not reheated and served; they are reworked to produce an entirely different dish.

Ritual law also includes doctrines that define the nature and extent of observances that pertain to the Sabbath and sacred festivals. The Sabbath extends from sundown Friday until the first star is seen on Saturday. No food is prepared by or for Orthodox Jews by others during this period. So, hot foods are limited to those that can be prepared in advance and kept hot. Yom Kippur (Day of Atonement) in September or October is a day of total fasting. Special foods are emphasized on each of the other sacred feast days. Some must be prepared according to specified rituals (see chapter references for descriptions) in relation to the following:

(a) Rosh Hashanah (New Year's Festival)—in September or October—Honey, honey cakes, and carrot tzimmes

(b) Sukkoth (Feast of Boths, a harvest festival)—in October—Kreplach, holishkes, strudel

(c) Channukuh (Festival of Lights)—in December—Potato latkes and kugel

(d) Chamise Oser b'Sh'vat (Arbor Day)—in January—Bokser which is carob fruit, fruits, nuts, raisins

(e) Purim (Feast of Esther)—in March—Hamantashen, nuts, raisins

(f) Pesach (Feast of Freedom as a result of the Passover)—in April—Specified Seder meals with unleavened bread, salt, bitter herbs, etc.

(g) Shevuoth (Feast of Weeks)—in May—Cheese and dairy foods

For the Orthodox Jew, the hazard of defilement by consumption of unfit food presents a challenge when away from home. Usually, it is resolved by refusal to consume food of unknown history. So, he/she provides his/her own food or may consume a kosher TV dinner if the foil has not been unsealed.

Secular.—An outgrowth of the religious necessity for paying close attention to details in food selection, preparation, and servce is an understanding of and appreciation for good food. The American Jewish community includes both those of Ashkenazic or eastern European and Sephardic or Spanish, Portuguese, and North African origins. The best food items from each have been adapted as necessary and adopted into the American Jewish cuisine. So, the array of foods includes the noodles and dumplings that are typical of German, Austrian, Polish, Hungarian, and Czechoslovakian cuisines; the thin pancakes rolled around various fillings and topped with various sauces that are typical of French and Russian fare; the steamed meat or cheese and vegetable mixtures in pasta envelopes typical of Italy and Russia; the pickled fish served with sour cream that are typical of Baltic countries and Russia; the beet and cabbage soup of Poland and Russia; the sour cream and vegetable mixtures typical of the Balkan States and the Middle East; and the pilafs that are typical of the Mediterranean area. So, a main meal is likely to include items of varied ethnic origin. Another distinguishing characteristic is that lunches and suppers often are eaten away from home at cafés and delicatessens in the European fashion.

Oriental Definitions of Food and Poison.—The central point of Oriental foodways is to elevate food and people interactions to a civilized pleasurable experience that transcends the utilitarian function of nourishing the body. By tradition, beliefs, attitudes, intentions, and behaviors are linked and focused in an integrated manner toward this end. Some underlying beliefs might be stated as follows:

(a) High quality ingredients are essential to final quality. Fresh fruits and vegetables at their peak quality are prized. High quality processed foods are used to good advantage.

(b) Food preparation requires close attention to details in order to enhance or develop desired colors, flavors, and textures and to mask or modify unwanted ones. Each dish is a creation. Ingredients are treated separately to develop individual qualities. Each of the ingredients in mixed dishes must be added at just the right time in cooking and in a prescribed sequence so that when cooking is completed, each will be at its optimum point.

(c) All of the equipment and furnishings in the dining area must be appropriate, creating a harmonious and restful atmosphere.

(d) The diners should conduct themselves with decorum, showing refined tastes, and acknowledging subtle differences in preparation that give distinction to what is presented. Gluttony is considered poor taste; children are admonished to eat until they are three-fourths full.

Chopsticks and a small bowl are basic eating equipment. Since there is no means by which the diner can gracefully divide larger pieces, foods are pre-cut.

Vegetables such as cauliflower, broccoli, and others that can be pulled apart are separated according to natural divisions. Stems are cut on the diagonal. Solid vegetables such as carrots and turnips are cut into bite-sized pieces. A variety of shapes are used, e.g., bias slices, diced, julienne. The pieces must be neat but not so uniform that they look machine-cut.

Meat is cut into natural and/or classic but manageable pieces. Cuts of meat, in the American sense, are unknown. Each piece of meat, of whatever part, is simply sliced in such a way that if it is tough the fibers will be so short that they provide little resistance in chewing. Small bones are not removed from the meat; they remain in the dish, adding flavor and nutrients.

Rice is the staple starchy food in southern areas; wheat and millet are common in northern areas. Many varieties of rice are grown. The concept of what is good, as defined by sensory qualities of odor, color, flavor, and texture varies according to the qualities of the predominant variety grown. Some prefer a short-grained sticky rice, others prefer one that is long-grained and less cohesive. Many varieties of wheat and millet are also grown. In northern areas, noodles and other kinds of pasta as well as flour products of the bread-biscuit type are common. Barley is also grown and used in many ways.

Food mixtures, food combinations, and food flavor blends dominate.

Rice appears to be the only food that is not prepared as a mixture; water is the only additive. Most entrées are mixtures of several vegetables with a meat and/or fish; nuts or fruits may be used as a garnish. Any food can be combined with any other if pretreated in such a way that harmony will be achieved; since few cooks are exceptional in selecting combinations, many menu combinations have evolved as a guide. Condiments, dipping sauces, and marinades are all blends. Condiments and dipping sauces are used by the diner to add a large-amplitude flavor note to suit individual tastes. On the other hand, the function of the marinade used in pretreatment is to enhance or potentiate the natural desirable flavors or to mask or modify undesirable ones.

In general, serving temperature of the food is not that important. The means of temperature control are not well developed. However, when a fragile flavor or texture quality is temperature-dependent, timing of preparation is controlled to ensure serving the dish at the desired temperature.

Tea is the common beverage. Many varieties and mixtures containing cinnamon, jasmine flowers and other flavorants are used. Water quality is important. Above all, it must not be "burned" by boiling. Rather, as soon as it comes to the boil it must be removed from the heat and immediately poured over the tea to initiate steeping. Boiling causes volatiles to escape, so the tea will be flat. Steeping time is precisely controlled according to the kind of tea and desired level of extraction.

The Chinese cuisine is the original Oriental cuisine. The others are similar, sharing many common features, but each is also unique in some respects. The common features are due to the overpowering regional influence of Chinese culture since time immemorial. Traditional and associated American adaptations of each of the major Oriental cuisines will be discussed in turn.

Chinese.—Two altogether different systems for presenting food are in common use. The first involves a succession of courses: appetizers, e.g., miniature egg rolls, miniature stuffed buns, jellyfish salad; steamed rice and a succession of entrées on serving platters or in serving bowls; soup. The second involves table self-selection and cooking of foods using a charcoal firepot. Raw and/or partially cooked meat, seafood, vegetables, noodles, and bean curd are arranged on a large platter. The diner selects and transfers an assortment of foods to an individual sieve which is immersed in the continuously simmering liquid in the firepot. When foods have cooked, the diner removes them to a personal bowl containing rice. These are consumed during the interval in which the next lot is cooking. When the last lot of food has been cooked and consumed, the liquid in the firepot which has now been flavored by the juices from the foods cooked in it is portioned among the diners and is consumed as the final soup course.

China covers an immense area; regional variation in the cuisine has evolved according to food availability and exposure to other peoples. With respect to food, there are no distinct boundaries to the various regions; indeed, scholars are divided in opinion as to whether there are four or five regions. Geographic basis is as valid as any in determining the number of regions, so four variations are distinguished:

(a) Peking—This region is in the north. Foodways are cosmopolitan since Peking has long been the major international and governmental center. Wheat is the staple, so steamed breads, noodles, dumplings, and pancakes are basic items of diet. Other features include wine sauces, meat pastries, and hot-pot dishes.

(b) Shanghai—This region is in the east and parallels the coast. Rice is the main staple. Fish and seafood are the other main source of protein. Foods are braised in a heavily thickened sauce containing an unusual amount of soy sauce. Many items are sweetened with white sugar, including the meat and fish dishes. Garlic is disliked as a seasoning.

(c) Szechwan—This region is in the west and is far inland. Rice is the basic staple. Ham is a favorite meat and many fungi are used. Noodle dishes are consumed as snacks. The food is spicy with hot pepper, garlic, ginger, and green onions.

(d) Canton—This region is in the south and much of it is coastal. Rice is the staple. Fish and many vegetables are characteristic. Roast pork is a favorite. Plum sauce and herbs are used as seasonings. Most foods are steamed and are lightly seasoned—just enough to emphasize the original flavors. *Dim-sum* (appetizers) originated in Canton and include chicken livers, dumplings, meatballs, and small pastries. Most restaurants in the United States serve food that is a reasonable facsimile of standard Cantonese fare.

Folk medicine is practiced widely; food is used as a medicine. More importantly, the principles of balance are extended to govern food consumption in general. Thus, *yin*, which is the feminine passive principle that represents darkness, coldness, and wetness, must be balanced with *yang*, which is the masculine active principle that represents light, heat, and dryness—positive factors.

Meals may have two general components, i.e., *fan* or grain-based foods and *ts'ai* or vegetable-based mixtures that contain meat or fish. The *fan* is the essential component, providing nourishment that is conceptualized as feeling full. *Ts'ai* is optional and provides sensory gratification, especially flavor. In addition, the *ts'ai* mixture must be balanced in terms of "hot" foods such as fatty meats, oily plants, and fried foods, and pungent and biting pepper must be compensated for by an equalizing quantity of "cold" foods such as water plants, crustaceans, and some beans. Separate sets of utensils are used for preparation and service of the *fan* and *ts'ai*, i.e., *fan* is prepared in a rice cooker and is served in a *kui* (bowl), whereas *ts'ai* is prepared in a *wok* and is served on a *tou* (platter).

Special diets have been stipulated for various medical, physical, and emotional conditions. Foods to be emphasized and avoided are specified as is the use of an herbal tea.

Chinese immigrants to the United States frequently have settled in concentrated groups in major cities such as Boston, Chicago, Los Angeles, New York, San Francisco, and Seattle. Despite the embargo on trade with Communist China, many of the traditional ingredients have continued to be available in these urban centers. Restaurants serving the regional variations also are available. Therefore, the recent immigrant and the Chinese-American often continue the traditional diet. Breakfast, lunch, or snack food items are changed first, when Americanization is initiated. Preferences for traditional entrées, seasonings, and methods of preparation are usually retained. Traditional dinner meals may be alternated with American-style ones. For social reasons, in public, traditional beliefs, attitudes, and practices are suppressed. They may be continued in the home. Assimilation is rare.

In suburbia, or in other areas of the United States, the immigrant and the Chinese-American usually consume the standard American diet and imitate the other foodways, to the extent possible. Often, imitation is mechanical since the underlying beliefs are not understood or accepted. American ways are necessary, in part, because of the difficulty of procuring traditional ingredients. When essential ingredients can be obtained, traditional items are prepared at irregular intervals and/or festive occasions such as Chinese New Year and weddings. Even so, the number of items that are prepared has diminished. So, skill in preparation is gradually lost. Instead, commonly available ingredients are prepared in quasi-Chinese style, e.g., vegetables are cut into bite-sized pieces and are cooked by the stir-fry method, meats and fish are marinated in soy sauce and are poached or braised.

Japanese.—The traditional Japanese cuisine is similar to the other Oriental cuisines in that a meal is defined as rice accompanied by one or more vegetable-based dishes, foods are pre-cut into bite-sized pieces, and food quality/aesthetics are important. It differs in that pickled vegetables, raw or broiled fish, and a sharp horseradish rather than mustard condiment is customary.

The artistic quality of the eating experience is of paramount importance. The selection and artistic arrangement of table appointments is integrated with the food for presentation as a harmonious whole. An elaborate set of considerations formally influences the design of a dish. These include color, texture, flavor appeal, harmony within and among individual items, variety—with emphasis on contrasts and appropriateness of the individual ingredients, the composition of the combination, and the serving utensil. Elaborate preparation techniques are followed systematically; cookery is rapid and controlled.

The Japanese cuisine has three altogether different systems for presentation of food. The first involves a succession of courses: appetizers such as pickled vegetables and soup; a succession of carefully planned and artistically arranged combinations of rice with entrée and accompaniments, all on separate plates. Each plate presented contains a combination that is a planned part of a total experience built around a gastronomic concept. The second system is designed to accentuate the qualities of tempura. The appetizer course is followed by presentation of assorted batter-fried seafood and vegetables accompanied by selected dipping sauces. The third employs hot rocks or a hibachi or grill and is for table cookery. While the diner consumes the appetizers, an attendant prepares the first portion of the main course. A large platter contains an attractive arrangement of assorted, individually portioned, raw, marinated and otherwise pretreated meat, seafood, and vegetables. The attendant prepares some of each item on the platter and serves a small portion of each item to each diner. All items are prepared in batches and are consumed immediately on completion of cooking. Thus, a continuous supply of hot just-done food is maintained throughout the meal.

Japanese immigrants to the United States have settled in Hawaii and the same mainland cities as the Chinese. Generally the new immigrants and first-generation Americans continue to follow foodways according to tradition. Second generation Americans are quite westernized. Although they consume rice and soy sauce more frequently than their neighbors, they usually eat standard American foods. Traditional items are prepared at irregular intervals as well as on festive occasions. The desire for artistic quality usually remains but time constraints usually preclude systematic expression. Third and fourth generation Americans appear to have totally accepted American foodways, including beliefs; Japanese dietary traditions are sneered at as "old fashioned."

Korean.—This cuisine is similar to other Oriental cuisines in that a meal is defined as rice or noodles accompanied by an array of vegetable-based dishes, foods are pre-cut into bite-sized pieces, and meat and fish are subordinate ingredients. It differs in that pickled vegetables are peppery and aged, spicing of entrées is dominated by garlic, hot peppers, and soy sauce, and vegetable dishes contain only one vegetable. Food is viewed in a more utilitarian way; it is prepared and served, not created. Having made some general decisions about what is to be served, the Korean cook will make a choice from ingredients available.

The Korean cuisine has three systems for presentation of food. All foods are placed on the table in appropriate sized serving dishes; some dishes may be very small, containing less than ½ cup. The diner serves himself a portion of rice or noodles into a personal bowl. Then, the diner reaches across the table to any desired dish and obtains one or more morsels which are placed in the personal bowl prior to consumption. A small quantity of each of one or more items is obtained in this way, from among the 6 to 50 side dishes available. Having obtained the desired subset of items, the diner proceeds to consume them. Then, he looks around for others that tempt, or he takes additional portions of the original subset. A second type of service is a method of table barbecuing. Thin slices of one or more kinds of meat are pretreated by marination in a standard mixture of sugar, green onion, pepper, and garlic. These are arranged on a plate or in a bowl for convenience. They are grilled on the top and sides of a charcoal-fired pot that is perforated on the top and sides so that juices drain away. Side dishes are placed here and there on the table. The diner takes a leaf, places meat, rice, soy sauce, and some self-selected assortment of other items on top. The leaf is then folded to form a package which is eaten from the hand. The third method uses a charcoal-burning hot-pot for table preparation of a thick soup of varied ingredients.

Like other Orientals, most Koreans have settled in the major cities. Since the concentrations are smaller, traditional ingredients are less likely to be available. Acceptance of many American foods is difficult, so the Korean usually just consumes a restricted array of foods. Traditions are maintained to the extent possible. American foods that are accepted appear to be consumed in addition to traditional foods.

Vegetarian Definitions of Food and Poison.—There are two distinct types of vegetarians. Type I vegetarians are only nominally vegetarian, i.e., by preference they are omnivorous, by economic necessity they are vegetarians. Thus, when meat is available, they consume it. Type II vegetarians are true believers, i.e., they have so much respect for animal life that they cannot sacrifice it in self-interest. Their beliefs may have either religious or philosophical bases. Some exclude all animal products. Others exclude meat, fish, and poultry. Some exclude only meat and poultry and some exclude only red meat.

In the United States, the most enduring group of conscientious vegetarians are Seventh Day Adventists, even though avoidance of meat is a voluntary individual expression of faith. The lacto-ovo vegetarian diet (milk, eggs, grains, and vegetables) diet is recommended. The amino acid content of the various grains, legumes, nuts, and seeds is known. Mixtures or combinations are selected so that the amino acid content of one component compensates for lack in another. Inclusion of the high quality protein of dairy products and eggs provides additional insurance.

Since 1965, a neo-vegetarian movement has gained an increasing number of adherents. Their beliefs, attitudes, intentions, and behaviors with respect to foodways are markedly different from those encountered in other times and places. For one thing, there is much variation in attitude toward consumption of flesh foods, social behavior (middling to deviant), and life-styles (typical for age to communal). For another, they are heterogeneous demographically, i.e., they are of all ages although the majority are young adults, of all levels of educational attainment, from middle and upper class backgrounds, of all ethnic groups, and they reside in practically every community.

Some few are individuals who practice a few restrictions according to a personal philosophy. For the most part, these individuals are not at nutritional risk.

Others avoid some flesh foods and are members of a group that has natural foods as its predominant focus. Some of these groups seek to improve health. A central belief is that fasting is used to clean out the system by allowing a period in which poisons can be eliminated. Since they are not replaced, the body will be purer and healthier. Others belong to groups of the counterculture that are engaged in passive protest against the agri-business system and the food processing establishment. Their main ecologic belief is that individuals should support increased efficiency in food production in order to meet world food needs by elimination of the need for red meat production. Red meat production is regarded as the most inefficient and wasteful food since 9 lb of grain are required to produce 1 lb of red meat. Individuals with these beliefs define various canned, dehydrated, and frozen foods—including TVP and soy milk—as poisonous because they are processed. Processing is regarded as bad and counterproductive because some nutrient decrease is inevitable, food additives are used for preservation, and it is energy-intensive. Members of these groups are not usually at nutritional risk.

Nutritionally, whether a person is a vegetarian or is omnivorous is irrelevant *per se*. Potentially, however, vegetarians are nutritionally vulnerable since they eliminate an entire category of rich sources of nutrients $1 \ldots n$. This increases the burden on the individual to accept personal responsibility for monitoring and control of nutrient intake.

Still others follow severely restricted diets and are members of cultist groups of the counterculture. These groups have established a comprehensive supporting belief structure, require strict adherence, and tend to limit social exposure of members to those of the same persuasion. Food cultism places its adherents at nutritional risk because strict adherence to extreme dietary strictures is required. When the number of foods avoided is extensive as in the more extreme forms, e.g., Zen Macrobiotics, nutritional adequacy may be impossible to achieve.

The Zen Macrobiotic diet engendered concern about the nutritional adequacy of vegetarian diets. Erhard (1973) described the philosophy and practices responsible for nutritional vulnerability and delineated the risky position of children subsisting on such diets. She cited the following cases:

(a) A 2½-year-old child at the 3rd percentile for weight/height with a bone age of 1¼ years and a 1-year-old child at the 3rd percentile of weight/height with a bone age of 3 months. Both suffered from rickets; neither crawled nor walked. Both were inactive, irritable, unable to speak, and scored low on the Denver Developmental Function tests. Assessment of nutrient intake, based on three-day diet records, revealed low intakes of kcal, calcium, iron, ascorbic acid, vitamin D, riboflavin, and fluid. The philosophy of the parents led them to accept such retardation as to be expected and perhaps a good thing. Medical opinion differed.

(b) A 2-year-old child that was starving, height 27½ in., weight 15 lb 10 oz, bone age 1 year, gross psychomotor retardation. Assessment of nutrient intake revealed that kcal and protein were somewhat low, half enough calcium and iron were provided and intakes of vitamin A (650%) and ascorbic acid (520%) were excessive. Hospitalization resulted in marked improvement. After discharge, the previous diet was resumed, physical deterioration recurred, and the child was readmitted. After physical rehabilitation, he was again discharged and again began slow starvation.

The preceding are among the few cases of severe malnutrition and rickets that have been reported among children of vegetarians. Stunted growth and anemia are more prevalent manifestations. Dwyer *et al.* (1978), who studied 119 vegetarian preschoolers, reported the following findings:

(a) Among those less than 6 months of age, all of whom were breast-fed, size was above the 50th percentile, i.e., normal.

(b) Among those between 6 and 17 months of age, size was below the 50th percentile in 50% of the cases; of those who were small, 50% were below the 25th percentile for weight.

(c) Among those over 18 months of age, size was below the 50th percentile in 50% of the cases.

(d) Energy intakes were appropriate on a per kilogram weight basis but were low for chronologic age because of small size.

(e) When the number of kinds of animal protein consumed were limited, the amount of animal protein consumed also was reduced.

The findings of Dwyer *et al.* (1978) support the contention that vegetarian diets are likely to be inadequate for children and to cause growth retardation and physical stunting. Pursuing this point, this group related child height to parental height and found that the abnormally large number that were short were unlikely to be short for genetic reasons. Also, they found that breast-feeding status, dietary group affiliation, and the extent of avoidance of animal foods were positively associated with observed size differences. Although the possibility exists that some factor not studied may account for small size, the data suggest that the vegetarian diet was the environmental variable that caused the observed growth stunting.

Some of the other groups of neo-vegetarians have adopted selected concepts from Oriental philosophy and folk medicine. The basic belief is that by controlling dietary intake so as to achieve a physiological state of equilibrium and digestive tranquility, the mind can be made free for peaceful meditation. To this end, *yin* (good) and *yang* (evil) must be balanced. Since *yang* represents aggressiveness and other unwanted traits that must be controlled, flesh foods that are *yang* in nature must be avoided. Selections are made among other foods so as to achieve balance according to quasi-religious precepts, as interpreted by the individual in light of his perception of his own needs. Oriental and/or Middle Eastern ingredients, spicing, and preparation methods are used to prevent contamination and/or diminution of effects. Thus, goal attainment is assured.

Information on the foodways of these various vegetarian groups, including foods consumed and preparation methods, is found in chapter references. A food guide for use with the lacto-ovo vegetarian diet has been developed by Smith. Food groups and serving sizes are shown in Table 16.6. Table 16.7 is a guide to the number of standard servings of the various foods that is necessary for nutritional adequacy.

Lacto-ovo vegetarian diets also can be planned to meet the nutritional needs of children (Vyhmeister, Register, and Sonnenberg 1977). The number of servings of foods from the four food groups differ for children of various ages (Table 16.8).

TABLE 16.6. FOOD GROUPS AND SERVING SIZES

Group I. Bread, Cereal, Pasta, and Rice
1 slice of whole grain or enriched white bread with butter or margarine
⅓–½ cup granola-type cereal
¾ cup cooked whole grain or enriched cereal
1 cup cold whole grain or enriched cereal
2–6 tbsp uncooked farina, cracked wheat, oatmeal, etc.
¾ cup cooked, enriched, whole grain or soy macaroni, noodles, etc.
1 of biscuit, muffin, pancake, slice of nut loaf, fruit bread, with butter or margarine
1 tbsp wheat germ
¾ cup cooked brown, converted or enriched rice
1 large cookie
3-4 crackers

Group II. Vegetable Protein Foods
TVP. This is a textured vegetable protein usually made from soybeans. It is available
in a dried form and needs reconstitution with water during preparation. TVP is used
mainly in casserole-type entrees in combination with foods from other groups. One 3-oz
package will be sufficient in a casserole to serve five. Check the label for serving information.
Legumes: 1 cup of cooked soybeans, chickpeas, brown or orange lentils, pinto, kidney or
navy beans, etc.
¼ cup of peanuts or peanut butter
6 oz soybean curd
Meat Analogues: These are usually canned or frozen meat-like foods derived from vegetable protein (often soy, gluten or nut protein). Three ounces of these imitation foods are
usually sufficient. These are available as chicken, beef, pork, sausage or bacon types.
They vary in many ways, so check the label for information.
Nuts and seeds: 1½ oz or 3 tbsp provides one serving. These are usually to be used as
snack foods or in combination with Group I or IV foods several times a week. To replace
legumes occasionally the quantity should be doubled or tripled. Nuts include cashews,
cashew butter, pignolias, pistachios, walnuts, brazils, pecans, among others. Sunflower,
sesame, pumpkin and squash seeds are the most readily obtained seeds in this country.

Group III. Milk and Eggs
Milk: The standard serving of milk is 1 cup of whole, 2%, skim (added vitamins A & D),
or other milk drinks. To substitute for 1 cup of milk you may use:
1¼ oz. cheddar cheese or processed cheese, etc.
1 oz. Swiss cheese
4 oz. cream cheese
4 tbsp. (¼ cup) cottage cheese
1 cup yogurt
1½ cups ice cream
Milk should be supplemented with vitamin D for all growing children and pregnant
women.
Eggs: 1½ eggs on the average are recommended by the Guide. This includes those used
in baked items, scrambled, fried, in omelettes, souffles, custards and casseroles, etc.

Group IV. Fruits and Vegetables

Whole, raw, baked, e.g., corn on cob, apple	1 medium
Leafy raw bulky vegetable, e.g., lettuce, bean sprouts	1 cup
Cooked, e.g., canned peas, cherries	½ cup
Large, e.g., grapefruit, melon (5″)	½
Small, e.g., grapes	15
plums	3–4
Juice, e.g., tomato, apple	½ cup (4 oz)
Dried, e.g., raisins, figs	2 tbsp

Fruits are numerous: apples, apricots, bananas, berries, melons, citrus (orange, grapefruit),
grapes, pears, peaches, plums, rhubarb, pumpkin and many more. Vegetables include:
asparagus, beans, bean sprouts, beets, cauliflower, carrots, celery, greens (lettuce, endive,
etc.), onions, parsnips, peas, potatoes, squash, tomatoes.

Reproduced with permission of the faculty of Home Economics, Univ. of Manitoba and the Manitoba Dept. of Health
and Social Development.

TABLE 16.7.   GUIDE TO NUMBERS OF STANDARD SERVINGS

Food Group	Adult Male	Adult Female	Pregnant Adult Female	18–19 Male	18–19 Female	13–15 Male	13–15 Female	10–12 Both	7–9 Both	4–6 Both	2–3 Both
I. Breads, cereals, pasta	8	6	6	9	5	7	5	5	4	3	3
II. Vegetable protein foods											
Legumes, meat analogues, TVP	1	¾	¾	1½	¾	¾	½	½	½	¼	⅛
Nuts and seeds	1	1	1	2	1	1	¾	¾	½	¼	⅛
III. Milk and eggs											
Milk	1½	1½	4	2–3	2–3	4	4	4	2	2–3	2–3
Eggs	1½	1½	1½	1½	1½	1½	1½	1½	1	1	1
IV. Fruits and vegetables	6	5	5–6	6	5	5	5	4	4	3	2
Extra foods[2]	no requirements										

Source: Adapted from *Vegetarian Food Guide*, with permission of the Faculty of Home Economics, University of Manitoba and the Manitoba Dept. of Health and Social Development.

[1] Amounts were determined by computer analysis of nutrients of test menus.

[2] These foods may provide calories, but few nutrients. They include sugar, jams, seasonings, beverages including alcohol, cream, pickles, foods used in garnishing, etc., and are useful mainly in providing flavor and color interest.

TABLE 16.8. NUMBER OF SERVINGS FOR CHILDREN PER DAY

Food Group	Standard Serving	1 to 3 Years	Ages 4 to 6 Years	7 to 12 Years
I. Milk and milk products	1 cup	2−3	2−3	3−4
II. Vegetable protein foods				
a. Legumes	1 cup	¼	½	½
Textured vegetable protein	20−30 g dry			
Meat analogues	2−3 oz			
b. Nuts, seeds	1½ tbsp	¼	½	¾
Peanut butter	4 tbsp			
III. Fruits and vegetables				
Total daily	½ cup cooked 1 cup raw ½ cup juice	2−3	3−4	4−5
Green leafy	daily	1	1	1
Vitamin C rich	daily	1	1	1
IV. Breads and cereals	1 slice whole wheat bread ½−¾ cup cooked cereal	3	3−4	4−5
V. Other				
Eggs	1	1	1	1
Fats	1 tsp	1−3	2−3	2−3

Source: Vyhmeister *et al.* (1977).

BIBLIOGRAPHY

General

BOYD, E.M., and BOYD, C.E. 1973. Toxicity of Pure Foods. CRC Press, Cleveland.

CAUL, J.F., and SJOSTROM, L.B. 1959. Consumer food product acceptance. Perfum. Essent. Oil Rec. *12*, 916−917.

SJOSTROM, L.B. 1959. Adding zest to foods. J. Am. Dietet. Assoc. *35*, 227−229.

Foodways of Blacks

ALEXANDER, M. 1968. The significance of ethnic groups in marketing. *In* Perspectives in Consumer Behavior. H.H. Kassarjian and T.S. Robertson (Editors). Scott, Foresman & Co., Glenview, Ill.

BAUER, R.A., CUNNINGHAM, S.M., and WORTZEL, L.H. 1968. The marketing dilemma of Negroes. *In* Perspectives in Consumer Behavior. H.H. Kassarjian and T.S. Robertson (Editors). Scott, Foresman & Co., Glenview, Ill.

BRADFIELD, R.B., and COLTRIN, D. 1970. Some characteristics of the health and nutrition status of California Negroes. Am. J. Clin. Nutr. *23*, 420−426.

COLTRIN, D.M., and BRADFIELD, R.B. 1970. Food buying practices of urban low-income consumers—a review. J. Nutr. Educ. *1*, 16–17.

CUSSLER, M.T., and DeGIVE, M.L. 1952. 'Twixt the Cup and the Lip. Twayne Publishers, New York.

DELGADO, G., BRUMBACK, C.L., and DEAVER, M.B. 1961. Eating patterns among migrant families. U.S. Public Health Rept. *76*, 349–355.

DICKINS, D. 1929. Negro food habits in the Yazoo Mississippi Delta. J. Home Econ. *18*, 523–525.

GRANT, F.W., and GROOM, D. 1959. A dietary study among a group of southern Negroes. J. Am. Dietet. Assoc. *35*, 910–918.

JEROME, N.W. 1968. Changing meal patterns among southern-born Negroes in a mid-western city. Nutr. News *31*, 9, 12.

JEROME, N.W. 1969. Northern urbanization and food consumption patterns of Southern-born Negroes. Am. J. Nutr. *22*, 1667–1669.

JEROME, N.W. 1975. Flavor preferences and food patterns of selected U.S. and Caribbean Blacks. Food Technol. *29* (6) 46, 48, 50–51.

MAYER, J. 1965. The nutritional status of American Negroes. Nutr. Rev. *23*, 161–164.

PAYTON, E., CRUMP, E.P., and HORTON, C.P. 1960. Dietary habits of 571 pregnant southern Negro women. J. Am. Dietet. Assoc. *37*, 129–136.

SANJUR, D., and SCOMA, D. 1971. Food habits of low-income children in Northern New York. J. Nutr. Educ. *2*, 85–95.

SCHUCK, C., and TARTT, J.B. 1973. Food consumption of low-income, rural Negro households in Mississippi. J. Am. Dietet. Assoc. *62*, 151–155.

WILSON, M.T. 1964. Peaceful integration: the owner's adoption of his slaves' food. J. Negro History *49*, 116–127.

Foodways of Jews and Muslims

ALEXANDER, M. 1968. The significance of ethnic groups in marketing. *In* Perspectives in Consumer Behavior. H.H. Kassarjian and T.S. Robertson (Editors). Scott, Foresman & Co., Glenview, Ill.

ANON. 1970. Kosher foods described. J. Am. Dietet. Assoc. *57*, 328.

KAUFMAN, M. 1957. Adapting therapeutic diets to Jewish food customs. Am. J. Clin. Nutr. *5*, 676–681.

KORFF, S.I. 1966. The Jewish dietary code. Food Technol. *20*, 926.

LEVIN, C.M. 1934. A study of Jewish food habits. Am. Dietet. Assoc. *9*, 389–395.

LEVIN, S.I., and BOYDEN, E.A. 1941. The Kosher Code of the Orthodox Jew. Herman Press, New York.

NATOW, A.B., HESLIN, J., and RAVEN, B.C. 1975. Integrating the Jewish dietary laws into a dietetics program. Kashruth in a dietetics curriculum. J. Am. Dietet. Assoc. *67*, 13–16.

SADOW, S.E. 1928. Jewish ceremonials and food customs. J. Am. Dietet. Assoc. *4*, 91—98.

SAKR, A.H. 1971. Dietary regulations and food habits of Muslims. J. Am. Dietet. Assoc. *58*, 123—126.

SAKR, A.H. 1975. Fasting in Islam. J. Am. Dietet. Assoc. *67*, 17—21.

SHAPIRO, M.L. 1919. Jewish dietary problems. J. Home Econ. *11*, 47—59.

Foodways of Latin Americans

ALEXANDER, M. 1968. The significance of ethnic groups in marketing. *In* Perspectives in Consumer Behavior. H.H. Kassarjian and T.S. Robertson (Editors). Scott, Foresman & Co., Glenview, Ill.

BRADFIELD, R.B., and BRUN, T. 1970. Nutritional status of California Mexican-Americans. Am. J. Clin. Nutr. *23*, 798—806.

BRUHN, C.M., and PANGBORN, R.M. 1971. Food habits of migrant farm workers in California. Comparisons between Mexican-Americans and "Anglos." J. Am. Dietet. Assoc. *59*, 347—355.

CLARK, M. 1959. Health in the Mexican-American Culture. Univ. of Calif. Press, Berkeley.

CRAVIOTO, R. *et al.* 1945. Composition of typical Mexican foods. J. Nutr. *29*, 317—329.

CZAJKOWSKI, J.M. 1969. Mexican Foods and Traditions. Univ. Conn. Coop. Ext. Serv. Bull. *64—64*.

CZAJKOWSKI, J.M. 1971. Puerto Rican Foods and Traditions. Univ. Conn. Coop. Ext. Serv. Bull. *70—17*.

DUYFF, R.L., SANJUR, D., and NELSON, M.Y. 1975. Food behavior and related factors of Puerto Rican-American Teenagers. J. Nutr. Educ. 7, 99—103.

FERNANDEZ, N.A., BURGOS, J.C., ASENJO, C.F., and ROSA, I. 1971. Nutritional status of the Puerto Rican population: master sample survey. Am. J. Clin. Nutr. *24*, 952—965.

HACKER, D.B. *et al.* 1954. A study of food habits in New Mexico (1949—1952). New Mexico Agric. Exp. Stn. Bull. *384*.

HACKER, D.B., and MILLER, E.D. 1959. Food patterns of the Southwest. Am. J. Clin. Nutr. 7, 224—229.

KIGHT, M.A. *et al.* 1969. Nutritional influences of Mexican-American foods in Arizona. J. Am. Dietet. Assoc. *55*, 557—561.

McGUIRE, L.M. 1954. "Mexico." *In* Old World Foods for New World Families. Dolphin Books, Garden City, N.Y.

ORTIZ, E.L. 1967. The Complete Book of Mexican Cooking. Bantam Books, New York.

PANGBORN, R.B., and BRUHN, C.M. 1971. Concepts of food habits of "other" ethnic groups. J. Nutr. Educ. 2, 106—110.

SANJUR, D., ROMERO, E., and KIRA, M. 1971. Milk consumption patterns of Puerto Rican preschool children in rural New York. Am. J. Clin. Nutr. *24*, 1320–1326.

TORRES, R.M. 1959. Dietary pattern of the Puerto Rican people. Am. J. Clin. Nutr. 7, 349–355.

YOHAL, F. 1977. Dietary patterns of Spanish-speaking people living in the Boston area. J. Am. Dietet. Assoc. *71*, 273–275.

Foodways of Orientals

ABIAKA, M.H. 1973. Japanese-American food equivalents for calculating exchange diets. J. Am. Dietet. Assoc. *62*, 173-180.

BAILEY, L.H. 1894. Some recent Chinese vegetables. N.Y. Agric. Exp. Stn. Bull. *67.*

BLASDALE, W.C. 1899. A description of some Chinese vegetable food materials. USDA Office Exp. Stn. Bull. *68.*

CHAN, S.L., and KENNEDY, B.M. 1960. Sodium in Chinese vegetables. J. Am. Dietet. Assoc. *37*, 573-576.

CHANG, C.D. 1969. Full Color Chinese Cooking. Shufunotomo Co., Tokyo.

CHANG, K.C. 1977. Food in Chinese Culture. Anthropological and Historical Perspective. Yale Univ. Press, New Haven.

CZAJKOWSKI, J.M. 1967. Chinese food and traditions. Univ. Conn. Coop. Ext. Serv. Bull. *67-64.*

FENG, C.D. 1954. The Joy of Chinese Cooking. Grosset & Dunlap, New York.

HARRIS, R.S. *et al.* 1949. The composition of Chinese foods. J. Am. Dietet. Assoc. *25,* 28-36.

HAWKS, J.E. 1936. Preparation and composition of foods served in Chinese homes. J. Am. Dietet. Assoc. *12*, 136-140.

HOH, P.W., WILLIAMS, J.C., and PEASE, C.S. 1933. Possible sources of calcium and phosphorus in the Chinese diet. The determination of calcium and phosphorus in a typical Chinese dish containing meat and bone. J. Nutr. 7, 535-546.

HOWE, R. 1969. China. *In* Robin Howe, The International Wine and Food Society's Guide to Far Eastern Cookery. Drake Publishers, New York.

JAFFA, M.E. 1901. Nutrition investigations among fruitarians and Chinese. USDA Office Exp. Stn. Bull. *107.*

JUDD, J.E. 1957. Century-old dietary taboos in the 20th century Japan. J. Am. Dietet. Assoc. *33*, 489-491.

POMERANTZ, Y. 1977. Food and food products in the People's Republic of China. Food Technol. *31* (3) 32-34, 38, 40-41.

WENKAM, N.S., and WOLFF, R.J. 1970. A half century of changing food habits among Japanese in Hawaii. J. Am. Dietet. Assoc. *57*, 29-32.

Foodways of Vegetarians

BERGAN, J.G., and BROWN, P.T. 1980. Nutritional status of "new" vegetarians. J. Am. Dietet. Assoc. *76* (2) 151-155.

BROWN, P.T., and BERGAN, J.G. 1975. The dietary status of "new" vegetarians. J. Am. Dietet. Assoc. *67*, 455-459.

CALVERT, G.P., and CALVERT, S.W. 1975. Intellectual convictions of "health" food consumers. J. Nutr. Educ. *7*, 95-98.

DWYER, J.T. 1980. Mental age and I.Q. of predominantly vegetarian children. J. Am. Dietet. Assoc. *76* (2) 142-147.

DWYER, J.T., KANDEL, R.F., MAYER, L.D.V.H., and MAYER, J. 1974A. The "new" vegetarians. Group affiliation and dietary strictures related to attitudes and life style. J. Am. Dietet. Assoc. *64*, 376–382.

DWYER, J.T., MAYER, L.D.V.H., DOWD, K., KANDEL, R.F., and MAYER, J. 1974B. The new vegetarians: The natural high? J. Am. Dietet. Assoc. *65*, 529-536.

DWYER, J.T., MAYER, L.D.V.H., KANDEL, R.F., and MAYER, J. 1973. The new vegetarians. Who are they? J. Am. Dietet. Assoc. *62*, 503-509.

DWYER, J.T. *et al.* 1978. Preschoolers on alternate life-style diets. Associations between size and dietary indexes with diets limited in types of animal foods. J. Am. Dietet. Assoc. *72*, 264-270.

ERHARD, D. 1973. The new vegetarians. Part I. Vegetarianism and its medical consequences. Nutr. Today *8* (6) 4-12.

FOOTE, R., and EPPRIGHT, E.S. 1940. A dietary study of boys and girls on a lacto-ovo vegetarian diet. J. Am. Dietet. Assoc. *16*, 222-229.

GULEY, H.M. 1977. A vegetarian program for students on a college bound plan. J. Am. Dietet. Assoc. *71*, 276-277.

HARDINGE, M.G., and CROOKS, H. 1964A. Non-flesh dietaries. 1. Historical background. J. Am. Dietet. Assoc. *43*, 545-549.

HARDINGE, M.G., and CROOKS, H. 1964B. Non-flesh dietaries. 2. Scientific literature. J. Am. Dietet. Assoc. *43*, 550-558.

HARDINGE, M.G., and CROOKS, H. 1964C. Non-flesh dietaries. 3. Adequate and inadequate. J. Am. Dietet. Assoc. *43*, 537-541.

HARDINGE, M.G., and STARE, F.J. 1954A. Nutritional studies of vegetarians. 1. Nutritional, physical and laboratory studies. Am. J. Clin. Nutr. *2*, 73-82.

HARDINGE, M.G., and STARE, F.J. 1954B. Nutritional studies of vegetarians. 2. Dietary and serum levels of cholesterol. Am. J. Clin. Nutr. *2*, 83-88.

JAFFA, M.E. 1901. Nutrition investigations among fruitarians and Chinese. USDA Office Exp. Stn. Bull. *107*.

JAFFA, M.E. 1903. Further investigations among fruitarians. USDA Office Exp. Stn. Bull. *132*.

MARSHALL, W.E. 1974. Health foods, organic foods, natural foods. Food Technol. *28*, 50-51, 56.

MIRONE, L. 1954. Nutrient intake and blood findings of men on a diet devoid of meat. Am. J. Clin. Nutr. 2, 246-251.

NEW, P.K.M., and PRIEST, R.P. 1967A. Food and thought: a sociologic study of food cultists. J. Am. Dietet. Assoc. 51, 13-18.

REGISTER, U.D., and SONNENBERG, L.M. 1973. The vegetarian diet. J. Am. Dietet. Assoc. 62, 253-261.

SCHAFER, R., and YETLEY, E.A. 1975. Social psychology of food faddism. Speculations on health food behavior. J. Am. Dietet. Assoc. 66, 129-133.

SIMOONS, F.J. 1961. Eat Not This Flesh: Food Avoidances in the Old World. Univ. Wisc. Press, Madison.

SMITH, E.B. 1975. A guide to good eating the vegetarian way. J. Nutr. Educ. 7, 109-111.

TABER, L.A.L., and COOK, R.A. 1980. Dietary and anthropometric assessment of adult omnivores, fish-eaters, and lacto-ovo-vegetarians. J. Am. Dietet. Assoc. 76 (1) 21-29.

TODHUNTER, E.N. 1973. Food habits, food faddism and nutrition. World Rev. Nutr. Diet. 16, 286-317.

VYHMEISTER, I.B., REGISTER, U.D., and SONNENBERG, L.M. 1977. Safe vegetarian diets for children. In Symposium on Nutrition in Pediatrics. C.G. Neumann and D.B. Jelliffe (Editors). Pediatr. Clin. North Am. 24 (1) 203-210.

WEST, R.O., and HAYS, O.B. 1968. Diet and serum cholesterol levels: comparison between vegetarians and non vegetarians in a Seventh Day Adventist Group. Am. J. Clin. Nutr. 21, 853-862.

17

Dietary Assessment: The Standard as a First Approximation

Quality of life is a pervasive concern; diet quality, including but not limited to nutritional quality, is part of the health-related aspect. A sense of nutritional well-being resulting from customary consumption of a diet with high nutritional quality is associated with good food ecology and good quality of life. How does one determine the nutritional quality of the diet of individuals and/or groups? The diet may be assessed, using the RDA as a guide. Dietary assessment is the process by which diet quality is determined and evaluated as a basis for correction. The RDA is the official standard for comparison of the expected and observed nutritional quality of the diet.

ASSESSMENT

The concept of dietary assessment is elastic and Parkinson's Law applies: "Work expands to fill the time available for its completion . . . ." Thus, a range from rapid but superficial assessment to a systematic and meticulous assessment is possible. Therefore, to reduce ambiguity, the nature and extent of tasks involved must be defined for each situation.

The concept of assessment is complex, with many implications and ramifications. To *assess* means to determine the importance, size, or value of and implies a critical appraisal for the purpose of understanding or interpreting or as a guide in taking action. The key terms associated with this concept are listed and explained as follows:

(a) importance—How important is nutritional quality to the individual/group? Is it important enough to motivate the individual/group to modify foodways?

(b) size—What is the size of the nutritional quality problem? One or many nutrients? Are the nutrients easy or difficult to obtain from dietary intake? Is the problem due to lack of awareness, dislikes, intolerances?

(c) value—Is food and/or nutrition education of value or must intervening variables of lack of time, energy, and/or money be controlled first?

(d) understand—What are the social, cultural, psychological, economic, and/or intake factors that create/maintain the food-related ecosystem of the individual/group? Is understanding of the implications and ramifications of these factors sufficient to enable appropriate suggestion of alternative food items?

(e) interpret—Does the individual/group have sufficient food and/or nutrition knowledge to interpret nutritional analyses, nutrition labels, advertisements? What are the signals of success/failure in dietary monitoring/control?

(f) guide in taking action—What is to be taught in what sequence and in what size increment? How much improvement in nutritional quality of the diet can be expected?

THE RECOMMENDED DIETARY ALLOWANCES (RDA)

The nutrient functions that define necessity for supply and the need for exogenous intake, as well as the expected effects of deficient or excessive intake, have been discussed in the preceding section. But, recommended quantities were not specified nor were outlines for deficient and excessive intake. This was deliberate, since understanding of nutrient functions and the RDA should precede its use in order to reduce the hazards associated with misinterpretation.

The RDA, prepared at approximately five-year intervals by the Food and Nutrition Board of the National Academy of Sciences, is the official authoritative statement of necessary nutrients to be supplied and estimated quantities likely to be appropriate for normal healthy Americans in various categories according to age, sex, and reproductive status. A summary table lists the nutrients and quantities recommended (Table 17.1). This table is the portion of the publication that is generally regarded as the RDA. In the 1980 edition, energy intake recommendations were separated from the summary table. These are listed in Table 17.2. The 1980 edition contained an additional listing of estimated safe and adequate intakes of other nutrients (Table 17.3). The text of the RDA publication reviews the purposes for which the RDA are intended to be used and summarizes research findings on which the allowances are based, nutrient by nutrient.

With each new revision of the RDA, to create awareness and to identify changes from the previous edition that may necessitate a redirection of nutrition education content, detailed papers are presented by designated spokesmen at the next regularly scheduled meeting of the major nutrition-oriented professional associations. These are published in their journals.

The RDA are intended for use by professionals—dietitians and nutritionists, nutrition educators, health professionals, food technologists, and food program administrators rather than the general consumer. Hence, reader sophistication in nutritional sciences is assumed. Summary discussions highlight important points that have served as the bases for decisions in setting the allowances. These are to remind the reader of pertinent considerations in using the table values. Use of the RDA by the uninitiated, especially when limited to use of the table values, has led to misunderstandings, and in some cases this is hazardous as comprehension of the implications and ramifications is absent or limited. Informed use is to be commended; uninformed use is to be condemned.

The Basic 4 Food Groups developed by the USDA are the food intake guide intended for general consumer use in planning an adequate diet. Unfortunately, the linkage between the Basic 4 and levels of intake of particular nutrients is unknown to consumers. Thus, they cannot relate dietary intakes based on the Basic 4 to need for supplements or to instructions with respect to changes in intake of particular nutrients for therapeutic purposes. Hence, consumers are confused and disquieted and a crisis in confidence has resulted.

Development of the RDA is delegated to the Committee on Dietary Allowances, a group of selected experts from the Food and Nutrition Board of the National Academy of Sciences. The process of developing the RDA involves review of the current edition, identification of new and/or special problems for consideration, review of the format and any problems associated with it, review of the world nutrition literature and selection of the most important papers to be used as a basis for revisions, review of and possible revision of the table values for each of the nutrients, and transmittal of a final draft to the Food and Nutrition Board for review prior to submission to the Assembly of Life Sciences of the National Research Council for final review (Comptroller General of the United States 1978).

In developing the RDA, two fundamental questions must be answered, namely: What is its purpose? And, why is it necessary? These seemingly trivial questions are of crucial importance. The intended uses of the RDA determine the cluster of factors that must be considered in developing each of the allowances, as well as their relative importance. As many answers as possible are generated. These are reviewed along with the food- and nutrition-related implications and ramifications—individually and collectively. Failure in this step might result in a value that is misinterpreted and might lead to widespread malnutrition. This is an outcome to be avoided at all costs.

TABLE 17.1. RECOMMENDED DIETARY ALLOWANCES, REVISED 1980[a]. FOOD AND NUTRITION BOARD, NATIONAL ACADEMY OF SCIENCES–NATIONAL RESEARCH COUNCIL

Designed for the maintenance of good nutrition of practically all healthy people in the U.S.A.

Sex Group	Age (Years)	Weight (kg)	Weight (lb)	Height (cm)	Height (in.)	Protein (g)	Fat-Soluble Vitamins Vitamin A (μg R.E.)[b]	Vitamin D (μg)[c]	Vitamin E (mg α T.E.)[d]	Water-Soluble Vitamins Vitamin C (mg)	Thiamin (mg)
Infants	0.0–0.5	6	13	60	24	kg × 2.2	420	10	3	35	0.3
	0.5–1.0	9	20	71	28	kg × 2.0	400	10	4	35	0.5
Children	1–3	13	29	90	35	23	400	10	5	45	0.7
	4–6	20	44	112	44	30	500	10	6	45	0.9
	7–10	28	62	132	52	34	700	10	7	45	1.2
Males	11–14	45	99	157	62	45	1000	10	8	50	1.4
	15–18	66	145	176	69	56	1000	10	10	60	1.4
	19–22	70	154	177	70	56	1000	7.5	10	60	1.5
	23–50	70	154	178	70	56	1000	5	10	60	1.4
	51+	70	154	178	70	56	1000	5	10	60	1.2
Females	11–14	46	101	157	62	46	800	10	8	50	1.1
	15–18	55	120	163	64	46	800	10	8	60	1.1
	19–22	55	120	163	64	44	800	7.5	8	60	1.1
	23–50	55	120	163	64	44	800	5	8	60	1.0
	51+	55	120	163	64	44	800	5	8	60	1.0
Pregnant						+30	+200	+5	+2	+20	+0.4
Lactating						+20	+400	+5	+3	+40	+0.5

[a] The allowances are intended to provide for individual variations among most normal persons as they live in the United States under usual environmental stresses. Diets should be based on a variety of common foods in order to provide other nutrients for which human requirements have been less well defined.
[b] Retinol equivalents. 1 Retinol equivalent = 1 μg retinol or 6 μg β-carotene.
[c] As cholecalciferol. 10 μg cholecalciferol = 400 I.U. vitamin D.
[d] α-tocopherol equivalents. 1 mg d-α-tocopherol = 1 α T.E.

Two general categories of intended uses of the RDA are: (a) a guide for use in planning dietary intake and (b) a standard for evaluation of the nutritional adequacy of exogenous nutrient intake, i.e., dietary intake, supplemented dietary intake, parenteral intake, etc. Specific uses include, but are not limited to, the following:

(a) A guide in planning for and obtaining food supplies for the American population as a whole and its subgroups, i.e., in planning for the allocation of resources in agricultural production and/or in trade arrangements for food imports

(b) A standard for comparison and interpretation of food consumption data for particular groups, in relation to assessment of nutritional status and/or need for dietary intake adjustments

(c) A guide in establishing standards for the size of payments in public assistance programs so that money available for food purchases will be sufficient to purchase a nutritionally adequate diet when used as intended

(d) A guide in evaluating the adequacy of food supplies on hand and planned in relation to meeting the aggregate nutritional needs of Americans

(e) A basis for developing nutrition education programs; it defines which nutrients must be included in presentations and content changes necessary as a result of new information

Water-Soluble Vitamins							Minerals			
Riboflavin (mg)	Niacin (mg N.E.)	Vitamin B₆ (mg)	Folacin (μg)	Vitamin B₁₂ (μg)	Calcium (mg)	Phosphorus (mg)	Magnesium (mg)	Iron (mg)	Zinc (mg)	Iodine (μg)
0.4	6	0.3	30	0.5	360	240	50	10	3	40
0.6	8	0.6	45	1.5	540	360	70	15	5	50
0.8	9	0.9	100	2.0	800	800	150	15	10	70
1.0	11	1.3	200	2.5	800	800	200	10	10	90
1.4	16	1.6	300	3.0	800	800	250	10	10	120
1.6	18	1.8	400	3.0	1200	1200	350	18	15	150
1.7	18	2.0	400	3.0	1200	1200	400	18	15	150
1.7	19	2.2	400	3.0	800	800	350	10	15	150
1.6	18	2.2	400	3.0	800	800	350	10	15	150
1.4	16	2.2	400	3.0	800	800	350	10	15	150
1.3	15	1.8	400	3.0	1200	1200	300	18	15	150
1.3	14	2.0	400	3.0	1200	1200	300	18	15	150
1.3	14	2.0	400	3.0	800	800	300	18	15	150
1.2	13	2.0	400	3.0	800	800	300	18	15	150
1.2	13	2.0	400	3.0	800	800	300	10	15	150
+0.3	+2	+0.6	+400	+1.0	+400	+400	+150	[h]	+5	+25
+0.5	+5	+0.5	+100	+1.0	+400	+400	+150	[h]	+10	+50

[e] 1 N.E. (niacin equivalent) = 1 mg of niacin or 60 mg dietary tryptophan.
[f] The folacin allowances refer to dietary sources as determined by *Lactobacillus casei* assay after treatment with enzymes ("conjugases") to make polyglutamyl forms of the vitamin available to the test organism.
[g] The RDA for vitamin B₁₂ in infants is based on average concentration of the vitamin in human milk. The allowances after weaning are based on energy intake (as recommended by the American Academy of Pediatrics) and consideration of other factors such as intestinal absorption.
[h] The increased requirement during pregnancy cannot be met by the iron content of habitual American diets or by the existing iron stores of many women; therefore the use of 30–60 mg of supplemental iron is recommended. Iron needs during lactation are not substantially different from those of non-pregnant women, but continued supplementation of the mother for 2–3 months after parturition is advisable in order to replenish stores depleted by pregnancy.
Reproduced from: Recommended Dietary Allowances, Ninth Edition (1980) with the permission of the National Academy of Sciences, Washington, D.C.

(f) A guide in formulating new foods; it defines which nutrients should be considered for inclusion and appropriate quantities

(g) A basis for setting guidelines for nutrition labeling; it defines which nutrients should be considered for inclusion and appropriate quantities

(h) A standard in regulating the nutritional quality of foods; it defines which nutrients should be present and expected quantities; comparison of expected and observed quantities allows for detection of unwanted changes and monitoring of progress in controlling deviations

The points that emerge from consideration of the preceding intended uses of the RDA address the questions of purpose and necessity. As a result, pertinent current operational concerns are brought to bear on various aspects of the review process.

Another portion of the task of developing the RDA is to determine the value for each of the allowances, i.e., the amounts to be supplied in fixed or regular quantities. Since the priorities in improving the nutritional status of the American population and/or its specific subgroups as well as the food and nutrition research findings available for use as the basis for discussion vary over time, the RDA must be revised periodically to reflect these differences.

TABLE 17.2.   MEAN HEIGHTS AND WEIGHTS AND RECOMMENDED ENERGY INTAKE

Category	Age (Years)	Weight (kg)	(lb)	Height (cm)	(in.)	Energy Needs (with Range) (kcal)	(MJ)
Infants	0.0−0.5	6	13	60	24	kg × 115 (95−145)	kg × 0.48
	0.5−1.0	9	20	71	28	kg × 105 (80−135)	kg × 0.44
Children	1−3	13	29	90	35	1300 (900−1800)	5.5
	4−6	20	44	112	44	1700 (1300−2300)	7.1
	7−10	28	62	132	52	2400 (1650−3300)	10.1
Males	11−14	45	99	157	62	2700 (2000−3700)	11.3
	15−18	66	145	176	69	2800 (2100−3900)	11.8
	19−22	70	154	177	70	2900 (2500−3300)	12.2
	23−50	70	154	178	70	2700 (2300−3100)	11.3
	51−75	70	154	178	70	2400 (2000−2800)	10.1
	76+	70	154	178	70	2050 (1650−2450)	8.6
Females	11−14	46	101	157	62	2200 (1500−3000)	9.2
	15−18	55	120	163	64	2100 (1200−3000)	8.8
	19−22	55	120	163	64	2100 (1700−2500)	8.8
	23−50	55	120	163	64	2000 (1600−2400)	8.4
	51−75	55	120	163	64	1800 (1400−2200)	7.6
	76+	55	120	163	64	1600 (1200−2000)	6.7
Pregnancy						+300	
Lactation						+500	

Source: from Recommended Dietary Allowances, Revised 1980. Food and Nutrition Board, National Academy of Sciences−National Research Council, Washington, D.C.

The data in this table have been assembled from the observed median heights and weights of children together with desirable weights for adults for the mean heights of men (70 in.) and women (64 in.) between the ages 18 and 34 years as surveyed in the U.S. population (HEW/NCHS data).

The energy allowances for the young adults are for men and women doing light work. The allowances for the two older age groups represent mean energy needs over these age spans, allowing for a 2% decrease in basal (resting) metabolic rate per decade and a reduction in activity of 200 kcal/day for men and women between 51 and 75 years, 500 kcal for men over 75 years and 400 kcal for women over 75. The customary range of daily energy output is shown for adults in parentheses, and is based on a variation in energy needs of ±400 kcal at any one age, emphasizing the wide range of energy intakes appropriate for any group of people.

Energy allowances for children through age 18 are based on median energy intakes of children these ages followed in longitudinal growth studies. The values in parentheses are 10th and 90th percentiles of energy intake, to indicate the range of energy consumption among children of these ages.

Essentially, the RDA for most nutrients are based on what is known about human requirements. These values are adjusted for differences in population groups from research control status, and a safety factor to cover what is unknown is added to that. This is a somewhat simplistic explanation and does not reveal the nature and extent of problems which are the cause of thoughtful deliberations. Some of the kinds of points at issue are presented for illustration:

(a) IF there is insufficient information on which to base a statement of requirement, THEN the mean intake value is used as a first approximation to an allowance. This is a "soft" allowance and will remain until better information is available. The values for vitamin E in the 1968 and 1974 RDA were of this type.

(b) IF information is available on the effects of zero intake AND the mean quantity necessary to restore/maintain the asymptomatic state is known, THEN the basis for the requirement can be stated and this can be used to derive an allowance. This is a "hard" allowance and probably will remain firm thereafter with only minor changes.

(c) IF information is available concerning the degree of risk of deficiency at the requirement level, given an estimate of individual differences in biological efficiency in digestion/absorption/metabolism of the nutrient, THEN a correction factor can be derived and applied to the requirement value.

(d) IF information is available concerning the distribution of the nutrient in foods, including but not limited to data such as sources of variability within each class of foods, sources of errors (and their magnitude) in composition values, and sources of variability in intake due to differences in bioavailability, THEN assessment of the expected effects will provide the bases for derivation of a correction factor and its application to the requirement value.

(e) IF precursors of the nutrient are commonly available in foods, THEN the efficiency of conversion must be evaluated in relation to need for an adjustment of the final value, given common supply sources.

(f) IF the information available is acknowledged to contain gaps, THEN the nature and extent of the gaps are assessed and a safety factor is applied.

The Comptroller General's report (1978) discussed some additional points that are public information:

> For most nutrients, judgment is required in extrapolating from requirements to allowances. Even for nutrients about which the greatest amount of direct information is available concerning human requirements, the knowledge is usually applicable only to infants and young adults. For very few of these nutrients is there enough information to permit calculation of a highly reliable estimate of variation among individuals. For most nutrient requirements, it must be assumed that variability is in the same range as that for the few nutrients that have been studied extensively. For nutrients that are not completely absorbed, values for efficiency of absorption tend to be highly variable. Also it is difficult to decide upon the appropriate criterion for determining when the requirements for some nutrients have been met. The criterion may be considered as an amount just in excess of that needed to prevent deficiency signs, it may be considered as an amount that ensures saturation of tissues, and it may be judged to be somewhere between these extremes and to be the amount needed to maintain a particular concentration in blood or a particular level of urinary excretion. Adequacy thus becomes a matter of judgment.[1]

The result of the long and involved deliberations by experts is derivation of a summary value to be published. At this point, the new value is

---

[1] From Comptroller General of the United States (1978).

TABLE 17.3. ESTIMATED SAFE AND ADEQUATE DAILY DIETARY INTAKES OF AD-
DITIONAL SELECTED VITAMINS AND MINERALS[a]

Category	Age (Years)	Vitamins			Trace Elements	
		Vitamin K (μg)	Biotin (μg)	Pantothenic Acid (mg)	Copper (mg)	Manganese (mg)
Infants	0−0.5	12	35	2	0.5−0.7	0.5−0.7
	0.5−1	10−20	50	3	0.7−1.0	0.7−1.0
Children	1−3	15−30	65	3	1.0−1.5	1.0−1.5
and	4−6	20−40	85	3−4	1.5−2.0	1.5−2.0
Adolescents	7−10	30−60	120	4−5	2.0−2.5	2.0−3.0
	11+	50−100	100−200	4−7	2.0−3.0	2.5−5.0
Adults		70−140	100−200	4−7	2.0−3.0	2.5−5.0

Source: from Recommended Dietary Allowances, Revised 1980. Food and Nutrition Board, National Academy of Sciences-National Research Council, Washington, D.C.
[a] Because there is less information on which to base allowances, these figures are not given in the main table of the RDA
and are provided here in the form of ranges of recommended intakes.
[b] Since the toxic levels for many trace elements may be only several times usual intakes, the upper levels for the trace
elements given in this table should not be habitually exceeded.

compared with the published value and a justification of the change,
based on the new information and/or considerations, is written for the
text of the RDA publication. When this has been completed for each
nutrient, the manuscript draft is submitted as noted above for the
mandatory reviews prior to publication.

PROBLEMS WITH THE RDA

The chairman of the Committee on Dietary Allowances and some
members of the committee, acting as spokesmen for the group, have
acknowledged publicly that there are some problems with the RDA that
result in misuse/abuse (Balsley 1977). These are listed because it is
important that professionals using the RDA understand the problems
and be able to discuss them:

(a) A customary intake that is less than the RDA is not necessarily
inadequate. Whether it is inadequate is an individual matter that depends on the individual's current need for the nutrient in question, as
established by biochemical tests. However, customary intake markedly
below the RDA increases the risk of deficiency. In setting the standard, a
safety factor is applied to ensure that the needs of those between the
median and 97.5% of the population are met (Fig. 17.1). The safety
factors which are added to all of the RDAs except calories are variable in
magnitude. Therefore, use of an arbitrary, although traditional, cutline
such as ⅔ or ¾ of the table value as a basis for the inference of whether
intake is inadequate may result in overstatement of the proportion of the
population whose diets are inadequate. Moreover, for simplicity, table
values are presented on a daily basis. Body stores or reserves enable it to

Trace Elements[b]				Electrolytes		
Fluoride (mg)	Chromium (mg)	Selenium (mg)	Molybdenum (mg)	Sodium (mg)	Potassium (mg)	Chloride (mg)
0.1−0.5	0.01−0.04	0.01−0.04	0.03−0.06	115−350	350−925	275−700
0.2−1.0	0.02−0.06	0.02−0.06	0.04−0.08	250−750	425−1275	400−1200
0.5−1.5	0.02−0.08	0.02−0.08	0.05−0.1	325−975	550−1650	500−1500
1.0−2.5	0.03−0.12	0.03−0.12	0.06−0.15	450−1350	775−2325	700−2100
1.5−2.5	0.05−0.2	0.05−0.2	0.1−0.3	600−1800	1000−3000	925−2775
1.5−2.5	0.05−0.2	0.05−0.2	0.15−0.5	900−2700	1525−4575	1400−4200
1.5−4.0	0.05−0.2	0.05−0.2	0.15−0.5	1100−3300	1875−5625	1700−5100

tolerate dietary inadequacy of short duration. Therefore, intakes are certainly acceptable when balanced so that a five- to eight-day mean is equivalent.

(b) The RDAs for some nutrients for members of some age groups, e.g., adolescents and the elderly, are not based on studies of requirements of persons in these age groups. Instead, they are extrapolations from other age groups. Their accuracy is unknown; the values serve as a first approximation until better values become available.

(c) RDAs have not been established for all nutrients known to be essential to man. This is because of lack of population data for many age/sex groups. Therefore, even consumption of the specified nutrients in the stipulated quantities does not imply dietary adequacy. For this reason, consumption of a variety of raw and fresh foods is still advised. In an effort to provide some guidance with respect to micronutrient intake, provisional ranges for 12 additional nutrients are given in the 9th edition (Table 17.3).

(d) Interactions between nutrients and other life-style factors and among nutrients are known to affect the requirement for some nutrients. Interactions complicate the problem of setting generally appropriate allowances, especially when insufficient information is available from which to state adjustment factors for expected kinds of variations. Interactions for which adjustment factors would be beneficial include, but are not limited to, the protein-calcium relationship, the iron-vitamin C relationship, effects of smoking, and the effects of stress of various types or levels. The RDA are designed for healthy people and not for special purposes; this limits the scope of the interactions that must be addressed. There is no information concerning the inflated demands imposed by disease, whether temporary or chronic. And, there is no adjustment for use of oral contraceptive agents, although the circulating levels of several nutrients are known to be affected. Similarly, there is no discussion of nutrients for their pharmacologic effects.

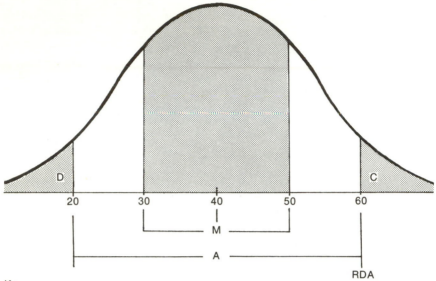

Key

M Mean requirement for nutrient X = 40U; ⅔ of the population requires the mean
   ± or 30 to 50 U.

A The mean ± 2 requirement for nutrient X = 20 to 60 U; 95% of the population group
   requires an amount within this range. The RDA is the upper value.

C A few, i.e., 2.5%, require more than the normal amount, i.e., more than 60U.

D A few, i.e., 2.5%, require much less than the normal amount.

FIG. 17.1. DISTRIBUTION OF POPULATION REQUIREMENTS OF HEALTHY
PEOPLE FOR NUTRIENT X, IN UNIT U, WHICH MAY BE MCG, MG, OR G, ETC.

Actual values vary with age, sex, activity levels, etc.

A recent report by the Comptroller General (1978) confirms the fact
that the criticisms of the RDA are a cause for concern. The three main
criticisms are:

(a) The RDA are an invalid guide because table values are based on
limited data, often based on samples of nutritional status of a few
subjects. The point is well taken since there is danger of under- or
overestimation of requirements due to the effects of individual differences which exert a heavy bias on small sample means. The expertise
of Committee members and the elaborate review process provide the best
assurance of mindful consideration of the implications and ramifications
of data deficiencies. Hence, the problem primarily reflects the fact that
scientific knowledge of human nutritional requirements is limited. Philo-
sophically, some basis is better than none. Similarly, some guide is better
than none.

(b) The RDA overstate the needs of most people. This is deliberate since to err on the side of somewhat more is of little consequence, whereas to err in the other direction may cause harm. The RDA are designed to meet the expected needs of 97.5% of the American population that is healthy.

(c) The RDA have not been developed for all essential nutrients—only for protein as 9 essential amino acids and for 16 other nutrients. There are no RDA for fat, CHO, and other nutrients of current importance in relation to degenerative diseases. This is to be expected, given the current set of purposes. To reiterate, the RDA are for healthy people. Consultation with a physician is warranted when adjusting diets for therapeutic purposes. Provisional allowances for additional nutrients have been developed, as noted above.

In summary, while the RDA are imperfect, they are useful. Because of limitations, they should be used with judgment.

Use of the RDA: The Way

A periodic reassessment of an individual's nutritional status is recommended because the demand for the various nutrients differs in the various stages of the life cycle. Changes in demand are more frequent and are greater in magnitude in the early years. The demand differs because of changes in:

(a) Body size

(b) Activity level

(c) Growth status—prepreparation storage build-up, acceleration, maintenance, repair, deceleration

(d) Reproductive status—prepreparation storage build-up, pregnancy and/or lactation, replenishment of stores

During a five-year period, one could very well move from one level of nutritional demand to another. Indeed, young women usually have demand changes of all four types to adjust to in a short period of time. Every time there is a major demand change of one of these types, or at least at five-year intervals, one should (a) monitor intake for a week and (b) compare intake to the appropriate RDA. This is the group norm and provides the most readily available basis for instituting appropriate changes.

The RDA are revised approximately every five years, after consideration of the new research findings available. A new approximation of optimal intake is produced and publicized. Therefore, publication of a new RDA can be used as a signal to trigger the recommended assessment.

The RDA are not intended for assessment of the nutritional status of individuals. They are intended for assessment of the nutriture of groups.

IF this is so, THEN can the RDA be used for individual assessment?

Yes, if one is well informed and adopts a reasonable rather than a "strict-constructionist" attitude when interpreting the findings. Individuals are members of population groups. Therefore, the RDA for the appropriate age/sex/reproductive status group can be used as a first approximation to the quantity that should be supplied.

Actual demand for any nutrient is unknown and unknowable. Laboratory tests are more indicative, i.e., they provide an index to the circulating level that can be compared to group norms, but they are not conclusive. This is because of individual differences in biological efficiency. Some individuals are metabolically sparing and others are metabolically wasting—with regard to utilization of any particular nutrient. But, at the present time this cannot be determined accurately for one nutrient, much less for all. For most people, the cost of an extensive set of more definitive but expensive biochemical analyses is prohibitive.

So, intake is monitored and mean values are compared with the appropriate RDA. Moreover, the individual must use himself/herself as a control, experimenting with changes and monitoring results. The procedure is:

(a) Collect intake data for a week and compute mean intake (procedures are discussed in the next chapter).

(b) IF the mean intake for a particular nutrient is somewhat low AND no symptoms are observed, THEN assume intake is sufficient but check it out—see (e) following.

(c) IF the mean intake of a particular nutrient is much greater than the RDA AND no symptoms are observed, THEN assume intake is not a problem but check it out—see (e) following.

(d) IF intake of a particular nutrient is close to the RDA value, THEN assume it is all right and direct effort to changes in intake of other nutrients where the results are likely to be greater.

(e) IF a check-out procedure is necessary, THEN adjust intake of the nutrient(s) to approximate the RDA[1] and ingest at this level for a month and observe.

-IF no changes are observed, THEN assume that intake level of that nutrient(s) is not that critical, i.e., some variability in intake can be tolerated, so narrow control is unnecessary.

-IF improvement is observed, THEN assume that intake of that nutrient(s) was somewhat inappropriate AND continued adjustment (increase or decrease, as indicated) or control is necessary. (This change in level of intake may need to be repeated several times in order to find the optimal personalized intake level.)

---

[1] IF megadose intake of addicting nutrients, e.g., ascorbic acid, has been customary, THEN a gradual reduction in intake is preferable to a sharp reduction to the RDA level. This is recommended in order to avoid symptoms of withdrawal.

-IF deterioration is observed, THEN assume that original intake was more appropriate and return to that level.

Adjustment of intake to the RDA can be achieved either by use of a supplement or by a conscious change in food choices. For testing purposes, use of a supplement for a month or so may be the easiest solution, if appropriate doses can be obtained. On a continuing basis, a change in dietary habits is recommended. This requires extensive knowledge of which foods are good and which are poor sources of each nutrient to be adjusted. Chapter 19 provides an extended treatment of this topic.

Abuse of the RDA

The RDA traditionally have been used in planning for and in assessment of the nutritional adequacy of the overall American food supply. This is a legitimate use. But, adequacy of the overall supply does not assure that the levels and distribution of effective demand for food will be related to the proportion of the population in each of the sectors of the American population. Nutritional surveys have documented the fact that nutrient intakes vary within and among the various population sectors. Hence, assurance of the adequacy of the overall supply with respect to any or all nutrients or the finding that the population mean intake of any or all nutrients approximates the RDA cannot be taken to mean that malnutrition has been eradicated; that would be a fallacious interpretation. Survey data on prevalence will show that some are malnourished; this estimate of magnitude of the social problem requires policy changes in other domains, since malnutrition is only a secondary problem.

BIBLIOGRAPHY

BALSLEY, M. 1977. Soon to come: 1978 Recommended Dietary Allowances. J. Am. Dietet. Assoc. *71* (2) 149-151.

BIERI, J.G. 1980. An overview of the RDAs for vitamins. J. Am. Dietet. Assoc. *76* (2) 134-136.

COMPTROLLER GENERAL OF THE UNITED STATES. 1978. Recommended Dietary Allowances: More Research and Better Food Guides Needed. Rept. CED-78-169. GAO, Washington, D.C.

MERTZ, W. 1980. The new RDAs: Estimated adequate and safe intake of trace elements and calculation of available iron. J. Am. Dietet. Assoc. *76* (2) 128-133.

MUNRO, H.N. 1980. Major gaps in nutrient allowances. The status of the elderly. J. Am. Dietet. Assoc. *76* (2) 137-141.

NATIONAL RESEARCH COUNC., DIV. BIOL. SCI., FOOD & NUTRITION BOARD. 1980. Recommended Dietary Allowances. 9th Edition. National Academy of Sciences, Washington, D.C.

18

Dietary Assessment: Diet History and Diet Record

The foodways of an individual evolve over time; they are always in a state of transition. The diet history of most people is an unknown, but it is not unknowable, just undefined. Most young people (you/they) eating away from their family home soon note that the food consumption habits and practices of eating companions differ from your/their own. And, you/they often make some changes in your/their own habits and practices as you/they encounter new situations. This is normal, and to be expected. What difference does it make nutritionally? That depends on the nature and extent of the change(s) and on the diet history of the individual. The same change may improve one person's diet and undermine the quality of another's. Documentation of the diet history of an individual is the fundamental task in laying the foundation for assessment and improvement.

A diet record is also an unknown; when required, it is often regarded as a bother. Conscientiously completed, it provides a valid basis for estimating nutrient intake. Otherwise, its use leads to an erroneous estimate of nutrient intake and inappropriate instruction that is rightly disregarded.

Both the diet history and the diet record are tools used to obtain data for use in preparing an estimate of (a) the individual's food-related problems to be dealt with in making dietary changes and (b) current food intake, respectively. The findings are used as the basis for assessing the tasks involved in making changes to improve dietary intake, likely obstacles, limitations that require retargeting of nutritional goals, and/or acceptance of the *status quo*.

ESTIMATE

The concept of an estimate is deceivingly simple. Its application to dietary assessment leads directly to a confrontation with the normal and natural complexity of an individual's foodways. An *estimate* is a rough or approximate calculation of the size, extent, or nature of some aspect of X and implies a judgment, considered or casual, that precedes or takes the place of actual measuring of X or testing it out. Aspects of an individual's foodways that might be estimated include, but are not limited to:

(a) Intolerances/avoidances of specific foods for reasons of health, religion, etc.—extent, and importance nutritionally

(b) Likes/dislikes—extent, and importance nutritionally

(c) Meal pattern—size of the meal, size of portions, importance of customary meal components, extent of control over eating frequency

(d) Approximate nutrient intake (actual intake can be obtained only by chemical analysis of a set of duplicate samples)

DATA COLLECTION: THE DIET HISTORY

Diet history data are usually collected from another person. The relationship is transient, but every effort should be made to make it functional. The image projected by the data collector should be pleasant, positive, and competent. A moderately strong approach is preferred, since it provides the greatest flexibility in responding to the personality encountered.

A friendly but impersonal manner is also essential. At the outset, a major point to be communicated is that an honest and complete answer is sought, so that sufficient understanding will result in selection of appropriate suggestions and points for instruction. Moreover, a non-judgmental attitude is imperative and must be projected. One must *not* respond with curiosity about interesting aspects of philosophical/religious beliefs or the like, shock at the revelation of grossly substandard living conditions, disgust at mistakes made, ridicule in relation to erroneous beliefs or faulty nutrition knowledge, etc. Any such responses are counter-productive since they prevent dietary improvement by terminating the relationship. (The interaction may continue or separation may occur.)

Diet history data are usually collected using a systematic procedure in order to control the nature and extent of data obtained. A written questionnaire and/or interview schedule (Fig. 18.1) is used for this purpose.

In some cases, a high frequency of negatives or blanks will indicate that a person's life-style is very different from the norm. In this case, some

Date: _____

Name: _____ Age: _____ Sex: _____ Household size: _____

Ht: _____ Wt: lb _____ Kilos _____ Ideal wt: lb _____ Kilos _____

Referral: _____

Diagnosis: _____

How much time do you spend in physical activity daily? _____

Occupational: sit _____ walk _____ heavy lifting/pushing _____

Recreational: sit _____ walk _____ jog _____ bike _____ other _____

Housework: sit _____ walk _____ stairs _____ mixed work _____

Other: walk to work _____ stairs _____

Do you eat at the same time every day? Yes No

Are there any foods you cannot/will not eat? What? _____

What kinds of foods do you eat at each feeding? _____

Food, Form[1] (Fill In)	Time	Place[2]	Serving Size[3]	Number Servings
Bread				
Jelly				
Margarine				
Cereal				
Sugar				
Milk				
Fruit (citrus)				
Juice				
Meat/substitute				
Green vegetable				
Yellow vegetable				
Other fruit/vegetable				
Salad				
Dessert				
Nuts				
Chips				
Candy				
Alcohol				
Soft drinks				
Legumes				
Vitamin supplements				
Mineral supplements				
Other food supplements				

[1] For example: canned and reheated; instant, reconstituted; fried; steamed and seasoned with fat and herbs; etc.

[2] For example: home—kitchen, dining room, living room; cafeteria; coffee shop; fast food take-out; etc.

[3] Household measures.

FIG. 18.1. SAMPLE ABBREVIATED DIET HISTORY FORM

leading questions are asked in an effort to elicit a description of the individual's foodways. Sample questions are listed in Table 18.1.

A high quality diet history will elicit necessary and sufficient information for making relevant suggestions for dietary change in an acceptable way. What are necessary data? That is a matter of professional judgment, given the objectives of dietary change. For example, questions regarding eating frequency and quantity consumed at a time may be very important in planning changes with an overweight person or a poverty stricken person or an ulcer patient, but interesting and irrelevant in the case of a heart patient. In the case of a heart patient, questions with respect to sodium and/or fat intake may be more pertinent.

IF a written questionnaire is used, THEN various predetermined subsets of questions, i.e., multiple forms, should be developed for each type of case, e.g., low income, unstructured life-style, ethnic, reduced calorie, cholesterol controlled, diabetic, ulcer. IF an oral interview strategy is used, THEN preparation should include review of the basic subset of questions to be asked, given the type of case. In any event, the basic subset of questions is identical; the only difference is that one is written and one is oral. However, the subset of questions asked is different for each type of case.

In developing the subset of questions for each type of case, a decision must be made to include/delete each question listed in the overall set. In making this decision, there are two questions to be answered: What is the purpose of asking question X in this case? Why is it necessary to have the answer to question X in this case? IF these questions cannot be answered immediately and satisfactorily, THEN the question should be omitted, since the data obtained will not be used in meeting an objective. Therefore, to ask the question would be a waste of valuable time.

What is sufficient information? Enough so that suggestions are acceptable; if too little is obtained, suggestions are too general and one feels hesitant about asking for specifics. Or the interviewer asks many questions that already should have been answered. One does not pursue an inapplicable point. IF a person is unable/unwilling to attempt/make dietary changes, THEN there is no justification for taking a diet history except when there is an immediate problem with food rejection. Moreover, there is no point in spending between half an hour and an hour obtaining in-depth answers to questions when only 15 minutes are allocated for diet instruction. The rule is: the amount of time allocated for taking a diet history is proportional to the instructional time allocation.

People are people. By taking thought, design of the questionnaire/interview schedule can take this into account so as to obtain reliable and useful data. Some common people problems are:

(a) People will tell you what they think you want to hear, e.g., IF you ask a person what he/she ate for breakfast, THEN the most likely answer comes from TV commercials—many people are reluctant (because of unacknowledged feelings of guilt?) to admit to a nutritionist that they do not eat breakfast.

TABLE 18.1. SAMPLE QUESTIONS TO EXPLORE IN A COMPLETE DIET HISTORY[1]

MEALS AND MEAL PATTERNS
a. Number of meals
  1. How many meals per day? 2, 3, 3 + snacks, continuous snacking
  2. Is the same number of meals consumed every day? Or does the number vary with the day of the week, weekend?
  3. Does the same pattern persist from week to week or is it variable?
b. Heaviness of meals BLD, BDS?
  1. Equally heavy or specific ones light and others always heavy or variable?
  2. Due to habit, spacing of meals or need?
c. Meal time - Is it fixed or variable according to activities or other factors?
d. Meal components - Are they fixed or variable? Day of week, week, season?
  1. What categories of foods are usually consumed at B? Fruit or juice; cereal (hot or cold); egg, meat or other entrée; bread; beverage; other?
  2. What categories of foods are usually consumed at the noon meal?
     (a) Soup, sandwich, dessert, bread, beverage?
     (b) Salad plate, bread, dessert, beverage?
     (c) Casserole, vegetable, salad, dessert, beverage?
     (d) Other pattern?
  3. What categories of foods are customarily consumed at the evening meal?
     (a) Whole meat - baked, broiled, fried; starchy food, vegetable, salad, dessert, bread, beverage, casserole, vegetarian entrée, entrée salad, soup, stew, organ meat.
  4. What categories of foods are customarily consumed as snacks?
     (a) CHO - FAT—carbonated beverage, soup, candy, cake, pie, cereals, chips, vegetables.
     (b) Proteins - hamburgers, eggnog
     (c) Non-caloric—coffee, tea, carbonated beverage

RITUAL OF EATING
a. Is food consumption a formal or informal activity? Is this relevant in determining amount and/or kind of food consumed?
b. Do you select your own food or is it selected for you?
c. Who decides the quantity of food consumed? Are you picky or do you clean the plate?
d. Do you eat alone or with a group? Is this a relevant factor in determining the amount and/or kind of food consumed?
e. Do you eat rapidly or slowly?
f. What utensils do you use in eating? Is this important?
g. What kind of table manners do you have? What are the main points, taboos, etc.?
h. Do you say grace before eating? What effect does this have on service and food quality?
i. Where do you eat? In dining room, at breakfast bar, in front of TV, while on the go (not sitting), etc. (With increased snacking and TV, this has altered patterns.)
j. Psychological reasons - why eat? (Like food, eat to live, etc.)

FOOD ITEMS AND COMBINATIONS
a. Are a variety of food preparation methods used? Or, does one predominate?
b. Are the same preparation methods used at all meals?
c. Which methods are used?
d. Are foods usually served with a sauce or gravy? What kind? Quantity?
e. Are condiments usually used? If so, what kind(s)? At what meal(s)?
f. What spices are customarily used? Are they used generally or only in specific dishes or with certain specified meats or vegetables? Are some spices always used in combination? If so, which ones?
g. Are individual foods served alone or are several foods usually combined in a dish? If combined, is the combination defined by tradition or is it the inspiration of the cook?
h. Are some foods customarily served together?

TABLE 18.1 *(Continued)*

ACCEPTABLE FOODS AND INGREDIENTS - WHAT DETERMINES?
a. Are you catholic in your tastes, i.e., do you eat whatever is presented?
b. Are you adventurous? Will you try new foods or do you only eat what is familiar?
c. Do you strongly prefer some foods or do you enjoy most foods about equally?
d. Have you had extensive experience with several cuisines other than your native cuisine? When was this? Was this exposure occasional or frequent? Was it over a short or long period of time?
e. Are aesthetics important to the palatability of food you eat? - color, texture, shape, contrasts?
f. How important is food quality? What quality do you eat?
g. What ingredients such as onions or celery or tomatoes are in many mixtures?

UNACCEPTABLE FOODS AND INGREDIENTS - WHAT DETERMINES?
a. Do you prefer familiar foods and combinations and preparation methods?
b. Do you strongly dislike some foods? Why? Color, texture, flavor, preparation method, etc.
c. Does frequent serving of a food cause you to reject it? Which foods do you respond to in this way?
d. Do you have a weight or health problem that causes you ro reduce the frequency with which you consume certain foods? Gas or indigestion?
e. Do you practice a religion that proscribes or forbids certain foods? Or sets certain fast or feast days? What are the proscriptions?
f. Are your dislikes variable depending on your companions and peer group pressure?
g. Do you avoid or reduce the frequency of serving a food because another member of your eating group dislikes it?
h. Do you not eat some foods that you enjoy because preparation takes too long, is too difficult, or you lack facilities?
i. Do you forego favorite foods because they are too expensive or are unavailable?

GENERAL QUESTIONS WHOSE ANSWERS MAY HAVE PERVASIVE EFFECTS
a. If you prepare your meals, do you plan your menus in advance or eat whatever?
b. Are preparation methods monotonous or variable?
c. Do the food items in your diet reflect seasonal availability?
d. Do you eat mostly fresh, frozen, or canned foods? Are some of these unacceptable?
e. What effects do food prices have on food items in your diet? Do you omit, consume less frequently, or ignore?
f. What are the effects of peer group pressure - nature and extent?
g. Has there been any change in your eating habits due to changes in what your mother prepared, changes in her skill, etc., that have had a strong effect?
h. Were the best foods served to your father? What effect did this have?
i. Did your mother restrict what was served to get around your father's dislikes?
j. What effect did your mother's disciplinary methods have on your food habits?
   - withhold when bad
   - bribe with food
   - prepare favorites when good
   - allow you to be picky or force you to clean your plate
   - force you to try new foods or just make available and encourage tasting
k. What effect does your geographic location have? Rural vs. urban
l. Do you frequently eat at fast food restaurants, specialty restaurants?
m Is dormitory food similar to what you normally eat? Do you expect it to change your eating habits? Long term or short term?
n. In short, are your food habits fixed or flexible? Do you adapt to the environment?
o. Do your food habits ensure a nutritionally balanced diet?
p. Dorm food—have you stereotyped it? Do you call it all starchy, greasy, etc., because that is all that is offered OR all that you select?

---

[1] Note: One can start most anywhere in selecting points to include in a definition and/or description of food habits. They are in a dynamic state of change, the degree of change being somewhat a function of personality and somewhat a function of circumstances, that is, food technology, food availability, stability of life-style, etc. Moreover, there are many interrelationships. This is *not* a questionnaire; it is to raise questions, any or all of which may be relevant to you.

(b) People will carefully answer the questions you ask, but they will not help you by indicating that other topics are more relevant; perhaps one should always conclude by asking whether there are any additional points that the individual wishes to offer.

(c) Most people eat as much as they want—not the amounts recognized as standard portions; they must identify a portion size and indicate fractions/multiples.

(d) Unless a man cooks, he may not know whether the meat was broiled or fried, etc.

(e) Busy mothers with several children become confused about whether Billy or Johnny dislikes carrots, has been eating well, is always hungry, etc. If the child is old enough, it is wise to ask the child whether he likes X,Y, Z, and Q, what he had for breakfast, etc.

(f) Unless people are asked specifically, they will talk only about the recent past—a month or so, but seasonal differences in intake become apparent only if one probes. In dealing with the food habits of the elderly, a brief review of foodways in each previous stage of the life cycle may be very revealing.

DATA COLLECTION: THE DIET RECORD

Diet record data are also usually collected from another person. Here again, while the relationship is likely to be transient, it needs to be functional.

At the outset, a major point to be communicated is that an honest and typical sample of food intake is sought. Therefore, IF the period for data collection is *not* typical because of illness, inconvenience, a special occasion resulting in feasting/fasting, or any other intervening variable, THEN discussion is necessary to determine whether to collect the data during the scheduled time period with appropriate notation or to come to mutual agreement on an alternate data collection period. This approach emphasizes the importance of typicality, the premise that underlies valid interpretation.

Given the temper of the times, many people feel that a diet record invades their privacy. So, a second point to be communicated is that one is *not* curious about the particular items/quantities eaten/not eaten with ill intent or to pry. The data are necessary and will be used to:

(a) Compute nutrient intake

(b) Determine which foods are consumed that are sources of nutrients that are either deficient or excessive, so that an adjustment in consumption frequency and/or alternatives can be suggested

(c) Determine the customary size of portions of various foods, so that an adjustment in quantity can be suggested, if necessary

(d) Identify the customary preparation methods used, in general and for specific items, so that alternate or modified methods can be discussed

(e) Identify the meal pattern and/or customary eating frequency with associated meal components; determine which classes of items are considered appropriate for a given meal component, e.g., gelatin, cookies, cupcakes, and tarts as lunch desserts and cakes, pies, and ice cream as dinner desserts

(f) Determine eating times and whether they are fixed or variable

Diet record data are usually collected by a systematic procedure in order to control the nature and extent of ambiguities and/or gaps. Explicit directions are given, usually both orally and in writing. Diet record forms are customarily used to control data arrangement for efficiency in retrieval and computation. Several different types of diet records have been devised. Each is described below:

(a) 24-hour recall—The individual lists/reports everything consumed in the preceding 24-hour period, except water, but including food supplements. This method provides the least information—which foods, which food groups, how much, which meal components, which food preparation methods, and when. Limitations: subject to memory errors and is least likely to be typical—does not provide any information on variation due to day of week, day of pay period, season, and the like.

(b) 3-day diet record—Usually three consecutive days are chosen, with or without a weekend day, since weekend eating habits have been shown to differ from weekday habits. All items consumed during the period, except water but including any food supplements, are recorded at the time of consumption. Brand names, recipes for home prepared mixed dishes, portion sizes, and time of eating are recorded. Limitations: less likely to be complete, does not provide any information on variation due to day of pay period, season, and the like. See samples, Table 18.2, Fig. 18.2.

TABLE 18.2. SAMPLE DETAILED DIRECTIONS FOR RECORDING DIET RECORD

1. Record at the time eaten. Record the exact amount of all food(s) you eat and all beverages you drink, except water.

2. Milk—Record the amount in cups or by carton size. List the kind(s), for example: whole milk, evaporated milk (diluted or undiluted), 2% milk, buttermilk, chocolate milk, nonfat dry milk (regular or instant), etc.

3. Fruit juice or drink—Record the amount in cups or by glass size. List the flavor, whether sweetened or unsweetened, and brand.

4. Fruit—Canned: record kind, amount, kind of syrup (light, etc.), amount of syrup used, note if home canned. Whole raw: record kind, number, and size. Frozen: record kind, amount, brand, sweetened or unsweetened or syrup pack, note if home frozen.

5. Vegetables—List name and how prepared such as baked, steamed, stir-fried, au gratin, etc. Cooked fresh: record number and size of pieces or half-cup portions. Frozen: number of half-cup portions, brand, note if home frozen. Canned: record number of half-cup portions of vegetable and juice separately, brand.

TABLE 18.2 *(Continued)*

6. Cereals—Cooked: record kind such as farina, oatmeal, rice, pasta, etc.; specify if whole grain or enriched; amount in tablespoons or cup portions after cooking. Dry: record kind, brand, amount in cup portions, sweetened or unsweetened, fortified or not.

7. Breads—Yeast: record kind; whether regular, sandwich, snack, hand sliced, etc.; amount; whether enriched or restored; brand or note if home made. Quick bread: record kind, size, number of portions, whether flour is enriched, note if home made, frozen, refrigerated, etc. Coffee cakes and pastries: record kind, portion size, number consumed, whether flour is enriched, note if home made, frozen, enriched, etc. Other: tortillas, etc.—list similar information.

8. Meats, poultry, and fish—Record kind, amount raw or as purchased, how prepared such as baked, broiled, fried. Fresh or frozen: record grade such as "choice," cut or piece such as chuck, hamburger, roast, steak, chop. Canned: indicate type of pack such as oil, water, tomato sauce, gravy. Sausages: type such as dry, smoked, "all-meat," "dry milk added," etc.

9. Cheeses—Record kind, amount in cups or size of piece or slice; whether natural or processed, whether regular or low-fat.

10. Fats, oils, shortenings—Record kind, amount in tablespoons or cups, brand, whether diet or regular, whipped or in cubes. Include cream, sour cream, non-dairy substitutes for cream and sour cream.

11. Desserts—Record kind, amount in half-cup portions or size of piece, note if home made.

12. Beverages—Record kind such as coffee, alcoholic, those made from beverage base mixes, etc.; amount in ounces or cups, accompaniments such as sugar, cream, lemon.

13. Nuts and peanut butter—Record kind, amount in fourth cup or tablespoon portions, brand, type such as regular or dry roasted or natural or homogenized or smooth or chunky, brand.

14. Eggs—Record size and number.

15. Legumes—Record kind such as dried beans, peas, and lentils; amount in cups after cooking; if canned brand and type of pack such as water, tomato sauce, molasses, etc.

16. Snack chips, pretzels, crackers, candy, etc.—Record kind, brand name, size package or number of pieces.

17. Miscellaneous—Record kind such as syrups, toppings, jams and jellies, pickles, condiments (chili sauce, ketchup, soy sauce, prepared mustard, mayonnaise, relish, vinegar, lemon juice), yeast. Specify types, amounts, and brands.

18. Food supplements—Record kind such as vitamin and/or mineral, yeast, bone meal, alfalfa meal, wheat germ, amount as pills or tablespoons, brand and attach label.

19. Home made items—Use recipe sheets to record ingredients, quantities, and number of portions.

(c) 7-day weighed diet record—Seven consecutive days are chosen. The quantity of all items served to the individual, except water but including any food supplements, is weighed or counted; plate waste is also weighed. Brand names, recipes for home prepared mixed dishes, portion sizes, and time of eating are recorded. Limitations: scales must be calibrated, may forget to weigh some items or may be unable to if items are eaten away from home, less likely to continue for the full data collection period, may plan food intake to minimize the number of ingredients/

Subject's Code Number: _____ (to be provided)
Interviewer's Code Number: ___ (to be provided)
Please RECORD all foods and beverages eaten on the following dates:
_____, _____, and _____. Thank you for your assistance and co-
operation.

Day 1 Time	Food Name	Amount Eaten	(Completed by Coder) Item No.	Weight g
Day 2				
Day 3				

FIG. 18.2. SAMPLE DIET RECORD

foods to be weighed; does not provide any information on variation due
to day of pay period, season, and the like.

Each of these can provide a valid but limited index to an individual's
food intake; the seven-day weighed diet record provides the most information but is most difficult and time-consuming. Although most foods
are available year-round in some form, i.e., fresh, frozen, canned, preference and/or price may result in differences in serving frequency among
the seasons. Therefore, repeated sampling may be advisable. IF one is
estimating the nutrient intake of a group of 50 or more individuals,
THEN the 24-hour recall will provide as good an index to intake as the 7-
day weighed diet record.

When three-day and seven-day diet records have been completed, they
should be reviewed immediately in order to answer any questions that
occur, fill in any gaps, etc. When this activity has been completed, the
next step in the assessment process can be initiated. This next step is to

estimate nutrient intake as a basis for determining which needs are met and which require adjustment, the basis for planning a program of action to correct any problems uncovered.

DATA INTERPRETATION: CONSIDERATIONS

The assessment process, like any other evaluative process, is based on selected premises. Since change is continual, the premises may become invalid and must be revalidated. Otherwise, resultant inferences will be irrelevant and/or unreliable. Therefore, check your premises! For example, IF it is true that since the standard three-meal pattern is infeasible given contemporary life-style imperatives and priorities AND that the meal manager tries to provide nutrients and quantities over a period of a week instead, THEN use of the 24-hour recall or 3-day diet record will result in invalid estimates of dietary intake since obtained values will be randomly high or low. Therefore, these methods cannot be used; they do not provide an index to typicality, the basis of assessment and subsequent action. Extending the length of the data collection period from three to nine days probably would solve the problem.

19

Dietary Assessment: Foods as Sources of Nutrients

Many men and women count calories; they know how many they ingest every day and can state the caloric content of a great number of foods on demand. But, beyond this many are not well informed and have misconceptions and/or erroneous beliefs in regard to the nutrient contributions of various foods. Analysis of an individual's diet intake data provides a basis for relevant food and nutrition education. A spectrum of responses to the opportunity is observed; some are eager, some indifferent, and some threatened.

METHODS OF COMPUTING NUTRIENT INTAKE

Several methods of computing nutrient intake are available. Each results in a different quality or level of accuracy of the estimate that is obtained. The decision to use/not use a particular method is determined by appropriateness, given objectives and limitations. The methods appropriate for the various levels are listed below:

(a) minimum level—IF all that is justified is a first approximation, as when the individual is relatively unable/unwilling to make diet changes or when instructional time is limited, THEN the Basic 4 or a nutrient score card (Table 19.1) is selected.

The Basic 4 can be used for a rapid but rough approximation. The Basic 4 pattern for adults includes: meat or meat substitute, two servings; milk and dairy products, two servings; breads and cereals, four servings; and fruits and vegetables, four servings. In addition, one should check for a source of ascorbic acid and vitamin A. This method can be used to make a gross check of intakes of protein, calcium, iron, thiamin, riboflavin, niacin, vitamin A, and ascorbic acid.

TABLE 19.1. DIETARY SCORE CARD SAMPLE

Food Class	Daily Need	Target Scores	Hits Scores
Dark green/dark yellow fruits and/ or vegetables (raw or cooked)	1 serving[1]	10	
Oranges, tomatoes, strawberries, cantaloupe, etc. (raw or cooked)	1 serving[1]	10	
Potatoes, corn and other vegetables and/or fruits (raw and/or cooked)	1 serving[1]	5	
Milk and/or other dairy products[2]	adults, 2 servings children, 3 servings teenagers, 3-4 servings	20	
Meat, poultry, and/or fish[3]	1 serving	15	
Legume or additional meat, poultry, fish[3]	1 serving	10	
Eggs	1 or 4/week	5	
Cereal (whole-grain or enriched)[4]	1 serving	5	
Bread (whole-grain or enriched)[4]	3-4 servings	5	
Fortified margarine or butter	1-2 tbsp	5	
Breakfast that includes milk, cheese or egg		10	
Total		100	

[1] A serving is ⅓ to ½ cup, except orange (1 sm), cantaloupe, ½.
[2] A serving is 1 cup or 1 oz cheese, etc.
[3] A serving is 2 to 3 oz cooked weight, lean.
[4] A serving is ½ cup cooked cereal, ¾ cup flakes, 1 slice of bread, ½ cup cooked noodles, macaroni, spaghetti.

(b) moderate level—IF a means of controlling intake of a few critical nutrients is desired, THEN use of the Exchange System will provide some structure and lists of comparable foods that allow variety with reasonable control and without the need for calculation of nutrient content.

The Exchange System (Caso 1950) was developed by a multidisciplinary team as a means for providing a moderate degree of control over the intake of critical nutrients in treating certain diseases. From experience, the patient care team members had recognized that not all diabetics would have the time and/or inclination to perform the calculations necessary for adequate intake control. This simplification was designed to provide control of protein, fat, CHO, and caloric intake. The concept also has been extended to provide energy-restricted but normal proportions of protein, fat, and CHO. Sodium and fat-controlled variations also have been developed. Copies of all of these may be obtained from the clinic dietitian at a local hospital.

The Exchange System uses a defined eating pattern as a means for general control of intake. The pattern defines the total number of servings of each class of food that is to be consumed daily and the distribution of food classes among feedings. For example, since control of eating frequency and quantity is desirable in dealing with some medical conditions, the pattern may call for five meat exchanges, one at break-fast and two each at lunch and dinner.

The Exchange System uses lists of foods in each food class that are approximately equivalent sources of the nutrient(s) controlled. The number of food classes varies with the particular version of the exchange system. For example, the 1976 Diabetic Exchange System includes lists for the following food classes: vegetables; fruits; breads and cereals; high, medium, and low fat meats/meat substitutes; fats; milk. To maintain within-class equivalence, foods must be prepared as stipulated and por-tions must be sized as stated. Composition of the lists, preparation method, and/or portion size vary among the different versions of the Exchange System, according to the needs of the condition for which it is designed.

The original Exchange System was designed to meet nutritional needs for all nutrients, to the extent possible, with the exception of a CHO restriction. The structure built in a B-vitamin and major mineral intake that is ordinarily adequate. Control of intake of iron, vitamin A, and ascorbic acid requires deliberate selection of items from the lists. The basic nutritional balance was necessary since the diet was expected to be followed lifelong.

Although the Exchange System was originally designed to control in-take for therapeutic purposes, the basic calorie-restricted version can be used by normal healthy people as well. However, the fact that intake of all nutrients is not controlled must be recognized. Therefore, deliberate selection and/or supplementation is necessary in addition.

(c) maximum level—IF the best estimate obtainable from food compo-sition data is desired and is justified by detailed data obtained from three-day diet records or seven-day weighed diet records, THEN the standard calculation method should be selected. This method is time-consuming since time is required to locate the specific food item from an array of approximately 4000 items and to calculate food values from recipe information, ingredient by ingredient. It is also subject to com-putational errors.

For general nutrient analyses, food composition values are obtained from: (a) USDA Handbook *8, Composition of Foods— Raw, Processed, Prepared*; (b) *Bowes and Church, Food Values of Portions Commonly Used;* (c) USDA Handbook *456, Nutritive Value of American Foods in Common Units;* or (d) USDA Home and Garden Bull. *72, Nutritive Value of Foods.* See Chapter 2 for description of these tables. The *Nutritive Value of Foods* is printed here as the Appendix.

Abbreviated lists of common sources of particular nutrients frequently are listed in magazine articles and popular books that focus public at-tention on the need for and sources of particular nutrients. These lists must be used with caution, as values may not be accurate or may be dated. For example, folic acid values obtained prior to 1974 are not regarded as accurate. When better analytical techniques became available in 1974, previous values were rejected. Therefore, relevance and reliability of sources and age must be verified. Sources also should be cited in the popular literature. Prior to use, details should be checked; when in doubt, it should be discarded.

Another example of a problem to watch for has developed with respect to statements of fiber content. Crude fiber values produced by the official and legal method for making fiber determinations are alleged to be inaccurate. The method was first developed in 1887 and has had only minor revision since. According to Van Soest (1977), who is an expert in fiber analyses, the crude fiber method produces values that are unrelated to the physiologically active fiber content of foods. So, until new tables are developed using values based on more accurate methods, assessment of fiber intake is meaningless. As of now, assessment should utilize common sense. For example, it is known that the fiber content of whole grains, fruits, and vegetables is greater than the fiber content of refined foods from which the natural fiber has been removed. It is also greater than the fiber content of puréed foods in which it has been mechanically broken down. For this reason, whole grains, fruits, and vegetables should be included daily.

For specialized purposes, use of supplementary tables may be necessary. Reliable tables for additional nutrients are listed as chapter food composition references. The information on the nutrient composition of ethnic foods is not as complete as that for the general population. Values for some foods are available; chapter ethnic food composition references provide a partial listing of sources.

The standard method of calculation is involved; it requires additional information and informed judgments. Salient points are:

(a) additional information

-table values in parentheses are *imputed*, i.e., inferred from the analytical values for similar foods—transcribe parentheses

-a zero value means that analyses have not detected any of that nutrient in the food—transcribe the zero

-a dash means that although the nutrient may be present, analytical values are not reliable enough, so no values have been announced yet—transcribe the dash

(b) bases of informed judgments

-IF a food item/ingredient is not listed, THEN the closest equivalent is used, e.g., natural apple juice is not listed so regular apple juice values must be used—add parentheses in red

-IF the food is a home-prepared item, THEN compute a value as the sum of ingredient values divided by the number of portions—add fat used in frying, etc. (Note: when one ingredient value is imputed, the computed value is indicated by red parentheses.)

IF the portion size differs from that listed, THEN adjust values by multiplying them by the appropriate fraction, e.g., ¼, ½, 1½. USDA Home Economics Research Report *41, Average Weight of a Measured Cup of Various Foods*, provides the gram weight values necessary for portion conversions for many foods. When portions are irregular in shape, information in the appendices of the USDA handbooks should be consulted.

To use the standard calculation method, one constructs a working table with the foods and their quantities on the left and the nutrients in table order across the top. The first step is to convert multiple portions of the same item to the same unit and sum the quantities; this saves computational time. Then the food item is located in the table or an imputed/computed value is obtained; this is entered in the appropriate portion of the working table. (Note: The number of digits listed in the table should be transcribed; computed values should be rounded to this number.) Then, when the nutrient values for all foods have been obtained, the columns are summed. A grand total for the period is computed when three-day or seven-day information is used; a mean is then computed. (The sums and the mean are only *estimates* because of errors in table values, the use of imputed values, and the lack of values as indicated by dashes.)

ASSESSMENT

Given the appropriate RDA and an estimate of intake of the various nutrients, obtained by one of the above methods, the assessment process can be initiated. The first step is to compare the expected (RDA) and observed (dietary, supplement, and total) intake values, and to identify those nutrients whose intake needs adjustment. The general procedure is outlined in Chapter 17. Additional discussion follows.

Comparison is one matter; interpretation is another. To aid comparison, compute the percent RDA for each nutrient—dietary, supplement, total—and the proportions of the total from dietary and supplement sources. Small differences between dietary intake and the RDA, defined as plus or minus 10%, should be ignored. Small differences are expected, since intake is only estimated, as noted above. Differences also may be due to a large number of inaccurate values, as when imputed values (table and derived, i.e., red parentheses) and/or dashes were used for more than 10% of the entries for any nutrient. In this case, too many unknowns make assessment impossible. Intake must be controlled and observations made.

NOMOGRAPH FOR BODY MASS INDEX (KG/M²)

Anthony E. Thomas,[2] Ph.D., David A. McKay,[3] M.D., and Michael B. Cutlip,[4] Ph.D.

ABSTRACT   The ratio of weight/height² emerges from varied epidemiological studies as the most generally useful index of relative body mass in adults. The authors present a nomograph to facilitate use of this relationship in clinical situations. While showing the range of weight given as desirable in life insurance studies, the scale expresses relative weight as a continuous variable. This method encourages use of clinical judgment in interpreting "overweight" and "underweight" and in accounting for muscular and skeletal contributions to measured mass.   *Am. J. Clin. Nutr. 29:* 302 304, 1976.

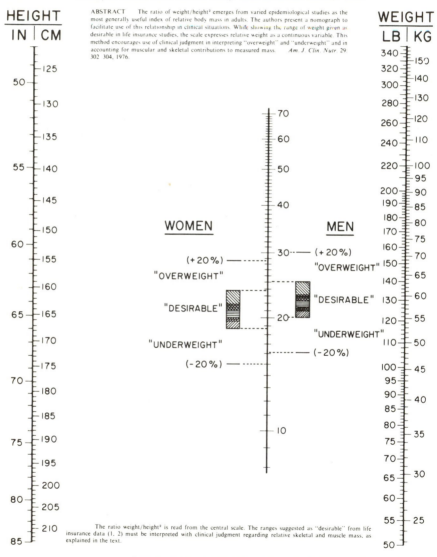

The ratio weight/height² is read from the central scale. The ranges suggested as "desirable" from life insurance data (1, 2) must be interpreted with clinical judgment regarding relative skeletal and muscle mass, as explained in the text.

A nomograph method for assessing body weight[1]

Anthony E. Thomas,[2] Ph.D., David A. McKay,[3] M.D., and Michael B. Cutlip,[4] Ph.D.

It has long been customary to include measurement of weight in clinical health assessments. Life insurance data have indicated an increased mortality risk for extremes of weight, and the insurance industry's tables showing desirable weights for height have become widely used (1, 2). However, these tables are somewhat cumbersome in practice and require an arbitrary and rather ambiguous classification of the patient by small, medium, or large "body frame."

The ratio of weight to various powers of height is often used in epidemiological studies. Data from diverse populations have indicated the superiority of weight/height[2] as the index of relative weight which is best correlated with other measures of obesity, such as skinfold thickness, and which is least correlated with height independent of weight (3–6). Sometimes designated "Quetelet's index," after an early proponent, this expression is being referred to with increasing frequency simply as the "body mass index" (BMI) (5). The division of weight by the square of height is, however, sufficiently demanding mathematically that this index has received little use in clinical settings. Yet it does offer the advantage of providing a continuous quantitative scale for relative weight which facilitates comparisons of individuals with population norms.

We have therefore developed a nomograph to ease the calculation and use of the body mass index in clinical settings (Fig. 1). It has been derived using the metric system, and the BMI scale units are thus in kilograms/square meter. Conversions to inches and pounds are given on the height and weight scales so that it can be used directly with measurement in those units. As an initial rough guide to BMI interpretation, we have indicated along the scale the approximate range corresponding to the life insurance tables' "desirable weights" and the points that are ±20% of the outside limits of this range. *Horizontal shading* has been used for "medium frame," *upper left to lower right diagonal shading* for "large frame," and *lower left to upper right* for "small frame." However, as no systematic method is available for classing individuals by "frame" (7), these distinctions are more suggestive than categorical and may serve best simply as a reminder to consider the skeletal contribution to relative weight. It is also important to assess clinically the individual proportion of muscle to fat before equating a high BMI

with obesity. Indeed, the clinician may prefer to make a preliminary judgment of weight status based on appearance alone before looking at the nomograph data.

Beyond this initial assessment, a photocopy of the nomograph may provide a useful display method for monitoring and encouraging weight control. Based on the index, and taking into account individual motivation and social support as well as body frame and muscularity, one can select an appropriate weight as a goal the individual can aim for in modifying eating and exercise behavior.

It has been suggested that the patient who looks fat usually is but that the diagnosis can be clinched by appropriate pinching (8). Skinfold calipers have been advocated as a way to quantitate the latter process, but the method has not gained general clinical acceptance. The assessment of relative weight is still widely relied upon and, with appropriate caution in interpretation, seems generally the best guide to nutritional status. While there are limitations implicit both in the body mass index (4) and in the life insurance tables (7), for the present a combination of these methods, as in our nomograph, seems to offer a reasonable approach for working with weight assessment and control.

References

1. METROPOLITAN LIFE INSURANCE COMPANY. New weight standards for men and women. Statist. Bull. 40: 1, 1959.
2. Build and Blood Pressure Study. Volume I. Chicago: Society of Actuaries, 1959.
3. KHOSLA, T., AND C. R. LOWE. Indices of obesity derived from body weight and height. Brit. J. Prev. Soc. Med. 21: 122, 1967.
4. FLOREY, C. V. The use and interpretation of ponderal index and other weight-height ratios in epidemiological studies. J. Chronic Diseases 23: 93, 1970.
5. KEYS, A., F. FIDANZA, M. J. KARVONEN, N. KIMURA, AND H. L. TAYLOR. Indices of Relative Weight and Obesity. J. Chronic Diseases 25: 329, 1972.
6. GOLDBOURT, U., AND J. H. MEDALIE. Weight-height indices. Brit. J. Prev. Soc. Med. 28: 116, 1974.
7. BROZEK, J. A review of Build and Blood Pressure Study. Human Biol. 32: 320, 1960.
8. MAYER, J. Overweight: Causes, Cost, and Control. Englewood Cliffs, New Jersey: Prentice-Hall, 1968.

[1] From the University of North Carolina, Chapel Hill, North Carolina, and the University of Connecticut, Storrs, Connecticut.
[2] Department of Anthropology, University of North Carolina.   [3] Department of Medicine, University of North Carolina.   [4] Department of Chemical Engineering, University of Connecticut.

The American Journal of Clinical Nutrition 29: MARCH 1976, pp. 302–304. Printed in U.S.A.

Caloric requirements are related to energy expenditure. The recommended allowance may be irrelevant for a given individual. It may be enough greater to result in unwanted weight gain. Appropriateness of body weight should be evaluated before any assessment of caloric requirement is made. (See insert, p. 380−381.)

A personalized estimate of energy needs may be calculated. First, an activity record (see Fig. 19.1) should be kept for the day(s) on which dietary intake was measured. Information on recording data is contained in table footnotes. Assessment involves comparison of energy supply with energy demand. Energy demand is calculated as follows:

(a) estimated resting metabolic need (kcal)—Use weight (desired weight, if overweight) in kilograms (pounds divided by 2.2) and a judgment of fatness to locate the appropriate table value (Table 19.2). Table values are computed for a 24-hour period.

(b) estimated physical activity output—Use of the information in Tables 19.3 and 19.4 to determine the level of energy expended for each activity. Record the number of minutes at the appropriate level (some activities may involve several levels; divide total activity time accordingly). To determine the number of calories used for each activity level, multiply the number of minutes times the rate for the level. Sum the calories for the levels used.

(c) total energy demand—Sum estimated resting metabolic need and estimated physical activity output. With even a 1% excess of intake over output, weight is gained over time.

There are no RDA for fat or carbohydrate (CHO). The U.S. Dietary Goal for fat intake is 35% calories. This is accepted for use as a standard for assessment purposes. The target CHO intake is computed by difference—it is the remainder after protein and fat calories have been computed. The method of calculation using physiological fuel values (protein, 4 kcal/g; fat, 9 kcal/g; CHO, 4 kcal/g) is:

(a) protein calories—X g protein (from RDA) × 4 kcal/g, e.g., 45 × 4 = 180 kcal from protein

(b) fat calories—35% × kcal divided by 9 kcal/g, e.g., 2000 × 0.35 = 700 kcal ÷ 9 = 77 g fat

(c) CHO calories—total kcal from protein and fat. Then subtract this value from kcal and divide by 4 kcal, e.g., 180 + 700 = 880 kcal; 2000 −880 = 1120 kcal from CHO; 1120 ÷ 4 = 280 g CHO. This quantity may seem high given recent low CHO fads, but it is a customary quantity.

Variation in nutrient intake among days is normal. Some nutrients, e.g., protein, fat, and CHO, are components of most foods so are ingested regularly. Therefore, 24-hour recall or 3-day diet records provide reliable estimates of intake. Other nutrients, e.g., vitamin A, are distributed irregularly in foods. Rich sources are ingested irregularly. Therefore,

TIME				LEVELS					
				0	I	II	III	IV	V
From	To	NO. OF MINUTES	ACTIVITY	At Rest Most of the Time (min)	Very Light Exercise (min)	Light Exercise (min)	Moderate Exercise (min)	Severe Exercise (min)	Very Severe Exercise (min)
TOTALS (Minutes)									

FIG. 19.1. SAMPLE ACTIVITY RECORD

24-hour recall and 3-day diet record data will tend to underestimate intake. Seven-day and, better yet, monthly intake will provide better estimates.

Some interactions among nutrients have marked effects on the efficiency of absorption. For example, IF ascorbic acid is ingested as a part of a meal containing iron, THEN absorption efficiency will be increased in relation to the quantity of ascorbic acid ingested. However, ingestion of ascorbic acid at other meals has no carryover effect, i.e., ingestion of a megadose in the morning has no effect on absorption of iron ingested at noon or evening meals.

A recent paper has indicated that tabulation of the iron content of foods does not provide a reliable index to the amount of iron available. Therefore, a new method has been developed (Monsen et al. 1978, 1980). For purposes of calculation of the amount available for a woman, iron stores are assumed to be 500 mg. (Those who have reason to suppose that their iron stores differ, especially men or those chronically anemic, should see Monson et al. 1978.)

To use this method of calculation, one lays out a working table as illustrated (Table 19.5). Total iron and ascorbic acid values are transcribed for each food from the general working table that was constructed for general assessment or directly from a handbook of food composition. The following procedure can be used to calculate iron availability for each meal (feeding).

TABLE 19.2. NORMAL RESTING METABOLIC ENERGY EXPENDITURE /24 HOURS[1]

| Sex Class | | Fat | Weight in Kilograms (lb) | | | | | | | |
M	F	(%)	45 (99)	50 (110)	55 (121)	60 (132)	65 (143)	70 (154)	75 (165)	80 (176)
Thin		5	—	1424	1526	1613	1714	1814	1901	2002
Medium		10		1359	1454	1555	1642	1742	1843	1930
Plump	thin	15	1181	1282	1382	1483	1570	1670	1771	1872
Obese	medium	20	1123	1210	1310	1411	1512	1598	1699	1805
	plump	25	—	1152	1238	1339	1440	1541	1627	1728
	obese	30	—	—	1166	1267	1368	1469	1555	1656

[1] Based on data from J.V.G.A. Durnin and R. Passmore (1967).

TABLE 19.3. ENERGY EXPENDITURE IN COMMON ACTIVITIES[1]

Level of Intensity	Activity[2]	Expenditure Rate (kcal/min) Females[3]	Males
Sedentary	eating handwork playing cards playing instrument studying typing	0.1-0.4	0.2-0.8
Light	bowling driving car ironing laboratory work personal care walking slowly	0.5-0.9	0.9-1.4
Moderate	cooking hand dishwashing hand laundry walking normally washing floors with mop	1.0-1.9	1.5-2.6
Heavy	cleaning vigorously gardening golfing making beds moving furniture playing ping pong playing volleyball walking upstairs washing car or windows	2.0-2.9	2.7-3.9
Strenuous	badminton bicycling dancing gymnastics horseback riding jogging playing tennis skiing swimming walking upstairs	3.0-5.0	4.0-6.0

[1] Based on data from J.V.G.A. Durnin and R. Passmore (1967).
[2] Other sports such as track, basketball, boxing, climbing, squash, etc., use more kcal during the active period (7-18 kcal).
[3] Energy expenditures are related to body size. They are reported for a female of 55 kg (121 lb) and a male of 65 kg (143 lb).

(a) ascorbic acid—Sum the values for the meal/feeding and record each total.

(b) Classify the meal/feeding re iron availability.

—High availability contains cooked/meat/fish/poultry prepared from a 3-oz lean raw portion OR at least 75 mg ascorbic acid OR a combination of cooked meat/fish/poultry prepared from a 1-oz lean raw portion AND between 25 mg and 75 mg of ascorbic acid.

—Medium availability contains cooked meat/fish/poultry prepared from a 1- to 2-oz portion OR between 25 mg and 75 mg ascorbic acid.

—Low availability contains cooked meat/fish/poultry prepared from

TABLE 19.4. ENERGY EXPENDITURE IN COMMON OCCUPATIONS[1]

Level of Intensity	Activity	Expenditure Rate (kcal/min) Females[2]	Males
Sedentary	office work retail sales	1.5-3.4	2.0-4.9
Light	drafting lab technician hairdressing hospital work auto repair aircraft pilot truck driver		
Moderate	building trades farm (partly mechanized) general labor lumbering steel mill coal mining	3.5-5.4	5.0-7.4
Heavy	farm labor lumbering steel mill coal mining garbage collection dock labor	5.5-7.4	10.0-12.4

[1] Based on data from J.V.G.A. Durnin and R. Passmore (1967).
[2] Energy is reported for a female of 55 kg (121 lb) and a male of 65 kg (143 lb).

a 1-oz lean raw portion OR less than 25 mg ascorbic acid.

(c) Estimate iron availability from meat/fish/poultry. Multiply the iron content by a factor determined by availability, and record the value.

—High availability, 14%.

—Medium availability, 12.2%.

—Low availability, 11%.

(d) Estimate nonheme iron availability from food other than meat/fish/poultry. Sum the values per meal/feeding. Multiply the obtained value by a factor determined by availability and record the value.

—High availability, 8%.

—Medium availability, 5%.

—Low availability, 3%.

To assess the adequacy of iron availability, sum the values for each meal. IF the absorbable iron total is greater than 1.5 for a woman of child-bearing age or greater than 1.0 for a man or an older woman, THEN intake is probably sufficient.

TABLE 19.5. SAMPLE CALCULATIONS OF ABSORBABLE IRON

Time	Food	Total Fe (mg)	MFP[1] Fe (mg)	Other Fe (mg)	Vitamin C (mg)	MFP Factor	Other Factor	Absorbable Fe (mg)
6:15	Toast (2)	1.0	0	1.0	0			
	Coffee (3)	0.3	0	0.3	0			
	Supplement (1)	18.0	0	18.0	60			
		19.3	0	19.3	60		0.05[2]	0.96
12:00	Cheddar cheese (2 oz)	0.8	0	0.8	0			
	Crackers (4)	0.1	0	0.1	0			
	Plums (2)	0.2	0	0.2	2			
	Cookies (3)	0.1	0	0.1	0			
		1.2	0	1.2	2		0.03	0.36
5:00	Beef patty (3 oz raw)	2.2	2.2	0	0	0.14		0.31
	Potato (1)	1.4	0	1.4	36			
	Zucchini (1 cup)	0.8	0	0.8	14			
	Peach (1)	0.6	0	0.6	8			
	Ice cream (1 cup)	0.1	0	0.1	0			
	Coffee (1)	0.1	0	0.1	0		0.08	0.24
		5.2	2.2	3.0	58			0.55
								1.87

Source: Adapted from Monsen (1980).
[1] MFP = meat/fish/poultry.
[2] Factors:
    —IF a meal/feeding contains MFP from a 3-oz raw lean portion OR at least 75 mg ascorbic acid OR a combination of MFP from a 1-oz lean raw portion AND 25 to 75 mg ascorbic acid, THEN it is *high availability* AND MFP factor is 0.14 and other factor is 0.08.
    —IF a meal/feeding contains MFP from a 1- to 2-oz raw lean portion OR 25 to 75 mg ascorbic acid, THEN it is *medium availability* AND MFP factor is 0.122 and other factor is 0.05.
    —IF a meal/feeding contains MFP from a 1-oz raw lean portion OR less than 25 mg ascorbic acid, THEN it is *low availability* AND MFP factor is 0.11 and other factor is 0.03.

BIBLIOGRAPHY

General References

CASO, E.K. 1950. Calculation of Diabetic Diets. Report of the Committee on Diabetic Diet Calculations, the American Dietetic Association. J. Am. Dietet. Assoc. *26*, 575-583.

DURNIN, J.V.G.A., and PASSMORE, R. 1967. Energy, Work, and Leisure. Heinemann Educational Books, Ltd., London.

MONSEN, E.R. *et al*. 1978. Estimation of available dietary iron. Am. J. Clin. Nutr. *31*, 134-141.

MONSEN, E.R. 1980. Simplified method for calculating available dietary iron. Food & Nutr. News *51* (4) 1-4.

VAN SOEST, P. 1977. Testimony. *In* Diet Related to Killer Diseases: Hearings. IV. Dietary Fiber and Health. Mar. 24-31, 1977. Select Comm. on Nutrition and Human Needs, U.S. Senate, GPO, Washington, D.C.

Food Composition References

ADAMS, C.F. 1975. Nutritive value of American foods in common units. USDA Agric. Handb. *456*. Washington, D.C.

CHURCH, C.F., and CHURCH, H.N. 1975. Bowes & Church Food Values of Portions Commonly Used. 12th Edition. J.B. Lippincott Co., Philadelphia.

CONSUMER & FOOD ECON. INST., AGRIC. RES. SERV. 1976. Composition of foods—raw, processed, prepared. USDA Agric. Handb. *8* (rev. sections). Washington, D.C.

ERDMAN, J.W., JR. 1979. Effect of preparation and service of food on nutrient value. Food Technol. *33* (2) 38, 40-41, 44-48.

FARROW, R.P., KEMPER, K., and CHIN, H.B. 1979. Natural variability in nutrient content of California fruits and vegetables. Food Technol. *33* (2) 52-54.

GODDARD, M.S., and MATTHEWS, R.H. 1979. Current knowledge of nutritive values of vegetables. Food Technol. *33* (2) 71-73.

HURT, H.D. 1979. Effect of canning on the nutritive value of vegetables. Food Technol. *33* (2) 62-65.

KAREL, M. 1979. Effect of storage on nutrient retention of foods. Food Technol. *33* (2) 36-37.

KRAMER, A. 1979. Effects of freezing and frozen storage on nutrient retention of fruits and vegetables. Food Technol. *33* (2) 58-61, 65.

LUND, D.B. 1979. Effect of commercial processing on nutrients. Food Technol. *33* (2) 28, 32-34.

USDA. 1977. Average weight of a measured cup of various foods. USDA Home Econ. Res. Rept. *41*, GPO, Washington, D.C.

Fatty Acids

ANDERSON, B.A. 1976. Comprehensive evaluation of fatty acids in foods. VII. Pork products. J. Am. Dietet. Assoc. *69*, 44-49.

ANDERSON, B.A. 1978. Comprehensive evaluation of fatty acids in foods. XIII. Sausage and luncheon meats. J. Am. Dietet. Assoc. *72*, 48-52.

ANDERSON, B.A., FRISTROM, G.A., and WEIHRAUCH, J.L. 1977. Comprehensive evaluation of fatty acids in foods. X. Lamb and veal. J. Am. Dietet. Assoc. *70*, 53-58.

ANDERSON, B.A., KINSELLA, J.E., and WATT, B.K. 1975. Comprehensive evaluation of fatty acids in foods. II. Beef products. J. Am. Dietet. Assoc. *67*, 35-41.

BRIGNOLI, C.A., KINSELLA, J.E., and WEIHRAUCH, J.L. 1976. Comprehensive evaluation of fatty acids in foods. V. Unhydrogenated fats and oils. J. Am. Dietet. Assoc. *68*, 224-229.

EXLER, J., AVENA, R.M., and WEIHRAUCH, J.L. 1977. Comprehensive evaluation of fatty acids in foods. XI. Leguminous seeds. J. Am. Dietet. Assoc. *71*, 412-415.

EXLER, J., and WEIHRAUCH, J.L. 1976. Comprehensive evaluation of fatty acids in foods. VIII. Finfish. J. Am. Dietet. Assoc. *69*, 243-248.

EXLER, J., and WEIHRAUCH, J.L. 1977. Comprehensive evaluation of fatty acids in foods. XII. Shellfish. J. Am. Dietet. Assoc. *71*, 518-521.

FEELEY, R.M., CRINER, P.E., and SLOVER, H.T. 1975. Major fatty acids and proximate composition of dairy products. J. Am. Dietet. Assoc. *66*, 140-146.

FRISTROM, G.A., STEWART, B.C., WEIHRAUCH, J.L., and POSATI, L.P. 1975. Comprehensive evaluation of fatty acids in foods. IV. Nuts, peanuts, and soups. J. Am. Dietet. Assoc. *67*, 351-355.

FRISTROM, G.A., and WEIHRAUCH, J.L. 1976. Comprehensive evaluation of fatty acids in foods. IX. Fowl. J. Am. Dietet. Assoc. *69*, 517-522.

POSATI, L.P., KINSELLA, J.E., and WATT, B.K. 1975. Comprehensive evaluation of fatty acids in foods. I. Dairy products. J. Am. Dietet. Assoc. *66*, 482-488.

POSATI, L.P., KINSELLA, J.E., and WATT, B.K. 1975. Comprehensive evaluation of fatty acids in foods. III. Eggs and egg products. J. Am. Dietet. Assoc. *67*, 111-115.

PRATT, D.E. 1975. Lipid analysis of frozen egg substitutes. J. Am. Dietet. Assoc. *66*, 31-33.

STANDAL, B.R., BASSET, D.R., POLICAR, P.B., and THOM, M. 1970. Fatty acids, cholesterol, and proximate analysis of some ready-to-eat foods. J. Am. Dietet. Assoc. *56*, 392-396.

WEIHRAUCH, J.L., BRIGNOLI, C.A., REEVES, J.B., III, and IVERSON, J.L. 1977. Fatty acid composition of margarines, processed fats, and oils. Food Technol. *31* (2) 80-85, 91.

WEIHRAUCH, J.L., KINSELLA, J.E., and WATT, B.K. 1976. Comprehensive evaluation of fatty acids in foods. VI. Cereal products. J. Am. Dietet. Assoc. *68*, 335-340.

Sterols

FEELEY, R.M., CRINER, P.E., and WATT, B.K. 1972. Cholesterol content of foods. J. Am. Dietet. Assoc. *46*, 134-148.

WEIHRAUCH, J.L., and GARDNER, J.M. 1978. Sterol content of foods of plant origin. J. Am. Dietet. Assoc. *73*, 39-47.

Major Minerals

FEELEY, R.M., CRINER, P.E., MURPHY, E.W., and TOEPFER, E.W. Major mineral elements in dairy products. J. Am. Dietet. Assoc. *61*, 505-510.

WONG, N.P., LACROIX, D.E., and ALFORD, J.A. 1978. Mineral content of dairy products. I. Milk and milk products. J. Am. Dietet. Assoc. *72*, 288-291.

WONG, N.P., LACROIX, D.E., and ALFORD, J.A. 1978. Mineral content of dairy products. II. Cheeses. J. Am. Dietet. Assoc. *73*, 608-611.

ZOOK, E.G. 1968. Mineral composition of fruits. I. Edible yield, total solids, and ash of 30 fresh fruits. J. Am. Dietet. Assoc. *52*, 218-224.

ZOOK, E.G. 1968. Mineral composition of fruits. III. Total solids, ash, nitrogen, and minerals of six dried fruits. J. Am. Dietet. Assoc. *53*, 588-591.

ZOOK, E.G., and LEHMAN, J. 1968. Mineral composition of fruits. II. Nitrogen, calcium, magnesium, phosphorus, potassium, aluminum, boron, copper, iron, manganese, and sodium. J. Am. Dietet. Assoc. *52*, 225-231.

Trace Elements

HAEFLEIN, K.A., and RASMUSSEN, A.I. 1977. Zinc content of selected foods. J. Am. Dietet. Assoc. *70*, 610-616.

MORRIS, V.C., and LEVANDER, O.A. 1970. Selenium content of foods. J. Nutr. *100*, 1383-1388.

MURPHY, E.W., WILLIS, B.W., and WATT, B.K. 1975. Provisional tables on the zinc content of foods. J. Am. Dietet. Assoc. *66*, 345-355.

PENNINGTON, J.T., and CALLOWAY, D.H. 1973. Copper content of foods. Factors affecting reported values. J. Am. Dietet. Assoc. *63*, 143-153.

SCHROEDER, H.A., NASAU, A.P., TIPTON, I.H., and BALASSA, J.J. 1966. Essential trace metals in man: Copper. J. Chron. Dis. *19*, 1007-1010.

Vitamins—Vitamin E

BIERI, J.G., and EVARTS, R.P. 1975. Vitamin E adequacy of vegetable oils. J. Am. Dietet. Assoc. *66*, 134-139.

KOEHLER, H.H., LEE, H.G., and JACOBSON, M. 1977. Tocopherols in canned entrées and vended sandwiches. J. Am. Dietet. Assoc. *70*, 616-620.

MCLAUGHLIN, P.J., and WEIHRAUCH, J.L. 1979. Vitamin E content of foods. J. Am. Dietet. Assoc. *75* (6) 647-665.

Vitamins—Folacin

DONG, M.H., MCGOWN, E.L., SCHWENNEKER, B.W., and SAUBERLICH, H.E. 1980. Thiamin, riboflavin, and vitamin B_6 contents of selected foods as served. J. Am. Dietet. Assoc. *76* (2) 156-160.

PERLOFF, B.P., and BUTRAM, R.R. 1977. Folacin in selected foods. J. Am. Dietet. Assoc. *70*, 161-172.

Ethnic Food Composition References

Chicano

CRAVIOTO, R., LOCKHART, E.E., ANDERSON, R.K., MIRANDA, F. DE P., and HARRIS, R.S. 1945. Composition of typical Mexican foods. J. Nutr. *29*, 317-329.

Chinese

CHAN, S.L., and KENNEDY, B.M. 1960. Sodium in Chinese vegetables. J. Am. Dietet. Assoc. *37*, 573-576.

HARRIS, R.S., WANG, F.M.C., WU, Y.H., TSAO, C.H.S., and LOE, L.Y. 1949. The composition of Chinese foods. J. Am. Dietet. Assoc. *25*, 28-36.

HAWKS, J.E. 1936. Preparation and composition of foods served in Chinese homes. J. Am. Dietet. Assoc. *11*, 136-140.

HOH, P.W., WILLIAMS, J.C., and PEASE, C.S. 1933. Possible sources of calcium and phosphorus in the Chinese diet. The determination of calcium and phosphorus in a typical Chinese dish containing meat and bone. J. Nutr. 7, 535-546.

LEUNG, W.T.W., BUTRAM, R.R., and CHANG, F.H. 1972. Food Composition Table for Use in East Asia, Part I. Proximate Composition, Mineral, and Vitamin Contents of East Asian Foods. DHEW Publ. (NIH) *73-465*, Washington, D.C.

RAO, M.N., and POLACCHI, W. 1972. Food Composition Table for Use in East Asia, Part II. Amino Acid, Fatty Acid, Certain B-Vitamin and Trace Mineral Content of Some Asian Foods. DHEW Publ. (NIH) *73-465*, Washington, D.C.

Filipino

FOOD AND NUTR. RES. CTR. 1968. Food Composition Table Recommended for Use in the Philippines. Handbook I (4th Rev.). National Institute of Science and Technology, National Development Science Board, Manila.

Native American

BOTKIN, C.W., and SHIRES, L.B. 1948. The composition and value of piñon nuts. New Mexico Exp. Stn. Bull. *344*.

CALLOWAY, D.H., GIAUQUE, R.D., and COSTA, F.M. 1974. The superior mineral content of some American Indian foods in comparison to federally donated counterpart commodities. Ecol. Food Nutr. *3*, 203-211.

KONLANDE, J.E., and ROBSON, J.R.K. 1972. The nutritive value of cooked camas as consumed by Flathead Indians. Ecol. Food Nutr. *1*, 193-195.

YANOVSKY, E. 1936. Food plants of North American Indians. USDA Misc. Publ. *237*, Washington, D.C.

20

Dietary Assessment: Food Management Practices and Nutrient Intake

"Conservation of natural resources," "environmental protection," and "doing your own thing"—all of these are contemporary slogans. They may be used as a battle cry or gathering word, or to express a position, stand, or goal of endeavor, or to make an impression. They are emotionally and psychologically loaded phrases, especially when applied to meal management.

Until now, meals have been served with reasonable regularity in most homes. To get them together took some doing. Contemporary life-styles result in individual activity patterns that are highly variable among family members and among days. Many conclude that the management of standard meals is infeasible. So, the traditional three-meal pattern may be defunct. But, the need to feed remains.

Some adaptation of the nutrition niche, i.e., the place where humans naturally or normally live and grow that must supply the nutrient factors necessary for human existence, is necessary. A nutritional Neanderthal, i.e., a person with primitive or rudimentary knowledge of nutrition, may fail to adapt. Dietary assessment is likely to reveal an uncontrolled intake. A member of the nutritional nutwing, i.e., a person who follows any fad mindlessly, may be caught in a trap. Dietary assessment is likely to reveal a badly unbalanced intake. One who is nutritionally noteworthy can adapt to and accommodate, as well as reconcile differences. This person has the nutrition notion and intake shows it.

CONSERVATION OF NATURAL RESOURCES (CNR)

Conserve, preserve, and *reserve* are three terms with distinct meanings that are at the heart of food management as related to nutrient ecology.

In this context, to *conserve*[1] means to take actions that result in careful preservation and protection of nutrient potency, especially by planned management of the natural or inherent supply; to prevent destruction by carelessness or neglect. To *preserve* means to protect from destruction, to keep free of decay, or to can, pickle, or similarly prepare for future use. To *reserve* means to set aside for future use.

All nutrients, even calories, can be lost from foods by discarding portions. In most countries, waste is largely due to destruction by molds, insects, rodents, and other pests. It reflects problems in storage and/or control of sanitation. The American food delivery system has solved these problems remarkably well. In affluent America, the throw-away society, the amount of food wasted is phenomenal and the loss is largely due to discard. A recent study of food waste at the University of Arizona (Harrison, Rathje, and Hughes 1975) revealed the following:

(a) The percentage of food wasted was between 9% and 10%.

(b) Straight waste, i.e., occasional discard of whole steaks, half loaves of bread, etc.

(c) The amount of food available and wasted varied by food group: meat/poultry/fish—less was available and less was wasted (12 to 4%); vegetables—less was available in 1974 but the percentage of waste increased; cereal products—more was available in 1974 but the percentage of waste decreased; sweets and packaged foods—availability was increased greatly but waste was low.

(d) The annual cost of food wasted was estimated for a two-person household as $80 to $100 (1974 prices).

The portion of the food purchased that is wasted is a portion of the food supply that could be utilized in the absence of customary income or sources of supply. The poor already appear to exploit this fact. The findings from the Arizona study support this point. They show that middle income people waste more than poverty level people, whose garbage is limited almost to plate scrapings. Garbage remains also indicated that those with less money for food reduced their intake of meat in 1974 as compared with 1973 when prices were lower. These trends continue into the 1980s.

Nutrients are lost by destruction. A few points in relation to specific nutrients follow:

(a) protein—It is destroyed by cooking at too high a temperature, e.g., IF the edges of a fried egg are frizzled, THEN the the protein in that part is destroyed.

(b) fat—It is destroyed by cooking at high temperatures, e.g., it forms a gummy, brown polymer film on surfaces of cookie sheets and it goes up in smoke when a piece of meat hits the hot frying pan.

---

[1]Definitions of italicized words in this chapter are adapted from Webster's Seventh New Collegiate Dictionary, 1969, G. & C. Merriam Co., Publishers, Springfield, Mass.

(c) carbohydrate—It is destroyed by dry heat cooking at high temperatures, e.g., sugar is caramelized and starch is toasted to dextrins.

(d) vitamin A—It is destroyed by oxidation, e.g., when the surfaces of carrot sticks turn white, oxidation has occurred.

(e) thiamin—It is destroyed by dry heat cooking at high temperatures, e.g., toasting destroys 25%, *and* by alkaline medium, e.g., when soda is added to the water in which peas are cooked.

(f) ascorbic acid—It is destroyed by oxidation, e.g., IF a fruit drink is opened and stored in the refrigerator for several days, THEN essentially all is destroyed.

Meal management involves the following activities: purchasing, storage, prepreparation, preparation, service, and use of leftovers. A variety of opportunities for conserving nutrients is associated with each of these aspects of meal management. Examples related to each aspect follow:

(a) purchasing—Processed items in bulk containers, such as large boxes of cereals, are less expensive per unit but are no bargain if they become rancid. If the food becomes rancid, it is discarded because of a disagreeable flavor and odor. (The oxidation of TG or fatty acids reduces their caloric value as well.) They should be purchased in lots that can be used in three months and stored in a closed container at refrigerator temperatures. Items in single-service containers have a high surface to volume ratio, so shelf-life is short.

(b) storage—Fresh and cooked items stored in the refrigerator are perishable. They should be stored in closed containers to prevent progressive dehydration, which results in discard, *and* used quickly before nutrient destruction occurs. Use of the crisper drawer helps to reduce wilting, but is only effective when an equilibrium moisture content is reached within the compartment. One small carrot has insufficient moisture for the compartment, so it becomes wilted in the process of reaching an equilibrium—it is asked to give more than it can give without harm. Sweet fresh vegetables lose their sweetness as sugar turns to starch, so are less appetizing. Moreover, the ascorbic acid content of broccoli and other low-acid/large surface vegetables is reduced to half in five days of refrigerated storage.

(c) prepreparation—The greater the surface area, the greater the rate of oxidation of vitamin A and ascorbic acid. Conservation of vitamins in fruits is optimized by serving them raw and whole. In vegetable cookery the tactic is to cook them immediately after paring, in as large pieces as is feasible.

(d) preparation—Water-soluble vitamins and minerals dissolve in water, especially when it is hot. Therefore, to minimize loss via this route the quantity of cooking water should be minimized and any excess reserved, i.e., set aside for future use as part of the liquid/flavoring in soups, stews, gravies, or sauces. To conserve vitamin A and ascorbic acid, fruits and vegetables should be cooked quickly in a minimum quantity of water. The water is brought to the boil, the fruit or vegetable is added, the water is returned to the boil, and the heat is reduced to the minimum that will maintain a simmering temperature. They should be served promptly or chilled and reheated, not held at serving temperatures for hours. The nutrient content of canned vegetables already has been reduced by an unwanted but unavoidable time-temperature outcome of the canning process. Further reduction can be minimized by heating the vegetable liquor and then adding the vegetables for quick heating. The thiamin content of cooked cereals is conserved by cooking them at simmering temperatures or by bringing them to the boil and removing them from the heat, to finish cooking on retained heat.

(e) serving—Plate waste—a few peas here, a spoonful of mashed potatoes and gravy there, three bites of meat—is estimated to be 40 to 45% of the total solid food waste. Given the number of items to be consumed at a feeding, plate waste is minimized when portion size is appropriate. To clean one's plate is of virtue in reducing waste only if it does not increase waist. Standard portion sizes have been developed for use in diet calculations and in institutions/commercial food establishments (Table 20.1). IF one consumes the standard meal components at a feeding, THEN these portion sizes are a reasonable first approximation for an adult. They must be reduced for children, invalids, etc. In households, plate waste is usually discarded; in institutions/commercial food establishments, it must be discarded for sanitary reasons.

(f) use of leftovers—Remainders and remains are generated in both preparation and serving. Recipes for many foods use half an egg, only the white (or the yolk), or part of a can of tomato sauce or condensed soup. Other recipes use the other part. Good management requires extensive knowledge of recipes so as to plan for use of the remainder. Otherwise, IF insufficient attention is given the remainder, THEN it deteriorates until it is unfit for consumption and must be discarded.

Recipes are usually adjusted to yield six servings, the quantity necessary for the average-sized family. When this quantity is greater than necessary for a meal, the remainder is reserved for another meal, preserved by freezing, extended, or incorporated into another dish.

Most experienced cooks will prepare just enough of items such as rice, macaroni, and potatoes most of the time, since quantity adjustments are easily made. However, when fresh fruits or vegetables are prepared, one usually prepares one-third, one-half, or the entire amount, with the result that a quantity too small to go around is left over. In this case, the remains might be incorporated into a macedoine, i.e., a fruit or vegetable mixture used as an ingredient in a sauce or jellied salad/dessert, or as a cocktail, salad, or garnish.

Leftovers always can be reserved or preserved. See standard cookbooks for suggestions.

TABLE 20.1. STANDARD PORTION SIZES

Bakery Items

Biscuits	1
Bread	1 slice
Cake, angel food	$\frac{1}{12}$th
Cake, layer	$\frac{1}{15}$th
Cake, sheet	2 in. square
Cookies	2
Crackers, graham	2
Crackers, soda	2
Pie, 8 in.	$\frac{1}{6}$th
Rolls	1

Beverages

Cocoa	6 oz
Coffee	6 oz
Juice or fruit ade	4 to 6 oz
Milk	8 oz
Tea, hot	6 oz
Tea, iced	10 to 12 oz

Cereal Products

Cereals, cooked	$\frac{2}{3}$ cup
Cereals, dry concentrated	$\frac{1}{4}$ cup
Cereals, dry flakes	$\frac{3}{4}$ cup
Cereals, dry puffed	1 cup

Dairy Products and Eggs

Butter/margarine	1 tsp
Cottage cheese	$\frac{1}{4}$ cup
Cream, coffee	1 oz
Eggs	1 to 2
Hard cheeses	1 oz
Ice cream or sherbet	$\frac{1}{2}$ cup
Yogurt	1 cup

Fruits

Canned	$\frac{1}{2}$ cup
Dried and cooked	3 oz
Fresh	
Apple, small	1 small
Banana, large	$\frac{1}{2}$
Berries	$\frac{3}{4}$ cup
Cantaloupe	$\frac{1}{6}$th
Grapes	$\frac{1}{4}$ cup
Pineapple	$\frac{1}{2}$ cup
Watermelon	$\frac{1}{2}$ lb

Meats, Fish, Poultry

Bacon	2 slices
Bologna and other luncheon meats	2 slices
Boneless, cooked (breakfast)	2 oz
Boneless, cooked (dinner)	3 oz
Canadian bacon	2 oz
Chicken, 2 to 2½ lb	$\frac{1}{4}$
Frankfurters	2
Lamb chops, 4/lb	2
Liver	2 oz
Pork chops, 3 to 4/lb	1

TABLE 20.1 *(Continued)*

Miscellaneous	
Dessert toppings	2 tbsp
Gelatin dessert	⅓ cup
Jam, jelly	1 tbsp
Nuts	1½ tbsp
Olives	3
Pickles, sliced	1 oz
Puddings	½ cup
Relish	1 oz
Syrup, honey	2 tbsp
Vegetables	
Canned or frozen	3 oz
Dried	4 oz
Fresh and cooked	3 oz
Lettuce wedge	⅙th
Potatoes	4 to 6 oz

ENVIRONMENTAL PROTECTION

The feeding environment which is often *the* personal nutrition niche is multifaceted with emotional/psychological, aesthetic, religious, socio-cultural, economic, physical, and territorial components. A range in quality of food experiences and/or food and people interactions results from the way these facets come together under various circumstances. Attainment of a high quality feeding environment that facilitates control of nutrient intake is a worthy goal. It can be attained, but its quality is fragile and needs protection. The implications and ramifications of protection of the environment of the nutrition niche are part of the larger concern with quality of life.

Environment is a word that means (a) the surroundings, i.e., the circumstances, conditions, and/or objects which accompany, condition, or determine status of a factor, in this case nutrient intake; (b) the complex of climatic and biotic factors that act on people or the environmental community and ultimately determine its nutritional form and probability of survival; and (c) the aggregate of social and cultural conditions that restrict or modify the food-related aspects of the life of an individual/group. *Protection* is a word that means to prevent injury or destruction by: (a) watching over with vigilance, (b) taking precautionary measures against possible dangers, (c) interposing a barrier to ward off what immediately threatens, and/or (d) taking actions to repel an attack. Survival requires a minimal supply of each of the nutrients. Good nutritional status requires that each of the nutrients be supplied at an optimal level. Meal management strategies are the means of control in the nutritional niche. The first goal is to get the person to eat. The second is for the individual to eat a nutritious combination of foods. The third is to get the person to adjust quantity ingested to needs.

Specifically, some illustrations in relation to meal management in the nutritional niche are:

(a) surroundings: circumstances—socio-cultural. Normally sharing of food is a primary means of facilitating a social interaction. Lack of mealtime companionship is frequently a problem for the ill or elderly. It sets up a degenerative spiral emotionally with the result that a person may lose interest in eating or may nibble continuously so as to fill time. Some appealing means to increase the frequency of food and people interactions is necessary in order to restore meaning, which is normally attached to everyday eating experiences. Meaning is a necessary prerequisite to caring enough about oneself to be mindful of intake. Preparing and serving food is a primary means of communicating a message of caring. A focus on creating rewards of sensual gratification through use of color, texture, flavor, and table appointments is also helpful. Above all, monotony must be avoided.

(b) surroundings: circumstances—economic. Poverty is a factor that conditions the eating experience by deprivation. Food ingredients as well as the facilities and equipment necessary for normal food preparation are usually lacking. In extreme cases, this sets up a degenerative situation in which reduced exposure causes many foods to be strange and rejected from an undefined fear of the unknown. Some enticing means of increasing exposure to nutritious foods is necessary so that all nutrients can be obtained. This is one of the necessary prerequisites to optimal utilization of the improved food availability resulting from government feeding programs. Training in or reconditioning of any or all aspects of meal management may be necessary in order to make a large enough impact on the food environment to correct nutritional deficits.

(c) surroundings: conditions. An unstructured life-style that results in eating whatever, whenever in a hurry from vending machines and/or fast food establishments. Intake analysis usually shows concentrating calories, fat, sugar, and salt and diluting intake of other nutrients. This sets up a degenerative situation in which unwanted weight gain and a systems slowdown coexist. IF one can predict which vending machines and/or fast food establishments will be utilized during a day, THEN knowing their wares and with a little forethought, one can compensate by carrying fruit, vegetables, cheese, and/or nuts, and the like. An ice chest stocked with individual cans of juice, yogurt, cheese, etc., is easily managed by those who travel extensively. Ingenious forethought is the prerequisite to good meal management under these conditions.

(d) surroundings: objects. Some people are trained to initiate feeding only when they are hungry. Others respond to external cues, i.e., objects and other aspects of their surroundings. This sets up a degenerative situation in which a person responding to cues eats when he/she is not hungry. Unwanted weight gain is the usual long-term result. Meal management efforts center on common techniques of behavior modification. Some objects that serve as cues may be removed from the environment; reduced exposure provides some relief. So, dishes of candy, nuts, and other pickup foods are eliminated. And, effort is directed to conditioning responses to elicit a diversion to rewarding non-feeding activity. So, one eats low-calorie meals and exercises.

(e) climatic factors. These include the prevailing mood/characteristic tone or the state of being of the food and people environment that characterizes the group or period. A pleasant, relaxed meal climate is a facilitating set-up factor. A tense and unpleasant meal climate sets up a degenerative situation and results in a variety of responses, e.g., it can take one's appetite away when one mentally escapes or it can induce anxious compulsive eating. A review of one's habits will help. What food(s) do you reject because even the thought evokes a painful memory? Who do you seek out/avoid at mealtime? Which restaurants do you patronize because of their environment and associated moods?

Everybody knows enough to manage the meal environment on special occasions, e.g., a dinner party. Guests are selected for congeniality, the house is cleaned and tidied, the best table appointments are used/displayed, precious ingredients and elaborate preparation methods as well as wine, candlelight, and music—all of these are used to create a rewarding festive mood. The care that goes into the success of the special occasion is impressive.

Generalized to the everyday situation, the same expression of caring via application of the same meal management techniques creates/maintains a positive supportive eating environment in which new foods are more easily introduced to children, therapeutic restrictions are more easily tolerated, and appetite is stimulated in the ill. Household policy decisions can be used to set-up/reinforce the means to meal management of climatic control. Traditional facilitating household policies were designed to evoke the desired mental set, e.g., the diners were to be grateful and express appreciation for the food and the labor of love by the provider and preparer which made the meal possible; mealtime was a time for shared enjoyment, so the diners were to display good manners and engage in pleasant problem-free conversation. Implementation of these household policies is a first step in protection of a high quality eating environment.

Contemporary informal eating territories and styles emphasize sensual gratification and sociability, often at the expense of nutritional and other values. It is awkward to create the right meal climate when one is part of an impatient line of people that finally gets a meal, only to disperse irregularly to crowded tables in a noisy room, car seats, or a cluster of people eating standing up. On an occasional basis it is harmless enough; on a daily basis, the effects might be something else.

(f) biotic factors. These are caused by living things, e.g., yeasts, molds, and bacteria. Food spoilage is wasteful and food poisoning is fearsome. Both are indicative of a degenerative situation. Food is rarely sterile. A few microorganisms usually cannot produce an infection since body defenses overwhelm and kill them; nor can an intoxication result, since too little poison is produced to be harmful. A variety of meal management activities are designed to protect the eating environment by controlling growth rate and/or conditions. Most control the level of contamination and use high or low temperature to retard growth rate. For example, if serving is delayed, hot foods such as meats, gravies and sauces, and soups should be kept at simmering temperatures (135° to 160°F) and cold foods such as chopped meat/egg/fish mixtures containing mayonnaise should be kept in the refrigerator (35 to 40°F); leftover meats, soups, and casseroles should be covered and refrigerated immediately *not* two hours later when they have cooled to room temperature; cream pies, puddings, and other creamy desserts should be stored in the refrigerator between meals; the remainder of canned juices, fruits, and vegetables should be left in the original container, covered, and refrigerated; the remainder of a package of frozen food that has been thawed should be cooked and *then* refrozen, if necessary.

The storage life of foods depends on storage conditions; at protective temperatures, foods can be stored for the length of time listed in Table 20.2. In any case, foods should be purchased in an appropriate sized container so that once opened it can be used up in a short period of time. Items such as jams and jellies, peanut butter, oil, shortening, catsup, and prepared mustard do not need to be refrigerated when used up within a month because their composition makes them antibiotic.

(g) socio-cultural conditions: restricting. Politeness demands that when we dine with others, we restrict our food choices to conform to the general pattern. IF everybody is having soup and a salad, THEN it is socially taboo for an individual to select a five-course dinner. This is a degenerative situation in which those individuals whose needs "deviate from the norm," e.g., those with ulcers, diabetes, or obesity, which necessitate intake control, regard the eating territory as hostile and are faced with restricted alternatives. They can conform and suffer physically. Or, they can deviate and suffer emotionally from embarrassment and/or socially from deprivation, when extent of participation is reduced. Meal management efforts can best be directed to the expression of caring via selection of an eating territory that minimizes exposure to temptation and maximizes opportunity to participate normally *and* by planning compensatory adjustments in intake around the social base.

TABLE 20.2. SAFE STORAGE CONDITIONS AND PERIODS

Food	Condition	Period
Fresh meats, pieces	Refrigerate 30−36°F	Loosely wrapped, 3−5 days Sealed, 1−2 days (becomes slimy)
Fresh meat, ground or cubed	Refrigerate 30−36°F	1−2 days; freeze otherwise
Variety meats	Refrigerate 30−36°F	Loosely wrapped, 1−2 days
Hams, partially cooked	Refrigerate 30−36°F	1 week for sure, perhaps longer
Hams, fully cooked	Refrigerate 30−36°F	1−3 weeks, 1 week for sure
Hams, smoked	Read label	Read label
Bacon, cured	Refrigerate 30−36°F	1−2 weeks; freeze otherwise
Coldcuts	Refrigerate 30−36°F	Loosely wrapped, variable -high moisture 3−5 days -dry 2−3 weeks -franks 1 week
Frozen beef, lamb	Frozen, 0°F	9−12 months
Frozen pork	Frozen, 0°F	6−9 months
Frozen veal	Frozen, 0°F	4−6 months
Frozen sausage, ham, bacon	Frozen, 0°F	1−3 months
Frozen beef liver	Frozen, 0°F	3−4 months
Frozen pork liver	Frozen, 0°F	1−2 months
Fresh poultry	Refrigerate 30−36°F	Loosely wrapped, 1−2 days
Frozen chicken	Frozen, 0°F	6−8 months
Frozen turkey	Frozen, 0°F	4−5 months
Fresh fish	Refrigerate 30−32°F	2−3 days
Fresh shellfish	Refrigerate in original closed container	1−5 days
Frozen fish	Frozen, 0°F	4−6 months
Frozen shellfish	Frozen, 0°F	3−4 months
Smoked fish	Refrigerate 30−32°F	3 days, then freeze
Canned goods	Ventilated, 50−60°F	1 year
Frozen precooked	Frozen, 0°F	3 months
Fluid milk	Refrigerate 36−40°F	3 days
Non-fat dry milk	Tightly closed, refrigerate	3 months
Hard cheeses	Refrigerate 36−40°F	Variable until moldy
Soft cheeses	Refrigerate 36−40°F	3−7 days

(h) socio-cultural conditions: modifying. Various aspects of the eating environment are subject to the influences of fashion, mode, fad, and craze. Effects can be transitory or permanent, trivial or major. But, in any case, they are difficult to measure. The nutritional intake estimate based on any sample is biased by the effects of the current fashion. It is not typical, and it may be unrelated to previous or future intakes. Meal management methods can be used to prevent development of a degenerative situation in such a way as to protect the environment of the nutritional niche.

Fashion means a prevailing custom, usage, or style during a particular time, the accepted usage by those wishing to be up-to-date. Recent fashions in food have emphasized Oriental, Middle-Eastern, vegetarian foods, and meal structures as well as unbalanced nutrient intake. Although human beings in all cultures have similar needs, these can be met by different foods and divisions of intake among meals. A person accustomed to a standard three-meal pattern that is nutritionally balanced customarily obtains certain nutrients from specific meals. A person accustomed to Oriental, Middle-Eastern, or other meal pattern that is nutritionally balanced customarily obtains the same nutrients but perhaps not at the same meal. The long-term substitution of Oriental dinners, for example, may unbalance intake by increasing intake of some nutrients and omitting others unless intake at other meals is adjusted to compensate. Of course, on an occasional basis, no harm is done.

Mode means the fashion of the moment that is followed by those who are anxious to appear elegant and sophisticated. Superficiality sets up a degenerative situation in which the nutrient intake of the nutritional Neanderthal is compromised because the individual is deceived with pseudo-intellectual rationale designed to justify the current mode. The nutritionally knowledgeable can follow the mode but use meal management strategies to rebalance intake in an unobtrusive way.

Fad means a practice or interest followed for a time with exaggerated zeal. It suggests caprice in taking up or dropping a fashion. The expected effects are determined by the type of fad.

As Alvin Toffler pointed out in *Future Shock*, the American culture is a throw-away culture in which constant replacement of material goods with "new improved" models is the prevailing custom. So, every year in preparation for the holiday season, a new fad in cookware is introduced. The "in" people rush out to purchase the new gimmick and a pattern of faddish usage is observed. Normally, the fad has only a short-lived effect on nutrient intake. In the old days, the new item was a mixer or a blender. The objective of purchase was to improve basic preparation capabilities. But, these markets became saturated. So, more exotic cookware items were created in order to expand markets. Some examples of fad-related cookware are fondue pots, popcorn makers, wine service, cheeseboards, crockpots, coffee brewing centers, and donut makers.

Exotic items have conversation value and appeal. So, they create desires in suburbia. The new cookware acquisition must be displayed and admired in order for the full benefit to be realized. To prove that one owns the latest gimmick, one ostentatiously uses it for food preparation on a social occasion. Therefore, everywhere one goes in a given season, one is served the same kind of food in some variant of the "in" cookware, while the suburbanite monitors responses. A high frequency of consumption of the "in" item introduces a uniformity into the intake pattern. To compensate, planned adjustment of the overall nutrient intake at other times is necessary.

Fad diets usually require consumption of special foods. These foods are infused with the magical virtues that are supposed to be necessary to deal with the health problem. In most cases, unless fad diets are followed for a long time, they are harmless but not very useful remedies. A fad diet is of no value in prevention or treatment of a chronic condition such as obesity because of its off-again, on-again nature. IF a fad diet is followed in public for social reasons, THEN compensatory adjustment in intake should be made privately so that nutrient intake remains balanced. Note: Assessment of dietary adequacy is not justified except in unusual circumstances when a person frequently follows fad diets. Interpretation rests on relevance and reliability of the sample of intake data. But, a sample of intake data will only be relevant to the current fad diet; it may be reliable. Hence, it does not serve as an index to typical intake. Repeated sampling would be necessary if one wished to assess intake over a period such as six months.

Craze means a transient infatuation, i.e., inspired with a foolish or extravagant love or admiration. A craze has two aspects that are manifested in eating behavior. First, there is the *binge* aspect which results in unrestrained indulgence in consumption of the "in" food. Secondly, there is the *jag* aspect which induces feelings of exhilaration in relation to consumption of the "in" food. Viewed objectively, the usual eating behavior is foolish since the "in" food has no intrinsic qualities that merit release of the normally inhibitory restraints. Children go through developmental stages in which food crazes are common. The best meal management strategy is to be accommodating. Since the effect is transient, it does not threaten the environment.

The meal management strategies discussed heretofore were directed to protection within the near environment. But, in contemporary American society, food availability and food quality are mainly determined by the far environment. This is because food is produced/processed/distributed according to aggregate demands. Meal management strategies to meet individual needs by reducing the effects of the far environment are also necessary. For example, the recent advent of nutrition labeling enables the buyer to select *for presence* of specific nutrients, e.g., vitamins, by comparing nutrient to price ratios among brands and *for absence* of specific nutrients, e.g., cholesterol, fat, sugar. The ability to "doctor" cake mixes, frozen entrées, etc., enables one to utilize convenience while protecting eating quality.

The foregoing is only a sample. In order to protect the feeding environment, one must know the following: what is of value; what is good; what aspects are vulnerable, especially those via *neglect*, i.e., destruction due to failure to pay attention to or carelessness in utilization; the state of the environment; and what is the estimated effect(s) of anticipated changes. All of these must be summarized and incorporated in a personalized environmental impact statement that guides protective household and away-from-home food-related policy decisions. Then, status must be monitored and adaptive strategies introduced. These should be flexible enough to enable one to adjust appropriately to changing realities, accommodate requirements, and reconcile differences so as to preserve the eating environment that will sustain the desired quality of life. Still, one must not become overinvolved in the activities of selection, preparation, and consumption of food. There is more to life than this.

PLANNING REWARDING FOOD AND PEOPLE INTERACTIONS

The technical definition of *reward* is something that is given in return for good or evil done or received and especially that offered or given for some service or attainment. The operational definition of what is rewarding, i.e., results in a desired return, depends on the perspective of an individual, given needs and values. Some alternative definitions are listed for illustration:

(a) Provides necessary and sufficient return, i.e., the rate of profit in the process of meal production per unit of cost (time, energy, and/or money)—perspective of the economy-minded meal manager who is simply a mercenary.

(b) Something given in repayment or reciprocation—family or guests perspective or of the meal manager who does it as a "labor of love."

(c) Evidence that a constraint has been lifted such that food and people interactions can *revert*, i.e., go back to their former state. All people experience this reward at some time or other, as when decreased purchasing power has forced them to eat less well until purchasing power was restored or when they have been ill and had to restrict food intake for a time.

(d) Evidence of a recurrence, i.e., a return of something that has happened or been experienced. All people experience this reward at some time or another, as when they become ill each time they eat X or when the season changes and they can again obtain X, etc.

(e) Evidence that the situation will *recrudesce*, i.e., there is a return to activity of something that has been suppressed, controlled, or lying dormant. The meal manager who takes advantage of a holiday to indulge himself/herself by allocating extra time, energy, and money to prepare special meals derives much satisfaction and a feeling of fulfillment. Lonely grieving elderly who rejoin a social circle and begin to eat with friends find the shared meals especially rewarding.

What is rewarding depends on the needs, values, and lovability (ability to give/receive) of the parties involved. Needs may include physiologic need for food, safety-security need, belongingness need, need for status and esteem, and need for self-actualization. See Chapter 16 with respect to these needs. Also, there is a difference according to whether one eats to live (the utilitarian value) or one lives to eat, which provides emotional/psychological and aesthetic rewards that transcend the utilitarian function of food.

Many people do not find food and people interactions that rewarding and do not give sufficient meaning to various levels of interaction. To make the food and people interactions more rewarding, one needs to clarify the individual's position:

(a) Ignorant—unaware of or uninformed of the value of X—They have no belief in the value of X, so it has no meaning.

(b) Rejecting—refuse to acknowledge, acquiesce in, or submit to; or to refuse to have, use, or take for some purpose; or refuse to hear, receive, or admit; or refuse to grant, consider, or accede to.

In the first case discussion of the value of X, exposure and discussion of response, vicarious exposure via films, etc., would be the mode for enrichment. In the case of rejection, some intervening variable such as lack of social skills must be dealt with. Once the cause of the unpleasantness is removed, then re-education via discussion, planned experiences, and the like can be implemented. A (re)definition of what is wanted, what is good, and what is appropriate should reinforce the perception of reward and lead to improved quality of life.

"DOING YOUR OWN THING"

Once one has grasped some of the basic concepts relating nutritional needs, conservation of natural resources, and environmental protection, one can begin to assess the effects of alternative food management practices on nutriture. It turns out that how persons "get their heads together" determines how they will "do their thing" in the food environment.

Food-use behavior is managed in one's head according to one's food-use ideology. (Remind yourself of what you know; see Chapters 14 through 16.) Based on one's subconscious and/or conscious beliefs and attitudes about what is appropriate/inappropriate food-use by certain persons in certain eating situations, one makes food-use decisions that result in "doing one's thing."

At any one point in time, IF a person is alive and well, THEN that person's food-use behavior based on his/her food-use ideology is normal—it is neither all right nor all wrong. But, at all times some aspects can be improved.

Dietary assessment, based on information provided by the diet history and diet record, results in identification of factors to work with in getting it together in a nutritionally improved way. Some questions that must be asked and answered fully and honestly are:

(a) How important is food and the eating experience to the person? (The answer provides the basis for determining how difficult it will be for the person to make changes.)

-Is food just a filler to allay hunger pangs?

-Is food the basis for socio-cultural and/or aesthetic experiences?

-Is food linked to the concept of the wife/mother role?

(b) Does the person value the consumption of nutritious meals?

(c) Does the person who prepares the food value serving nutritious meals?

-How does that person define nutritious? (Does inclusion of steaks, roasts, and chops weekly and vegetables three to four times a week satisfy the definition?)

-Does that person think that meals should consist of whatever is desired or available?

-Does that person take pride in knowing that the usual diet is nutritious and projects a sense of well-being as a result?

The data provided by the diet history and diet records do not answer these questions. But, the data collected using these tools provide the basis for making inferences on the following aspects:

(a) Extent of time spent in planning, shopping, preparing

(b) Size of food budget in relation to the number to be fed

(c) Extent of interest/involvement in the food domain—perfunctory to optimal, convenience to scratch preparation

(d) Nature and extent of knowledge/skills in food and nutrition—various areas—may give a pretest, if unsure

The answers on these points lead to information on the time, energy, money, and knowledge resources that one can work with. (Direct questions usually cannot be asked without offending.)

Given this definition of another aspect of the overall problem and what one has to work with, one can define the nature and extent of action to be taken. Several levels of program have been identified. Typical ones are outlined below:

(a) the minimum program for management of improved nutriture— Anybody can do it, even if only slightly interested; even this little bit would improve many diets. *Deliberate* selection of the best alternative, i.e., iodized salt, fortified margarine (vitamin A), fortified milk (vitamin D), and enriched breads and cereals (iron, some of B vitamins), is simple and does not require a change in price, eating quality, or life-style.

(b) the moderate program for management of improved nutriture— This requires some motivation but brings modest improvement in most cases. *Deliberate* selection of the best alternative, as outlined above plus consumption of regular meals and control at the level of the Basic 4. Implementation of a regular meal schedule is necessary for prediction.

Predetermined components result in built-in control which can be verified by checking, using the Basic 4. This means willingness to develop a habit, which requires some adjustment of life-style so that one can plan for food availability; one cannot do whatever, whenever. In assessment, one seeks to determine whether there is any pattern to eating times within and among days, items eaten at the various eating times, availability of on-the-fly-drive-ins or vending machines—and whether the individual knows the Basic 4.

(c) the major program for management of improved nutriture—This requires long-term motivation but brings rewarding improvement in most cases. *Deliberate* selection of the best alternative, consumption of regular balanced meals, as outlined above, plus careful planning, purchasing, and serving is based on detailed food and nutrition knowledge—nutrition labeling, portion control, and eating environment control. This level means valuing nutritional well-being enough to allocate time, energy, and money to do it right. It becomes a cornerstone or feature of life-style. In assessment, one seeks to determine whether the person knows the fundamentals of menu planning, knows how to make shopping lists, knows prices, knows how to save food money wisely, knows nutrient content of alternative items, is familiar with nutrient labeling, knows preparation methods that conserve nutrients, knows food storage techniques for conservation and/or environmental protection, and knows serving techniques and portion control.

Once the necessary information is available and the program level has been identified, one applies the standard education principles in getting the learning task accomplished. Discussion of these is beyond the scope of this book.

BIBLIOGRAPHY

ANON. 1976. The garbage fact sheet. *In* Family Economics: Resources and Security in an Era of Scarcity. Proc. 16th Conf. Western Reg. Family Economics—Home Management Educ., Nov. 18-20, 1976, Provo, Utah. Brigham Young Univ. Press, Provo.

HARRISON, G.G., RATHJE, W.L., and HUGHES, W.W. 1975. Food waste behavior in an urban population. J. Nutr. Educ. 7 (1) 13-16.

21

Dietary Assessment: Food Ecology— Nature, Nurture, and Nutriture

Every point in time can be regarded as a point of transition, since change is always occurring. This transition can be seen with peoples, places, and things—including man's relationship in the United States to his food environment. Observations of American food intake are made periodically and changes are recorded. From these reports inferences are drawn about the expected effects of these changes. These expected effects are related to published data in the areas of food production, food processing, public food and nutrition education, health, etc. The inferences reflect what is known about the expected effects at a given time, i.e., they are a corrected approximation, based on past history.

For example, nutrition survey data prior to 1975 suggested that there were suboptimal intakes of calcium, iron, vitamin A, and ascorbic acid among several segments of the American population. Results from more recent observations by the National Center for Health Statistics suggest some changes in intake:

(a) Thiamin and riboflavin intakes were at least adequate in all poverty, race, sex, and age groups studied.

(b) Calcium intakes of adult Black women were consistently lower than the RDA, irrespective of income group.

(c) Mean vitamin A intakes were below the RDA among white adolescents and young adult women in low income groups, and among female Black adolescents, irrespective of income.

(d) Mean protein intakes were below the RDA for adolescents, Black and white women, older men in low-income groups, older Black men irrespective of income, and high-income white females.

(e) The mean intake of iron was below the RDA in most population subgroups.

ECOLOGY—NATURE OF CURRENT FACTORS

The food ecosystem is subject to a variety of forces. These come together variously and result in dynamic interactions which frequently have repercussions in nutrition. IF one is weak, THEN one is vulnerable and one's nutritional status is bent out of shape in first one direction and then another, according to the force applied to the system. IF one is strong, THEN one can resist the impact of the various forces, individually and collectively, and will manage to consume a well balanced diet whatever the circumstances. To cope effectively, one must accept personal responsibility for making continuous adaptive adjustments that appropriately accommodate and/or reconcile differences, as necessary. So, one must be mindful rather than mindless. This requires that one (a) expand his/her consciousness of nutritious food alternatives so as to minimize the "never think of it" excuse, (b) pay close attention to detail, and (c) reach out and overcome limitations of time, energy, money, knowledge, etc., especially since everything in the food ecosystem is in a dynamic state of change.

A person's ability to cope with change depends in part on being able to anticipate and assess the impacts of the various forces on the food ecosystem and make compensating counter-moves. In this process, knowledge is power. Are Americans in the know?

By law, the Secretary of Agriculture is obligated to set up a situation in which it is possible for Americans to be well nourished. To accomplish this mission, necessary and sufficient food must be available and people must know how to select a nutritious diet. Accordingly, the national food supply/demand situation is carefully monitored and controlled, and various food and/or nutrition education programs have been developed.

As a basis for the food and/or nutrition education programs, various aspects of food acceptance and nutrition have been studied, e.g., food consumption patterns, food purchases, food shopping behavior, nutrient needs, etc. A recent study by Fusillo and Beloian (1977) was designed to investigate the nutritional knowledge of those who do at least half the food shopping for the household. The five areas of knowledge investigated and the associated findings were:

(a) how easy/difficult it is to obtain selected nutrients from selected common foods—Shoppers knew that protein, fat, and carbohydrate are easily obtained from foods but were wrong or unsure about vitamins and minerals.

(b) storage of ten nutrients—Shoppers knew that fat is stored but most were wrong or unsure about the others, although about half knew about storage of calcium and ascorbic acid.

(c) nutrients supplied by indicator foods from the four food groups—*Milk*—Shoppers knew that it is a good source of vitamin D, calcium, and riboflavin, as well as protein and fat, but did not know that it was a poor source of iron, thiamin, vitamin A, and ascorbic acid. *Bread*—They knew that it is a good source of carbohydrate, thiamin, and ribo-flavin, but did not know that it is a good source of iron, and many were wrong or unsure of its content of other nutrients. *Beef*—Shoppers knew that it is a good source of protein and fat, more than two-thirds knew that it is a good source of iron, but only half knew that it is not a good source of ascorbic acid and most did not know that it is a good source of vitamins and minerals. *Tomatoes*—Most knew that they are a good source of ascorbic acid, but more than half did not know that they are a good source of vitamin A and were unsure about content of other vita-mins and minerals.

(d) role of selected nutrients on health of various tissues—Shoppers' knowledge was poor as to which of the four indicator foods would supply nutrients for building body tissues, strong teeth and bones, blood cells, healthy skin, nervous tissue function, vision, and fighting infection. They were largely wrong but also unsure.

(e) foods that are approximately equivalent sources of selected nutri-ents—Shoppers knew which foods could be substituted for bread and meat, although they did not know that pork and beans are a meat (pro-tein) substitute. They did not know that potatoes and tomatoes are sub-stitutes for each other except for the carbohydrate, or that milk is similar to meat and meat substitutes in protein, vitamin, and mineral content.

Despite the recent popular interest in nutrition, this study shows that while there are some people who are knowledgeable, most people have only minimal knowledge of nutrition. Their knowledge is not specific with regard to even the ten most widely recognized nutrients. Therefore, the conclusion is that the American people do *not* possess the knowledge basic to making food and/or supplement choices.

One of the attributes of a responsible adult is that he/she is a "good provider," i.e., supplies (procures or prepares) what is necessary for sus-tenance in advance. Procurement is the first aspect. According to a USDA survey (1978), food shoppers are one of three identifiable types or are atypical:

(a) "self-actualizing"—39% find satisfaction in buying and preparing food. Characteristics: They buy favorite brands although cost is higher, generally like to shop and experiment with new food products or recipes for sensory appeal, and allocate time for food preparation as an enjoyable activity.

(b) "utilitarian"—32% shop so as to save time and money. Charac-teristics: They regard shopping as a necessary but not particularly enjoyable chore, aim at minimizing time and effort in shopping, aim at minimizing costs (adhere to budget and select for low unit cost). Price is the critical variable in selection.

(c) "careful or prudent"—18% are mindful of various aspects of the process of providing food. Characteristics: They plan menus, prepare shopping lists, take advantage of advertised specials, compare prices among brands, evaluate nutritional contribution, consider food additives, etc.

(d) The remaining 11% show mixed characteristics.

Another factor is the increasing consumption of fast food meals whose main component is a hamburger, fish and chips, fried chicken, pizza, tacos, etc. In the past 20 years, consumption of fast food meals has increased from an occasional to a frequent occurrence. The frequency of consumption is expected to increase further, at least into the 1980s.

Nutritionists have been concerned with the nutrient composition of the individual items and various assortments of items commonly consumed as meals, but only limited information on composition is available. The nutritional impact depends on (a) the assortment of items selected, (b) frequency of consumption, and (c) nutrients needed/not needed versus those supplied by other meals. IF fast foods were utilized primarily as snacks, THEN the objective would be to minimize calories. IF they are utilized to replace traditional meals, THEN expected assortments should be nutritional equivalents or at least of reasonable nutrient density.

Nutrient content data are available for all of McDonald's products and from analysis of selected items by some other chains. The general effect of McDonald's products has been assessed. Important points that have emerged are:

(a) In general, the food items are as nutritious as those prepared at home but cost twice as much.

(b) The impact for those consuming fast food meals one to three times per week is not of major concern. The impact for those consuming six or more fast food meals per week *is* of concern.

(c) The nutritive value of the meal or snack depends on the assortment of items selected.

(d) Five out of seven common assortments contain $\frac{1}{5}$ or more of the United States RDA of protein, thiamin, riboflavin, and ascorbic acid. None contain a significant amount of vitamin A and $\frac{1}{5}$ of the calcium is provided only if the assortment contains a milkshake.

(e) The caloric content is high (mean reported as 600 to 1200 in 2 different studies).

(f) The mean nutrient density per 100 kcal, according to Greecher and Shannon (1977), was: protein, 4 g; iron, 0.5 mg; thiamin, 0.05 mg; and ascorbic acid, 2 mg—acceptable levels for these nutrients, especially good for protein. However, calcium and vitamin A levels were low.

Those whose life-style involves increasing consumption of fast food meals need to assess the nutritional impact of these meals on their nutritional intake. Then they need to plan for necessary adjustments in other meals.

The salt, sugar, and fat contents of fast foods also have been recognized as a cause for concern. There is some evidence of high sodium content; individual items contained 100 to 500 mg. Cantor (1977) has summarized the sugar and fat situation as follows:

. . . affluence in life-style is frequently reflected as richness of diet as well as in "eating out." Moreover, richness in diet can be associated with fat and sugar in the diet, and "eating out" with fast foods and snack foods consumed "on-the-go." The latter also are not only identified with high fat and high sugar but reflect "fast" as part of the life-style and, in some respects, reinforce fast living. This matrix of change incorporates an increasing incidence of degenerative and stress-related diseases, which in turn are associated with overconsumption and the affluent diet that again signifies high fat and sugar consumption.

Another factor that may have a positive or negative impact on nutritional status is customary consumption of snacks/meals from vending machines. The nutritional effect cannot be evaluated out of context. It must be related to individual nutrient needs, given other foods consumed and likely to be consumed during the day.

Vending machines were introduced at about the turn of the century and have their place in providing food. They permit expansion of the eating territory by permitting foods to be sold in times and places where they could not otherwise be sold economically. Until the 1950s, vending machines supplied pre-packaged items, e.g., bottled soft drinks, candy, peanuts, and gum. Then machines that could provide (a) heated foods, e.g., coffee and hot chocolate, and (b) refrigerated foods, e.g., fruits and juices, sandwiches, and ice cream novelties, were developed. Even more recently, machines that provide entrées to be reheated in microwave ovens have appeared. Clearly, at this time technology is adequate for provision of nutritious foods and complete meals via vending machines. When the array of foods provided is planned in relation to the expected nutritional needs of the local consumers, vending machines are a valuable means of providing nourishment.

Nonetheless, junk foods are the items that are most available from vending machines, earning them a poor reputation nutritionally. This is a matter of consumer demand. Vending machines are sized to hold a quantity of food that can be profitably stocked and sold at a pre-determined rate, which is the basis for the supply route. Prepackaged, non-perishable items are safe. New stock is placed behind leftovers and is sold in a short time before it can deteriorate. Any item that does not sell most of the time at a given location is replaced. The more nutritious foods such as milk, sandwiches, and hot foods have a short shelf-life. Therefore, they can be supplied only to locations where demand is sufficient to warrant frequent, usually daily, delivery. This is the factor that prevents a better array of foods in most locations.

Availability should be investigated and appropriateness of the offerings should be assessed in relation to individual needs. In relation to nutriture, customary consumption of vended foods is neither good nor bad, *per se*. It is only more or less appropriate in relation to nutrient needs. When natural or standardized items such as fruit, juice, milk, and ice cream novelties, or branded items such as soups, stews, macaroni and cheese, pork and beans, and spaghetti are available, their nutrient composition can be estimated from standard tables of food composition. When non-standard items such as sandwiches are available, their nutrient content must be estimated from the values for their components.

Another factor that has a major impact on food consumption is price/availability. During the 1970s the effects became particularly evident with respect to consumption of sugar (sucrose) and animal products. Between 1909 and 1965, per capita sucrose consumption rose to between 100 lb and 110 lb, which provided 20 to 24% of calories consumed, i.e., 400 to 500 kcal/day. Intake remained in this range up through 1974, when the combined effects of commercial introduction of an alternative low cost sweetener and high consumer price caused consumption to drop sharply and continue the downward trend. In 1975, per capita consumption was 87.5 lb. At the same time, increased use of other sweeteners and sugars caused total per capita intake to rise slightly to 120 lb. Moreover, while total carbohydrate intake has been decreasing since 1909, the fraction from sugars has been increasing, which has prompted the "McGovern Committee" to recommend that sugar intake be reduced to not exceed 10% of caloric intake.

The effect of food price/availability is related to household size and composition as shown by a recent study by Salathe and Buse (1978). These investigators, using the 1965 household food consumption survey data, developed "adult equivalent scales" which express the consumption of food of individuals of various ages and sexes as a proportion of that consumed by an adult male, aged 20 to 55 years. In assessing food consumption, foods were classified into six food classes: total food, vegetables, grain products, beef and pork, dairy products excluding butter, and fruits. Findings were:

(a) Total food intake is less so food expenditure is lower for children than adults, elderly than middle-aged adults, and females than males. Compared with the adult male, infants and elderly females cost only about half as much to feed. Adult females and elderly men cost about ¾ as much to feed.

(b) For a household of a given size, food expenditure can be expected to be greater with older rather than younger children, be greater at any given age if the child is male, and be lower if members of the household are elderly rather than younger.

(c) Household composition affects expenditures for the various food classes. As compared to the adult male, male children add less to expenditures for vegetables, beef, and pork, add more for grain products, and are equivalent for dairy products and fruits. Compared to an adult female, a female child adds less to expenditures for vegetables, beef, pork, and fruits, and adds more for grain products and dairy products. As compared with an adult male, an adult female adds less to expenditures for grain products, beef, pork, and dairy products, adds more to expenditures for fruits, and is the same for vegetables. The elderly add less to expenditures in all food classes except fruits.

Since the quantities of food consumed vary with household food composition, the amount of money budgeted for food needs to vary accordingly. Any figure such as $10/person is oversimplistic. Instead, a scale using $10, for example, for the adult male and proportionate amounts (Fig. 21.1) for other household members would be more realistic.

Other factors that have been associated with recent changes in animal product consumption include, but are not limited to:

(a) consumers' perception of the fat content of milk products—A major study shows that many consumers have misconceptions that affect their choices when they attempt to reduce fat and/or cholesterol intake, i.e., about half appear to think that the fat content of whole milk is between 5% and 50%, more than 60% appear to think that low-fat milk contains between 2% and 20% fat, about half appear to think that non-fat milk contains 1 to 4% fat, and a third appear to think that non-fat dry milk contains 1 to 2% fat (43% correctly thought that it contained less than 1% fat). Panel evaluations have demonstrated that consumers can distinguish small differences in fat or solids-non-fat content. The problem lies in their misconception of fat content.

(b) grade of meat and acceptability—About half of the meat produced is graded, of which 80% is graded Choice. Stated preferences of consumers is for lower grade meat with less marbling and finish. Measured preference is for the familiar Choice grade meats.

(c) use of soy protein extenders and Textured Vegetable Protein (TVP) meat analogs—These have been accepted and are expected to replace about 10% of meat consumption within the decade.

Since early times, food additives have been used in food preservation processes and have changed man's relation to his food supply. In the

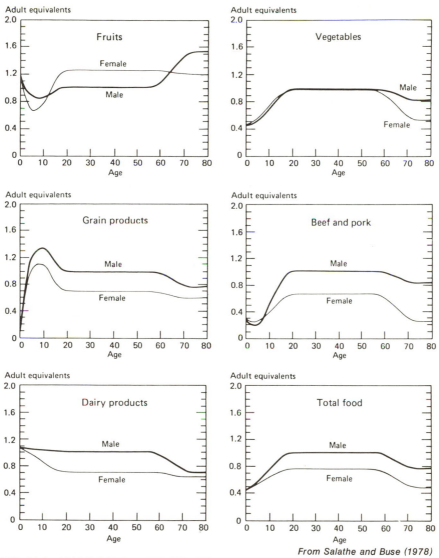

FIG. 21.1. ADULT EQUIVALENT SCALES

From Salathe and Buse (1978)

beginning and to a great extent until very recent years, food additives were crude natural mixtures of inorganic and/or organic chemicals, e.g., honey, molasses, vinegar, and saltpeter. All of these, like the medicinal herbs in common use at the time, were known to contain an "active principle." The major objective of the sciences of inorganic and organic chemistry was to identify, extract, purify or isolate, and synthesize the "active principle," since it was more potent and more controllable.

Once the "active principle" was identified, its chemical name was used. This was the point where the American public became uncertain about what was added to foods. Sugar and salt were familiar; sucrose and sodium chloride, however, were unheard of.

There was really nothing new but the food additives had been transformed from the familiar and had been given strange new identities (see Chapter 16). The food processing industry was totally unprepared for the wave of criticism and condemnation generated by consumer activists (Fig. 21.2).

Overreaction has had two kinds of effects that have nutritional implications. (1) Many people stopped eating some or all processed foods. In some cases, home-prepared equivalents were substituted, resulting in only a small nutritional effect. In other cases, items or categories of foods were eliminated and replaced with greatly expanded consumption of a few items, resulting in a major imbalance in intake. Between these two extremes, there were many gradations of effect. (2) The food processing industry began to produce items without preservatives. Shelf-life was shorter, so prices were increased, ostensibly to cover the cost of the quantity that had to be discarded or sold at discount outlets.

NURTURE

When viewed by someone else, a person's relation to his/her food ecosystem appears to be relatively stable and resistant to change. However, man's relation to his food environment is in a dynamic state of change as each person makes small adaptive changes and/or deliberate major changes in relation to a continuous set of perceived alterations in his/her food environment. Consequently, dietary intake may become maladjusted in relation to needs, so it may be necessary for a health care professional to intervene in the change process—to modify the nature, extent, direction, and/or speed of changes.

People are resistant to changes imposed by others. In order to nurture, i.e., further the development of, one must overcome a number of obstacles or kinds of resistance. Usually, these are related to people problems. As a result, the task is to create a support structure within which to nurture nutritional well-being.

The diet history provides the information necessary for nurturing productive changes. The critical variable is the person's food ideology, i.e., the beliefs and attitudes that underlie his personal food practices. Assessment involves aspects such as:

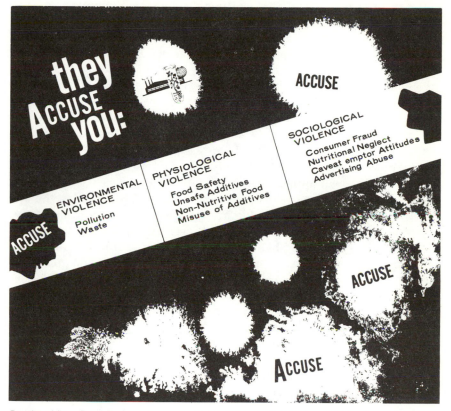

Reprinted from Food Technology, cover, 24 (8). 1970. Copyright © by Institute of Food Technologists

FIG. 21.2. CHARGES AGAINST THE FOOD DELIVERY SYSTEM THAT RESULTED FROM A CREDIBILITY GAP AND CREATED A CRISIS IN CONFIDENCE

(a) What is the classification system that underlies the personal definition of what is food/not food?

(b) What is the definition of what is food/not food—items, attributes/quality, seasoning, preparation method?

(c) How important is variety? Is rapid development of monotony a problem? What items are accepted as staples for daily use?

(d) Does the person feel secure that the food he/she consumes is safe, wholesome, nutritious, and properly controlled? Or is he/she susceptible to fads and quacks? Is he/she fearful and rejecting?

(e) Does the person feel that his/her diet is socially acceptable or is there embarrassment because of lack and deprivation?

(f) Is skill in food preparation/service linked to self-esteem or self-actualization needs? Is the food domain the major or only feasible domain in which these needs are met?

(g) What factors determine the accept/reject decision for items and combinations?

(h) What are the effects of who the person eats with, what is eaten at the same feeding, when food is eaten and the cues initiating feeding behavior, where the person eats (what is available in the eating territory), how the person eats (rate, ritual, etc.)?

Some elements will stabilize and some will destabilize the food/nutrition ecosystem. These need to be known and classified. IF one has the answers to questions such as these in mind, THEN one is cognizant of the important elements in the person's food ideology and can identify what one has to work with and what one has to avoid. It is counter-productive to initiate a change in one aspect of a person's food and nutrition ecosystem that creates a drag of one or many new problems. Understanding of the particulars of the individual ecosystem is necessary to avoid this outcome. The starting point for change is an aspect with a high probability of payoff (it may not be the element that has the biggest possible payoff, since one may need to lead up to it). Success at the outset is essential as a motivation and morale builder.

It is not easy to nurture. One must have the wide-angle view of what the problem is and anything might turn out to be the critical variable. Consider the expected effects of this contemporary concern. The particular problem has been very negative and counter-productive. When trying to intervene to get the nutritional job done, one does not need this problem as one already has enough to do; but it will not go away. Indeed, if not dealt with, it may become more of a problem.

The problem derives from the effect of man's ignorance of contemporary food technology coupled with man's inhumanity to man. Traditionally, food-getting activity was a central behavior associated with the adult role of man and animals. Adults knew all about it. Increasingly, since the turn of the century, American adults have been freed from any but selection activities; production is not a part of the food-getting role. Underexposure to food production problems and realities has resulted in progressively less knowledge about them so that now man seems to fear the unknown. But when one is not involved in something, it becomes an unknown. The vast size and complexity of the food chain from producer to consumer are overwhelming as well as full of unknowns, so fear has led to distrust.

Man's inhumanity to man is well known—greed, lies, cheating, thievery, etc. All of these fuel fear and distrust. When individuals are involved in production, others involved are known and regarded as nice people. When others are unknown, they may possibly be regarded as predators in a jungle who are ready to pounce. So when underexposure and fear of the unknown coincide with cynicism, a degenerative pathway of disillusion, declining trust, detachment, and separation are the usual outcomes and may be voiced in confrontation as "I accuse" and "Ain't it awful." Fear, distrust, and defensiveness may predominate. To restore normality to the nutritional niche requires knowledge. Knowledge is power. With the answers to "What is food's purpose?" and "Why is food necessary?" one can begin to nurture.

BIBLIOGRAPHY

APPLEDORF, H. 1974. Nutritional analysis of food from fast-food chains. Food Technol. *28* (4) 50, 52-55.

BREELING, J.L. 1970. Are we snacking too much today? Today's Health *48* (1) 48-50, 52.

CANTOR, S.M. 1977. Ideals and realities in food systems. *In* Food and Nutrition in Health and Disease. N.H. Moss and J. Meyer (Editors). Ann. N.Y. Acad. Sci. *300*, 262-265.

DONOVAN, W.P., and APPLEDORF, H. 1973. Protein, fat, and mineral analyses of franchise chicken dinners. J. Food Sci. *38*, 79-80.

FUSILLO, A.E., and BELOIAN, A.M. 1977. Consumer nutrition knowledge and self-reported food shopping behavior. Am. J. Public Health *67* (9) 846-850.

GILLIE, R.B. 1971. Endemic goiter. Sci. Am. *224*, 93-106.

GREECHER, C.P., and SHANNON, B. 1977. Impact of fast food meals on nutrient intake of two groups. J. Am. Dietet. Assoc. *70*, 368-372.

ISOM, P. 1976. Nutritive value and cost of "fast food" meals. Family Econ. Rev. (Fall) p. 10-13. Consumer & Food Econ. Inst., Agric. Res. Serv., USDA, Washington, D.C.

PEARSON, A.M. 1976. Some factors that may alter consumption of animal products. A review. J. Am. Dietet. Assoc. *69*, 522-530.

SALATHE, L., and BUSE, H. 1978. The relationship between household food expenditures and household size and composition. *In* National Food Review, January. Economics, Statistics and Cooperatives Service, USDA, Washington, D.C.

SHANNON, B.M., and PARKS, S.C. 1980. Fast foods: a perspective on their nutritional impact. J. Am. Dietet. Assoc. *76* (3) 242-247.

USDA. 1978. Food shopping behavior. *In* Service: USDA's Report to Consumers. USDA Publ. *153*. Washington, D.C.

22

Nutritional Risk and Life Expectancy: Life–style, Eating, and Health Care

In the past ten years, the relationship among these three factors has become a focus of concern. The mounting costs of health care have become a hotly debated political issue. All factors related to costs have come under intense scrutiny.

The overall costs of preventive health care appear to be less than the costs of treatment once disease has become manifest, especially if later years must be spent in a nursing home at public expense. Recent studies have suggested that seven health-related behaviors have a greater impact on health than do the amount and quality of medical care *per se*. Therefore, since these are amenable to change, they are the targets of educational efforts in prevention programs. The nutrition-related behaviors associated with good health are: (a) limited alcohol consumption, (b) consumption of three meals per day, unsupplemented by between-meal snacking, (c) consumption of breakfast, and (d) control of weight at the normal level.

The United States Senate Select Committee on Nutrition and Human Needs conducted a series of hearings on "Diet and Killer Diseases." The views of eminent scientists, medical experts, spokesmen for professional societies such as the American Dietetic Association, representatives of the food industry and its trade associations, and other interested parties were entered in testimony. The testimony is a matter of public record.

Topics discussed included diet and cardiovascular disease, diet and obesity, diet and diabetes, dietary fiber and gastrointestinal disease, and nutrition and the elderly. As a result of these hearings, more attention has been focused on the importance of life-style, eating, and health care.

The tumultuous hearings were remarkable because of the mixture of scientific fact, empirical observations, beliefs, attitudes, opinions, intentions, and behaviors. The indiscriminate mix of points was bewildering. Still, the short-run effects were positive, i.e., press coverage created public awareness and interest, and the government recognized the importance of the nutriture of Americans in health care cost containment. The controversial Dietary Goals, original and revised versions, evolved from the testimony given at these hearings and the committee's need to make some policy in response. The long-run effects are still unknown; legislation is still pending and response to the Dietary Goals, other than debate, has not been measured.

This same committee investigated a number of topics with respect to nutrition and health. In the forward to a report, Senator McGovern (1976) made the following statements:

My appraisal of the handling of U.S. food policy over the last four years leads me to conclude that one of the most important, if not the most important, guides in the management of the food system is nutritional health. Most would agree that the final objective of any food system is the maintenance and improvement of nutritional health of the population. It is only natural that nutritional health be among the key measures applied to food policy decisions.

I fully recognize that there are those who think that nutritional health concerns are irrelevant to the hard economic choices that must be made in governing a system of such weighty and complex elements as the food system.

It is precisely because of the unpredictability and intractability of our food situation that we must view it in terms of its impact on people. It is all too easy, as we are seeing now, to have the weakest and the least organized of our number of (sic) take up the slack when the plans of the powerful misfire.

The remedies will not all be obvious, or easy; they demand the rethinking of established economic patterns and assumptions . . .

We have ample warning of the need to change the direction of our food economy, both for our physical and economic well-being. And we have in the history of the evolution of food-policy making in this century ample guidance on the ways of altering the system. We ignore this history at our peril.

THE PHYSICAL HEALTH PREDICAMENT: RIGHTS AND RE-SPONSIBILITIES

Until the 1950s, the cost of medical treatment and hospitalization was comparatively low, i.e., $40 per day for routine hospital care (Culliton 1978). Then, available methods of treatment were relatively simple.

Since then, advancing medical science and technology have developed powerful methods for diagnosis and treatment of catastrophic illnesses. Another factor is that the health care industry is a conglomeration of big systems and numerous small private enterprises operating in an unco-ordinated decentralized way, i.e., each part is optimizing for itself with little or no responsibility for the whole. And, each part purchases the "best" rather than appropriate services. So, the overall costs often far exceed what would be necessary or desirable. Critics seriously question whether this is appropriate to the needs of the trusting bewildered patient who is not in a position (emotional or technical) to make decisions, so goes along with recommendations. Costs have risen to a level beyond the means of more than a few. At the same time, the right to good medical care for all has been reaffirmed.

To extend the availability and benefits of medical advances to a large portion of the populace, an attitudinal shift in terms of who covers the costs was necessary. IF everybody contributed a portion of the costs by means of a general assessment, THEN the costs could be covered. So, the costs of this type of health care have become a societal responsibility. Medicare (for the elderly) and Medicaid (for the poor) were created in 1965, and kidney dialysis/transplant cost coverage in 1973. These programs are funded from the income taxes.

But, the costs of these programs have skyrocketed. They and other medical costs now account for 10% of the GNP (Culliton 1978), and are rising faster than costs in any other sector of the American economy. As a result, medical care costs have become a major political issue with much pressure for containment.

Methods of containment can be focused on either the curative or preventive medicine portions. Until now medicine has been primarily curative. Preventive measures have more potential for cost containment, so they are being re-emphasized. They usually include control of dietary intake, so nutrition has become an important concern of medicine. At most, experts only hope to interest and involve 50% of the populace.

The concept of disease prevention is not new. But, most individuals do not seem to worry about their health until they lose it. So, they are irresponsible and are not conscientious in implementing preventive measures. It is difficult to live with many constraints, so health-compromising rather than health-enhancing ways are followed. As a result, the incidence, prevalence, and severity of major illnesses are greater than natural. And, the costs are probably greater than society will afford.

In his discussion "Responsibility for Health," Knowles (1977) said:

Prevention of disease means forsaking the bad habits which many people enjoy—overeating, too much drinking. . .it means doing things which require special effort—exercising regularly, improving nutrition. . . .The idea of individual responsibility flies in the face of American history, which has seen a people steadfastly sanctifying individual freedom while progressively narrowing it through the development of the beneficent state . . . the idea of individual responsibility has given way to that of individual rights—or demands, to be guaranteed by government and delivered by public and private institutions. The cost of private excess is now a national, not an individual, responsibility. . . .The next major advances in the health of the American people will be determined by what the individual is willing to do for himself and for society at large. If he is willing to follow reasonable rules for healthy living, he can extend his life and enhance his own and the nation's productivity.[1]

In this domain, as in so many others, the slogan "If you're not part of the solution, you're part of the problem" clearly applies. The problem is multifaceted. Only a few facets will be discussed within the context of this discussion.

An emerging concept is that preventive medicine appears to require a delicate balance of responsibility between collective and individual efforts. For example, the most effective measures in preventive medicine have been the public health management of the quality of water, air, food, and sewage; drug regulation; and mandatory immunization programs. The collective measures have been managed for some time in the public interest. They have been updated and upgraded recently, given new concerns and capabilities. The individual must manage a number of aspects, among them nutrient intake, weight control, and exercise. These areas of individual responsibility are the current focus of activity. Activity has increased markedly since the Ten State Nutrition Survey, and reports of subsequent surveillance activities revealed significant prevalence of deviant nutrient intake.

The incongruity between the result of a sequence of events and the normal expected result is ironic. Traditionally, within a given culture, the affluent have had better general health and greater longevity than the poor. So, affluence has long been popularly associated with good health. Most Americans are affluent but their health is suboptimal. What is the problem?

Affluence removes food cost as a limiting factor affecting basic food consumption. The American economy is based on bigness and continuing growth—a high rate of production and a high rate of consumption, on a *per capita* basis. So, people are encouraged to eat more or at least food that requires more steps. And advertising is supportive. It is deliberately designed to create for any given product:

(a) awareness of the social value of high consumption

(b) a need or desire for it that encourages impulse buying

(c) a climate of permissiveness in regard to excess consumption

In short, advertising entices. But, advertising is not the only culprit. The automation that made affluence possible reduced physical energy output, and, therefore, caloric need. It also added the stress of time discipline, new kinds of frustration, and boredom. So, the degenerative

---

[1]From J. Knowles (1977). Copyright 1977 by the American Association for the Advancement of Science. Quoted with permission of the author and AAAS.

diseases such as obesity, hypertension, and cardiovascular disease have increased—both in incidence and prevalence. This is the irony of affluence.

As a people, we emotionally evade the fact that our eating habits are not optimal in terms of our health, given our life-style. It is true that one should eat for health; it is also true that eating is an activity to be enjoyed. So, limits must be set. At the same time, it is inappropriate for normal people who are free of disease to allow negative admonitions to permeate their consciousness in such a way as to become the basis for a severely restricted food array. What is needed is the wisdom to select the right amount of a balanced diet.

THE PHYSICAL HEALTH PREDICAMENT: BELIEFS

From time immemorial, health-related beliefs about what food(s) a person should/should not eat under certain circumstances, i.e., pregnancy, lactation, illness of one kind or another, have been followed. Some were followed for short periods of time, e.g., a few days, and had no noticeable effect on nutritional status. Others were followed for long periods of time, with little effect on nutritional status. Others were central and controlling factors in food consumption, often having severe nutritional outcomes. In this century, and in our American culture based on science, we pride ourselves on rational thought. So, we have generally rejected traditional health-related food ideology as "old wives' tales."

It turns out that traditional beliefs have been replaced with a new set, which may be equally invalid, being based on a variety of misinterpreted facts and half-truths. Today's reality is that nearly every family will have one member on a therapeutic diet for treatment of some medical condition. Therefore, an understanding of their effects is necessary. This is especially so in regard to beliefs that create resistance to necessary dietary change—these must be modified or eliminated. Beliefs that are useful in treatment need to be reinforced.

If one were to do a study of people's knowledge of what foods to eat/not eat for ulcers, heart disease, diabetes, etc., one would find that general knowledge is faulty and that there are many misconceptions and gaps. In short, the model for the common wisdom is a piece of swiss cheese—it has holes of random size and depth at random intervals. Beliefs follow a continuum from popular to those based on scientific fact. People tend to sort out into the following classes:

(a) people who are ignorant of basic facts, who follow practices of family and friends

(b) people who know basic facts but are out-of-date, so select food inappropriately

(c) people who know but who are inconsistent. They may follow scientific or popular beliefs or some combination thereof

(d) people who know basic facts and follow them in a reasonable way

(e) people who know basic facts but overcompensate

Remnants of traditional belief systems survive today. Until recently, health care professionals dealt only with traditional beliefs when working with new immigrants from less developed countries or members of some American subgroup cultures who had little exposure to our health care delivery system. So, understanding of these traditional belief sets and their implications were poorly understood. The anti-establishment movement which rejected modern medicine revived traditional beliefs and practices and applied them out of context with some unusual results.

Traditional Beliefs: Food as Medicine

Traditional health-related aspects of food ideology have their roots in ancient Egyptian and Babylonian medicine but have undergone continuous change over time. The traditional belief structure provides a list of what is food for each recognized illness, a statement of what "foods" are taboo, an explanation of why (may be myth), and usually a ritual to be observed in order to bring about the desired change in well-being. Moreover, IF a person breaks some taboo, THEN some evil will follow. This is the mechanism for control leading to social conformity.

The list of foods allowed/proscribed for a given medical condition varies among cultures. Latin Americans and others may classify foods as "hot" and "cold"—which has to do with their effect in balancing body humors, a concept that goes back from the Middle Ages to Greek and Roman times. Orientals classify foods as "yin" and "yan(g)," a similar concept. Some foods, usually staples, are in a class that allows *ad libitum* consumption. The list of foods to be eaten is composed usually of those that are rare or costly. Therefore, if they are sacrificed in getting rid of the illness the benefit is clear. The list of foods proscribed usually includes many items that are available and desired. Therefore, if they are not eaten, this sacrifice will bring a benefit.

The explanation of why a food should or should not be eaten may be based on observations or myths. For each category of food, a set of beliefs evolves that defines who, what, and when X,Y, Z, and Q can be eaten in relation to various illnesses. The set of beliefs defines what is suitable for individuals and categories of people to eat in certain times and conditions, e.g., a man works hard so he is given the best choice of "hot" items such as beef in the largest portions available, a man should eat heart and liver so he will be strong like a lion, on hot summer days one should eat only "cold" foods, when sick one should eat chicken soup because it is strengthening, when pregnant it is expected that one will crave odd combinations of foods that may be difficult to obtain such as pickles and strawberries in mid-winter, one should fast intermittently to clean out the poisons from the system, etc. (The preceding are examples of beliefs; merit is not implied.)

The ritual has two avowed purposes. The first is to appease the gods who are angry (song and dance). This shows that the person acknowledges that a sin has been committed, that he/she repents, asks for forgiveness, and gives praise that he/she is forgiven. This is often accompanied by a bribe—money, food, or sacrifice. The second purpose is penance. Some people are slow learners and public involvement in a ritual reinforces the learning. The person gives valuable time as reparation for past injustices, i.e., one must pay the price. One engages in long involved food preparation techniques that are tedious and one follows the details exactly in order to demonstrate that one is no longer rebellious.

All of this defines *what is good*, and therefore, *what is wanted*, under special conditions. IF one accepts these beliefs and follows the prescribed procedures conscientiously, THEN all will be well, in theory. IF a gap develops between what is and what is wanted, THEN fear, anxiety, and evil will result. But, as in all things, cultural transmission of all of the concepts is imperfect, meaning is lost, and rituals become empty and are finally abandoned. This is especially likely to occur when a more credible belief system is available.

Contemporary Beliefs

The contemporary health-related ideology has a scientific base, even though cultural transmission has garbled parts of it. The public health "Establishment" continually beams informational messages at the public. At first glance, one might think that the result would be an informed public. But, change in food habits comes slowly—slowly, if at all and certainly not universally. This is because the information flow is according to the gossip model. People select, magnify, and transmit what they want to hear and what they think their listener wants to hear, and not everybody gets the intended message. Most people are fairly rational and will do what is wanted, if they get the message. But usually they will agree and do nothing since they do not identify with it that much, i.e., they do not get the message. When fear takes over, people become irrational and do whatever they wish, e.g., follow quacks or fad diets. So, people eat rightly/wrongly for health.

"Being good" all of the time is not easy and most people do not have that much self-discipline in relation to eating. The human factor is counter-productive and undercuts any effort to change people from eating what they like to eating what they should.

Contemporary beliefs regarding eating and health are diffuse. A few of these are:

(a) Freedom from incapacitating illness, but not necessarily good health, is highly valued. This is achieved by means of surgery/drugs. Diet is not that important, so it can be ignored or at least does not have to be adhered to rigorously.

(b) Megadoses of vitamin C will cure the common cold.

(c) Vitamin E will prevent heart attacks.

(d) Alcohol and spices are "bad" for ulcers; the diet is strict and must be followed for a year.

(e) Eat right (however that is defined) and you will feel good, you will get "psyched up" and be euphoric. Reject incongruous foods; body signals will tell you when you are not eating correctly.

(The above are examples of beliefs; merit is not implied.)

THE PHYSICAL HEALTH PREDICAMENT: CUMULATIVE AND AGGREGATE EFFECTS

As one reaches middle-age, health concerns begin to appear in a large, indistinct, and distorted form—as a shadow or reflection—and uneasiness results. At age 20, the wise ones would view the *prospects* of physical health at 50, 60, and 70, *given* several alternative combinations of current health, habits, or biological make-up, when life-style and eating patterns X, Y, Z, and Q are continued. And, they would make necessary adjustments so that these factors are likely to come together for good health in later life. This takes vision, i.e., an unusual ability to discern and foresee the outcomes. And, it takes discipline and perseverance. Few individuals are of this type. More common are those who do not worry about their health until they lose it. Then they review their combination in *retrospect*, play "blame," "if only. . . ," and "poor me," and seek the fountain of youth. Hindsight is better than foresight—an old but true saying.

Permissiveness has been in vogue for a generation; still the meaning of the concept of allowing discretion seems to be confused with freedom. But, permissiveness and freedom are not the same thing. It is one thing to tolerate or allow discretion. It is another to allow freedom, with the implication that one can do whatever, whenever, with no consequences. To clarify, the quality of *discretion* has several aspects which must be considered in regard to protecting/preserving health:

(a) having or showing discernment or good judgment in conduct of X

(b) being circumspect, i.e., carefully considering all circumstances and possible consequences

(c) having ability to make responsible decisions

(d) having earned the right and power necessary for making individual choices or judgments

Freedom means that one has no obligation or commitment, i.e., one is set loose from restraints or constraints, so that the course of action is determined by the actor. This concept implies that there is no cost to the actor, irrespective of the course chosen. This is a fallacy; freedom is not free. There is always a price; it may mean a sacrifice.

Science has been able to elucidate many points in the relationship among life-style, eating, and health. Still, the available information is insufficient for predicting the exact outcomes associated with the myriad possible combinations of these multifaceted variables. Negative effects from some incompletely defined combinations of these variables have been observed. Risk factors associated with the etiology of some of the major diseases have been identified. Still, in no case has the cause and effect relationship been identified. For this reason, a conclusive argument cannot be presented. Unfortunately, an indicative one does not seem strong enough to persuade and/or overcome the normal resistance to change from the self-deluding easy way.

Moreover, many people appear to succeed with their unhealthy way. But, lest anyone be misled, the following point must be acknowledged: everybody is made with certain tolerances, i.e., relative capacity to endure or adapt physiologically to an unfavorable environmental factor. At the same time, one must acknowledge a corollary concept: the tolerance, i.e., the allowable deviation from the physiological standard is unknown and unknowable for any individual. So, for a given individual, effects may not appear to be hazardous at any specific point in time. Who can tell how close he/she is to the limit of his/her tolerance or what the cumulative and aggregate might be? What then is the best course to follow?

How it will come out is an unknown: there are many sources of uncertainty for any individual along the way. Many points seem obscure; others are only dimly perceived. Still, we are the most enlightened generation although we only grope toward the light. Review of a few scenarios is thought-provoking.

Life-style and Eating

The cumulative and aggregate effects of life-style can be startling and frightening. A few sketches of people-types illustrate the over-thirty life-style as it relates to eating and health:

(a) The vigorous, active, healthy you. You bike to work, walk your bike upstairs, and stow it in the far corner of the office. You work all day at your pencil-pusher job and then bike home. Then, it's off to the pool or the tennis courts for an hour or so before dinner. Then, you eat right and light, but the food is good and you enjoy. You work two hours on whatever is pressing—job or personal or community. You turn in and sleep well.

(b) The nervous, upright, uptight you. You jump into your car and frustrate your way through a maze of city traffic to work. You take the elevator up. You work all day at your pencil-pusher job. You eat intermittently throughout the day. A doughnut and coffee in the morning, a heavy lunch, coffee and ice cream in the afternoon. You jump into the elevator and quickly descend, just ahead of the mob. You scurry to the car, jump in, and pull it away. You have made it so far; now to negotiate the traffic. Home at last, you pour yourself a drink and flop until dinner. It is heavy—steak, baked potato, gelatin salad, rolls and butter, apple pie with cinnamon sauce, and coffee. Then, you scan the paper, watch a few television shows, and flop into bed where you toss and turn, complaining about the rat-race. You weigh 250 lb but are only 67 in. tall. You are on your way!

(c) The exercising-to-compensate you. You exercise as soon as you arise and eat a reasonable breakfast. Then, you ride to work, walk up the stairs, and work all day at your pencil-pushing job. Intermittently, you make up reasons to walk around some. You take black coffee only at breaks, decaffeinated coffee when you remember. Lunch is light—a sandwich only. After a nerve-racking day you ride home, go to the pool or the courts, eat a light dinner while you work, and continue working until 2 a.m. when you fall into bed super-exhausted. This cannot continue!

Once again the scene has changed; the over-60 view. The sequelae:

(a) Older, more mature, slower now, but still vigorous and healthy, you walk to work and up the stairs and work all day. You take the breaks just to be sociable—coffee sometimes but no snack unless there is fruit. You walk home and dine moderately, but with enjoyment. Then, you go out for a walk. Physical labor on Saturdays. Swim and ski in season. Bowl and tennis frequently.

(b) Older and more harried than ever. You are up and at the exercises before breakfast, you drive to work, rush into the office, and continue to rush. Then you sit and fret over all the new problems. Meanwhile, your secretary keeps your coffee cup full. You lunch in the cafeteria with your peers—a sandwich and dessert. After lunch, it is more of the same until quitting time when you rush home, grab a drink to relax, and eat quickly and mechanically while you brood on the problems of the day. Then it is a quick walk for health and back to work until 2 a.m. Then, tired and hyper, you take your ulcer to bed.

(c) Old and sick—slower, still heavy, uptight about mild diabetes and high cholesterol, and nervous. You exercise in the morning, eat a light breakfast, ride to work, push a pencil all morning but arrange to walk around some. You have coffee and saccharin at the a.m. break, a low cholesterol lunch, tea at the p.m. break. You ride home, grab the one drink that is allowed and sip it slowly, trying to make it last. Then, a low cholesterol dinner and a walk for health. Then, you scan the paper, and go to bed exhausted.

That was a heavy confrontation. The quality of life portrayed in some scenarios leaves much to be desired. To avoid these unwanted outcomes requires positive action based on acceptance of personal responsibility.

Diet and Disease

In the old days, disease was treated by manipulation of diet and/or use of herbal teas. Then, improved methods of chemical extraction resulted in isolation of the "active principle." Advances in pharmacology allowed incorporation of these compounds into a vast array of tablets and capsules. Thus, drugs became available for treatment of disease and soon were the preferred treatment. But then, the spectre of side-effects surfaced. Growing concern has resulted in position statements by two major medical groups. These groups encourage Americans to utilize dietary treatment to the extent possible:

(a) The American Diabetes Association—Wood and Bierman (1972), speaking for this group, stated

Some of those treating diabetics appear to have their therapeutic priorities mixed up. The physician and the dietician should never forget that careful control of the food the diabetic eats is still the basic treatment of mild and moderately severe cases of diabetes . . . .It is not that insulin and oral drugs lessen the need for modification of the patient's diet. It's the other way around: diet might lessen the dependence upon drugs. Many cases can and should be controlled by diet alone.[1]

(b) The Heart and Lung Institute—Robert Levy (1977), speaking as director of this group, stated in response to a question concerning availability of drugs to deal with excesses

. . . the behaviorists . . . have convinced us that the American would prefer to take one pill a day, and do whatever they wanted to do. The problem is that we don't have that one pill, and the problem is that the evidence is clear that all or any drugs have some side effects associated with them. And if we can get away

---

[1]From Wood and Bierman (1972). Reproduced with permission of *Nutrition Today*, 101 Ridgely Avenue, Annapolis, Md. 21404. © May/June, 1972.

from drugs by using nutritional concepts, by using diet, that will be far better for the American public in the long run.

Nutriture and Cancer.—Cancer is a major public health problem in the United States. It is the second leading cause of death. The relationships between nutriture and cancer risk, development, and control are complex and not well understood. Nutriture probably does not cause cancer but it may create/maintain the physiological conditions that modify its growth potential. Different kinds of cancer appear to respond differently to different states of nutriture. In 1974, the National Cancer Institute was mandated to study the relationships between nutritional variables and cancer. Study of these with respect to many nutrients has begun. A number of points have emerged:

(a) calories—Restriction of calories, especially from carbohydrates, appears to reduce the incidence of and delay the onset of breast, lung, and skin tumors in rats. It increases the incidence of hepatic tumors and has no effect on the incidence of adrenal adenomas. A variety of plausible explanations for these varying effects has been proposed; none have been verified.

(b) fat—Animal studies have indicated an association between fat content of the diet and incidence of some kinds of tumors. In humans, increased fat intake is associated with increased mortality from breast cancer. Animal studies also show that the kind of plant/animal source of the fat is a factor. There is conflicting evidence with respect to whether diets high in PUFA increase the risk of cancer. A number of possible mechanisms have been proposed; none have been verified.

(c) cholesterol—An epidemiological association between prevalence of CHD and leukemia, breast, and colon-rectum cancers has suggested that cholesterol may be a common etiologic factor. Case control studies of circulating cholesterol levels have not confirmed this relationship.

(d) protein and amino acids—No consistent patterns have surfaced; responses are highly variable. Deficiency of some amino acids appears to suppress tumorigenesis, perhaps by depressing antibody production so that cell-mediated immune responses are more effective in defense.

(e) vitamin A—Animal studies have demonstrated an association between deficiency and development of tumors at a number of sites in oral and gastrointestinal tissues. Vitamin A excess depresses tumor growth but has limited usefulness in treatment because it is toxic. A number of explanations for the mode of action have been given; none have been verified.

(f) B vitamins—Riboflavin retards the growth of liver tumors. Folic acid and B_{12} enhance induction of tumors by chemical carcinogens.

(g) ascorbic acid—It may have a protective role in minimizing the carcinogenicity of nitrosamines. A powerful reducing agent, it reduces nitrite to nitrous oxides.

(h) minerals—Some minerals that are not nutrients and are not usual dietary constituents are known carcinogens. Those minerals that are nutrients, including Zn, Na, K, Ca, Mg, Se, and Cu, may or may not have an effect on tumor growth; contradictory results have been reported. Iodine deficiency predisposes one to thyroid cancer.

Thus, a movement to utilize dietary management of food and nutrient intake as the main treatment modality in control of selected diseases has begun. In this century, diet management has not been notably successful. However, nutritional awareness has increased greatly during the past few years. Perhaps now, with the encouragement and support engendered by the temper of the times, more people will find the strength to implement preventive and therapeutic diets.

BIBLIOGRAPHY

ALCANTARA, E.N., and SPECKMAN, E.W. 1976. Diet, nutrition, and cancer. Am. J. Clin. Nutr. *29*, 1035-1047.

CULLITON, B.J. 1978. Health care economics: the high cost of getting well. Science *200* (4344) 883-885.

KNOWLES, J. 1977. Responsibility for health. Science *198* (4322) 1103.

LEVY, R. 1977. Testimony Before the Select Committee on Nutrition and Human Needs, U.S. Senate. Diet Related to Killer Diseases, II. Part I, Cardiovascular Disease (Committee Print). GPO, Washington, D.C.

MCGOVERN, G. 1976. Forward. *In* Select Committee on Nutrition and Human Needs, U.S. Senate. Nutrition and Health II. Nutrition and Health Revised with a Study of the Impact of Nutritional Health Considerations on Food Policy (Committee Print). GPO, Washington, D.C.

SELECT COMM. ON NUTRITION AND HUMAN NEEDS, U.S. SENATE. 1975. Index to publications on nutrition and human needs. (Committee Print). GPO, Washington, D.C.

WOOD, F.C., and BIERMAN, E.L. 1972. New concepts in diabetic dietetics. Nutr. Today 7 (3) 4-10, 12.

23

Nutritional Risk and Life Expectancy: Hunger and Malnutrition

Some people are hungry and malnourished. Since the year one, this has been so and it will continue to be so until the end of time. Each generation must confront this problem and seek its own solution(s) according to the times. This is as true in America as anywhere else.

Previous American solutions, though increasingly less functional in combatting the problems, sufficed as far as the American public was concerned until 1968. Until then, the problems of middle-class Americans overshadowed the effects of nutritional deprivation of the poor. Then a documentary film hit the prime-time slots of the major television networks. It was shocking and evoked an immediate response. It showed that in affluent America, some people were suffering hunger and/or malnutrition as severe as that seen in the less developed countries. People had a rude awakening that expanded their consciousness of how the less fortunate live.

What did they see that was so upsetting? Incredible as it may seem, scenarios like the following:

(a) Poor families of Blacks and whites in the rural South—free-living in their own shanties. Several children, who look retarded and are dirty as well as ragged, are clustered around a rickety table that is covered with worn-out oilcloth. They are eating biscuits and red-eye gravy (made by adding water to the frying pan in which ham has been cooked) from mismatched chipped dishes. Some are whining for more, but are told sharply that that is all there is. An interview with an adult reveals that this is a typical meal. On payday there will be peas, meat, and cornbread; this may last a few days. But, most of the time the children are hungry. The father has no regular job, and there never is enough money.

(b) Black migrant workers in a camp in Florida. Meals are cooked twice a day when they are working. There is a heavy meal in the morning and leftovers go to the field for later. A boiled meal of peas has cooked all day and is ready at night. There is a communal atmosphere. Meals are eaten out in the open as the shack barely has sleeping room. An interview with an adult reveals that they work all month at times and occasionally make as much as $400, but most of the time they work less and make about $200. Because they move around, participation in the Food Stamps Program is impossible.

(c) Poor whites of European extraction in Appalachia are seen in the next scenario. There is the father in his baggy bib-top coveralls and corncob pipe, the frazzled mother in an ill-fitting worn housedress, and several dirty, barefoot ragged children that are dull and listless. The family is clustered around a rickety table eating stew that is mostly potatoes and gravy from mismatched, cracked and chipped dishes under the glare of a bare bulb. Bread is used to sop up the gravy. An interview with the father reveals that the family lives on welfare, has Food Stamps, and purchases potatoes, cabbage, celery, onions, beets, carrots, hamburger, stew meat, some franks and sausages, noodles, and white bread. These, with a few staples such as flour, sugar, and coffee, make up the diet.

(d) Native American Indians (Navajos) are shown in traditional dress in front of a shack in a desolate expanse of desert. Shots of children herding sheep and hoeing corn, beans, and squash are shown. The pot of beans is cooking on a fire in front of the shack. An interview with the adults reveals that cash income is almost nil; they do not participate in Food Stamps or other government programs because they live too far from town to deal with office visits, forms, and food delivery. Almost no foods are purchased except a few items at the trading post. They grow corn, beans, squash, tomatoes, and chilis. They purchase flour, sugar, salt, and some other staples. Coffee, cookies, etc., are purchased occasionally as a treat.

(e) Mexican-American braceros in California are shown in a migrant worker camp in front of a worn-out stucco building. The family eats typical Chicano foods supplemented with soft drinks. Everybody is wearing colorful assorted ragged clothes. The interview with the adults reveals that annual income is $4100 for a family of 6. They bring home fruits and vegetables from the field, in season. They may participate in government feeding programs. Breakfast is coffee, beans, and tortillas. Lunch is beans and/or tortillas, stew, and a beverage which may be soft drinks, Kool Aid, or beer. Dinner is beans and/or meat, rice or potatoes, tortillas, and the same assortment of beverages as at noon; a dessert may be served.

These stereotypes reflect the fact that poverty is a bad situation. These were class representative families, carefully selected to get the points across. Points were:

(a) The mean income was too low; there was no way to obtain a decent assortment of foods so as to supply all of the nutrients.

(b) The needy poor did not participate in the government feeding programs because of lack of access. They were too mobile, the distances were too great, or some other factor made the mechanism too difficult.

(c) The diet was too limited. Whole classes of foods were absent, meat was provided in token amounts, fruits and vegetables were few, and dairy products were almost nonexistent.

(d) The diets were too high in salt, starch, sugar, and fat.

(e) The meal climate was drab and depressing. Table appointments were atrocious and scarce.

(f) Family cooking facilities were poor. There was insufficient storage, refrigeration was lacking, and the range might be wood or coal-burning.

All of these points were well taken. As a result of the impact of this documentary film and its sequelae, Americans became aroused.

THE WHITE HOUSE CONFERENCE ON FOOD, NUTRITION, AND HEALTH

The fact that many Americans suffered from hunger and/or malnutrition was distressing, especially in the midst of material abundance and wealth. This was embarrassing and intolerable. So, the White House Conference was called to address the problem. The remarks of the President at the opening session are quoted in part:

This meeting marks an historic milestone. What it does is to set the seal of urgency on our national commitment to put an end to hunger and malnutrition due to poverty in America. . .

At the same time, it marks the beginning of a new, more determined and more concerted drive than ever before, to reduce malnutrition that derives from ignorance or inadvertence. . .

Until this moment in our history as a nation, the central question has been whether we as a nation would accept the problem of malnourishment as a national responsibility. . .

That moment is past. . . Speaking for this administration, I not only accept the responsibility—I claim the responsibility. . .

. . .There is a moral imperative. . . we must because we can. . . This Nation cannot long continue to live with its conscience if millions of its own people are unable to get an adequate diet. . .

A child ill-fed is dulled in curiosity, lower in stamina, distracted from learning. A worker ill-fed is less productive, often absent from work. The mounting costs of medical care for diet-related illnesses; remedial education required to overcome diet-related slowness in school; institutionalization and loss of full productive potential; all of these place a heavy economic burden on society as a whole.[1]

---

[1]From Nixon (1970).

From this text, it is clear that the Nixon administration had been well primed. The statements set the tone, but allowed for news coverage which, as a result of sensationalism, became an exposé.

There were several important outcomes of this conference. The first was recognition of the need for continuing surveillance and evaluation of the nutritional status of Americans. The second was a set of guidelines for nutriture of nutritionally vulnerable groups. The right to an adequate diet was affirmed as was the right to tactful handling to avoid stigmatization.

The outcomes of the WHC were expansion and strengthening of the federal food assistance programs so as to reach more of those at nutritional risk, an increase in the nutrition education component so as to upgrade the knowledge of those receiving assistance so that wise nutritional choices could be made, and continued attention to the nutritional vulnerability of some segments of the American population.

A commitment has been publicly reaffirmed, some mechanisms have been strengthened, and some new approaches added. Still, the problems of hunger and malnutrition remain and do not seem any nearer to solution.

INTERVENTION: POINTS TO PONDER

Undeniably, hunger and malnutrition are risky as well as unpleasant. In America, few actually starve to death but many suffer from reduced mental and physical capacity. Life expectancy is probably reduced as well.

Most of the federal monies spent to improve the nutritional status of the American people is spent on the poor, with few indications of improved nutriture. The poor are a heterogeneous group; low income is probably the only basis of commonality. Therefore, many kinds of assistance may be necessary to remedy and/or relieve various aspects of the multifaceted problem that creates/maintains nutritional risk. Some understanding is a necessary prerequisite to a functional relationship. Consider the following:

(a) Some of the poor have had a limited food experience because cost has been a severely limiting restriction. Therefore, they may not be very receptive to new items or combinations unless accepted by someone they know and respect. This presents a challenge in utilization of foods as sources of nutrients. An informal leader and word of mouth may do what a formal approach cannot.

(b) Some of the poor are powerless to improve their nutriture with the food money they have. They are relatively unskilled in knowledge of the nutrient composition of foods and do not know how to use nutrition labeling to good advantage.

(c) Some of the poor feel deprived of the normal satisfaction of food needs. Therefore, they are not motivated to make the best nutritional choices they might; other aspects related to foods are more important.

(d) Some of the poor are in an insecure position; on a continuing basis, demands exceed income. So, they go from crisis to crisis. Therefore, since they must meet fixed expenses for home, transportation, etc., they often use money earmarked for food for these purposes. IF by chance they do have a few dollars available, THEN they may spend the money for a feast. They probably will not purchase extra staples to raise the usual intake by a smidgen.

(e) Some of the poor show anomie, i.e., conventional social standards or concepts related to eating behavior have no influence on their beliefs, attitudes, intentions, or behavior. A different set of norms applies. A non-judgmental attitude is necessary to bridge this gap.

(f) Some of the poor are isolated in self-defense, so that they are difficult to reach with an offer of assistance. They take a position that translates, "No one is going to care that much about what happens to you when you get right down to it." Therefore, anyone who tries to intervene is viewed with suspicion, i.e., this translates to "What's in it for them?" Therefore, the first step is to create a trusting relationship and to avoid meddling.

(g) Some of the poor are resigned to the fact that most foods are beyond their reach. In defense, they tend to deny the existence of desired but unobtainable items. This defense is effective. Otherwise, their raw nerve endings would signal deprivation to such a degree that they would become frustrated and angry and would be likely to act in a socially unacceptable manner, such as steal or riot. Thus, it is not only cruel but dangerous to tantalize them with off-again, on-again programs.

(h) Some of the poor are inadvertently poor; they have the same background, values, and attitudes as middle-class people. They are easily offended by denigrating circumstances or encounters.

Limited Access

Until the late 1960s, relief programs were structured to deal with problems of poverty on a walk-in basis. This definition of responsibility meant that no matter how many needy families there were in American society, only those that sought help were of interest or concern. But, at that time it became apparent that for undefined reasons those who needed help most were reluctant to seek it. Investigation showed that the problem was one of limited access.

Access has two sets of meanings, i.e., permission or ability to enter or communicate with or to make use of and a way or means of approach. In relation to the food and people interaction, limited access means:

(a) permission to enter a food assistance program—This is given only if a person meets stated criteria and can fill in the forms. This depends on ability and presents a problem to many of the poor because the criteria, while uniformly applied, do not always make sense and the bureaucrat uses a procedure where judgment is required. Needy people are excluded in this way. Moreover, the forms are very complex and tedious. The ideas are sometimes beyond the capacity of people with low mentality or who are senile. The forms are often unreadable; uneducated people cannot deal with the long legal terms and the elderly who have limited vision can only read large print, but the text is in fine print. In an effort to prevent/control cheating, questions are asked in such a way that people with some pride are offended and refuse to answer. For any or all of these reasons, permission to enter a program is denied.

(b) ability to communicate with—Poor people and minorities have difficulty in communicating needs to authorities, so they get no help. This seems to be because people in power positions cannot relate to the needs of poor people so they fail to provide a channel for communication; defensive attitudes such as anomie, powerlessness, suspicion, and distrust interfere. So, for these reasons, when the poor fill in the forms they do not give the whole story or it does not fit what is wanted in some way, so access is denied.

(c) ability to make use of—The program may be there and the person/ family may qualify, but some intervening variable may prevent its use to good advantage. For example, with the Food Stamps program, the purchase of food stamps requires possession of cash at the place and time where the food stamps are dispensed. To use all of the food assistance programs requires many trips to the office for interviews with the caseworker. This takes time and transportation, which many poor do not have. What does one do with three pre-school children while one waits two or more hours in line at the office? What if your health is not up to the trip plus the two-hour wait? Commodities are given out at fixed intervals in quantities that will last the interim. How much food can one carry home in a shopping cart? What if one does not have enough refrigerated storage to handle the quantity? What if meals are delivered at home and one does not like the food served? What if one cannot eat some/all of the items for health or religious reasons? What if the meals are good at the congregate meal sites but one is too embarrassed to go because his/her clothes are not good enough? What if one just is not up to making the effort to get dressed and go? What if one does not like or is offended by the other people at the site? What if one makes the effort and then is unable to eat the food?

(d) a way or means of approach—The WIC program provides money and supplemental foods for infants and mothers. But, if the mother spends the money and cooks the food, can she refuse to share it with other family members? The School Lunch program is set up to meet one-third of the nutritive needs of a 9- to 12-year-old. But, is this much help to teenagers? The School Lunch is provided 5 days a week and meets one-third of the needs of a 9- to 12-year-old—but, IF the family can predict that the child will receive this meal, THEN no other food may be provided for the child. Is the child better or worse off?

The problems are very complex. Other aspects also are noted by nutritionists. For example, the programs are funded in the short run. This limits access; it is a limited approach since most people must eat several times a day, every day, for a lifetime. And, IF a family qualifies for only one program, but needs a combination of all of them in order to meet the varying needs of all family members, THEN single programs are only a limited approach to the problem.

MALNUTRITION

Major urban medical centers in the United States have reported a small number of patients admitted for malnutrition. Often such cases are limited to children or the elderly who are suffering from the severe forms of malnutrition that are life-threatening. Protein-calorie malnutrition (PCM) is the general term for starvation-related emaciation. *Kwashiorkor* is the type that occurs when protein intake is deficient. Its prevalence is greatest among children one to four years of age. It occurs even when caloric intake is sufficient. Visible manifestations are retarded growth and development, irritability, lassitude, edema, muscular wasting, depigmented hair and skin, and scaly skin texture. Other manifestations are hypoalbuminemia, fatty liver, decreased pancreatic enzyme secretion, anemia, hypokalemia, and hypernatremia. *Marasmus* is the type that occurs when both protein and calorie intake are chronically insufficient. Visible manifestations are gross emaciation—wasted fat and muscle tissue, retarded growth and development, and shriveled facial aspect. Unlike kwashiorkor, in marasmus there is usually little or no edema, depigmentation of the hair or skin, or scaly skin changes. Other manifestations are low serum protein and reduced liver function due to protein depletion. Senile starvation is the adult form of PCM that is suffered by some of the elderly.

BIBLIOGRAPHY

NIXON, R.M. 1970. Message of the President to the Congress of the United States. *In* White House Conference on Food, Nutrition, and Health. Final Report. GPO, Washington, D.C.

24

Nutritional Risk and Life Expectancy: Preventive Diets

Recently, the concept of eating for health has been expanded to accommodate a preventive aspect. The notion of a preventive diet is an outgrowth of research concerning the etiology of killer diseases. *Prevent* is one of a class of words which mean to stop something from occurring. Specifically, it implies taking advance measures against X, which is a possible or probable effect or event. It differs from *preclude*, which implies the shutting out of every possibility of X happening or taking effect—an impossible dream.

Preventive measures can be implemented in a variety of ways for varying levels of control. On the one hand, the strictures can be so limiting that the diet is austere and unlikely to be followed on a continuing basis. Or, they may be so mild that they are ineffective in reducing risk.

Advocacy of specific preventive diets is highly controversial, since none has yet been demonstrated as effective for the entire population and no comprehensive study of the economic and other effects has been conducted. Nonetheless, the concept of a preventive diet has merit and is gaining support. What is at issue needs to be understood so that one can take an informed position.

THE DIETS

The basic diets for prevention of obesity and cardiovascular disease have been designed for adults. These are presented below.

Obesity—The Diet-Exercise Regime

In order to implement a preventive weight control diet, one's beliefs, attitudes, intentions, and overt behavior must be integrated around a focus of appropriate weight as something of remarkable value. Appropriate weight should be regarded as a commendable asset reflecting the height of physical thriving and achievement.

As a preventive diet, a *fixed regimen* with numerous strictures *cannot work.* Lack of harmony between a fixed energy supply and a variable demand creates a continuous stress. This affliction is aggravated by imposition of restrictions and leads to rebellion. What is necessary is to govern intake and accommodate variation in the availability of food to bodily needs that are created as the tissues serve their special purposes. An internalized monitoring and control system with a governor is the only mechanism by which an optimal solution can be achieved.

A weight control diet to be followed for 40 years differs from one designed to be followed for 40 days on a crash basis. It is a "free" diet with no strictures and no gimmicks. It is no easier and no less difficult than a corrective diet, but it is different.

The governor should be set for an eating input of at least 1800 calories. This is the minimum recommended on a continuing basis under normal circumstances. IF this level of caloric input exceeds caloric output, THEN increased physical activity is less hazardous than additional caloric restriction. This is because the likelihood of meeting needs for the other nutrients is much less at lower caloric intake levels. Nutrient density in ordinary foods is just not sufficient, and wise selection for increased density would be restrictive and impossible in the long run. The resulting monotony and inconvenience would lead to abandonment. Of course, specified nutrients can be supplied by carefully selected supplements. But, not all nutrients are available in supplement form.

A "free" diet is ideal. It allows for the following:

(a) Unlimited choice in terms of eating frequency and the quantity of food consumed at a particular feeding. This flexibility facilitates maintenance of normal food and people interactions, which reduces the probability of rebellion.

(b) Unlimited choice of eating territory, since no special items are necessary and there is no item that is restricted. Again, this flexibility reduces the probability of rebellion.

(c) Unlimited choice with respect to which items and combinations may be consumed, within and among days. Thus, one may at a particular feeding consume the same subset of items as one's companions; this avoids awkwardness.

(d) Unlimited choice in terms of which items will be consumed in limited quantity and the extent of the limitation.

The cumulative and aggregate caloric intake must be regulated at the level at which the governor is set. A "free" diet requires that choices be made as a positive action. Thus, freedom is not free. Choices must be made within and among days in respect to the following:

(a) which feeding(s) will be eliminated or reduced in size

(b) which eating territory will be utilized with reduced frequency

(c) which items or combinations will be consumed with the quantity and/or frequency adjusted

One may opt for maximum freedom of choice, which requires that one keep a running total as a basis for decision. Or, one may predetermine some aspects as a matter of simplification. In this case, one selects a meal pattern or a cluster of patterns that can be followed in random order. Meal components are defined and limit the caloric intake accordingly. One of these methods is not better than another in any absolute sense; effectiveness is related to appropriateness for a particular individual. Those whose work-life is structured may prefer the running total option and the accompanying challenge to think through the "best" selection each time, utilizing a game approach. Others, whose work-life demands decisiveness all day may be relieved of the responsibility for details by using a pattern(s) of self-selected choices.

A corrective diet requires a sharp reduction in caloric intake. As this results in physiologic stress, medical supervision is wise. Dietetic counseling also has merit; information on modified food preparation techniques, nutrient density, and food products can build confidence, aid in adjusting habits, and reduce frustration. A variety of alternatives including fasting, liquid formula diets, diet pills, and special fad diets is available. But, these are *not* recommended under normal circumstances since they usually cannot be utilized for more than six weeks, which is insufficient for more than a small weight loss. They also may lead to complications. Since they do not retrain habits, even if they do result in weight loss, it is likely to be temporary. The preventive diet outlined above would be a necessary sequel for long-term success. More drastic measures are not warranted except in life-threatening cases.

Cardiovascular Disease—The Prudent Diet

There are no proven ways to prevent atherosclerosis, a major form of cardiovascular disease. Therefore, the need for implementation of a preventive diet is a matter of controversy among experts. As usual, some experts are rash and were early advocates of drastic dietary changes, others are more moderate and advocate the Prudent Diet, and still others are even more cautious and advocate no dietary changes until more is known. So, each individual must take a position.

A recent paper (Reiser 1978) provides a statement of the points against the 300 mg cholesterol limit. The basic difficulty with this recommendation is that while it might be advisable for hyperlipidemic individuals, there is no evidence that justifies generalization to normolipidemic persons. Moreover, some hyperlipidemics who need medical care may be misled and may develop a false sense of security. And, implementation of this recommendation by the majority who are normolipidemics would deprive them of traditional, nutritious desired foods such as eggs, dairy products, liver, beef, and pork. Unless these restrictions can be demonstrated to reduce the risk of a heart attack, it appears to be an unjustified and possibly harmful recommendation.

Like the cholesterol limit, each of the other Prudent Diet recommendations has been criticized. The thrust of each point is fairly well accepted; the stipulated level is more controversial.

The Prudent Diet, which is advocated by the American Heart Association and other groups, is based on a concept that derives from the old Puritan idea of avoiding excess. The idea of prudence is to show caution as to danger or risk. The means is to govern and discipline oneself in relation to diet intake by use of reason. Within this framework of prudence, a rationale has been developed that supports implementation of the following goals for the American population:

(a) to encourage individuals to reduce their caloric intake so as to maintain ideal weight

(b) to decrease the national mean lipid intake from 42 to 45% calories to 35%

(c) to change the ratio of polyunsaturated fatty acids to saturated fatty acids to 1

(d) to decrease the national mean dietary cholesterol intake from 800 to 300 mg per day

(e) to decrease the national mean dietary sugar intake from 1½ cups per day to between ¼ cup and ½ cup; to increase intake of starch and fiber

(f) to increase the proportion of calories from protein by increasing intake of fish and/or vegetable proteins

(g) to decrease salt intake from a national mean of 15 g/day to 5 g/day

(h) to decrease consumption of alcoholic beverages to one serving per day

Not all people need to make such extensive dietary changes. Nonetheless, each individual is encouraged to adjust food consumption as follows:

(a) High saturated fat meats, e.g., beef, lamb, and pork—intake to be decreased to 4 4-oz portions per week (cooked weight).

(b) Moderately high saturated fat meats, e.g., veal, chicken, and turkey—intake to be increased to 4 4-oz portions per week (cooked weight).

(c) Fish—intake to be increased to 6 4-oz portions per week (cooked weight).

(d) Super-high saturated fat meats—e.g., liver, heart, brain, and shell-fish—intake to be limited to 1 4-oz portion per week (cooked weight).

(e) Eggs—intake to be decreased to 4 per week (all uses).

(f) High fat/cholesterol dairy products, e.g., hard cheese, whole milk, butter, ice cream—intake to be eliminated; items to be replaced with modified low-fat/low cholesterol non-dairy substitutes.

(g) Shortening—to be replaced by oil.

(h) Standard gravies and sauces to be eliminated or prepared without fat.

(i) Salt—intake to be decreased by limiting use of salt-cured foods, salty snack foods, and elimination of table salting.

(j) Sugar—intake to be decreased by severe restriction of candy and desserts.

(k) Starch and fiber intake to be increased by systematic inclusion of whole grain bread and cereal products. Fruit and vegetable consumption to be continued at current or expanded levels.

The above guide to the number of servings of particular critical kinds of foods to be limited is applicable to men consuming diets of more than 2500 kcal. It is inappropriate for women consuming 1800 kcal diets or less, as the number of servings of meat of the stipulated portion size would result in a protein intake greatly exceeding the recommended 45 g or 12 to 15% kcal. Fat intake also would exceed 35% kcal, unless all other fat were omitted from the diet. The simplest approximation would be to halve the portion sizes.

In order to implement this preventive diet, a very different set of beliefs, attitudes, intentions, and eating behavior is necessary. The Prudent Diet is the basis for a set of food habits that are expected to be followed for 40 years or so. It is moderate in the sense that meats and eggs are not eliminated. Nevertheless, it is very difficult for free-living adults to follow consistently. Shopping is extra time-consuming and often there is frustration as well as additional expense associated with purchase of fat-modified food products. Modified food preparation methods must be learned. Fish and meats not customarily consumed must become the usual fare. And, the frequency of eating in restaurants must be minimized because of lack of control of fat and salt content of foods.

On the absolute scale, it is a moderate diet and is prudent as well. Relative to customary indulgence resulting from affluence, abundance, and variety, it seems austere. But, it is much easier to accept than is one of the therapeutic fat-controlled diet plans, which are similar in nature but more severe in extent. The choice becomes prevention versus taking the risk of care.

IF the concept of prevention is to bear fruit, THEN a dietary assessment should be a routine part of the annual physical examination. At the outset, the concepts of risk and prevention should be explained. Next, expected outcomes related to varying levels of compliance should be outlined as a basis for choice. Then, a typical sample diet intake should be evaluated against the standard of the goals outlined above to identify areas for improvement. A review of the goals and implications should be presented as a basis for motivation. Finally, one (or more) area(s) for improvement should be selected to start with (goal setting) toward the first approximation to the Prudent Diet. This approach is less threatening; it does not overwhelm a person. Subsequent annual assessments should review progress, reinforce points, and retarget goals for increasingly closer approximations to the Prudent Diet. Interim follow-up consultations should be scheduled as necessary to facilitate progress toward goal attainment.

DISCUSSION

People dread the killer diseases; to develop one is a major catastrophe. There is *no cure for damaged vital tissue* since it does not regenerate. Once the damage is done, symptoms may be reduced in severity by compensation or replacement but the effects cannot be eliminated nor can the original condition be restored. Therefore, the notion that prevention is better than cure is a misconception. *Prevention is a necessity, not just the best alternative.*

Obesity and cardiovascular disease are mass maladies that are prevalent to an excessive degree in the American population at the present time. Like all epidemics, they surfaced as a result of disturbances in the human culture. In vulnerable individuals, the capacity to cope was overtaxed.

Diet-related aspects of life-style appear to be critical variables that could be manipulated in reducing the risk. In recognition of this fact, preventive diets are advocated. And, implementation in childhood is the ultimate goal.

Implementation in childhood is advocated since lifelong eating habits and other aspects of adult lifestyle at least have their antecedents in, and may be developed in, childhood. Moreover, the cumulative and aggregate effects as a preventive measure are greater.

Nonetheless, the wisdom of implementing these dietary changes in childhood has been challenged by questioning whether such changes might result in decreased myelinization of brain and CNS tissue, decreased absorption and/or transport of fat-soluble vitamins, and/or in early development of gall bladder disease. An acknowledged medical expert, Antonio M. Gotto, Jr., testified to the "McGovern Committee" that at the present time no hazard has been demonstrated with respect to these conditions, and even the potential hazard is small. Thus, fears seem unjustified.

This is not to imply that these changes can be implemented mechanically. In making the necessary dietary substitutions, care must be exercised so that the supply of all nutrients is maintained at an adequate level. Intakes of fat, cholesterol, sugar, salt, and alcohol must be controlled on a lifelong basis. However, with the exception of alcohol, intake quantities need to be adjusted to needs that vary with the physiological demands associated with the various stages of the life cycle. Adjustment is particularly important during the periods of growth and development, i.e., infancy, childhood, adolescence, pregnancy, and lactation. The adjustments provide a challenge but are not impossible. The hope that such an achievement brings makes the effort worthwhile.

CHEATING ON DIETS AND OTHER ABERRATIONS

A preventive diet is meant to be followed consistently as a lifelong habit. Consistency is the key to hope of benefit. But, most people lack sufficient discipline and have a need for structure and sanctions to help them deal with temptations. Otherwise, they cannot adhere to a diet over time. At the same time, they tend to rebel against whatever structure is proposed/provided. Hence, the phenomenon of cheating on diets occurs.

To cheat means to violate the rules using trickery that escapes observation. Society cannot pursue all of the cheats in every domain, for the possibilities are endless. So, people have learned that they may get by or they may be called to account.

One can cheat only if one is following a set of rules on what to eat/not eat that is imposed by somebody else who is in an authority position. Unless one is engaged in self-delusion, one cannot escape oneself and self-observation. This means that any acts of non-compliance are not cheating but are deliberate and irresponsible. The threat of being exposed when one must explain one's beliefs, attitudes, intentions, and/or behavior is a powerful deterrent. It is for this reason that individuals must be held personally responsible and individually accountable, if only to themselves.

Acceptance of personal responsibility is a "safe" course of action. IF a person accepts personal responsibility for control of dietary intake, THEN preventive diets are "free" within the constraints of designated caloric and fat (or other nutrient) levels. Therefore, the decisions governing what and how much an individual may eat in a particular instance are a matter of discretion. Any food may be eaten in some quantity, as long as its contribution is counted in the daily accounting. Therefore, eating some portion of any food is not cheating, so long as it is taken into account.

The challenges associated with adhering to a diet in the long run may require all of the strength one can muster. Consider the problem of food binges. Some people are subject, intermittently, to a strong and compelling force that drives them to eat food X recklessly with no restraint. Given an opportunity and a weakness that facilitates gratifying one's desires, a food binge can result when (a) a mood or whim initiates it or (b) there is a felt need to escape from a situation that requires excessive compliance. Some people respond to the urge by eating in general. They just have to eat something and are not particular about what. Others, e.g., "chocoholics," respond to the urge by eating a particular food.

Undeniably, this kind of deviation is counter-productive. It must be acknowledged and dealt with. Otherwise, erosion sets in and the individual soon develops an "it doesn't matter" attitude and abandons the diet effort. Any strategy that helps an individual to resist the urge should be encouraged.

BIBLIOGRAPHY

REISER, R. 1978. Oversimplification of diet: coronary heart disease relationships and exaggerated diet recommendations. Am. J. Clin. Nutr. *31*, 865-875.

25

Nutritional Risk and Life Expectancy: Pregnancy

In the United States, we often agree and do nothing—up to a point. Then, moral indignation brings immediate attention to the problem. Recently, moral indignation regarding the problems of hunger and malnutrition of pregnant women manifested itself. The following statement was published in the proceedings of the White House Conference on Food, Nutrition, and Health (1970):

There must be a national affirmation that every woman has the right to high quality and high standard health care. This includes a food intake that will prepare her for and carry her through a healthy pregnancy and childbirth and permit her infant to flourish. It affirms that the right to adequate nutrition is an inseparable part of the basic right to health care and that women require and are entitled to sufficient amounts of nutritious food.

The implications and ramifications of this statement are far-reaching. Pregnancy inflates nutritional needs, making the pregnant woman and her unborn infant vulnerable. In a family with limited food availability (quantity and/or quality), they are affected first and suffer most. The condition of the infant at birth and the possibility of complications for the mother are increased by malnutrition. Thus, both are at risk when malnourished. Risky situations are to be avoided and risk is to be reduced to the extent possible.

Despite general affluence and advanced medical care, neonatal and infant morbidity and mortality rates have been higher than expected for some time. The United States ranks 15th out of 40 nations rated (1969 ranking, latest available). As a result, in 1966 the National Research Council created a Committee on Maternal Nutrition which made recommendations for study of causes and remedies.

PREGNANCY: NORMAL SUPPLY AND NORMAL DEMAND

Pregnancy, a biologically normal state for a woman who is physiologically mature, inflates the physiologic demand for *all* nutrients. Increased supply of all nutrients is necessary to (a) support growth and development of both maternal and fetal tissues and (b) build normal maternal and fetal reserves of selected nutrients. So, nutriture is a critical variable in the outcome of a pregnancy.

The influence of the quality of prematernal nutrition on conception and the outcome of pregnancy was first documented systematically during World War II in Holland where rations from October 1944 to May 1945 were limited to 1000 kcal, including 30 to 40 g protein. Observed effects were:

(a) babies conceived prior to the hunger period—As the proportion of the gestational period during the hunger period increased, the length and/or birth weight of the baby tended to decrease. There was no increase in the rate of stillbirths, prematurity, or malformations.

(b) babies conceived during the hunger period—The rate of conception decreased as did size, as noted above.

Next, Burke and co-workers confirmed and expanded information on the effect of diet quality on the condition of the newborn. Using the then current standards for evaluation of dietary quality they showed that babies born to mothers consuming diets rated good to excellent were in good to excellent condition at birth. In contrast, those born to mothers consuming diets rated poor were likely to be rated poor (stillborn, premature, died within three days of birth, had congenital defects, or were functionally immature).

Subsequent work has demonstrated that because growth and development are most rapid during this stage of the life-cycle, nutrient demand is greatest. Moreover, the fetus is fragile; this vulnerability leads to the greatest consequences.

The physiological demands for the various nutrients differ according to the anabolic activities associated with the point in the pregnancy. During some stages, the demands exceed usual capacity to supply from current intake. Therefore, needs are met, to the extent possible, from maternal reserves. Normally, maternal needs for nutrients other than calories are met from pre-pregnancy stores, so previous nutriture is important as a prepreparation. Normally, part of the caloric needs is met by early-stage increases in adipose tissue storage. Because the normal food supply for a human infant is human milk, which is not a good source of iron, fetal storage of iron is induced during the later stages of prenatal development. Thus, some depletion of maternal iron reserves is normal. In a woman who has been well nourished, this does not present a health hazard, although the reserves do need to be replenished if there is a possibility of additional pregnancies.

The inflated demand for all nutrients is unquestionable. However, the average requirement for all nutrients has not been determined. Therefore, recommendations for daily intake and rationale pertain only to selected nutrients. Therefore, also, the need to rely on foods as sources of unspecified nutrients is even greater.

At the present time, the normal range for weight gain during pregnancy is 20 to 25 lb. IF weight gain is 24 lb, THEN this weight, in pounds, is distributed as follows: (a) the infant, 7.7; (b) placental tissue, 1.4; amniotic and other body fluids, 4.5; (d) uterine tissue, 2.0; (e) mammary tissue, 0.9; (f) blood, 4.0, and (g) adipose tissue, 3.5. Anabolic processes involved in producing these various components create the demands. Current recommendations for supply and a summary of accepted rationale follow:

(a) calories—The estimated mean energy intake necessary for a normal pregnancy is 80,000 kcal. For an average length pregnancy, this is a mean intake of 300 kcal/day above the fixed non-pregnant allowance. The basal metabolic demand is increased in order to supply the extra tissues as well as growth and development needs; half of the extra calories are necessary to meet this need. During the first trimester, caloric needs are about 150 kcal above usual, so the difference is stored. During the remainder of gestation, demands are about 350 kcal/day so normally some of the adipose stores are used. Reserve energy stores are also utilized during labor.

Activity level determines the variable portion of the energy requirement. The other half of the recommended intake covers this need and includes an allowance for individual differences. IF physical activity is reduced during the last trimester of pregnancy, THEN caloric intake must be adjusted accordingly or unwanted weight gain will occur. Usual caloric intake may suffice. Norms for weight gain have been established; the pattern of an individual's weight gain needs to be monitored and compared with the norms. Too rapid, too slow, or any sharp change calls for correction in intake.

The recommended minimum caloric intake is 1800 to 2000 kcal, irrespective of maternal size. This recommendation recognizes that the possibility of fetal nutritional deprivation should be avoided and that below this intake level nutritional adequacy is unlikely. IF overweight, THEN weight is not corrected unless absolutely necessary, and then only under medical supervision.

(b) protein of high biologic value—The gross mean protein requirement is 925 g, which is used for growth and development of accessory maternal tissue and fetal tissue, both of which have a sizeable protein base. This is the basis for a recommended mean increase of 30 g above the non-pregnant allowance, and assumes an energy intake above 36 kcal/kg to spare protein from energy usage.

(c) calcium and phosphate—The mean quantity of calcium deposited in the bones and teeth of the fetus, primarily during the last two months of gestation, is 28 g. To meet this need, an increase of 400 mg/per day is recommended. The usual recommendation to maintain the 1:1 calcium to phosphate ratio also applies.

Physiologic changes affect maternal calcium metabolism and possibly the requirement also. Only a partial explanation is presently available. The efficiency of absorption is increased, but not enough to meet the increased demand. Therefore, intake should be increased. During pregnancy, 25 g Ca are deposited in fetal tissue and 500 mg are dispersed in the placenta and amniotic fluid. An additional quantity is deposited in maternal tissues in preparation for lactation. Given the mean absorption level, the estimated requirement is a total of 350 g, to be supplied during the third trimester. This demand can be met from maternal bone stores since it is only 2.5% of the mean stored quantity. However, this is not recommended since the cumulative effect of repeated depletion associated with multiple pregnancies is osteomalacia. Dietary intake can be adequate. Use of calcium salts is unnecessary unless dietary intake is chronically low.

(d) iron—The mean quantity required for fetal blood supply and storage is 370 mg and for a 25% or more expansion of maternal blood supply plus what is lost on delivery is 290 mg—a total of 660 mg. The recommended intake is the sum of normal plus gestational needs. The normal needs are reduced for this period by 120 mg, the amount "saved" by cessation of menstruation. Therefore, the mean requirement is 540 mg. Given a 10% absorption norm and a high frequency of prematernal insufficiency, the recommended intake is an increase of 30 to 60 mg/day.

(e) iodine, sodium, magnesium, and zinc—The iodine requirement increases to support an increased metabolism; the recommended increase is 25 μg; which is provided by a normal iodized salt intake. Given the expanded blood volume, the sodium requirement is increased in order to maintain normal osmotic pressure; no recommendation has been made because the need is customarily met by normal salt intake. A recommended 150 mg increase in magnesium intake has been made, although recent research findings to support this are unavailable. A 5 mg increase in zinc intake is recommended in order to provide for fetal stores since human milk appears to supply less than the required amounts during the first few months of life.

(f) vitamin A—This requirement increases about 20 to 25%. This is necessary to meet needs for cell growth in accessory maternal as well as fetal tissues and tooth and bone formation. Mean fetal stores accumulated are 7000 μg.

(g) B vitamins—Metabolic processing associated with growth and development requires extra energy. The requirements for thiamin, riboflavin, and niacin are inflated accordingly. The recommendations have been increased by 0.4, 0.3, and 2 mg, respectively, per 300 kcal above non-pregnant intake. During pregnancy, the circulating folic acid levels of some women fall, which has been interpreted by some to mean that either a dietary deficiency or a metabolic alteration occurs. Until the point is resolved, the recommended intake is twice the non-pregnant level. During the third trimester of pregnancy, both the circulating and urinary excretion levels of pyridoxine fall. Here again, this finding may be attributed to deficient supply and/or metabolic alteration, so until this point is resolved, the recommended intake is increased by 0.6 mg. Limited evidence from studies of fetal content of B_{12} (stores of 50 to 100 μg) is the basis for a recommended intake increase of 1.0 μg.

(h) ascorbic acid—The requirement for ascorbic acid is increased by expanded utilization in forming intercellular cement and in increased iron absorption/utilization to support normal hemoglobin concentrations. The recommended intake increase is 10 mg.

From the above, it is clear that necessary increases for most nutrients are only modest. These are summarized in Table 25.1. A common rule is: IF protein needs are met, THEN all other nutrient needs are likely to be met, with the exceptions of vitamins A, C, and D. A corollary is: IF protein needs are not met, THEN intakes of calcium, phosphate, iron, and the B vitamins are likely to be low, since these nutrients are usually obtained from foods that supply protein. Indiscriminate self-medication with vitamin and/or mineral supplements is hazardous and routine prescription is not justified; both lead those with poor diets to a false sense of security, since all nutrients are not available in supplements.

PREGNANCY: DEFICIENT SUPPLY OR INFLATED DEMAND

Undernourishment can result from an absolutely deficient intake (poverty and/or ignorance) or a relatively deficient intake due to concurrent maternal growth and development demands in individuals who are not yet physiologically mature. Deprivation widens the gap between supply and demand, depleting any maternal stores and retarding growth and/or development of the fetus. Inflated demand depletes any stores and may retard maternal and/or fetal growth and/or development; the specific outcome depends on timing and magnitude of the gap.

Prenatal nutrition is inversely related to the probability of complications such as toxemia for the mother and poor condition at birth for the

TABLE 25.1. RECOMMENDED NUTRIENT INTAKE ALLOWANCES DURING PREGNANCY

FOOD AND NUTRITION BOARD, NATIONAL ACADEMY OF SCIENCES–NATIONAL RESEARCH COUNCIL RECOMMENDED DAILY DIETARY ALLOWANCES,[a] REVISED 1980

Designed for the maintenance of good nutrition of practically all healthy people in the U.S.A.

Category	Age (Years)	Weight (kg)	Weight (lb)	Height (cm)	Height (in.)	Protein (g)	Fat-Soluble Vitamins			Water-Soluble Vitamins		
							Vitamin A (μg R.E.)[b]	Vitamin D (μg)[c]	Vitamin E (mg α T.E.)[d]	Vitamin C (mg)	Thiamin (mg)	Riboflavin (mg)
Females	11–14	46	101	157	62	46	800	10	8	50	1.1	1.3
	15–18	55	120	163	64	46	800	10	8	60	1.1	1.3
	19–22	55	120	163	64	44	800	7.5	8	60	1.1	1.3
	23–50	55	120	163	64	44	800	5	8	60	1.0	1.2
Pregnant						+30	+200	+5	+2	+20	+0.4	+0.3
Lactating						+20	+400	+5	+3	+40	+0.5	+0.5

[a] The allowances are intended to provide for individual variations among most normal persons as they live in the United States under usual environmental stresses. Diets should be based on a variety of common foods in order to provide other nutrients for which human requirements have been less well defined.
[b] Retinol equivalents. 1 Retinol equivalent = 1 μg retinol or 6 μg β-carotene.
[c] As cholecalciferol. 10 μg cholecalciferol = 400 I.U. vitamin D.
[d] α-tocopherol equivalents. 1 mg d-α-tocopherol = 1 α T.E.
[e] 1 N.E. (niacin equivalent) = 1 mg of niacin or 60 mg of dietary tryptophan.

baby. Classic research studies have demonstrated that poor diet is associated with greater than normal prevalence of infants that are stillborn, premature, or die within three days, are functionally immature, and/or have other congenital defects.

A larger number of the infants born to teenagers who are not physically mature are low-birth-weight babies. The largest percentage of such babies is born to the nonwhite under-15-years age group. This is of concern since these babies are high-risk babies. Expected outcomes are discussed in Chapter 26.

Toxemia of pregnancy is a dreaded hazard suffered by more than 5% of pregnant women. It accounts for the majority of both maternal and fetal deaths. Recent clinical evidence has demonstrated that the liver damage which is the immediate cause results from malnutrition, especially the type resulting from poverty. Common clinical symptoms are hypertension, edema, and albuminuria. Rarely are convulsions and coma seen. The optimal treatment is nutritional therapy. A high protein/vitamin/mineral diet is used to correct these deficits. Protein intake is especially important to restore circulating plasma protein levels, which is necessary to eliminate the edema and albuminuria. To use a restricted sodium diet and/or a diuretic is to treat the clinical symptoms and not the problem. Such treatment also adds to the problem and endangers both maternal and fetal health by causing potassium loss.

Anemia is a complication, i.e., a problem factor that makes a successful outcome of pregnancy more difficult to achieve. It is common among, but not limited to, the poor. A combination of poor iron stores and deficient intake results in iron-deficiency anemia. Placental transfer of iron usually results in supplying fetal needs at maternal expense, manifested

Water-Soluble Vitamins				Minerals					
Niacin (mg N.E.)[i]	Vitamin B$_6$ (mg)	Folacin[j] (μg)	Vitamin B$_{12}$ (μg)	Calcium (mg)	Phosphorus (mg)	Magnesium (mg)	Iron (mg)	Zinc (mg)	Iodine (μg)
15	1.8	400	3.0	1200	1200	300	18	15	150
14	2.0	400	3.0	1200	1200	300	18	15	150
14	2.0	400	3.0	800	800	300	18	15	150
13	2.0	400	3.0	800	800	300	18	15	150
+2	+0.6	+400	+1.0	+400	+400	+150	[h]	+5	+25
+5	+0.5	+100	+1.0	+400	+400	+150	[h]	+10	+50

[i] The folacin allowances refer to dietary sources as determined by *Lactobacillus casei* assay after treatment with enzymes ("conjugases") to make polyglutamyl forms of the vitamin available to the test organism.

[g] The RDA for vitamin B$_{12}$ in infants is based on average concentration of the vitamin in human milk. The allowances after weaning are based on energy intake (as recommended by the American Academy of Pediatrics) and consideration of other factors such as intestinal absorption.

[h] The increased requirement during pregnancy cannot be met by the iron content of habitual American diets or by the existing iron stores of many women; therefore the use of 30–60 mg of supplemental iron is recommended. Iron needs during lactation are not substantially different from those of non-pregnant women, but continued supplementation of the mother for 2–3 months after parturition is advisable in order to replenish stores depleted by pregnancy.

by the anemia. Oral therapy, 200 mg/day, is the most common mode of treatment. It is continued three to six months following restoration of normal circulating levels of hemoglobin in order to replenish depleted stores. A megaloblastic anemia results from a deficient folic acid intake, reflecting negligible intakes of green vegetables and animal proteins. Supplementation is used in correction.

PREGNANCY: EXCESS SUPPLY AND DECREASED DEMAND

Traditionally, a woman was expected to gain weight during pregnancy and a fat baby usually was considered to be a healthy baby. So, given American living conditions at the turn of the century, a sizeable number of babies weighed 15 to 18 lb at birth. To reduce maternal weight gain to a reasonable level and to produce smaller babies that would be easier to deliver was an attractive and appropriate goal. Unfortunately, the means that evolved were not appropriate. This goal was achieved by imposition of a semi-starvation diet that was low in calories, protein, carbohydrate, water, and salt. Supporting notions were: (a) the "parasite theory"—the fetus will obtain what it needs from maternal stores and (b) the "maternal instinct theory"—IF the stores are insufficient, THEN the mother will crave and consume suitable foods to supply what is needed. In retrospect, this seems absurd.

Obesity is not considered desirable, so excessive weight gain during pregnancy is undesirable. The difficulty is that the necessary and sufficient amount appears to vary on an individual basis. The mean weight gain of 24 lb can be used only as a guide. A person who is very thin should expect to gain more than this in order to have a sufficient energy reserve.

One who is of normal weight might use this amount as a target. One who is above normal weight might be better off to gain somewhat less, i.e., 3 to 4 lb less.

During pregnancy is *not the time* to follow a rigorous weight reduction diet. First, low calorie diets tend to be less nutritious—undesirable at a time of inflated nutrient need. Secondly, the use of an alternative metabolic pathway for supply of energy during a period of greater than normal utilization is a physiologic insult.

Excessive intake of other nutrients is also to be avoided. There is no value in ingesting a quantity that creates stress. Placental transfer is efficient and IF the maternal circulating level of some nutrient is within toxicity range, THEN the possibility of fetal harm should be a consideration. At the present time, there is some evidence that suggests that routine ingestion of megadoses of ascorbic acid by the pregnant woman creates nutritional risk for the neonate by shifting its circulatory setpoint upward. The diet of the neonate, whether human milk or formula, is a poor source of ascorbic acid. The sharp drop in circulating level that results within a few days of birth is not well tolerated; the neonate goes through withdrawal.

PREGNANCY: FOOD ECOLOGY, NUTRITIONAL RISK, AND LIFE EXPECTANCY

From time immemorial, food-related beliefs, attitudes, intentions, and behavior during pregnancy have been one focus of interest and concern. Each culture has devised some means of control for the purpose of ensuring maternal and fetal health. In earlier times, a great body of folklore provided guidance and direction for feeding practices. As scientific knowledge became a more important basis for clinical advice, the common wisdom was replaced by supposition based on clinical observation. This in turn has given way to a newer approximation of the optimal diet which is based on research findings. Still, residuals of older belief systems and traditional practices remain and are adhered to by some American women.

Increasingly, nutritional risk has been recognized as one cumulative and aggregate effect of a complex of factors that include, but may not be limited to, psychosocial status, previous health, health practices, quality of health care received, dietary practices, motivational status, and exposure to environmental hazards. The number of combinations in which these can come together is almost infinite; the same effect can result from various combinations. The observed effects can be summarized as points along a continuum from high nutritional risk to low nutritional risk. High risk is associated with a high probability of complications or mortality for both the mother and infant.

Folk Beliefs and Dietary Practices

Since earliest times, the diet of a pregnant woman has been considered as an important factor in determining the physical, mental, and temperamental attributes of the infant. To ensure development of desired attributes, diet usually has been monitored and controlled according to elaborate sets of rules and rituals. The belief systems explicitly defined (a) which foods must be eaten and conditions for consumption—who, when, where, and how much; (b) which foods might be eaten on an optional basis or given specific circumstances; (c) which foods must not be eaten; and (d) which people, places, and things (including foods) must not be touched lest they become contaminated.

Although the intention of dietary control was to ensure consumption of an optimal diet, because the bases for beliefs were subject to error, some of the beliefs and practices that evolved were counter-productive. In large part, this probably was due to development of belief structures that reduced flexibility in adapting to changes in the common diet. For example, in the beginning, if the common diet of a poor people on subsistence level was primarily carbohydrates, then beliefs might encourage increased consumption of meat and/or milk but as affluence and abundance resulted in an increased customary intake of protein, the advice to consume more meat and/or milk might have become inappropriate.

Since the scientific era began, such beliefs/practices have been rejected by most people as superstitions, i.e., resulting from ignorance, fear of the unknown, or trust in magic or chance. Thus, the class of beliefs of the type that food X must not be eaten because it will cause a facial birthmark, a mongoloid, or other malformation was rejected. Similarly, the class of beliefs of the type that food X should be eaten because it will cause the baby to be strong, courageous, agile, etc., was rejected. Still, some of these beliefs persist and may be followed in addition to or instead of newer concepts.

Bizarre cravings for (a) specific items, e.g., watermelon in December, or (b) combinations, such as strawberries and dill pickles, are tolerated and indulged in in consideration of the woman's "condition." The origin of these beliefs is obscure. But, since they appear to make sense within the context of the "maternal instinct theory," indulgence is common.

Nutritional importance is a function of the item craved and the frequency of consumption. The appropriate response varies with the degree of nutritional effect. In most cases, the indulgence(s) is nutritionally unimportant. Acknowledgement, accompanied by an accepting attitude, will be the most productive strategem. (Any implication of nonacceptance and ridicule will terminate the relationship.) Otherwise, a nonthreatening but positive and constructive corrective action is necessary—for example, in the case of pica, a craving for starch, clay, soot or other practically inedible substance. Pica is a special case since such substances may be consumed in a large quantity on a daily basis, displacing nutritious foods.

Nausea and Vomiting

"Morning sickness" is a misery that many pregnant women complain of. The symptoms of nausea and vomiting are usually transitory and occur most frequently during the first trimester. Symptoms are attributed to hormonal changes and/or psychologic discomfort concerning the pregnancy which affects the nerves, activating the smooth muscles of the intestinal wall. Except in extreme cases, which may require hospitalization, no nutritional risk results. Dietary treatment suffices; small dry meals are alternated with beverage intake at frequent intervals. The items to be consumed should be selected carefully for acceptability and easy digestibility.

Other Food and People Interactions

Specific individual intolerances also may develop, e.g., radishes and cucumbers may result in heartburn, onions or green pepper may cause belching or hiccups, deep fat fried foods or carbonated beverages including beer may cause a stuffed feeling. Simple elimination of the offending item(s) is preferable to treatment with antacids, since these affect absorption of nutrients.

Recommended Food Additions

As previously indicated, it is difficult for a woman to meet her nutritional needs from regular table food since she requires a higher nutrient density than other family members. However, if her customary diet is nutritionally adequate, it should be continued. In meeting the inflated needs due to the pregnancy, the best alternative is the addition of 1 glass of skim milk (12 g CHO, 8 g protein, 90 kcal) and 2 oz meat (about 21 g protein and 190 kcal). This combination provides about 300 calories, increases B vitamin intake, and provides the additional calcium and phosphorus that are necessary. A serving of fruit or vegetable can be selected to provide the necessary amounts of vitamins A and C. IF her diet is not usually adequate, THEN the material presented in the previous section will be useful in planning a base diet.

THE SPECIAL SUPPLEMENTAL FOOD PROGRAM

The text of the 1975 Women, Infants and Children Nutrition Act states that Congress has found that pregnant women are at nutritional risk because of poor or inadequate nutriture. Factors creating nutritional risk were stipulated. These include, but are not limited to:

(a) potential or known inadequacy of customary nutrient intake pattern resulting from low income

(b) anemia

(c) prematurity or miscarriage

(d) abnormal maternal growth, i.e., undernutrition, obesity, or stunting

(e) maternal age under 18 years

(f) high frequency of pregnancy

The Special Supplemental Food Program for Women, Infants and Children (known as the WIC Program) was created as a remedy. Under this program, the nutrients to be supplied to a qualified pregnant woman (based on the 1974 RDA) are: protein, 46 to 76 g which is 60 to 100% of the RDA; calcium, 720 to 1200 mg which is 60 to 100% of the RDA; iron, 10.8 to 18 mg which is 60 to 100% of the RDA for non-pregnant women; vitamin A, 3000 to 5000 IU which is 60 to 100% of the RDA; ascorbic acid, 36 to 60 mg which is 60 to 100% of the RDA; and calories, 600 kcal which is 25% of the RDA (Select Comm. on Nutr. and Human Needs).

This program, like all other federal food programs, has been criticized for its limitations and failures in implementation. Still, its purpose has been achieved to the extent that some women who needed and consumed the foods made available under this program benefited. This intervention in their food ecosystem has a real effect for participants even if it is not reflected in published statistics.

Nutritional Risk and Life Expectancy

Research during the 1930s and 1940s scientifically confirmed the common sense idea that good nutritional status is related to the probability of a good outcome of pregnancy. Research during the 1950s demonstrated that maternal malnutrition was associated with life-threatening or mortal maternal and/or fetal outcomes. Research during the 1960s and 1970s revealed that even if dietary adequacy is achieved only through intervention during pregnancy, the outcome probabilities are greatly improved. Hence, the current emphasis is on decreased nutritional risk via modification of one or more aspects in the individual's food ecosystem.

BIBLIOGRAPHY

ANON. 1970. Report of Panel II-1 Pregnant and Nursing Women and Infants. *In* White House Conference on Food, Nutrition and Health. Final Report. GPO, Washington, D.C.

SELECT COMM. ON NUTRITION AND HUMAN NEEDS, U.S. SENATE. 1975. WIC Program Survey—1975. GPO, Washington, D.C.

26

Nutritional Risk and Life Expectancy: Infancy

Every person is an individual and assessment of status/progress must be on two bases, namely (a) *ipsative*, i.e., using the person as his own control, and (b) *normative*, i.e., using the appropriate reference group norms as a standard for comparison. Recent research has demonstrated that observed status/progress is the effect of the particular combination of a variety of factors that evolve. As both the number of factors and their combinations are innumerable, definite predictive statements of cause and effect that are generalizable are impossible. However, some common patterns can serve as a basis for discussion or for illustration. Nutriture and food ecology are two of the critical variables in the nurture of an infant, and they may determine whether the infant grows and/or develops according to the genetic potential with which it is endowed.

Growth rate and development rate are major parameters in evaluation of the effects of nutriture and food ecology on the status/progress of the infant. *Growth rate* refers to the rate of multiplication of cells, which determines organ size. *Development rate* refers to the degree of complexity of function of the organ, which determines the quality of its function. While growth and development norms (Fig. 26.1, 26.2) have been prepared from statistical observation and summarization, they should be used only as a standard for comparison. On an ipsative basis, a problem is indicated, for example, when a baby that ranks in the 50th percentile at birth on any parameter drops to the 40th by 3 months and to the 35th at 5 months. Similarly, a baby that ranks at the 50th percentile at birth on a parameter such as weight, ranks in the 60th and 75th percentiles at the 3rd and 5th months, respectively. When making a normative comparison, care must be used to avoid creating anxiety and/or guilt. IF an infant is otherwise healthy and growing at a reasonable rate on the ipsative scale, THEN there does not seem to be any

461

NCHS PERCENTILES*   NAME_____ _____ RECORD #_____

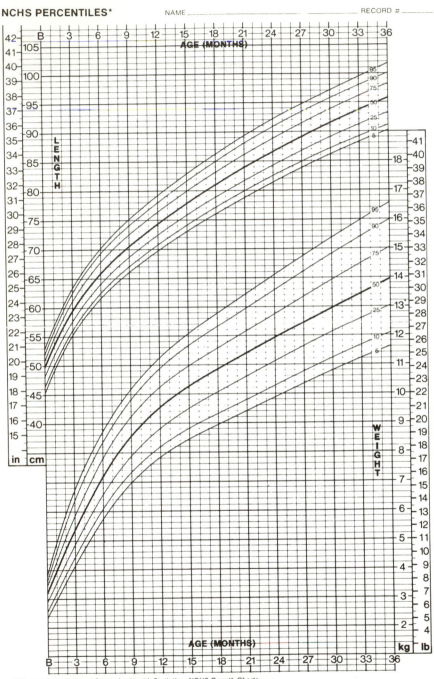

*Adapted from: National Center for Health Statistics: NCHS Growth Charts,
1976. Monthly Vital Statistics Report. Vol. 25, No. 3, Supp. (HRA) 76-1120.
Health Resources Administration, Rockville, Maryland, June, 1976.
Data from The Fels Research Institute, Yellow Springs, Ohio.

FIG. 26.1. SAMPLE RECORDING CHART OF PHYSICAL GROWTH BETWEEN BIRTH
AND 36 MONTHS OF AGE (GIRLS)

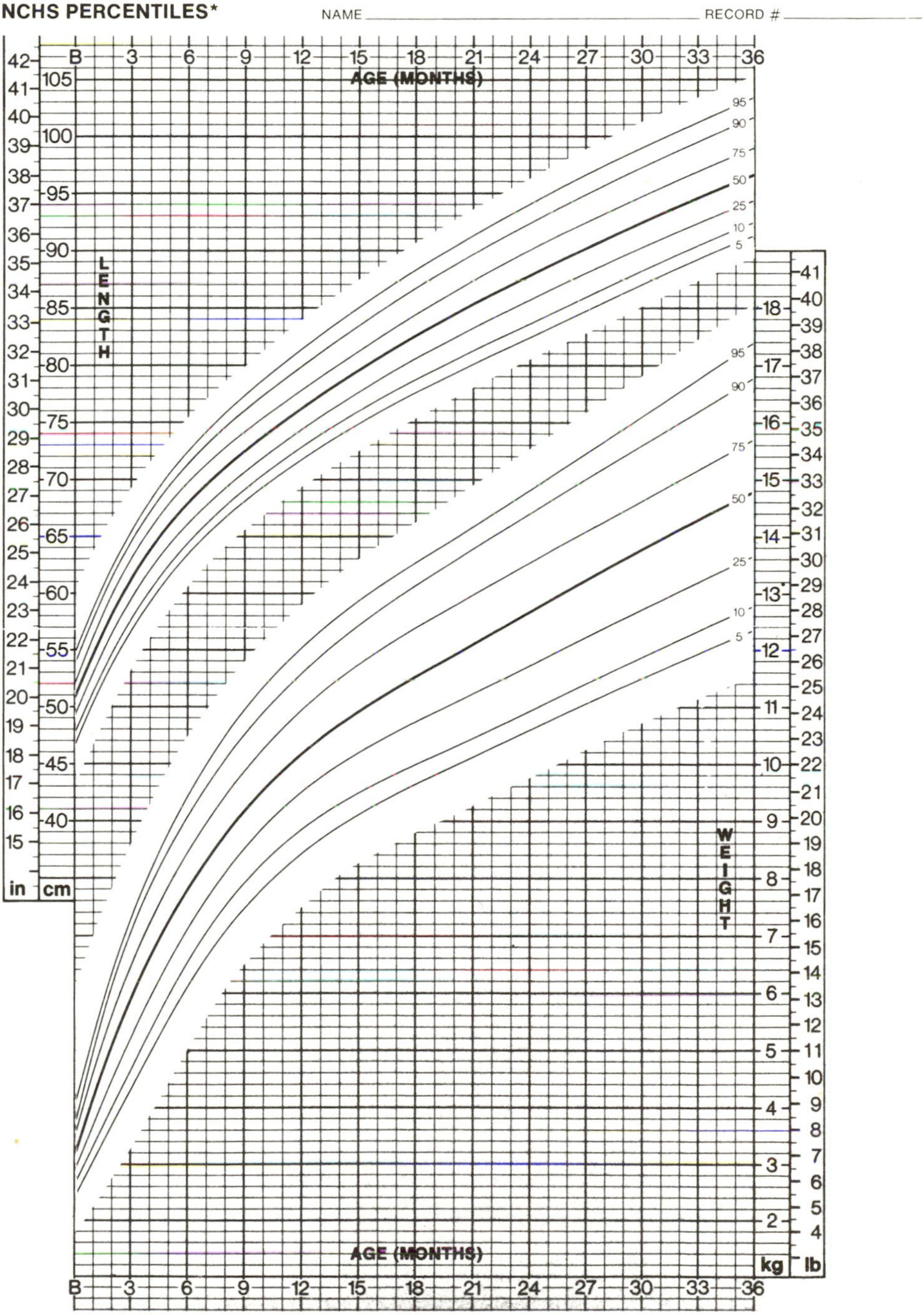

FIG. 26.2. SAMPLE RECORDING CHART OF PHYSICAL GROWTH BETWEEN BIRTH AND 36 MONTHS OF AGE (BOYS)

* Adapted from: National Center for Health Statistics: NCHS Growth Charts, 1976. Monthly Vital Statistics Report. Vol. 25, No. 3, Supp. (HRA) 76-1120. Health Resources Administration, Rockville, Maryland, June, 1976. Data from The Fels Research Institute, Yellow Springs, Ohio.

cause for concern with respect to level of physiological capacity. Widdowson (1977), in discussing the effects of smallness, said:

All the evidence goes to show that babies born small for their gestational age, for whatever cause, do not grow particularly rapidly after birth. . . Does this matter? How much of a disadvantage is it to the individual to be undernourished *in utero* and therefore small at birth and small in later life? A small newborn baby or animal has greater problems over thermal regulation and maintenance of blood sugar than a large one, but, once the immediate postnatal period is past and so long as nutrition and the environment become satisfactory, there seems no particular disadvantage in growing along the 40th rather than the 60th percentile. It is true that the organs of a small individual are small, and if taken out of the body and analyzed they might be condemned as having fewer cells in them than those of large ones, but as far as we know these small organs are quite capable of performing their proper physiological functions in the small individual to which they belong.[1]

This is not to imply that there are no psychological or social challenges; they are simply different sets of problems in other domains. On the other hand, big is not necessarily better for health. Recent research indicates that over-feeding an infant increases the number of adipose cells, increasing the probability of a lifelong weight control problem.

INFANCY: NORMAL SUPPLY AND NORMAL DEMAND

An infant requires the same array of nutrients as does any older human being. However, the nutrient density necessary to meet needs differs since surface-to-volume ratio, absorption, and metabolic efficiencies, etc., differ. The need for all of the various nutrients is unquestionable, but requirements for most have not been established; in some cases a first approximation is available. The RDA (Table 26.1) is based on the composition of human milk, which the Food and Nutrition Board admits is the optimal food source, when available. What is known about nutrient requirements is summarized below.

Calories

The caloric requirement for an infant is high in relation to weight and is unknown. Using mean intake data as a first approximation, recommendations of 120 kcal/kg at birth gradually decreasing to 100 kcal/kg at 1 year have been made. Using some information on energy costs, the

---

[1] From Widdowson (1977). Quoted with permission of the author and the New York Academy of Sciences.

proportions utilized in the fixed and variable portions have been estimated. The fixed portion is utilized in basal metabolism (60 kcal) and in
specific dynamic action (5 kcal). The variable portion is utilized for
growth (15 kcal) and physical activity (35 kcal). Fecal loss commonly
amounts to an additional 5 kcal. Since the physical activity level varies
widely, for the same infant over time and among infants, rate of weight
gain in relation to length and bone structure must be monitored and
adjusted accordingly. Normally, birth weight triples during the first 10 to
12 months. Although calories should be provided by a combination of
protein, fat, and carbohydrate sources, the best ratio for infants has not
been determined. A number of ratios have been proposed and have been
supported with some plausible explanation.

Protein

A high proportion of the protein requirement is necessary to supply
needs for tissue growth of normal infants growing at a normal rate; the
remainder is necessary for tissue maintenance. Fomon (1974) reports
that 1.6 g protein/100 kcal appears to be adequate to support growth,
i.e., it is the requirement, for the first 6 weeks. Thereafter, during the
first year, since growth rate is decreased, the requirement is estimated to
be 1.4 g protein/100 kcal. Breast milk provides high Biologic Value (BV)
protein at this level. Other sources of milk do not, and when beikost, i.e.,
other foods, are added to the diet, the protein quality is likely to be reduced. Therefore, Fomon (1974) recommends 1.9 g/100 kcal and 1.7 g/
100 kcal for the first 6 weeks and the remainder of the first year, respectively.

The true requirements for essential and nonessential amino acids are
unknown. A first approximation of the requirement is now available from
work by Fomon (1974). The essential amino acid requirements are determined by the cumulative and aggregate needs for tissue growth and
maintenance. For each essential amino acid, the nature, i.e., the amino
acid composition of the protein portion of the growing tissues, and the
extent, i.e., the rate of tissue extension and turnover with release of
amino acids that can be recycled into the anabolic processes of tissue
protein production, determine the overall value which is expressed as its
requirement. Based on studies in which the supply of calories and other
nutrients was adequate and protein of high BV was fed at levels ap-
proximating adequacy, Fomon (1974) deduced some preliminary estimates of amino acid requirements (mg/100 kcal): histidine, 26; isoleucine, 66; leucine, 132; lysine, 101; phenylalanine, 57; methionine, 24;
cystine, 23; threonine, 59; tryptophan, 16; and valine, 83. Since the non-

TABLE 26.1. RDA FOR INFANTS

FOOD AND NUTRITION BOARD, NATIONAL ACADEMY OF SCIENCES–NATIONAL RESEARCH COUNCIL RECOMMENDED DAILY DIETARY ALLOWANCES,[a] REVISED 1980

Designed for the maintenance of good nutrition of practically all healthy people in the U.S.A.

Category	Age (Years)	Weight (kg)	Weight (lb)	Height (cm)	Height (in.)	Protein (g)	Fat-Soluble Vitamins			Water-Soluble Vitamins	
							Vitamin A (μg R.E.)[b]	Vitamin D (μg)[c]	Vitamin E (mg α T.E.)[d]	Vitamin C (mg)	Thiamin (mg)
Infants	0.0–0.5	6	13	60	24	kg × 2.2	420	10	3	35	0.3
	0.5–1.0	9	20	71	28	kg × 2.0	400	10	4	35	0.5

[a] The allowances are intended to provide for individual variations among most normal persons as they live in the United States under usual environmental stresses. Diets should be based on a variety of common foods in order to provide other nutrients for which human requirements have been less well defined.
[b] Retinol equivalents. 1 Retinol equivalent = 1 μg retinol or 6 μg β-carotene.
[c] As cholecalciferol. 10 μg cholecalciferol = 400 IU vitamin D.
[d] α-tocopherol equivalents. 1 mg d-α-tocopherol = 1 α T.E.

essential amino acids are produced from excess/recycled essential amino acids and/or nonprotein nitrogen, no estimates are available for them.

Fat

The optimal proportion of fat in the infant diet is unknown. Experience is largely limited to effects within the range of 30 to 55% of calories. Intakes in this range are necessary in order to provide sufficient calories within the volume limits the infant can handle.

Linoleic acid has long been recognized as the essential fatty acid. A major function appears to be as a precursor to prostaglandins, which, with cyclic AMP, modulate hormonal control of water and electrolyte balance across membranes. Arachidonic and linolenic acid are also precursors of prostaglandins but can be supplied by biosynthesis so are not essential fatty acids. Four other odd-numbered fatty acids, i.e., 8, 11, 14−19:3ω5; 5,8,11,14−19:4ω5; 8, 11, 14−21:3ω7; and 5, 8, 11, 14−21:4ω7, are also precursors of prostaglandins (Schlenk 1972).

The absolute requirement for linoleic acid or some equivalent combination of the other five fatty acid precursors of prostaglandins is unknown. The ratio of fatty acids with three and four double bonds has been determined for heart, liver, and serum tissues. It was demonstrated to correlate well with the manifestations of essential fatty acid deficiency. Using available data on circulating levels obtained at selected levels of fatty acid intake and a curve-fitting procedure, a first approximation of the infant requirement was estimated to be 1% of the caloric intake. Since the amount of fat necessary to supply calories greatly exceeds this level, the requirement for essential fatty acids is easily met except in very unusual circumstances. However, essential fatty acid deficiency in infants has been reported.

The circulating cholesterol levels of infants are lower than those of

Water-Soluble Vitamins					Minerals					
Riboflavin (mg)	Niacin (mg N.E.)[r]	Vitamin B_6 (mg)	Folacin[f] (μg)	Vitamin B_{12} (μg)	Calcium (mg)	Phosphorus (mg)	Magnesium (mg)	Iron (mg)	Zinc (mg)	Iodine (μg)
0.4	6	0.3	30	0.5[g]	360	240	50	10	3	40
0.6	8	0.6	45	1.5	540	360	70	15	5	50

[r] 1 N.E. (niacin equivalent) = 1 mg of niacin or 60 mg of dietary tryptophan.
[f] The folacin allowances refer to dietary sources as determined by *Lactobacillus casei* assay after treatment with enzymes ("conjugases") to make polyglutamyl forms of the vitamin available to the test organism.
[g] The RDA for vitamin B_{12} in infants is based on average concentration of the vitamin in human milk. The allowances after weaning are based on energy intake (as recommended by the American Academy of Pediatrics) and consideration of other factors such as intestinal absorption.

adults and appear to vary according to the milk source. Because of current interest in cholesterol level with respect to adult coronary heart disease (CHD), a number of hypotheses have been proposed in relation to the significance of the dietary cholesterol content of the infant diet. The hypothesis receiving research support holds that an exogenous source of cholesterol is necessary to the infant in order for development of feedback control mechanisms. The hypothesis is that biosynthesis is limited and without an exogenous source would have to be greatly augmented. The exogenous supply induces liver enzyme systems necessary for biosynthesis and catabolism of cholesterol in response to variations in supply and demand.

Carbohydrate

There is no known requirement for carbohydrate. The optimal proportion of carbohydrate in the infant diet is unknown. When the diet is entirely milk or formula, the range in carbohydrate intake is 35 to 55% calories. The breast-fed infant ingests carbohydrate as lactose (glucose and galactose). The formula-fed infant ingests carbohydrate as lactose (glucose and galactose); sucrose (glucose and fructose); fructose, if honey is used; and variable quantities of indigestible mixtures of polysaccharides depending on the dextrose equivalent value (DE) of the corn syrup used. The types of carbohydrate included in the infant diet are further extended when other foods are added to the diet, e.g., cereals, which contain amylose (maltose), amylopectin (maltose and isomaltose), and modified starches (maltose, isomaltose, and perhaps indigestible portions with a variety of chemical substituents, since infant ability to degrade these has not been established), and meats (glycogen).

The α-amylose activity of pancreatic juice is low in infants less than six months of age. It is insufficient to degrade starches to maltose and glucose so starch absorption is low. This has been confirmed by demonstration of insignificant increase in the circulating glucose level following starch ingestion. Starch remains in the chyme and is degraded by colon bacteria for their own metabolic supply.

Water

Water requirements are unknown. Fomon (1974) has reviewed the literature and has provided the following estimates (ml/day): age 1 month—growth, 18; evaporation, 210; fecal loss, 42; and urinary excretion, 56; and age 1 year—growth, 6; evaporation, 500; fecal loss, 105; and urinary excretion, 182. In warm weather, warm climates, or when water is lost due to fever or diarrhea, additional water intake is necessary to prevent dehydration.

Renal capacity to concentrate urinary solutes, primarily urea and sodium, does not reach its potential in infancy so urine volume is relatively large. The renal solute load in millosmoles (MO) is determined by the quantity of urea and electrolytes to be excreted. Fomon (1974) has developed a basis for prediction of the renal solute load: each gram of dietary protein yields approximately 4 MO and each milliequivalent (mEq) of Na^+, K^+, and Cl^- yields 1 MO. Normal infants can concentrate urine to approximately 600 MO/liter. Many infant foods are about 95% water (approx. 28.5 ml/oz) and formula at 100 kcal/100 ml is about 90% water (27 ml/oz). Therefore, IF the infant ingests 1 liter of whole milk formula (900 ml water) AND has normal growth, evaporation, and fecal losses (270 ml), THEN a urine volume of 630 ml must dilute (protein solutes 33 g × 4 MO= 132 MO + Na^+ solutes 25 mEq × 1 MO = 25 MO + K^+ solutes 39 mEq × 1 MO = 39 MO + Cl^- solutes 29 mEq × 1 MO = 29 MO = 225 MO) 225 MO, a concentration of approximately 350 MO/liter urine. Thus, need for additional water intake can be determined.

Minerals

Estimated requirements are the sum of the amounts necessary for tissue formation and replacement of evaporative, urinary, and fecal losses, adjusted for absorption efficiency. Estimated mineral requirements are based on data from the 1950s, the most recent available. The calcium requirement is relatively high in order to meet needs for skeletal and dental deposition on top of other basic needs. The estimated requirement is 388 mg for the first 3 months and 299 mg from the 4th to the 12th month. The phosphate requirement is estimated to be 132 mg during the first 3 months and 110 mg during the remainder of the first year. The Mg requirement has been estimated as 16 mg and 13.5 mg during the first 3 months and the 4th to 12th months, respectively.

The iron endowment of an infant at birth depends on the circulating red cell mass at birth and on the liver stores, so it is highly variable among infants. IF iron intake is deficient, THEN liver iron stores are depleted in three to four months and the circulating level falls. The mean amount of absorbed iron is estimated to be 0.7 mg/day during the first year. Absorption efficiency is affected by concomitant meat and ascorbic acid intake, but the magnitude of the effect has not been established in infants. So, using the old absorption value of 10%, the requirement has been estimated as 7 mg/day.

The copper endowment of an infant at birth is sufficient to meet needs for several months. The requirement has not been established.

The Zn requirement has not been established, but plasma and hair levels in some American infants are less than those of infants in other areas of the world. This finding has stimulated further study. Breast milk is a good source of Zn but some of the commercial formulas are not, which may account for the finding.

All other trace minerals are required by the infant. Little information is available, as requirements have not been established.

Vitamins

All of the fat-soluble vitamins are needed by the infant although little is known concerning infant needs, metabolism, etc. The accepted requirement for vitamin A is 30 IU/kg/day, since studies have demonstrated normal weight gain and dark adaptation at levels of 25 to 35 IU/kg/day. The requirement for vitamin D is unknown; an accepted estimate is 100 to 200 IU. The circulating plasma level of vitamin E is maintained at 1 mg/100 ml if intake is 0.4 mg/g PUFA (polyunsaturated fatty acids), so this level is accepted as the first approximation to a requirement. The estimated vitamin K requirement is less than 5 μg/day. Because some infants develop a hemorrhagic disease within the first few days, a single parenteral dose of 0.5 to 1.0 mg vitamin K_1 is given almost universally as a preventive measure.

All of the water-soluble vitamins are needed by the infant, but requirements are not clearly defined. The estimated ascorbic acid requirement of 10 mg/day is a first approximation based on a very limited set of data. Human milk is a good source of ascorbic acid, so the circulating ascorbic acid level of breast-fed infants has been demonstrated to be 0.6 mg/100 ml. This is a level several times above that at which scurvy develops in an adult. In adults, a mean intake of 10 mg will maintain serum levels one-third to one-half that value, so 10 mg is assumed to be adequate for the infant.

The thiamin requirement is 0.2 mg/1000 kcal. In the absence of definitive data, requirements have been estimated to be approximately equivalent to levels in breast milk.

A small baby will have smaller requirements than a larger one on an absolute basis, though they may be relatively higher. Moreover, a small baby will not catch up to normal weight for a long time. Widdowson (1977) has discussed what is known:

> The reason the small baby does not grow very rapidly is because it is not hungry enough to take enough food to enable it to do so . . . We have suggested that if the individual has been retarded in growth and is therefore small at the age when appetite centers are developing in the hypothalamus, then the appetite will be "set" at a level appropriate to the size and rate of growth at the time . . . Appetite control comes into play immediately after birth. A small size at this time is inevitably associated with an appetite geared to the small size and hence the baby grows slowly and remains small.[1]

INFANCY: DEFICIENT SUPPLY AND INFLATED DEMAND

Failure to thrive is a syndrome observed in malnourished infants. They do not gain weight as rapidly as expected and may show various other deficiency symptoms as well. Points with regard to deficient supply of specific nutrients follow.

Calories

When caloric intake is deficient, weight gain may slow down or cease and/or physical activity level may be reduced. A thin and listless baby is the result. Moreover, when calories are insufficient, muscle protein will be degraded and the liberated amino acids will be deaminated and degraded to provide energy. Protein-based growth and development needs will be unmet, resulting in retardation. The nature and extent of retardation will vary, depending on the timing and severity of caloric deficit. The kidneys are not fully functional until the end of the first year. Muscle catabolism results in increased urea production. The renal solute load thus may exceed renal capacity, adding complications due to an elevated blood urea nitrogen (BUN) level.

---

[1] From Widdowson (1977). Quoted with permission of the author and the New York Academy of Sciences.

Protein

Essential amino acids are necessary for formation and maintenance of muscle and nervous tissues, bone matrix, and hormones, enzymes, and other secretions. A slowdown in muscle growth results in a smaller muscle mass for age and may be accompanied by retarded muscle development. If so, this is manifested in decreased muscle coordination; the observed effect is that the infant is slow to crawl, grasp, sit, etc.

Minerals

The neonate is less able to tolerate an abnormal calcium to phosphate ratio than are older infants. Hypocalcemic tetany has been observed during the first week of life when an improperly diluted cows' milk formula has been given. A calcium to phosphate ratio of 2:1, the ratio in human milk, is the optimal ratio. The imbalance resulting from a ratio of 1.2:1, the ratio in cows' milk, creates a deficient circulating level of calcium, probably because of failure to absorb the calcium phosphate salts.

The incidence and prevalance of anemia used to be high. Anemia is more likely to develop in premature infants or twins, because their iron stores are not likely to be optimal. Anemia may appear before six months because humans' and cows' milk are both inadequate sources of iron. Breast-fed babies and those fed home-prepared formulas are normally given a supplement starting at an early, but variable, age. Commercially prepared formulas are routinely fortified with iron at a level of 8 to 12 mg/qt so additional supplementation is unnecessary. Iron-fortified cereals are also available.

Deficient iodine and zinc intakes have been observed in breast-fed infants whose mother's intakes were deficient. Growth retardation and poor appetite were the clinical manifestations observed. Fluoride supplementation to reduce the level of dental caries at later stages has been advocated as a preventive measure. Supplementation is recommended to be equivalent to 1 ppm in water.

Vitamins

Few cases of vitamin deficiency in infants have been reported; however, more may exist. Only limited information on symptomology is available.

Premature infants fed a formula containing much greater than normal quantities of polyunsaturated fatty acids and iron have been known to develop a vitamin E deficiency. In these cases, observed symptoms were anemia, reticulocytosis, and thrombocytosis. In premature infants, the need for dietary vitamin E may be greater than in full-term infants because body stores are likely to be underdeveloped, growth rate may be greater, and fat absorption is likely to be impaired. A supplement of 0.5 mg/kg/day has been recommended as a safety measure.

Infants borne and breast-fed by poorly nourished mothers or who are fed formulas that have been heat processed have sometimes developed a pyridoxine (vitamin B_6) deficiency with consequent impairment of protein metabolism. High protein formulas have caused some infants to develop ascorbic acid deficiency. An intake of vitamin C as high as 50 mg/day proved to be necessary to avoid tyrosinemia and tyrosinuria.

INFANCY: EXCESSIVE SUPPLY

Inadvertently, toxic and even fatal doses of some nutrients have been fed to some infants. Such an outcome is to be avoided. Discussion of nutrients where the hazard exists follows.

Energy

This is the nutrient most likely to be supplied in excess since a common misconception avers that a fat baby is a healthy baby. While the effects of excess caloric intake are not fatal in the short run, they may be in the long run. Recent research has demonstrated that there are three periods when the number of adipocytes (fat cells) is expanded to accommodate an increasing need for energy storage. One of these is in infancy. The theoretical explanation of the effects of hypertrophy and hyperplasia are discussed in Chapter 7.

The relative number and lipid content of adipose cells in obese and non-obese infants have been determined (Knittle *et al.* 1977). Between ages 4 and 12 months, both fat cell number and lipid content increase. Then the pattern changes. From 12 to 24 months, the lipid content of adipose cells in obese infants increases. Cell size expands and reaches adult cell size in order to accommodate the stored lipid. During the same period, the lipid content decreases to less than the amount at 12 months in non-obese infants. Heredity and/or the effects of over-nutrition may cause a decreased response to epinephrine, resulting in reduced lipolytic activity per cell with consequent compensatory increase in cell numbers. This aspect is under investigation.

An infant that has become overweight or obese is *not* placed on a reducing diet. The treatment objective is to reduce the rate of weight gain. Over time, in a non-harmful way, the correct weight/height relationship can be (re)established. To achieve this goal, the recommended caloric intake is 110 kcal per kg for infants 0 to 6 months of age and 90 kcal per kg for infants 6 to 12 months of age. Limiting milk consumption to 30 oz, with replacement of fluid volume by water, allows introduction of other foods within the caloric allowance.

Hypervitaminoses A and D

Thousands of cases are reported annually. Usually, excessive intake is inadvertent, reflecting misunderstanding or carelessness in use of a concentrated supplement. Supplements are available as fish liver oils or as water-miscible preparations. These are available in a variety of concentrations. Prescribed dosage needs to be verified.

Toxicity has been observed with an intake of 75,000 IU for 3 months when an oil supplement was taken. The water-miscible preparations are more toxic. Toxicity has been observed at intakes of 18,000 IU for 3 months and 22,500 IU for 142 months.

Clinical manifestations of vitamin A toxicity include lack of appetite, growth retardation, drying and cracking of skin, long bone pain, and bone fragility. Hypercalcemia, nausea, diarrhea, weight loss, and frequent urination are common manifestations of vitamin D toxicity, given an intake of 10,000 to 30,000 IU/day. No maximum "safe" level has been determined, although daily ingestion of 1600 IU has been reported with no apparent effect on growth rate.

INFANCY: FOOD ECOLOGY, NUTRITIONAL RISK, AND LIFE EXPECTANCY

The mother supplies the infant's food either directly or indirectly and is personally responsible for its nutritional adequacy. Thus, she is the key factor in the food ecosystem. Initially, there are three alternative food sources for the infant. Later, a variety of food sources and intake patterns is possible.

Human milk or a nearly equivalent milk substitute is the sole source of nourishment initially. Breast-milk, a home-prepared formula, or a commercially prepared formula are the three alternative food sources. Each is "best" under some circumstances and each has its proponents and opponents. None is uniformly appropriate.

Human Breast Milk

IF this food source is to be utilized optimally, THEN several adjustments in the dietary intake of the mother are necessary. These ad-

TABLE 26.2. RECOMMENDED NUTRIENT INTAKE ALLOWANCES DURING PREGNANCY

FOOD AND NUTRITION BOARD, NATIONAL ACADEMY OF SCIENCES–NATIONAL RESEARCH COUNCIL RECOMMENDED DAILY DIETARY ALLOWANCES,[a] REVISED 1980

Designed for the maintenance of good nutrition of practically all healthy people in the U.S.A.

							Fat-Soluble Vitamins			Water-Soluble Vitamins	
Category	Age (Years)	Weight (kg)	(lb)	Height (cm)	(in.)	Protein (g)	Vitamin A (μg R.E.)[b]	Vitamin D (μg)[c]	Vitamin E (mg α T.E.)[d]	Vitamin C (mg)	Thiamin (mg)
Females	11–14	46	101	157	62	46	800	10	8	50	1.1
	15–18	55	120	163	64	46	800	10	8	60	1.1
	19–22	55	120	163	64	44	800	7.5	8	60	1.1
	23–50	55	120	163	64	44	800	5	8	60	1.0
Pregnant						+30	+200	+5	+2	+20	+0.4
Lactating						+20	+400	+5	+3	+40	+0.5

[a] The allowances are intended to provide for individual variations among most normal persons as they live in the United States under usual environmental stresses. Diets should be based on a variety of common foods in order to provide other nutrients for which human requirements have been less well defined.
[b] Retinol equivalents. 1 Retinol equivalent = 1 μg retinol or 6 μg β-carotene.
[c] As cholecalciferol. 10 μg cholecalciferol = 400 IU vitamin D.
[d] α-tocopherol equivalents. 1 mg d-α-tocopherol = 1 α T.E.
[e] 1 N.E. (niacin equivalent) = 1 mg of niacin or 60 mg of dietary tryptophan.
[f] The folacin allowances refer to dietary sources as determined by *Lactobacillus casei* assay after treatment with enzymes ("conjugases") to make polyglutamyl forms of the vitamin available to the test organism.

justments are necessary to maintain the mother's nutritional status and to produce the quantity and quality of milk essential to meet the infant's nutrient needs. All of the nutrients required by humans are required by the lactating mother, but are required in greater than normal quantities, the levels of some being inflated to their maximum level as listed in Table 26.2.

Caloric and fluid intakes need to be carefully monitored and controlled so that the necessary volume of milk can be produced. The mean quantity produced per day is 30 oz. The milk has a mean caloric value of 20 kcal/oz. So, the caloric value of the milk produced averages 600 kcal. To produce this quantity of milk, approximately 400 kcal is expended. Hence, the mother's caloric requirement is increased by an average of 1000 kcal/day. Normally 4 to 8 lb fat (14,000 to 28,000 kcal) is stored during pregnancy against this need. Therefore, endogenous and exogenous sources of calories can be utilized.

The cost of extra food for the mother is significant and may exceed the cost of formula feeding. Using the USDA thrifty and liberal food plans, Peterkin and Walker (1976) imputed the value of additional food required by the lactating mother in 1976. The weekly costs were $3 and $5, respectively. The weekly cost of the vitamin D supplement that is customarily given to the breast-fed infant was an additional $0.50.

The nutrient profile of human milk differs markedly from that of other mammalian milks. It is also highly variable according to point in the lactation cycle, time of day, point in the feeding, and among women. The basic composition is genetically determined such that the upper limit for

Water-Soluble Vitamins					Minerals					
Riboflavin (mg)	Niacin (mg N.E.)	Vitamin B$_6$ (mg)	Folacin (μg)	Vitamin B$_{12}$ (μg)	Calcium (mg)	Phosphorus (mg)	Magnesium (mg)	Iron (mg)	Zinc (mg)	Iodine (μg)
1.3	15	1.8	400	3.0	1200	1200	300	18	15	150
1.3	14	2.0	400	3.0	1200	1200	300	18	15	150
1.3	14	2.0	400	3.0	800	800	300	18	15	150
1.2	13	2.0	400	3.0	800	800	300	18	15	150
+0.3	+2	+0.6	+400	+1.0	+400	+400	+150		+ 5	+25
+0.5	+5	+0.5	+100	+1.0	+400	+400	+150		+10	+50

[g] The RDA for vitamin B$_{12}$ in infants is based on average concentration of the vitamin in human milk. The allowances after weaning are based on energy intake (as recommended by the American Academy of Pediatrics) and consideration of other factors such as intestinal absorption.

[h] The increased requirement during pregnancy cannot be met by the iron content of habitual American diets or by the existing iron stores of many women; therefore the use of 30−60 mg of supplemental iron is recommended. Iron needs during lactation are not substantially different from those of non-pregnant women, but continued supplementation of the mother for 2−3 months after parturition is advisable in order to replenish stores depleted by pregnancy.

a particular nutrient is one that a normal infant can tolerate. Below the upper limit, composition varies somewhat with maternal nutriture and other factors. The nutrient profile of breast milk from well nourished women is incomplete, being limited to only a few nutrients. Per 100 ml, human milk appears to contain mean quantities as follows: protein, 1.1 g; fat, 4.2 g; lactose, 7.2 g; ascorbic acid, 4 mg; and calcium, 34 mg. It also contains a water-soluble vitamin D conjugate.

Variability in composition can be summarized as follows:

(a) protein—In the short run, it is not affected by maternal intake (quantity or quality) since it is maintained at maternal expense. In the long run, it is affected by maternal intake (quantity or quality) since it tends to be reduced with increasing duration.

(b) fat—Fatty acid composition varies on a diurnal basis, being greater in the early morning; within the feeding, being greater at the end; and among women, according to dietary intake, being higher in saturated fatty acids when a high carbohydrate diet is consumed.

This variability has been rationalized as necessary to meet the infant's need to break the nightly fast with a first feeding of above-average caloric density and to become satiated so as to terminate each feeding when sufficient nutrients have been ingested. IF this rationale is correct, THEN fat content may function in self-regulation of food intake by the infant.

(c) minerals—Composition is highly variable among women, but the levels of calcium, iron, copper, fluorine, etc., have not been demonstrated to vary with maternal intake.

(d) vitamins—The levels of fat-soluble vitamins A, D, and E have not been demonstrated to vary with intake. The levels of water-soluble vitamins vary directly with maternal intake.

The mammary contractile response in humans differs from that in other mammals. It is a sustained response and is maintained by a series of milk-ejection responses. Suckling provides the immediate thermal and tactile stimuli. The circulating level of the hormone *oxytonin* is a primary factor in readying the mammary tissue for secretion. It is under the control of the hypothalamus. As pregnancy progresses, the quantity required to elicit the milk-ejection response decreases progressively. So, immediately after birth, the threshold is low and a very small quantity elicits the response. At the same time, the circulating level normally begins to increase. It increases in relation to the infant's growing need for milk. However, the release of oxytonin can be blocked by CNS activity in response to cold, emotional conflict, and pain. So, it is necessary that the mother be confident, comfortable, and relaxed so that she can release a sufficient quantity of milk to nourish the infant adequately.

The food selection of the mother also needs to be monitored and controlled so as to maximize the purity of her milk. Any impurity that reduces the quantity ingested, causes vomiting or diarrhea, or interferes with the feeding relationship is likely to have a negative impact on infant nutriture, so is of concern. Recent research has confirmed some of the observations that are a part of the folklore that surrounds breastfeeding. For example:

(a) Consumption of chocolate by the mother can cause adverse reactions in the infant such as diarrhea, constipation, eczema, irritability, and fretful sleeping. It turns out that theobromine, which is a stimulant similar to caffeine that is contained in all cacao products, stimulates CNS and heart muscle action, induces diuresis, and causes smooth muscle relaxation. It passes freely into breast milk. Therefore, a mother who consumed 4 chocolate bars/day could expose the infant to 10 mg theobromine/day. This quantity has been demonstrated to cause adverse effects in sensitive infants.

(b) Consumption of onions, cucumbers, and members of the cabbage family by the mother can cause colic in the infant. These are "gas-formers" for infants as well as adults.

Pesticide and drug residues have been detected in human milk. Journalistic exploitation of this has created a public furor that now appears to be subsiding somewhat. The number of investigations of pesticide and drug residues in human milk is small. And although greater than expected levels of some pesticides have been detected, evidence of immediate hazard to the infant is not available. Rather, effects, if any, appear to be similar in nature and extent to those attributed to environmental contaminants. Kroger (1974), in discussing the topic of general contaminants in human milk, stated, "It can be inferred that all drugs administered to lactating mammals will appear in their milk; this includes caffeine, nicotine, analgesics, sedatives, opiates, ethers, and chloroform among others."[1] To avoid the possibility of side effects, the lactating mother should avoid taking drugs, including the relatively innocuous over-the-counter ones.

Home–Prepared Formula

IF this food source is to be utilized optimally, THEN a different set of dietary adjustments is necessary so that the mother's nutritional status can be maintained and her weight reduced to the pre-pregnancy level. The mother's caloric intake should be reduced to the non-pregnant level. Intakes of minerals and vitamins might be continued above the non-pregnant level for some time to assure replenishment of maternal stores, especially if additional pregnancies are a possibility. During pregnancy 4 to 8 lb fat were laid down in preparation for lactation. Since these caloric stores are unnecessary, they should be eliminated. The added activity in caring for the infant may be sufficient to effect a slow weight loss toward the pre-pregnancy weight. IF not, THEN a reduced calorie diet and/or increased exercise may be necessary.

Satisfactory infant formulas can be prepared from fresh whole or evaporated cows' milk, goats' milk, and other mammalian milks. According to current medical opinion, skim milk (fresh or powdered) should not be used unless an adjusted formula is used. Vegetable oil can be added to return the fat content to a level that provides the infant with sufficient calories.

The composition of other mammalian milks differs from that of breast-milk, so modification is necessary in order to meet an infant's needs. Cows' milk contains approximately twice the protein, six times the minerals, and two-thirds the lactose of human milk. Therefore, the basic modification is dilution with water to reduce protein and mineral content to appropriate levels and addition of sugar, e.g., sucrose, corn syrup, or dextrimaltose, to increase the carbohydrate content. Starch cannot be used as a source of carbohydrate since the infant's amylase production is insufficient during the first several months. Therefore, since the infant cannot degrade the starch to absorbable simple sugars, it is not nourishing.

Nutrient density requirements and tolerances are highly variable for one infant over time and among different infants. Therefore, a wide variety of formulas have been devised.

---

[1] From Kroger (1974). Quoted with permission of the author and the New York Academic Press.

The solute and caloric density of the formula may be related to feeding frequency, "need" for early introduction of solid foods, and excessive weight gain. According to Taitz (1977),

> ... observation gave rise to a hypothesis that would explain excessive weight gain. ... It was suggested that since babies tend to adjust their volume of intake to the caloric density of the feed, the daily water intake of babies fed overconcentrated feeds was reduced. This made infants particularly vulnerable to changes in external water balance, and also made them unable to tolerate long periods without feeding, giving rise to the common complaint that the infants never seemed to be satisfied. Since the obvious response to crying, fretful babies was to offer them more overconcentrated feed, a vicious cycle was created with two possible effects. First, babies would be overfed. It is easy to see that the temptation to introduce solids early would be very powerful. Second, it may be no coincidence that a disturbingly high rate of hypertonic dehydration was reported. ... It has long been known that gross mistakes in formula preparation may lead to hypernatremia, but this was a situation in which relatively small but repeated and widespread mistakes were being made.[1]

When the early introduction of solid foods and proper formula concentration was implemented, weight gain fell to a normal level for breast-fed infants. This finding tends to support this hypothesis.

Gastrointestinal and renal function do not reach full capacity until nearly the end of infancy. Therefore, osmolality of the formula is an important consideration in preventing diarrhea and/or diuresis. As discussed in Chapter 8, concentrations of amino acids, sugars, and salts are involved. Osmolar load is a limiting factor in relation to nutrient density. Research has shown that, typically, premature infants can tolerate a protein content of only 16% calories, with a total concentration of solids equivalent to 24 kcal/oz. Some experimentation may be necessary to find the optimal formula for the particular infant.

The composition of goats' milk also differs from that of human milk. Therefore, special formulas are necessary if goats' milk is to be used as a base.

The cost of home-prepared infant formulas was computed by Peterkin and Walker (1976). These costs were less than the cost of the additional food that would be consumed by a lactating mother. The weekly July 1976 cost in Washington, D.C. for an infant consuming five 6-oz bottles/day was:

(a) $2.81 for a whole milk formula made from regular fluid pasteurized milk fortified with vitamin D and sugar. Assumptions were that the milk was purchased in ½-gal. cartons and that the infant also was fed juice

---

[1] From Taitz (1977). Quoted with permission of the W.B. Saunders Co.

or was given an ascorbic acid supplement which cost $0.50/week.

(b) $2.88 for an evaporated milk formula made from diluted evaporated milk fortified with vitamin D and sugar. Assumptions were that the evaporated milk was purchased in 13-fl oz cans and that the infant also was fed juice or was given an ascorbic acid supplement which cost $0.50.

Commercially Prepared Formulas

IF this food source is to be utilized optimally, THEN the dietary adjustments that are necessary for the mother are the same as in the preceding case and appropriateness is the criterion in selection of a formula.

A number of milk-based and soybean-based formulas are commercially available in powdered and concentrated liquid form. These have been carefully formulated according to the RDA and are fortified to supply additional quantities of iron. The fatty acid composition may be altered by substitution of PUFA for some portion of the saturated fatty acids normally found in mammalian milk. Lactose-free formulas are also available to meet the needs of those infants that develop a lactose intolerance. The osmolality of commercially prepared formulas is closely adjusted to a level that most infants can tolerate.

The cost of commercial infant formulas was computed by Peterkin and Walker (1976). Costs were less than, equal to, or greater than the cost of additional food consumed by a lactating mother depending on the type of formula used. The weekly July 1976 cost of commercial formulas in Washington, D.C. for an infant consuming five 6-oz bottles/day was:

(a) $4.77, if made from concentrated formula purchased in 13-fl oz cans
(b) $5.01, if made from powdered formula purchased in 1-lb cans
(c) $6.50, if purchased in ready-to-use 32-fl oz cans

Introduction of Solid Foods (Beikost)

Infant feeding practices with respect to the introduction of solid foods are highly variable among regional, ethnic, and socioeconomic groups in the United States. Recent studies of infant feeding practices have focused on topics that include, but are not limited to:

(a) choice of foods
(b) timing of introduction of various foods
(c) source of information of feeding practices
(d) folk beliefs associated with infant feeding practices
(e) resultant nutrient intake

Some definitive and some comparative studies have provided a limited amount of information. The generalizations that follow were derived from selected studies related to these topics and are meant only to provide an overview. To work effectively with mothers of infants, one must study the prevailing practices and make an assessment of their expected effect on infant nutriture. In every individual case, general premises must be checked before any inference is drawn.

Choice of Foods.—Home-prepared and commercial baby foods are alternatives. Each is the "best" alternative in some circumstances.

A variety of simple foods can be prepared satisfactorily, given time and a blender. Batch preparation and frozen storage of individual portions are generally recommended. Care must be taken to minimize bacterial contamination during preparation and storage. Home-prepared baby foods continue to be less expensive than similar commercial items. According to Peterkin and Walker (1976),

. . . baby foods prepared by using proper procedures at home are as nutritious as commercially prepared ones; some are more nutritious. Because of the low total solids content of some commercially prepared baby foods and the addition of sugar or starch to many, concentrations of protein, vitamins, and minerals are likely to be less than for corresponding foods prepared in the home. Beef and chicken puréed at home provide more of most nutrients than commercially strained beef and chicken—chiefly because they contain less water. Home-prepared beef and chicken with broth added would provide less nutrients and lose less than home-prepared beef and chicken without broth.

The number of commercial baby foods available is enormous; it is reported to be approximately 400 items. The salt content has been voluntarily limited to not more than 0.25%, as recommended by a special committee of the National Academy of Sciences-National Research Council. The recipes used in the formulation of these products change frequently, and nutrient composition changes accordingly. The reader is cautioned to check the date whenever nutrient content is reported as statements are soon obsolete.

The appropriateness of consumption of any given class of infant foods cannot be judged on presumptive evidence. At the very least, it depends on the composition of the total diet. As pointed out by Anderson (1977), for example: IF an infant receives 40% of the caloric intake from whole milk (cows'), THEN protein needs are met and use of strained meats to provide protein is unnecessary. On the other hand, on the same caloric basis the breast-fed infant will receive less protein and might need the added protein.

Timing of Introduction of Solid Foods.—Breast milk or formula is all that is fed initially. Then, according to a study by Purvis (1973), as early as sometime during the first month, the white middle-class infant is switched to whole, 2%, or skim milk and a variable but increasing number of other foods. These supplementary foods, including juices, fruits, vegetables, infant cereals, eggs, meats, and table foods are introduced at variable times.

In general, with the exception of iron nutriture, infants appear to be well nourished, even over-nourished. Highlights of findings by Purvis (1973) are:

(a) calories—The intake was usually sufficient and was supplied in variable proportions by the various food groups.

(b) protein—The intake varied on the average between 1½ and 2½ times the recommended allowance.

(c) calcium—Intake was largely a function of milk and/or formula intake, as expected.

(d) iron—The intake was variable but low, with 58% not ingesting the recommended quantity. Adequacy of intake was related to consumption of iron-enriched infant cereals and/or formulas, so tended to be more adequate the first six months when these foods were fed. During the second six months, these foods were usually replaced with foods of low iron density.

(e) sodium—The intake was highly variable, but related primarily to intake of table foods. There is no RDA for this essential nutrient. Intake is usually expressed in mEq.

(f) vitamin A—Intake was usually adequate from baby foods and/or table foods. Supplementation was customary, but probably unnecessary in most cases.

(g) B vitamins—Mean intakes of thiamin, riboflavin, niacin, and B_6 were adequate. Infant cereal was the primary source of riboflavin and niacin.

(h) ascorbic acid—Although the mean intake was more than twice the recommended quantity, a number of infants ingested inadequate amounts. It may be that awareness was the critical variable, since those that consumed significant quantities from foods also ingested supplements that contributed to excessive intakes.

Source of Information on Feeding Practices.—The set of infant feeding practices recommended by health care professionals undergoes frequent revision. However, at any given point in time, the practices actually followed tend to differ within and among population subgroups, as documented by numerous research reports. These show that "practical" information on feeding practices is customarily obtained from mothers, neighbors, friends, and other such informal sources. This common wisdom, or folk beliefs, is regarded by many people as having great authority, so that it may be followed instead of or in addition to recommended practices.

Folk Beliefs Associated with Infant Feeding Practices.—Health care workers involved with low-income ethnic subgroups have reported persistent folk beliefs and practices that are notably different from prevailing contemporary patterns. Often these are (a) based on recommendations that were made a quarter of a century earlier and/or (b) similar to those reported from anthropological field studies of isolated groups, e.g., "hot-cold" syndrome, dosing with herbal teas and tonics. For the most part, descriptions of subgroup folk beliefs have been included on an occasional basis in the discussion sections of reports of food intake or nutritional status. Hence, the literature is diffuse.

With acculturation, subgroup folk beliefs are replaced with the prevailing contemporary folk beliefs. Recent studies have reported some patterns that include, but are not limited to:

(a) United States-as-a-whole—According to the mother's preference, infants should be breast and/or bottle fed on demand to age six months. They should be weaned to solid foods between the first and sixth month; items and order of introducing foods are not so important and so should be a matter of the mother's preference. Weaning from the bottle to a cup should occur between the 9th and 15th month, although a night bottle might be continued for 24 months.

(b) North-central Blacks—According to the mother's preference, infants should be breast and/or bottle fed to 18 months, on demand. A bottle should be continuously available as a supplement. Solid foods should be introduced starting in the second week; items and order are unimportant so should be according to mother's preferences.

(c) Hispanics—After the first 2 to 3 days, according to the mother's preference, infants should be breast and/or bottle fed on demand or on a schedule to age 18 months. Solid foods generally should be introduced between the second and sixth month. However, meats and eggs should be delayed until the third to sixth month. Fats should be introduced at one year. Some groups adhere to the "hot-cold" system of beliefs. See p. 326.

(d) Native Americans—According to the mother's preference, infants should be breast or bottle fed on demand to age 18 months. Solid foods should not be introduced until one year, so these pre-school children may not be used to chewing meats and other chewy foods.

The "best" infant feeding practices are unknown. In any case, they probably vary among infants. The current recommendations are a combination of fashion and fact. Therefore, the fact that folk beliefs and practices differ from the conventional pattern is interesting but may be irrelevant. IF the aim is a happy, healthy growing infant, THEN unusual beliefs and practices should be accepted if they also promote interest in a variety of foods and serve as antecedents for good physical and mental health in later years.

Resultant Nutrient Intake.—Maslansky *et al.* (1974) surveyed infant feeding practices of low income Black and Puerto Rican families in New York City. Nutrient intakes were similar to those summarized above, but cultural influences were pervasive factors in selection, timing, and source of nutrients.

Bowering *et al.* (1978) reported findings from a study of infant feeding practices among low income Blacks and Puerto Ricans. Findings were compared with those of Purvis (1973) and Maslansky *et al.* (1974). Both similarities and differences were found, e.g., at 1 year these infants still received 50% of their kcal from milk unlike the others who received only 35% kcal from milk at this age; solid foods were also likely to be introduced earlier than recommended; Black infants did not consume as much vegetable as previously reported. Moreover, feeding practices for infants under one year were found to differ greatly between Blacks and Puerto Ricans, thus casting doubt on the frequent suggestion that ethnic differences do not occur until one year of age or so.

Since the findings reported by Bowering *et al.* (1978) are newer than those of Purvis (1973) and Maslansky *et al.* (1974), reported differences may be due to time-related changes in availability of infant foods as the net effect of a variety of socioeconomic factors and in diffusion of the common wisdom with respect to the "best" infant feeding practices, etc. Therefore, findings of Bowering *et al.* (1978) represent a newer approximation with some points that bear watching.

A subsequent nationwide study by Purvis *et al.* (1978) reported the following:

(a) Infant feeding practices changed considerably during the 1970s. Food sources changed, so the mean nutrient intakes also changed.

(b) Mean overall caloric intake remained about the same between 1972 and 1977 (Fig. 26.3).

(c) By 1977, the mean percentage of calories ingested from baby foods had decreased from 34 to 26% among babies 3 to 9 months of age (Fig. 26.4).

(d) By 1977, the mean percentage of calories ingested from table foods had increased from 10 to 17% among babies 3 to 9 months of age.

(e) By 1977, skim milk and partially skimmed milk had replaced whole milk in many cases. The overall use of milk had decreased; this decrease was offset by increased use of commercial formula. Breast feeding had increased from 4.5 to about 17%.

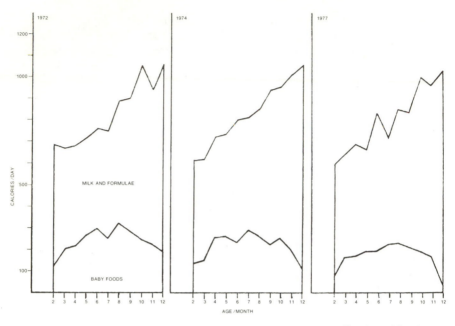

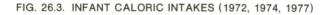

Courtesy of G.A. Purvis

FIG. 26.3. INFANT CALORIC INTAKES (1972, 1974, 1977)

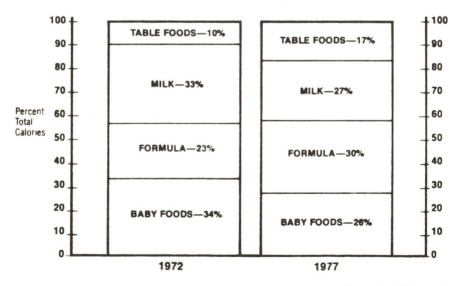

Courtesy of G.A. Purvis

FIG. 26.4. DISTRIBUTION OF FOOD INTAKE FOR A 3–9 MONTH OLD INFANT'S DIET

(f) By 1977, the sodium content of baby foods had been sharply reduced by removal of salt from them. However, increasing use of salted table foods partially offset the effect.

(g) The percentages of calories from fat and carbohydrate changed (Fig. 26.5). The percentage of calories from protein was already extremely high in 1972 and continued to rise.

(h) By 1977, infant cereal, which is fortified at a lower level than previously as the result of a 1974 nutrition labeling regulation, had ceased to be the predominant source of iron. The apparent effect is that between 80% and 90% of the infants studied were not provided with iron at the level of the RDA (Fig. 26.6).

Nutritional Risk

The text of the Women, Infants and Children Nutrition Act of 1975 states that Congress finds many infants are at special risk of physical and mental health due to poor or inadequate nutriture. Nutritional risk for children includes, but is not limited to, deficient patterns of growth, nutritional anemia, and known inadequate nutrient intake patterns. To remedy this problem supplemental foods are made available to qualified lactating mothers and infants. Foods for lactating mothers are to supply: protein, 40 to 66 g, which is 60 to 100% of the RDA; calcium, 720 to 1200 mg, which is 60 to 100% of the RDA; iron, 10.8 to 18 mg, which is 60 to 100% of the RDA for non-pregnant women; vitamin A, 3600 to 6000 IU, which is 60 to 100% of the RDA; ascorbic acid, 48 to 80 mg, which is 60 to 100% of the RDA; and calories, 650 kcal, which is 25% of the RDA. Foods for infants are to supply: protein, kg × 2.0 g, which is 100% of the RDA; calcium, 540 mg, which is 100% of the RDA; iron, 15 mg, which is 100% of the RDA; vitamin A, 1800 IU, which is 90% of the RDA; ascorbic acid, 35 mg, which is 100% of the RDA; and calories, 100% to age 3 months and 75% thereafter to age 1 year.

Although this federal food program has its limitations and failures in implementation, it has undoubtedly benefited participants to the extent that they consumed the food supplied. Normal growth, freedom from nutritional anemia, and adequate intake of stipulated nutrients should be demonstrable.

Food Ecology

This is the other aspect of nurture that is within the scope of this discussion. In addition to the basic biological need for and drive to obtain food, an infant has safety-security needs. These are associated with the

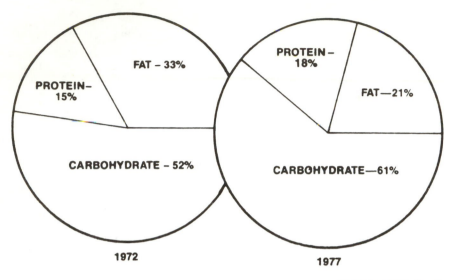

Courtesy of G.A. Purvis

FIG. 26.5. DISTRIBUTION OF CALORIES IN THE TOTAL DIET OF 3–9 MONTH OLD
INFANTS (1972–1977)

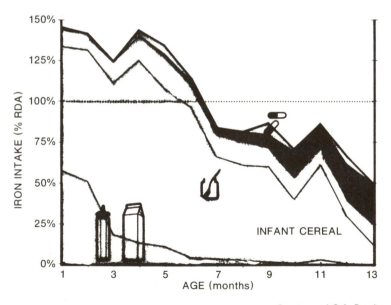

Courtesy of G.A. Purvis

FIG. 26.6. IRON INTAKE OF INFANTS

Effect of Reduced Infant Cereal Iron Level.

central developmental task of infancy which is to establish *trust-mis-trust relationships* (Erikson 1950). Thus, the food and people inter-actions at this stage of development are a fundamental part of later psycho-social development, especially in relation to food ecology. This fact has long been recognized and the importance of the quality of the relationship in nurturance has been a customary focus in educational programs.

An environmental factor in the nutrition niche, the aggregate effect may be characterized as some more or less positive point along the pleasure-pain continuum. At the pleasure extreme, feeding is a highly satisfying experience that is equated with love, pleasure, protection, and comfort. The infant's slightest wish is responded to as a command. So, because food-getting is too easy, the child often fails to become peppy and demanding, tends to lack initiative, perseverance, drive, curiosity, etc.

At the other extreme, feeding is an unsatisfactory experience that is equated with indifference and inappropriate schedule (force feeding or unavailability), unpleasant interaction (anxiety, tenseness, irritability, etc.), illness as a result of intolerance, or discomfort. These result in frightening experiences of frustration and/or pain. So, because food-get-ting is difficult and/or dangerous, the child may become a picky, fussy eater. The following scenarios are revealing:

(a) the normal infant—The first-time mother is insecure for the first few days but then gains confidence and radiates love, security, and pleas-ure which evoke positive responses from the infant, who is willing to try new foods and is secure as he/she learns to master eating techniques.

(b) the premature infant—The mother goes home and waits while the infant remains in an unstimulating atmosphere for a month or so. By the time the baby comes home, the mother tends to be nervous and insecure. She radiates tension, fear, anxiety, and shame which evoke negative re-sponses from the infant, who becomes fussy. As the mother anxiously introduces new foods, the infant learns to hesitate and becomes picky— the basis for attention and power struggles.

(c) the fat infant—The mother is happy and proud, at first associating fatness with health. But, this infant is always hungry and is heavy. The mother at first radiates pleasure but this turns to displeasure; the baby responds with frantic efforts to regain a pleasant interaction, becoming more demanding and overeating, if possible, which aggravates the prob-lem. A suspicious, insecure response develops.

(d) the allergic infant—The mother is panic stricken and tends to be over-anxious and over-protective. She radiates tension and fear to the infant who responds with fussiness and pickiness. This infant tends to be non-cooperative when the mother carefully and anxiously introduces new foods; this infant learns to be suspicious and to distrust unfamiliar foods.

(e) the malformed infant—The mother has fear, anxiety, and guilt feelings compounded with frustration in coping. She radiates these to the infant who also may suffer from fear and/or frustration in mastery of feeding techniques. This infant may try all kinds of games for power, especially if such behavior is reinforced.

Infants learn food-getting/food consumption behavior and food ideology continuously, either because of or in spite of the situation. Any unwanted effect probably can be modified if detected early enough, even malnutrition. For example, until recently, expert opinion was that irreversible mental retardation was the inevitable result. However, as a result of further examination of available data, some researchers had an inkling that the observed retardation might be due to the fact that a listless baby does not command or hold attention so it may not receive a normal amount of stimulation. Hence, it would be functionally isolated from a normal environment and would be retarded as a result of deprivation. By pursuing this line of reasoning, some researchers demonstrated that if an enriched environment was provided prior to age three, the retardation might be largely overcome. Thus, as of now, it does not appear that malnutrition *per se* has a permanent effect on learning ability. Therefore, ecological balance in the nutritional niche is most important.

Traditionally, infant feeding practices have been a blend reflecting home learning, parental instruction/guidance, peer experiences, and/or some formal instruction. The aggregate pattern has changed only by a slow process of diffusion. Observed differences in practices have been related to socioeconomomic status and/or cultural background, which had long been identified.

Recently, the rate of change in infant feeding practices has accelerated and the practices, themselves, have become highly variable. Changes have been observed as a response to media coverage of nutritional issues that may or may not pertain. Recent studies reviewed and summarized earlier in this chapter have documented the nature and extent of some of the changes that are occurring. They have demonstrated that the mean intake of many nutrients does not approximate the RDA. Although these studies provide only an estimation of what is happening, they do serve as a weathervane.

The most rational inference is that one should not respond to any current nutrition issue by following a crisis model of adjusting infant feeding practices. The objective is to provide the infant with a diet which provides a nutrient profile that approximates the RDA, the best guide to meeting the infant's needs. The media report the aggregate pattern. In cases of major deviance from the pattern, intensive effort should be directed at the critical nutrient intake(s), but it should supplement, not replace, instruction with respect to other nutrients. One must continually be aware of the practices advocated by the media and of the anticipated effects of overreaction, misinterpretation, etc., in the general public.

BIBLIOGRAPHY

ACOSTA, P.B., and ARANDA, R.G. 1972. Cultural determinants of food habits in children of Mexican descent in California. *In* Practices of Low-Income Families in Feeding Infants and Small Children, Proceedings National Workshop. S.J. Fomon and T.A. Anderson (Editors). DHEW Publ. (HSM) 72-5605, GPO, Washington, D.C.

ANDERSON, T.A. 1977. Commercial infant foods: content and composition. *In* Symposium on Nutrition in Pediatrics. C.G. Neumann and D.B. Jelliffe (Editors). Pediatr. Clin. North Am. *24* (1) 37-47.

BOWERING, J. *et al.* 1978. Infant feeding practices in East Harlem. J. Am. Dietet. Assoc. *72*, 148-155.

ERICKSON, E.K. 1950. Childhood and Society. W.W. Norton, New York.

FOMON, S.J. 1974. Infant Nutrition. 2nd Edition. W.B. Saunders Co., Philadelphia.

HAHN, P., and KIRBY, L. 1973. Immediate and late effects of premature weaning and feeding a high fat or high carbohydrate diet to weaning rats. J. Nutr. *103*, 690-696.

HAMBRAEUS, L. 1977. Proprietary milk versus human breast milk in infant feeding. *In* Symposium on Nutrition in Pediatrics. C.G. Neumann and D.B. Jelliffe (Editors). Pediatr. Clin. North Am. *24* (1) 17-36.

JELLIFFE, D.B., and JELLIFFE, E.F.P. 1978. The volume and composition of human milk in poorly nourished communities. A review. Am. J. Clin. Nutr. *31*, 492-515.

JEROME, N.W., KISER, B.B., and WEST, E.A. 1972. Infant and child feeding practices in an urban community in the north central region. *In* Practices of Low- Income Families in Feeding Infants and Small Children, Proceedings National Workshop. S.J. Fomon and T.A. Anderson (Editors). DHEW Publ. (HSM) 72-5605, GPO, Washington, D.C.

KNITTLE, J.L., GINSBER-FELLNER, F., and BROWN, R.E. 1977. Adipose tissue development in man. Am. J. Clin. Nutr. *30*, 762-766.

KRAMM, K.M., and OWEN, G.M. 1972. Nutritional studies on U.S. preschool children: dietary intake and practices in food procurement, preparation, and consumption. *In* Practices of Low-Income Families in Feeding Infants and Small Children. Proceedings National Workshop, DHEW. S.J. Fomon and T.A. Anderson (Editors). DHEW Publ. (HSM) 72-5605, GPO, Washington, D.C.

KROGER, M. 1972. Insecticide residues in human milk. J. Pediatr. *80*, 401-405.

KROGER, M. 1974. General environmental contaminants occurring in milk. *In* Lactation, a Comprehensive Treatise, Vol. III, Nutrition and Biochemistry of Milk/Maintenance. B.L. Larson and V.R. Smith (Editors). Academic Press, New York.

KROGER, M., and WATROUS, G.H. 1973. Inhibitory substances in human milk. J. Milk Food Technol. *36*, 140-142.

MASLANSKY, E. *et al.* 1974. Survey of infant feeding practices. Am. J. Public Health *64*, 780-785.

MASOVER, L. Unpublished thesis material. *Cited in* SENATE SELECT COMM. ON NUTR. AND HUMAN NEEDS, U.S. SENATE. 1977. Dietary Goals for the United States, 2nd Edition. GPO, Washington, D.C.

PETERKIN, B., and WALKER, M.S. 1976. Food for the baby. . . Cost and nutritive value considerations. Fam. Econ. Rev., Fall. p. 3-9. Consumer & Food Econ. Inst., Agric. Res. Serv., USDA, Washington, D.C.

PURVIS, G.A. 1973. What nutrients do our infants really get? Nutr. Today *8* (5) 28-34.

PURVIS, G.A., WALLACE, R.D., SKEBERDIS, J.H., and STEWART, R.A. The role of the diet in the nutrition of U.S. infants. Presented XI International Congress of Nutrition, 1978, Rio de Janeiro. (personal communication).

REISER, R., and SIDELMAN, Z. 1972. Control of serum cholesterol homeostasis by cholesterol in the milk of the suckling rat. J. Nutr. *102*, 1009-1016.

SCHLENK, H. 1972. Odd-numbered and new essential fatty acids. Fed. Proc., Fed. Am. Soc. Exp. Biol. *31*, 1430-1435.

SHAEFER, A.E., and JOHNSON, O.C. 1969. Are we well fed?. . . The search for the answer. Nutr. Today *4* (1) 2-11.

SIMS, L.S. 1978. Dietary status of lactating women. I. Nutrient intake from food and from supplements. J. Am. Dietet. Assoc. *73*, 139-146.

SIMS, L.S. 1978. Dietary status of lactating women. II. Relation of nutritional knowledge and attitudes to nutrient intake. J. Am. Dietet. Assoc. *73*, 147-154.

TAITZ, L.S. 1977. Obesity in pediatric practice: infantile obesity. *In* Symposium on Nutrition in Pediatrics. C.G. Neumann and D.B. Jelliffe (Editors). Pediatr. Clin. North Am. *24* (1) 107-115.

WIDDOWSON, E.M. 1977. Prenatal nutrition. Ann. N.Y. Acad. Sci. *300*, 188-196.

Nutritional Risk and Life Expectancy: Childhood

Intermittently, public attention focuses on child nutrition, which becomes an issue of national concern. In recent years, problems related to both under- and over-nutrition have been identified. A number of intervention programs had been implemented in an effort to reduce the incidence of various types of cases.

The data available on the nutritional status of children are rather limited. Surprisingly, there have been only three national population surveys of the nutritional status of American children. Sporadically, there have been local/regional studies. About 20 of limited age range, from a particular socioeconomic group, and/or some minority group, have been reported.

The three national population surveys were the Preschool Nutrition Survey, 1968-1970; the Ten State Nutrition Survey (TSNS), 1968-1970; and the Health and Nutrition Examination Survey (HANES), 1970-1974. In all, more than 10,000 children were evaluated.

Owen and Lippman (1977) reviewed the findings from the three national studies. They found that the prevalence of severe deficiency among young children was low:

(a) enlarged thyroid gland, less than 1%

(b) oral lesions associated with riboflavin and niacin deficiency, less than 1%

(c) vitamin A deficiency, between 1% and 2%

(d) vitamin D deficiency, between 1% and 2%

For children over age six years, the findings were somewhat different. For example:

(a) enlarged thyroid gland, 3 to 4%

(b) oral lesions associated with riboflavin and niacin deficiency, 3 to 4%

(c) vitamin A deficiency, 5%

(d) vitamin D deficiency, 1 to 2%

The prevalence of deficiency appears to be low. Other findings of interest also surfaced. The Preschool survey found that low income was correlated with small size of white children, and the TSNS found that with increasing income, children were heavier, taller, and had more mature skeletal and dental development. These three studies found that the mean size of Black children was less at birth and did not reach the mean for whites until between ages two and three. From age three to early adolescence, Black children grew more rapidly and were taller and heavier but not fatter than white children. The Preschool survey and TSNS found that siblings of the same age/sex groups were similar in height, weight, and degree of fatness. The TSNS also found great similarities in degree of fatness between children and their parents.

Dietary intake and biochemical findings were considered together. Findings from the three studies, except where noted, were similar:

(a) IF age, sex, and race are held constant, THEN caloric intake increases with income.

(b) Protein intake at each age was 1½ to 2 times the appropriate RDA.

(c) Vitamin A intakes were generally acceptable, although at each age Black children had lower median intakes and serum levels. Spanish-American children had the lowest vitamin A intake levels; 20 to 30% had unacceptably low intakes.

(d) About one-third of the children had dietary ascorbic acid intakes of about 20 mg, or half the RDA. When total intakes, including supplements, were compared with biochemical findings, the estimate was revised to a prevalence of 10 to 15%.

(e) The median calcium intake approximated the RDA. However, 20 to 30% of the Black children had intakes below half that of the RDA.

(f) Twenty to thirty percent ingested less than 5 mg iron per day. The Preschool survey reported the prevalence of anemia in Blacks as, 12%; Spanish-Americans, 10%; and whites, 7%. The HANES findings were 20 to 33%.

Many children are obese. However, the mean caloric intakes of the fat and lean children are approximately the same so a difference in energy expenditure may be the main problem.

The early reports of the TSNS that sampled groups expected to be at risk implied that the prevalence of malnutrition was substantial and that cases of malnutrition as severe as those seen in the less developed countries were observed. When the findings were aggregated with those of two other national samples, the proportions of those with deficiency were found to be lower. Reinterpretation of the findings using the median rather than the mean also presents a different picture.

Local/regional studies of particular groups report similar findings but greater severity in many cases. They support the position that anemia is a problem, although the prevalence varies with the group and the technique(s) used in measurement. (Hemoglobin and hematocrit values are not reliable indexes; serum iron and total iron binding capacity also need to be measured.) Vitamin A and ascorbic acid intakes are inadequate among scattered groups of minority children from low income families. Suboptimal Zn nutriture has been reported in one study. This finding has created much speculation with respect to the prevalence of Zn deficiency and possible implications.

Childhood nutriture is important to growth and development in relation to expression of genetic potential and later health. Food and feeding related beliefs, opinions, attitudes, intentions, habits, and practices are established during this period and have a lifelong impact on nutriture. Since no meals are provided and/or there is an abundance of empty-calorie snack foods in many homes, many children are nutritionally vulnerable.

CHILDHOOD: NORMAL SUPPLY AND NORMAL DEMAND

Nutritional needs of children are somewhat high in relation to their size. Both demands to support growth-related metabolic activity and demands to support a relatively high activity level inflate needs. Generally, height and weight changes follow a typical pattern. But, individuals differ in the time of commencement of and duration of the active growth period, so chronological age is only a first approximation in estimating needs.

Caloric intake is a critical variable in relation to growth rate. In constructing the RDA, the Food and Nutrition Board uses averages. To meet individual needs, the recommended intake should be adjusted to maintain the usual percentile weight or to modify weight in the appropriate direction.

The nutritional needs of toddlers aged one to three years differ from those of infants. During the toddler stage, the growth rate is reduced; appetite often lags accordingly and in the short run should be ignored. All nutrients are needed; those for which RDA have been established are listed in Table 27.1.

Protein requirements are relatively high in order to meet the needs for muscle mass development. Muscles in the back, buttocks, and thighs must develop in order for the toddler to stand and walk. The protein needs should be met with a protein combination of high biologic value; the essential amino acids must be supplied in order for muscle protein to be produced.

Mineral requirements are also relatively high. In order for the skeleton to bear the increasing weight, hardening by deposition of mineral salts is

TABLE 27.1. RDA FOR CHILDREN OF VARIOUS AGES

FOOD AND NUTRITION BOARD, NATIONAL ACADEMY OF SCIENCES–NATIONAL RESEARCH COUNCIL RECOMMENDED DAILY DIETARY ALLOWANCES,[a] REVISED 1980.

Designed for the maintenance of good nutrition of practically all healthy people in the U.S.A.

								Fat-Soluble Vitamins			Water-Soluble Vitamins	
Category	Age (Years)	Weight (kg)	(lb)	Height (cm)	(in.)	Protein (g)	Vitamin A (µg R.E.)[b]	Vitamin D (µg)[c]	Vitamin E (mg α T.E.)[d]	Vitamin C (mg)	Thiamin (mg)	Riboflavin (mg)
Children	1–3	13	29	90	35	23	400	10	5	45	0.7	0.8
	4–6	20	44	112	44	30	500	10	6	45	0.9	1.0
	7–10	28	62	132	52	34	700	10	7	45	1.2	1.4
Males	11–14	45	99	157	62	45	1000	10	8	50	1.4	1.6
	15–18	66	145	176	69	56	1000	10	10	60	1.4	1.7
	19–22	70	154	177	70	56	1000	7.5	10	60	1.5	1.7
Females	11–14	46	101	157	62	46	800	10	8	50	1.1	1.3
	15–18	55	120	163	64	46	800	10	8	60	1.1	1.3
	19–22	55	120	163	64	44	800	7.5	8	60	1.1	1.3

[a] The allowances are intended to provide for individual variations among most normal persons as they live in the United States under usual environmental stresses. Diets should be based on a variety of common foods in order to provide other nutrients for which human requirements have been less well defined.
[b] Retinol equivalents. 1 Retinol equivalent = 1 µg retinol or 6 µg β-carotene.
[c] As cholecalciferol. 10 µg cholecalciferol = 400 I.U. vitamin D.
[d] α-tocopherol equivalents. 1 mg d-α-tocopherol = 1 α T.E.

necessary. Additional teeth develop and are mineralized during this period.

The needs of the preschool child, aged four to six years, are somewhat greater than those of the toddler. They are approximately the same for both sexes. The RDA are shown in Table 27.1. Growth continues, but at a lesser rate. Periods of intense physical activity are interspersed with periods of inactivity. Needs vary with the daily pattern of activity. All nutrients continue to be necessary. The protein requirement remains relatively high to meet demands for increasing muscle mass and development. The mineral requirement continues to be high to support continued mineralization of bones and teeth.

The needs of the seven- to ten-year-old child are a little greater but not much different; the RDA are adjusted accordingly (Table 27.1). Growth during this stage is normally slow but highly variable. During this stage, body stores are accumulated to support the pre-pubertal growth spurt. Mineralization of bones and teeth continues.

CHILDHOOD: DEFICIENT SUPPLY OR INFLATED DEMAND

Growth retardation and iron-deficiency anemia are the two manifestations of malnutrition that are prevalent in the United States at this time. Individual cases of classic deficiency diseases may be seen occasionally.

Individual differences in the timing and duration of growth spurts are well known. So, whether growth is stunted or just delayed a little is somewhat difficult to determine unless the height-weight of a child differs markedly from the age-sex norm. The exact magnitude of the calorie deficit that will result in significant growth retardation has not

	Water-Soluble Vitamins					Minerals			
Niacin (mg N.E.)[1]	Vitamin B$_6$ (mg)	Folacin[2] (μg)	Vitamin B$_{12}$ (μg)	Calcium (mg)	Phosphorus (mg)	Magnesium (mg)	Iron (mg)	Zinc (mg)	Iodine (μg)
9	0.9	100	2.0	800	800	150	15	10	70
11	1.3	200	2.5	800	800	200	10	10	90
16	1.6	300	3.0	800	800	250	10	10	120
18	1.8	400	3.0	1200	1200	350	18	15	150
18	2.0	400	3.0	1200	1200	400	18	15	150
19	2.2	400	3.0	800	800	350	10	15	150
15	1.8	400	3.0	1200	1200	300	18	15	150
14	2.0	400	3.0	1200	1200	300	18	15	150
14	2.0	400	3.0	800	800	300	18	15	150

[1] N.E. (niacin equivalent) = 1 mg of niacin or 60 mg dietary tryptophan.
[2] The folacin allowances refer to dietary sources as determined by *Lactobacillus casei* assay after treatment with enzymes ("conjugases") to make polyglutamyl forms of the vitamin available to the test organism.

been determined, but there is some evidence that it is small, e.g., 250 kcal. However, this is a sizeable percentage of the child's allowance which is in the range of 1300 to 2400 kcal depending on age, sex, and size. IF caloric intake is less than needs, THEN the labile body proteins will be degraded to supply energy. Therefore, they will be unavailable for muscle mass development and muscle wasting also may occur. Therefore, the muscle mass of the child will be underdeveloped so he/she will lack stamina and endurance. Lacking energy, this child will be less alert and will show symptoms of lassitude.

In recent years there has been a continuing effort to determine whether protein or energy is the growth-limiting factor in protein-calorie malnutrition which affects some American children and many children in less developed countries. Payne (1975) stated the position that IF the diet of 2- to 3- year-olds contains even 5% of the calories as protein, from vegetable and/or animal sources, THEN the protein level is "safe" and energy is probably the limiting factor. Thus there is no protein problem.

Concern with preschool malnutrition has increased because of the TSNS findings of Schaefer and Johnson (1969) that the same kinds and prevalence of malnutrition exist among American children as in the less developed countries. For example, out of approximately 13,300 children of up to age 6 years, there were 8 cases of extreme vitamin A deficiency and 7 severe cases of kwashiorkor and marasmus—totally unexpected findings. In addition, there were the following:

(a) 490 cases of vitamin D deficiency (3 to 7%) including 18 cases of rickets

(b) 532 to 665 (4 to 5%) with general protein-calorie nutrition and 465 cases of severe growth retardation

(c) 665 (5%) with goiter

(d) 532 cases of scorbutic gums

In discussing the small number of cases of extreme deficiency, Schaefer and Johnson (1969) stated that in fact in this country this many cases was unexpected. The lesser forms seen represent "hidden hunger" which puts the children at nutritional risk should they be stressed. General health of these children was better than that of children in less developed countries because water, food, sewage, and medical care are better than that abroad. Because these general conditions are better, such children are not stressed except by common childhood diseases. Hence, frank starvation, beriberi, palagra, and advanced scurvy are not seen.

The text of the 1975 Women, Infants and Children Nutrition Act (WIC) states that Congress finds that many children are at special risk of physical and mental health impairment due to poor or inadequate nutriture. Poor growth rate or attainment, anemia, and inadequate nutrient intake are the nutritional risks of childhood. In an attempt to reduce the risk for children aged 1 to 4 years, the supplemental foods program provides foods to supply the following nutrients, based on the 1974 RDA, to qualified participants: protein, 23 to 30 g which is 100% of the RDA; calcium, 800 mg which is 100% of the RDA; iron, 10 to 15 mg which is 100% of the RDA; 2000 to 2500 IU vitamin A which is 100% of the RDA; ascorbic acid, 40 mg which is 100% of the RDA; and calories, 66% of the RDA. Participating children undoubtedly have benefited; a program limitation is the number of children that can participate. Since preschool children cannot effectively fend for themselves, especially in competition with older siblings, this program is especially important.

CHILDHOOD: EXCESSIVE SUPPLY

Many children gain extra weight between growth spurts, but then they thin out again and stay thin. Others gain weight and continue to gain. These latter cases are cause for concern.

Childhood is a second period in which the body pool of fat cells may be expanded. IF a child chronically ingests more calories than are necessary, THEN the excess will be stored AND when the cells in the pool become filled to the set-point, pool size is expanded in order to increase storage capacity.

The relative number and lipid content of adipose cells in obese and non-obese children, aged 2 to 16 years, have been determined. The patterns are very different and provide a partial explanation of the problem. Findings (Knittle, Ginsberg-Fellner, and Brown 1977) that pertain to non-obese children are:

(a) Mean cell size and number remain approximately the same between ages 2 and 10; then they increase.

(b) Mean cell size attains adult size at about age 12; thereafter, mean cell size is approximately the same as that of obese children.

(c) Mean cell number stabilizes between ages 14 and 16.

Findings that pertain to obese children (Knittle, Ginsberg-Fellner, and Brown 1977) are:

(a) Mean cell size, which already has reached adult size by age 2 years, remains approximately the same thereafter.

(b) Mean cell number is greater than in non-obese children at all ages between 2 and 16.

(c) Mean cell number stabilizes between ages 14 and 16.

Thus, the obese child has larger adipose cells and a greater number of cells at all ages. The causes of these differences are not well understood. Heredity and/or the effects of over-nutrition may be involved. Lipolytic activity induced by epinephrine is decreased. This may cause cell proliferation as a compensatory mechanism It would allow sufficient fatty acids to be released; a small amount from a larger aggregate would suffice. This is under investigation.

Childhood obesity is not a new phenomenon. What is new is recognition of the fact that generation of extra adipose cells at this time increases the probability of lifelong obesity. Therefore, since obesity is a major problem of adulthood that has its roots in childhood, preventive and remedial efforts are directed to this age group.

Weight control, i.e., reduced rate of weight gain, is the goal for children of preschool and school age who are overweight or obese. If the rate of gain can be reduced, in the long run the proper weight to height relationship can be (re)established. The recommended caloric intake is 60 kcal/kg for the weight the child would have at the 50th percentile norm. The recommended distribution of calories from a normal mixed diet is 20% from protein and 40% each from fat and carbohydrates. This distribution will allow gradual reduction in fat deposits without sacrificing growth in height or lean body mass.

High intakes of vitamin supplements by preschoolers have been reported recently (Kramm and Owen 1972; Crawford, Hankin, and Huenemann 1978). In most cases, the use of supplements was unrelated to need. In many cases, supplementation was unnecessary and resulted in excessive intakes.

Toxic intakes of vitamins A and D have been reported for a number of years. These are reported to and are summarized by the National Center for Disease Control. Such intakes are usually inadvertant, resulting from ingestion of high-potency drops in low-potency quantities after a supply change. The adult simply does not perceive that a different quantity might be necessary.

Excessive intakes of some foods, e.g., milk, have been reported to result in excessive intakes of calcium, phosphorus, and protein. Overconsumption of milk results in displacement of other foods, especially fruits and vegetables, and may cause a secondary deficiency. Particular problems due to the higher calcium and phosphorus intakes have not been reported. The effects of the elevated protein intakes are not well defined. Calcium absorption is reduced and there may be a possible relation to circulating cholesterol levels.

CHILDHOOD: FOOD ECOLOGY, NUTRITIONAL RISK, AND LIFE EXPECTANCY

For the purposes of establishing nutritional requirements and mean nutrient intake, the nutriture of children has been viewed out of context. But, in order to intervene successfully, the child's nutritional status has to be regarded as an outgrowth of his environment. The child lives in a family or institution, in American society, at a particular point in time, and under a particular set of conditions. All of these determine the array of foods available to the child. The child, reacting to some or all of these factors, consumes some or all of the foods presented and over time achieves the observed nutritional status. This summarizes the systems view.

Ecologically speaking, the overall initial goal is to sustain an eating environment which creates and reinforces a positive, accepting attitude toward food, eating, and food and people interactions in general. IF the child enjoys what he eats, THEN he has the prerequisites for acquiring beliefs, attitudes, opinions, intentions, and behaviors necessary for healthy functioning in the food environment. Nothing should be allowed to mar this positive feeling; manners, etc., are not critical variables during early childhood.

IF the eating environment radiates warmth and good cheer and is free from distractions and pressure, AND the child is assisted in using utensils or the food is pre-cut AND only small immediate objectives such as tasting food G or finishing X are set, THEN a hungry child will eat, all other things being equal. Until taught quantity and time discipline, a toddler or preschooler tends to respond naturally to physiological needs. The amount of physical energy expended by a child is highly variable within and among days; appetite varies accordingly. Thus, observed eating behavior with respect to quantity and eating frequency tends to be erratic and exasperating. The child should not be forced to eat a fixed quantity. IF the daily intake is uniformly too little or too much, THEN presence of some problem that requires medical attention may be indicated.

Spacing of meals is quite important. A child may play hard, exhausting immediate energy supply and creating a high demand for withdrawal from storage and processing that exceeds short run capacity. Therefore, symptoms of semi-starvation—weakness, irritability, and inattention—

will develop. The resulting behavior is both unnecessary and undesirable. A good breakfast is a good start, but lack of appetite or time may intervene. To compensate, the child should carry some nutritious food that can be consumed *ad libitum*. Later meals should be of reasonable but not compensatory size. Otherwise, poor habits result. A child is nutritionally vulnerable because of limited ability to deal with intervening variables such as excitement, fatigue, or minor illness. The child should not be forced to eat in spite of these conditions. Rather, since the child is dependent, the adult is personally responsible for minimizing this level of hazard; prevention is the best approach to control.

Each of the three stages of childhood confronts a child with a new set of developmental task-related challenges in every domain, including the eating experience. Observed behavior reflects the nature and extent of resolution, as well as its general quality.

The central developmental task confronting the toddler is to resolve the conflict among *autonomy* and *shame* and *doubt* (Erikson 1980). The toddler is striving for mastery over people, places, and things encountered as he/she establishes a basic identity; mobility and curiosity support this drive. When thwarted, the child accumulates a burden of failure and shame. Therefore, since the child is dependent, the adult is personally responsible for adjusting the size of obstacles in the eating environment to an appropriate size that facilitates positive development.

The central developmental task confronting the preschool child is to resolve issues concerning *initiative* and *guilt* (Erikson 1950). The preschool child is engaged in experimentation with situations and evaluating his response to them. He is curious, adventurous, and imitative. In this context, he is aware of others' responses to foods and food and people interactions. The preschool child is receptive to learning simple task-oriented techniques/strategies associated with various aspects of food preparation and service; he excels in the "assistant-to" role. Since the child is dependent, the adult is personally responsible for creating/maintaining an atmosphere of honest attitudes, intentions, and overt behavior.

The central developmental task confronting the school-age child is to resolve issues concerning *industry* and *inferiority* (Erikson 1950). The school-age child is involved in observation of alternative ways of doing things and in activities to develop competence, confidence, and independence. At this stage, a youngster may be interested in learning about roles of nutrients, foods as souces of nutrients, and how to monitor intake. Physical limitations, food intolerances, etc., are especially burdensome. Since the child is becoming independent, he/she increasingly shares responsibility for food selection, the quality of the eating experience, and smoothness of food and people interactions.

Children's food preferences are highly variable. They evolve in response to a continuously changing set of experiences which include (a) exposure to new people and their foodways, eating territories, foods, utensils, etc.; (b) positive associations due to enjoyable company, celebration of a festive event, excitement of exotic but pleasurable meals, and oral gratification due to color, flavor, and texture appeal; and (c) negative associations due to illness, bad manners, monotony, and painful physical experiences—too sour, bitter, biting, hot, cold, etc.

The information available concerning children's food preferences is very meager; we do *not* have a data base collected according to age cohort across all population subgroups. Therefore we cannot say whether observed changes in food habits are age-related, a function of general population trends, or a result of differential exposure. Five common assertions are discussed briefly:

(a) Children dislike spicy foods. This statement is misleading. Children like the style of cooking that they are used to and may not accept foods of other cultures. They are more sensitive to temperature, bite, etc., and will reject what is painful. However, Chicano children like the hot spicy corn-bean-tomato-chili dishes that they are exposed to. Similarly, Italian-American children become accustomed to the spicy Italian sauces, sausages, peppers, etc.

(b) Children prefer finger foods. Children aged one to four years may prefer these since they are engaged in exploring texture and are not yet proficient in use of eating utensils. At some point in the preschool period, children usually will limit acceptance of finger foods to those consumed by adults in the household.

(c) Children prefer raw vegetables to cooked vegetables. This depends on how they are cooked. They are well accepted if cooked only to the just-done stage but they are especially enjoyed raw if the noise of chewing attracts attention and/or annoys other members of the household.

(d) Children dislike mixtures. The like-dislike response depends on exposure. A Chinese-American child accepts numerous meat-vegetable mixtures but may hesitate over a stew with an unfamiliar flour gravy. And, a child used to a sandwich lunch and a solid meat-potato-vegetable dinner would be likely to reject a casserole or stew because it is unfamiliar.

(e) Children prefer familiar foods. This is true; however, in a situation where everybody else is eating and enjoying unfamiliar foods, most will try the foods.

The approach to and techniques used in rearing the child are an important factor in food acceptance. Consistency magnifies the effect(s). The observed effects depend on the exact way all factors come together, but a few generalizations have emerged from research. In summary:

(a) A permissive approach does not always lead to an open, accepting attitude toward eating and food and people interactions. There is some evidence that when a child is urged and coaxed but allowed the choice, erratic response leads to fussiness.

(b) A laissez-faire approach which minimizes direction and interference but encourages experimental sampling of people, places, and things is most likely to lead to an open-minded, flexible approach. Moreover, the child will be unlikely to reject a food or eating experience simply because it is an unknown.

(c) An authoritarian approach which compels a child to try everything, eat most of every portion, etc., may lead to an openness as a result of extensive exposure but it is more likely to result in rebellious rejection of numerous items.

The points that are related to and affect a child's relation to his food are innumerable. A few points about common concerns follow. A small number of dislikes is natural and normal. Dislike for a particular food should be ignored; a nutritionally equivalent item should be substituted. Categorical dislike for a class of foods such as meats is more serious since one may encounter difficulties in supplying some nutrients; causes for rejection and a remedy should be sought. Preference for empty-calorie snack foods that crowd out more nutritious foods is serious; retraining is necessary. Categorical rejection of unfamiliar foods may lead to problems in adjusting to changed food availability; encouragement and support for experimentation are necessary.

The nutritional and psychosocial consequences of the overall pattern of a child's eating habits need to be assessed and corrections implemented so as to balance the effects around optimality, however that is conceived. Whether nutritional risk and a threat to life develop depends on how the various factors come together in a particular case. Few die, but many perform suboptimally. Correction of marginal deficits can be expected to result only in small improvements, but every little bit counts.

BIBLIOGRAPHY

CRAWFORD, P.B., HANKIN, J.H., and HUENEMANN, R.L. 1978. Environmental factors associated with preschool obesity. III. Dietary intakes, eating patterns, and anthropometric measurements. J. Am. Dietet. Assoc. 72, 589-596.

ERIKSON, E.K. 1950. Childhood and Society. W.W. Norton, New York.

KNITTLE, J.L., GINSBERG-FELLNER, F., and BROWN, R.E. 1977. Adipose tissue development in man. Am. J. Clin. Nutr. 30, 762-766.

KRAMM, K.M., and OWEN, G.M. 1972. Nutritional studies on U.S. preschool children: dietary intake and practices in food procurement, preparation, and consumption. In Practices of Low-Income Families in Feeding Infants and Small Children, Proceedings National Workshop, DHEW S.J. Fomon and

T.A. Anderson (Editors). DHEW Publ. (HSM) *73-5605*. GPO, Washington, D.C.

OWEN, G., and LIPPMAN, G. 1977. Nutritional status of infants and young children: U.S.A. *In* Symposium on Nutrition in Pediatrics. C.G. Neumann and D.B. Jelliffe (Editors). Pediatr. Clin. North Am. *24*, 211-227.

PAYNE, P.R. 1975. Safe protein-calorie ratios in diets. The relative importance of protein and energy intake as causal factors in malnutrition. Am. J. Clin. Nutr. *28*, 281-286.

SCHAEFER, A.E., and JOHNSON, O.C. 1969. Are we well fed? . . . The search for the answer. Nutr. Today *4* (1) 2-11.

28

Nutritional Risk and Life Expectancy: Adolescence

Adolescence is characterized by utter confusion and/or extreme agitation—the nature, extent, and duration of such turmoil is highly variable among individuals. In the general confusion, nutriture *per se* is often neglected, although hunger may be assuaged. So, a great and continuous risk of harm and small chance of successfully avoiding disaster characterize these years. This is especially true for the teenage girl who limits caloric intake in an attempt to control her developing shape. IF she is malnourished and becomes pregnant, THEN her life and that of her infant may become endangered.

Examination of a few positions is revealing and brings into perspective some expected outcomes. IF a teenager was well nourished as an infant and a child, THEN other things being equal, he/she is physiologically set up to cope with the physiological demands of physical maturation. IF a teenager was poorly nourished in infancy and/or childhood, THEN the stress of rapid growth and development accentuates the effects of the previous nutritional history. For example, IF caloric intake (protein, fat, or carbohydrate) was low, THEN fat stores will be suboptimal and musculature may be undersized and/or underdeveloped. The body responds slowly to growth hormone and the sex hormones, so growth is stunted and sexual maturation is delayed. The time is not right; supply is out-of-phase with demands so problems that can never be corrected develop. Social and psychological problems are likely to develop and compound the problem. IF the teenager becomes interested in diet and starts to correct the deficits, THEN he/she will begin to grow, but since the time is past for some aspects to grow and develop they can never come together so as to reach genetic potential. The parts growing in the current stage will be overdeveloped in relation to those developed earlier, and, the end of the growth period will come before potential is reached, so the individual will be stunted in one or more aspects.

ADOLESCENCE: NORMAL SUPPLY AND NORMAL DEMAND

The nutrient needs of teenagers are highly variable. In general, needs for all nutrients are somewhat greater in the period that precedes the pubertal growth spurt and markedly higher during the growth and development period. They then taper off to the adult levels in the post-growth period. Since individuals mature at different rates, the greatly inflated and diminished demand points occur at various chronological ages. So, the RDA (Table 28.1) can be used only as a first approximation. Girls usually mature during the 11 to 14 years period and boys during the 15 to 18 years period. The RDA reflect these differences.

During adolescence, sexual maturation rate (SMR) varies among individuals. SMR is a more accurate guide to nutritional needs than is chronologic age. Therefore, individuals of a particular age group who are precocious would be likely to require nutrient supply at the next higher level. And, those whose development is checked for some reason, other than nutritional, would be likely to require nutrient supply at the next lower level. To avoid false security with respect to supply/demand status, this assessment of SMR to supply level should be repeated periodically.

Peak nutrient demands are met from a combination of endogenous and exogenous sources. A well-nourished teenager will have significant body stores of most nutrients. These can be drawn upon temporarily to meet peak needs. However, the stores do need to be replenished, especially by teenage girls in preparation for pregnancy. Dietary sources should be consumed at a level that meets usual demand and replenishes stores. Specific points with respect to need for particular nutrients follow.

Calories

The BMR is increased during the pubertal growth spurt and then it drops to adult levels based on final body size. BMR establishes the fixed portion of the energy demand. The magnitude of the variable portion depends on the nature and extent of physical activity engaged in. This portion of the total energy demand can be calculated using the charts in Chapter 7. Research has demonstrated that while teenagers are busy, actual energy expenditure may be low.

Protein

The demand is increased by growth requirements for production of additional muscle, skin, bone, blood, and hair tissue as well as hormones and enzymes. To meet this need, the RDA approximate adult levels which are about 25% greater than childhood levels.

Minerals

The demand for calcium, phosphate, and magnesium is increased due to need to mineralize the lengthening skeleton. The onset of menstruation increases the adolescent girl's need for iron. Moreover, as a future pregnancy would require additional iron, liver stores are accumulated against this need. Use of a supplement is probably necessary to meet a level of need of this magnitude.

Vitamins

The demand for the B vitamins is generally increased in conjunction with caloric needs. The need for vitamin A and ascorbic acid increases to normal adult levels.

ADOLESCENCE: DEFICIENT SUPPLY AND INFLATED DEMAND

During the pubertal growth spurt, the teenager attains adult stature. A deficiency of any nutrient will retard growth rate, and hence, ultimate size. When no other cause is present, general symptoms of suboptimal functioning such as dry skin, dull hair, irritability, and fatigue may imply a lesser deficit. Specific overt manifestations of major deficiency, other than anemia, are not often observed.

ADOLESCENCE: EXCESS SUPPLY OR DECREASED DEMAND

Two classes of nutrients are likely to be supplied in excess by the unwary teenager: calories and vitamins. In every way, the causes and effects differ.

Obesity, or at least overweight, is the effect of continued intake of an excess of calories. In the general population, it is most likely to result from individual cases of maladaptation. However, there are some cultural subgroups with high prevalence of obesity in which early maturation of the female is often followed by early and continued obesity.

Studies of the food intake and energy expenditure patterns of teenagers show that the overweight and normal weight teenagers consume about the same number of calories. The critical variable is energy expenditure. The overweight and obese teenagers are less active. For whatever reason(s), they select less demanding activities, are less active participants, and/or engage in physically demanding activities for a shorter time span and probably less frequently. As a result, their muscle mass is also less developed. Thus, their BMR is somewhat less and the variable portion of their energy demand is much less. So, their total energy demand is less

TABLE 28.1. FOOD AND NUTRITION BOARD, NATIONAL ACADEMY OF SCIENCES-
NATIONAL RESEARCH COUNCIL RECOMMENDED DAILY DIETARY ALLOWANCES[a]
FOR ADOLESCENTS, REVISED 1980

Category	Age (years)	Weight (kg)	Weight (lb)	Height (cm)	Height (in.)	Protein (g)	Fat-Soluble Vitamins			Water-Soluble Vitamins		
							Vitamin A (μg R.E.)[b]	Vitamin D (μg)[c]	Vitamin E (mg αT.E.)[d]	Vitamin C (mg)	Thiamin (mg)	Riboflavin (mg)
Males	11–14	45	99	157	62	45	1000	10	8	50	1.4	1.6
	15–18	66	145	176	69	56	1000	10	10	60	1.4	1.7
Females	11–14	46	101	157	62	46	800	10	8	50	1.1	1.3
	15–18	55	120	163	64	46	800	10	8	60	1.1	1.3

[a] The allowances are intended to provide for individual variations among most normal persons as they live in the United States under usual environmental stresses. Diets should be based on a variety of common foods in order to provide other nutrients for which human requirements have been less well defined.
[b] Retinol equivalents. 1 Retinol equivalent = 1 μg retinol or 6 μg β-carotene.
[c] As cholecalciferol. 10 μg cholecalciferol = 400 I.U. vitamin D.
[d] α-tocopherol equivalents. 1 mg d-α-tocopherol = 1 αT.E.
[e] 1 N.E. (niacin equivalent) = 1 mg of niacin or 60 mg of dietary tryptophan.

and they store the excess. Thus, they are maladapted because they have
not adapted their appetite to low energy demands. Since many feel
compelled to eat for social reasons, they consume more than they need.

Others eat to compensate and are only vaguely aware of the quantity of
food that they consume. Some are bored; they eat for something to do.
Some are apprehensive or frustrated; they eat compulsively to ease their
anxiety. This mode of alleviating the symptoms by means of comfort,
solace, or reassurance creates more problems than it solves. Hence, it is
maladaptive.

A large number of the female members of some cultural subgroups seem
to become obese in their early teens and remain so for the rest of their
lives. No satisfactory explanation for this phenomenon has been provided. Low income and consumption of high carbohydrate diets are
associated, but whether the cultural pattern results in decreased physical
activity or unnecessarily increased consumption is unclear.

When the lipid content of adipose cells approaches capacity, reaction
kinetics creates opposition which slows the rate of accumulation and
triggers other responses. The number of adipose cells is a critical variable
in weight control, controlling the aggregate amount of lipid that can be
stored. See Chapter 7. The pubertal growth period is the third, and
seemingly final, period in life when the number of adipose cells can be
increased. Therefore, control of the energy supply/demand relationship
during this period is of fundamental importance to adult weight control.

Excessive intake of vitamins varies from trivial to toxic levels. Usually,
the intake is deliberate but based on misconceptions of need and expected effects. Frequently, excessive intake patterns are faddish and short-
lived, so should be ignored because they are probably harmless. When
chronic, high doses can be hazardous. In the case of vitamin A, therapeutic doses are given in the treatment of acne and create a risk of
side effects unless carefully monitored. The B vitamins, being water-

Water-Soluble Vitamins				Minerals					
Niacin (mg N.E.)[r]	Vitamin B₆ (mg)	Folacin[f] (μg)	Vitamin B₁₂ (μg)	Calcium (mg)	Phosphorus (mg)	Magnesium (mg)	Iron (mg)	Zinc (mg)	Iodine (μg)
18	1.8	400	3.0	1200	1200	350	18	15	150
18	2.0	400	3.0	1200	1200	400	18	15	150
15	1.8	400	3.0	1200	1200	300	18	15	150
14	2.0	400	3.0	1200	1200	300	18	15	150

[f] The folacin allowances refer to dietary sources as determined by *Lactobacillus casei* assay after treatment with enzymes ("conjugases") to make polyglutamyl forms of the vitamin available to the test organism.
[g] The RDA for vitamin B₁₂ in infants is based on average concentration of the vitamin in human milk. The allowances after weaning are based on energy intake (as recommended by the American Academy of Pediatrics) and consideration of other factors such as intestinal absorption; see text.
[h] The increased requirement during pregnancy cannot be met by the iron content of habitual American diets or by the existing iron stores of many women; therefore the use of 30–60 mg of supplemental iron is recommended. Iron needs during lactation are not substantially different from those of non-pregnant women, but continued supplementation of the mother for 2–3 months after parturition is advisable in order to replenish stores depleted by pregnancy.
Reproduced from: Recommended Dietary Allowance, Ninth Edition (1980) with the permission of the National Academy of Sciences, Washington, D.C.

soluble, are not retained to a significant excess beyond need. A high circulating level of vitamin D can disturb calcium, phosphate, and magnesium metabolism, resulting in mineralization of soft tissues. Although a toxicity syndrome has yet to be associated with mega-dose ingestion of vitamin E, high consumption is not recommended since it is accumulated in seemingly limitless quantity. The hazard of excess consumption of ascorbic acid in relation to conditioned deficiency and other manifestations was delineated in Chapter 12.

ADOLESCENCE: FOOD ECOLOGY, NUTRITIONAL RISK, AND LIFE EXPECTANCY

Adolescence is a period of turmoil and the teenager's relation to his food reflects this. From the inside view, his relation to his food is under control—his own. He asserts his right to eat whatever, whenever, and however. From the outside view, it seems to be out of control since the structure of regular planned consumption is uncommon. And, unfortunately, a small percentage of teenagers become malnourished and require medical treatment. The percentage is small but represents thousands. So, nutritional risk causes concern. Characterization of a few cases clarifies the nature and extent of some common aspects.

Busy Bee Blewett

Bee is popular. She engages in constant and frantic activity associated with school, clubs, music, dance, and spectator sports. Hurry, hurry, hurry—she runs from one activity to another. Her schedule is impossible.

She drags out of bed late, grabs an instant breakfast or a glass of milk if she can, and rushes off. Between morning classes she grabs a snack from the vending machine and hopes for time to eat it before class. At noon she goes to a meeting, passing by the vending machine again for more munchies. After school she has more activities or work; she grabs a carbonated beverage for a pick-up during the break. At 10 p.m. she staggers in famished and fatigued, she forages in the refrigerator and gulps down whatever she can find, then flies to her room to study half the night. Since Bee is popular, weekends follow a similar pattern of activities.

Nutritionally, the diet intake pattern associated with this life-style is deplorable. Bee does not pay mindful attention to her nutritional needs; whether due to ignorance, neglect, or disdain, the effect is the same. Hunger is assuaged by consumption of empty-calorie foods that are rich in fat, sugar, starch, and/or salt. Protein, vitamins, minerals, and bulk are missing or short. Bee is busy but not physically active so she gains weight.

To the casual observer, she may seem normal. But, she is not quite up to par and has no reserves to draw on in case of illness, injury, or pregnancy. She is vulnerable.

Atlas Athlete

Atlas makes a cult of the body. He is engaged in constant and frantic physical activity in an attempt to build his physique and prowess. His schedule allows time for consumption of the strict training diet imposed by his coach. He rises at dawn, runs two miles, and sits down to a heavy training meal and an array of dietary supplements. Then he goes to school and gets through the morning; no snacking is allowed. He eats his planned training lunch, based on one advocated by an Olympic star. Then he gets through the afternoon classes and works out until dinner time. Dinner is a heavy red meat and vegetable meal. Afterward, he flops in front of the television or half-heartedly attempts to study. The weekend workouts are strenuous and eating is heavy.

Nutritionally, the diet pattern associated with this life-style is likely to be adequate because of the quantity of food consumed. However, the quantity of food consumed is much greater than normal. It is necessary, given energy outputs. It programs appetite, so the habit of overeating is established. Thus, when Atlas slows down, he will gain weight rapidly.

In the hope of improving physical performance, the dietary and training regimens of stars are imitated. When little or no improvement in performance results, a degenerative response pattern often develops— disillusion, erosion, indifference, and finally abandonment. Ingestion of some assortment of nutrients is intensive but transitory. Therefore, the effect is unlikely to be harmful.

Fat Faddy

Fat Faddy makes a cult of her body—she desires the striking sleek and slender look. She is engaged in constant and frantic dieting efforts. Her eating pattern is two to three weeks on strict diet A, about three weeks of eating whatever she desires, two to three weeks on strict diet B, etc. Hunger is not assuaged and the diet is not satisfying, so the degenerate pathway is followed: disillusionment with the diet, erosion of belief in its value, indifference in following it, then abandonment. As customary food habits have not been affected, they are revived and hunger disappears. Eating again becomes a pleasure. But, then weight starts to increase again, so another diet is sought and implemented.

Nutritionally, the erratic eating pattern associated with this style of weight control is disastrous. Deficits of some nutrients are aggravated by excesses of others; stress results. But, it is only temporary since a new pattern is soon implemented. The new pattern may alleviate or exacerbate the stress. Fat Faddy has no reserves to draw on in case of illness, injury, or pregnancy. Her general nutritional status is marginal and she is exceedingly vulnerable.

Health Trip Hoozit

Hoozit makes a cult of his/her body. He/she is engaged in a continuing and balanced schedule of eating and physical activity. Hoozit's typical weekday schedule is to rise at dawn, and to jog two miles before sitting down to enjoy a leisurely, planned, and well prepared breakfast. He/she walks/bikes to school, attends classes, and consumes a fruit snack between classes. After joining friends in the milk line and consuming a sack lunch with the group, he/she attends afternoon classes and walks/bikes home. Then, he/she joins the group for a workout at the gym, and later takes a short rest before sitting down to a leisurely dinner. It is planned and well prepared. He/she utilizes the evening for work, television, and/or study. Hoozit follows a different schedule on weekends. Saturday he/she rises at dawn, jogs two miles before sitting down to a quick but planned breakfast, and then, bikes to work. He/she consumes a snack at both breaks and purchases lunch, selecting an acceptable but nourishing assortment of items. He/she bikes home after work, does the chores, and joins friends for an evening out. Sunday, he/she sleeps in, consumes a leisurely planned brunch, and then joins a group for some combination of outdoor activities, e.g., biking, jogging, tennis, volleyball, or swimming. Eating time and place are variable, but are selected carefully.

The planned diet-exercise regimen is intended to create/maintain optimal physical health. In relation to nutriture, IF knowledge of nutritional needs and food sources of nutrients is sound AND Hoozit uses reason to guide choices and set limits, THEN the health trip is a positive action for health. IF misconceptions exist in regard to nutrient needs/sources or IF food fads are followed, THEN the effects of dietary inadequacy are added to nutritional needs inflated by high physical demand AND nutritional disaster may ensue. Therefore, Health Trip Hoozit may be nutritionally vulnerable.

This brief view of four cases reveals the inherent bases for nutritional vulnerability that are associated with these styles. The socio-cultural matrix of a given local area is one factor that determines which type of case predominates. And, the "temper of the times" is a predisposing factor.

In addition, teenagers as individuals have tasks confronting them as a result of their basic human needs. These needs are manifested in every domain, in this case in respect to food: physiological demand for food; safety-security in relation to food, the eating experience, and food and people interactions; belongingness with respect to food and people interactions; status in food and people interactions; and self-actualization through relations to food, the eating experience, and/or food and people interactions. Chapter 16 contains a detailed discussion of these needs. Suffice it to say that if Busy Bee has an underlying need for belongingness, she may overdo eating of the "in" foods in order to ensure group acceptance. This may further decrease her nutrient intake if the "in" foods are empty-calorie foods. Or, if any of the case types have an underlying safety-security need, they may opt for organic foods; the nutritional effect is unpredictable. Or, if the need is for belongingness and love, and they lack this in specific relationships, they may accept a philosophy that focuses on love and respect for all living things; vegetarianism would result. How these underlying problems are dealt with is reflected as a deviation from the typical model for their case. Many variations result.

All teenagers are confronted also with the central developmental task. According to Erikson (1950), at this stage of development it is to resolve the conflict between *identity* and *role diffusion* or *confusion*, i.e., a disorientation that results in diffuse actions. Formerly, one's position was determined by birth and the father's occupation. Class differences determined the beliefs, attitudes, intentions, and overt behaviors that were instilled in childhood. Therefore, grave difficulties were encountered if one's nature caused one to be a misfit and seek another position.

Ostensibly, in America, an individual can attain any level of position that is desired. Middle-class beliefs, attitudes, intentions, and overt behaviors are the norm. But these are in a continuous state of change and many cultural subgroups have their own ways.

Of course, individuals do not all respond in the same way. But, some pattern appears to have emerged. Resolution of the identity crisis requires that the teenager experiment with a variety of foodways as part of the process of growing up. Efforts are diffuse; the teenager tries many different foodways as a means of gaining experience. As other aspects of his/her position become clear, out of this confusion of foodways evolves an individual set that will be in harmony with other aspects of the person's identity. Thereafter, this set will be a part of his/her identity.

The turmoil of adolescence thus appears to result from diffuse efforts to resolve the identity crisis, which is a preliminary to adulthood. Because of the turmoil, the teenager is potentially at nutritional risk. Fortunately, growing boys have appetites proportional to their needs. So, they are unlikely to become malnourished. Teenage girls have sufficient appetite but they attempt to control it to limit their weight and may become malnourished. If they then become pregnant, life may be threatened.

BIBLIOGRAPHY

ERIKSON, E.K. 1950. Childhood and Society. W.W. Norton, New York.

FRANKLE, R.T., and HEUSSENSTAMM, F.K. 1974. Food zealotry and youth. Am. J. Public Health *64*, 11-18.

HAMPTON, M.C., HUENEMANN, R.S., SHAPIRO, L.R., and MITCHELL, B.W, 1967. Caloric and nutrient intakes of teen-agers. J. Am. Dietet. Assoc. *50*, 385-396.

HAMPTON, M.C. *et al.* 1966. A longitudinal study of gross body composition and body conformation and their association with food and activity in a teen-age population. Am. J. Clin. Nutr. *19*, 422-435.

KAUFMANN, N.A., POSNANSKI, R., and GUGGENHEIM, K. 1975. Eating habits and opinions of teen-agers on nutrition and obesity. J. Am. Dietet. Assoc. *66*, 264-268.

LEVERTON, R.M. 1968. The paradox of teen-age nutrition. J. Am. Dietet. Assoc. *53*, 13-16.

SCHORR, B.C., SANJUR, D., and ERICKSON, E.C. 1972. Teen-age food habits. J. Am. Dietet. Assoc. *61*, 415-420.

Nutritional Risk and Life Expectancy: Young Adulthood

From the perspective of the young adult, i.e., the inside view, his/her foodways appear to be an outgrowth of those that evolved during adolescence. In part, this is true. But it is also true that a young adult may be unaware of the magnitude of changes that may have occurred.

The young adult is aware that he/she has moved from the family home into another living arrangement. However, frequently he/she does not perceive the series of small changes in the array of foods consumed, eating frequency, number and class of meal components, etc., that occur in response to an ever changing set of situational imperatives. A sharp difference in food availability is necessary in order to claim attention given other needs/demands. Even then, complaints rather than awareness of nutritional implications are a frequent outcome.

From the perspective of concerned parents and professionals, i.e., the outside view, young adults often appear to subsist on a nutritionally inadequate diet. A variety of factors is involved. They differ somewhat according to college student or non-college student status:

(a) College students are engrossed in academic and extracurricular activities or are employed. For many, food and nutrition management means to assuage hunger with whatever is at hand. Those living in apartments would appear to be most vulnerable. Some do not have time and energy to manage well on a limited budget. Others lack necessary knowledge/skills, never having been involved with food and nutrition management considerations before.

(b) Those who are employed full-time or are starting a home are engrossed in establishing job- and/or social position-related activities. Due to limits of time, energy, and/or money that are imposed by these circumstances, or lack of knowledge/skill in food and nutrition management, their diet is often poorly controlled.

The diets of young adults feature coffee, starchy foods, and snack foods (Jakobovits *et al.* 1977). In addition, meal skipping and fad diets are common. As a result, a balanced intake of all nutrients is unlikely in many cases.

Observation reveals that IF a constraint (e.g., time, energy, money, knowledge/skill) is imposed for a long time, e.g., throughout the college years, THEN the change in foodways may become permanent. IF there are intermittent periods when more time is available or when food gifts are received, THEN a personalized version of family foodways is likely to be continued.

During this stage of the life cycle, nutritional risk is related more to income than to age *per se*. Prevalence of frank malnutrition is lower in this age group than in others and consequences are not as grave, except in the case of pregnancy.

YOUNG ADULTS: NORMAL SUPPLY AND NORMAL DEMAND

Maintenance of tissue integrity and appropriate weight for height are the nutritional objectives for this stage in the life cycle. Since full growth has been attained, physiologic demand is based on a combination of basal metabolic and activity-related needs.

More is known about the nutriture of young adults than of any other age group. This is probably attributable to the fact that most human nutrition research is done by faculty using student subjects.

The reference man and woman developed by the Food and Nutrition Board as models for nutrient needs are young adults, aged 25 years, living under standardized conditions that are presumed to be typical for Americans at this point in time The nutrient needs associated with these male and female reference standards are used (a) for evaluation of the nutritional status of the young adult population, (b) as a basis for planned decreases in caloric intake in later years (by age decade), and (c) as a standard for maintenance needs. The discussions of normal supply and demand in Chapters 3 through 13 were based largely on the research findings and theoretical explanations derived from studies in this age group. They are not repeated here.

All nutrients are needed by the young adult for maintenance and repair of tissues. However, the overall demand is only moderate and is lower than in teenage years, e.g., caloric need may be decreased by 500 kcal/day. Therefore, when caloric intake is adjusted to control weight appropriately, the necessary nutrient density presents a challenge. IF the individual remains physically active, THEN the challenge is more easily met without compromise. This is because the greater the caloric intake the greater the number of alternative ways in which other nutrient needs can be met. Specific points with respect to supply and demand of each class of nutrients follow.

Calories

The BMR for males and females of different sizes is shown in Table 7.1. It represents the demand for energy created by life-sustaining functions. Physical activity creates a variable demand that is superimposed on the BMR. The size of this demand varies according to nature, intensity, and duration parameters. IF weight is appropriate and stable, THEN caloric intake is adjusted to output. Otherwise, since one tends to slow down physically to a noticeable degree by age 30, one should monitor intake and output monthly and adjust caloric intake appropriately.

Reasonable proportions of protein, fat, and carbohydrate have been stated as 15%, 35%, and 50%, respectively. Research related to etiology of the killer diseases, coronary heart disease in particular, has demonstrated that in men serum lipid levels rise and atherosclerosis appears and develops during late teens and twenties. Therefore, since a causal relationship between diet and disease development is generally accepted, emphasis on control of the proportion of fat intake during this stage seems to be appropriate. This is especially so since at the present time, once the damage is done it cannot be reversed.

Minerals

IF the recommended proportions of protein, fat, and carbohydrate are implemented, THEN the quantity of meat consumed would be less than current mean intakes and the quantity of cereals consumed would be greater. The most noticeable effect on mineral nutrition would be decreased iron uptake due to ingestion of a lower total quantity and a lower proportion of heme iron, which is the most absorbable type. This is a matter of concern, although a mean intake of 12 mg on a continuing basis would be adequate and might be provided. However, IF a documented past history of a woman's iron intake were unavailable so that the extent of her liver iron stores were unknown, THEN because monthly menstrual losses are significant AND the iron cost of a pregnancy is high, AND because absorption is somewhat variable according to need, the 18 mg intake recommended by the Food and Nutrition Board is more desirable. It is sufficient for maintenance and provides for some excess to allow for replenishment of stores. Young women usually do not require an intake of more than 2000 kcal. Since the mean iron content of the current American diet is 6 mg/kcal, supplementation is necessary.

Intake of other minerals, e.g., Zn and Cu, also might be marginal since meat is a major source. However, cereals do contain some so consumption of a greater quantity would increase their importance as a source.

Vitamins

The thiamin, riboflavin, and niacin needs are related to carbohydrate and/or caloric intake. Therefore, IF the planned proportion of carbohydrate is obtained from whole grain or enriched products, THEN intake of these vitamins will be adequate. A positive action is usually required in order to ingest a sufficient quantity of vitamin A and ascorbic acid since these vitamins are distributed unevenly in foods.

YOUNG ADULTS: DEFICIENT SUPPLY AND INFLATED DEMAND

Deficient supply of any nutrient is a possibility. However, at the present time, iron is the only nutrient that is likely to be undersupplied unless there is an intervening variable. And, the undersupply situation is confined to women. IF a woman consumes a diet that provides less than the mean amount of iron, THEN development of iron-deficiency anemia is a likely outcome, all other things being equal. Compensatory supplementation is the recommended solution.

Use of one of the oral contraceptive agents (OCA) creates a pseudo-pregnant metabolic state. Therefore, the demand and supply relationships are altered. By law, a package insert must call attention to this fact. The need for vitamin B_6 is inflated to an important degree; compensatory supplementation is advocated.

YOUNG ADULTS: EXCESS SUPPLY AND DECREASED DEMAND

Energy is the nutrient most likely to be supplied in excess. When the former college and/or high school athlete accepts employment in a sedentary position, the downward readjustment of food intake presents a formidable problem since intake must be halved. IF the level of physical activity can be reduced to a normal level over a two-year period or so, THEN excessive weight gain during the period of dietary readjustment can be avoided.

Others face the same problem in adjusting to a sedentary worklife, but it is usually less severe. For this reason, it may be unrecognized until a significant gain has been made.

Excess of any other nutrient is also a possibility. The effects of excessive supply were covered in Chapters 3 through 13.

YOUNG ADULTS: FOOD ECOLOGY, NUTRITIONAL RISK, AND LIFE EXPECTANCY

The young adult is confronted with (a) the general problems of creating a desirable work-centered/leisure-centered life-style, and (b) according to Erikson (1950), resolution of the conflict between *intimacy* and *isolation*. The way in which these are dealt with affects food ecology, which determines nutritional risk and may affect life expectancy.

Historically, when an individual left school at some age between 12 and 18, adult responsibilities for job, house, family, etc., were assumed immediately. The transition was quite abrupt. Because expectations and demands were less, most appeared to function adequately. Advice, assistance, and other forms of support also were available from the family who lived nearby.

The current situation is different for about 75% of American teenagers. Most continue their education at the community college or college level. Hence, they do *not* assume the burden of adult responsibilities until four to six years later. During the interim, teenage foodways may be continued and reinforced or new food habits and practices may develop.

When the young adult has completed his/her education, then the adult role is assumed. This presents a variety of challenging tasks associated with development of some type of work-centered/leisure-centered lifestyle. The stresses that occur frequently result in a configuration of priorities with food and nutrition close to the bottom. This creates nutritional risk for the young woman. Four common aspects of the new role are: the provider role, the new work situation, intimate group relationships, and decreased physical activity.

Acceptance of Personal Responsibility as a Provider

At this stage one is expected to assume full adult responsibility for determining the degree of importance of and priority associated with provision of food, food experiences, and food and people interactions. If one does not, importance and priority are determined by chance, since "not to decide is to decide." Goals and objectives evolve accordingly and determine choice, knowledge and skills required, etc. The amount of food expenditures, the amount of time and other resources allocated to purchasing and preparation as well as other related tasks, the quality of kitchen and dining facilities selected/maintained, etc., are a function of the nature and extent of responsibility assumed, given opportunities.

Adjustment to New Situation

The job is a major factor in determining identity and status. For most people, co-workers set norms for beliefs, attitudes and opinions, intentions, and habits or practices in relation to food and food experiences, as well as food and people interactions. The individual must identify with these in order to fit in and be accepted. Status is usually accorded to older established members and must be earned by the newcomer by developing skill in a unique and valued aspect that enriches group potential.

Establishing Intimate Group Relationships

Marriage or any other shared living arrangement requires that divergent beliefs, attitudes, preferences, and intentions, as well as habits and practices with respect to choice of foods, food experiences, and food and people interactions, become an issue. Whether acceptance and enrichment or tension and conflict result depends on the degree of divergence and the degree of flexibility of the individuals involved. During this stage, income is low in relation to demands on it, so nutriture may be suboptimal. If a pregnancy occurs, the young woman and her unborn child are at nutritional risk.

Adjustment to Decreased Physical Activity

The usual interpersonal, productivity, and/or time-discipline requirements of the majority of occupations create anxiety and frustration which result in nervous fatigue. In the interests of production efficiency, mechanical aspects are performed by machine. So, the physical demands are low and are frequently insufficient for utilization of the adrenalin secreted in response to nervous stimuli. The result is a sedentary lifestyle; little physical energy is expended at work and one is too enervated to expend much on leisure-time activities. This tendency must be overcome in the interests of weight control and physical fitness.

Within this framework, a number of other factors contribute to the pattern of relations to the food environment that evolve. Alone, or in combination, they may create nutritional risk.

The food habits developed by a young adult usually are similar to those followed in the late teens, all other things being equal. Thus, the four types described previously, i.e., Busy Bee, Atlas Athlete, Fat Faddy, and Health Trip Hoozit are often continued by young adults. The strength of these food habits grows and they become more resistant to change.

Also, the cumulative and aggregate effects of marginal or imbalanced intake may become manifest.

Another factor that shapes a young adult's relation to his/her food environment reflects the degree of resolution of developmental tasks in previous stages and whether further development or regression has occurred. For example, an infant may have learned to trust all aspects of the food and people interaction. While a strong relationship will be resistant to change, a major or continuing set of negative experiences can result in erosion of trust. Therefore, if this has occurred, trust may need to be re-established or bolstered. Or, feelings of general inferiority compounded with lack of focus during the teenage years may have infiltrated and undermined an otherwise healthy food ecosystem. This would need attention. Thus, the unfinished business of other stages may be an intervening variable with extensive ramifications. For health, correction is necessary.

Permeating this stage of the life cycle, as all others, are the basic human needs. These may be satisfied in a vast number of ways at an almost infinite number of levels. These needs, discussed in Chapter 16 in moderate detail, are physiological needs, safety-security, belongingness, status, and self-actualization. Satisfaction of these needs is in a dynamic state of change and is always relative. Depending on assumptions, one can visualize a wide array of outcomes.

As a result of all these forces, the observed food habits at the beginning of young adulthood may be inconsistent. However, as one settles the pattern becomes more distinct. IF the ecological effect is improved as challenges are met, THEN nutritional risk is reduced. IF it continues to be marginal, the cumulative and aggregate effect may be suboptimal nutritional status that verges on pathology. IF poor habits continue, THEN the setup for definite pathology exists.

Reporting of the foodways and nutrient intakes of young adults has been sporadic, resulting in a fragmented view that has created popular concern. Since the early years of this century there have been intermittent reports of selected aspects from Maine, New York, Florida, Iowa, Montana, California, Oregon, and other states. No nationwide studies limited to this age group have been reported, although the group is included in the sample when most stratified sampling plans are used. Because of differences in temporal, regional, situational (dormitory or free-living), age, sex, and methodological variables, the studies are not comparable. Hence, the fragmented view results.

To an unknown extent, the foodways and nutrient intakes of young adults nationwide may be similar. IF so, THEN findings of Jakobovits *et al.* (1977) with respect to college women may be generalized. This group of investigators compared 1974 findings with those from a study 30 years earlier and of investigations at other times and places. Using the 1974 RDA as the standard for evaluation, some findings of general interest were:

(a) Mean intakes from diet and supplements of ascorbic acid were very high, mean intakes of protein and vitamin A were high, and mean intakes of iron were low. Mean intakes of riboflavin, preformed niacin, calcium, calories, and thiamin approximated the standard. The range of intake means was wide and reflected a few individual means rather than flat distributions.

(b) Mean intakes of calories and eight other nutrients studied were similar to those obtained earlier in this locale. The RDA had changed so nutritional interpretation and implications differed.

(c) Approximately one-third utilized at least one nutrient supplement, usually a multivitamin with iron.

(d) The amount of money spent for food was unrelated to nutritional adequacy.

(e) Mean eating frequency was greater than five, reflecting a habit of snacking in addition to consuming meals.

(f) Meal skipping patterns were discernable. Lunch was the meal most often skipped (75% of subjects). This was attributed to a scheduling problem: lack of a defined lunch period and insufficient time between a series of class periods. Breakfasts were consumed by more than 50% of the subjects.

Undoubtedly, the cumulative and aggregate effect of poor nutrition in this stage poses a threat to life expectancy. Until this stage, concern was with immediate effects in regard to growth and development and long-term effects which were not well understood were omitted. But, in this stage, the focus shifts to health maintenance for the duration. IF one fails during this stage, THEN the damage is done even though pathology does not often become manifest or an immediate threat until later. Therefore, it behooves one to control dietary intake, to the extent possible, in this stage. No amount of care in a subsequent stage can reverse effects of poor nutrition, although the rate of progression and/or misery might be reduced somewhat by means of a strict therapeutic diet.

BIBLIOGRAPHY

ERIKSON, E.K. 1950. Childhood and Society. W.W. Norton, New York.

HOSKINS, M.D. 1976. Reassessment of food practices and preferences of some university students. New Mexico Agric. Exp. Stn. Bull. *640*.

JAKOBOVITS, C. *et al.* 1977. Eating habits and nutrient intakes of college women over a thirty-year period. J. Am. Dietet. Assoc. *71*, 405-411.

OSTROM, S., and LABUZA, T.P. 1977. Analysis of a seven-day diet survey of college students. Food Technol. *31* (5) 69-71, 74, 76.

SCOULAR, F.I., and DAVIS, A.N. 1968. Balance studies of young college women consuming self-selected diets. North Texas State Univ., Denton.

30

Nutritional Risk and Life Expectancy: Middle Age

Killer degenerative diseases such as diabetes, heart disease, stroke, and cirrhosis pose an increasing threat to life expectancy, starting in middle age. In addition, debilitating and disabling degenerative diseases such as arthritis and osteoporosis add to the total of those who survive but are disabled by the killer diseases. Obesity has been identified as a common contributing factor.

With the exception of coronary heart disease, research has not demonstrated a cause and effect relationship between dietary intake and life expectancy. The incidence (number of new cases), prevalence (total number of cases), and severity of these chronic conditions, with the very recent exception of CHD, are rising. That prevalence is increasing is not surprising since rising life expectancy has resulted in a larger proportion of the American population in the older age cohorts. But, incidence and severity imply lack of solution. A longer duration portends a longer period of debility and disability as the cumulative and aggregate effect of physiological insult. In recent years, the medical profession has increasingly recognized the fact that preventive diets in middle age might delay the onset of degenerative diseases and/or decrease their severity. Therefore, interest in the foodways and nutriture of this group has been revived.

Nutritional vulnerability or risk is relative and a function of the criteria applied. IF the cumulative and aggregate effect of food intake during middle age is degenerative disease, THEN one is clearly open to damage, be it loss or injury.

The foodways of the middle-aged are an outgrowth of those practiced in young adulthood. But, they also may differ somewhat due to modifications in response to expanded potential, because of accumulated knowledge and skills as well as released time and funds.

MIDDLE-AGE: NORMAL NUTRIENT SUPPLY AND NORMAL DEMAND

Tissue maintenance and repair create most of the metabolic demand for the various nutrients during this stage of the life-cycle. All nutrients are necessary, but the range of requirements has not been defined. So, the RDA are not specific for this age group.

Aging is a continuous process that is usually associated with positive outcomes up to and including young adulthood and thereafter with increasingly negative outcomes. It is accompanied by a decreasing total number of functional cells. The nature and extent of cell decrease vary among cell types and among individuals in a way that is not well understood. Cells of the liver, gastrointestinal mucosa, skin, and hair (except for those genetically programmed for baldness) appear to sustain their population size. Those of muscle, nerve, and kidney tissue decrease in number and result in progressive reduction in functional capacity. Other types of cells decrease in number but loss of functional capacity has not been detected. Because of the gradual decrease in total cell number, basal metabolic rate is decreased as well. For this reason, the demand for all nutrients is progressively reduced somewhat. However, the only recommendation that has been generally accepted is that caloric intake should be decreased by 5% for each decade beyond age 25.

At the same time, the collagen content of tendons, ligaments, skin, and blood vessels increases. These tissues become less elastic, which interferes with functional capacity. As a result, metabolic demand is less. In addition, decreased functional capacity affects stamina and endurance, so inclination for participation in vigorous physical activity decreases. Given the typical middle-aged sedentary life-style, total caloric needs are not appreciably greater than metabolic needs.

Another factor, which affects the nutritional needs of women, is the menopause. Menstruation ceases naturally at some point between ages 35 and 60, or it may be caused artificially by oophorectomy. In either case, the reduction in estrogen secretion induces profound metabolic changes and concomitant changes in the circulating levels of various nutrients (Tables 30.1 through 30.3). The following points have been taken from discussions by Wilding (1974) and Gallagher and Nordin (1974).

Calcium

Postmenopausal osteoporosis appears to result from estrogen deficiency, which causes parathyroid hormone-induced negative calcium balance by mobilizing calcium from bone. The circulating Ca level has been reported to be 0.13 mg/100 ml above normal in women between 50 and 60 years.

TABLE 30.1. SERUM CONSTITUENTS WITH KNOWN SIGNIFICANT PATTERNS OF CHANGE AT THE MENOPAUSE[1]

Constituent	Changes in Mean Values From 5th to 6th Decades	Level of Significance (Relative to Males)
Urea	+ 2.26 mg/100 ml	$p<0.025$
Uric acid	+ 0.45 mg/100 ml	$p<0.001$
Inorganic phosphate	+ 0.22 mg/100 ml	$p<0.001$
Calcium	+ 0.13 mg/100 ml	$p<0.001$
Alkaline phosphatase	+ 2.12 KA Units	$p<0.001$
Cholesterol	+26.61 mg/100 ml	$p<0.001$
Total lipids	+ 0.21 g/100 ml	$p<0.001$
Sodium	+ 0.74 mmole/liter	$p<0.025$

[1] From Wilding, Rollason, and Robinson (1972). With permission of the author and the Elsevier/North-Holland Press.

TABLE 30.2. MEANS AND STANDARD DEVIATIONS FOR 17 BIOCHEMICAL CONSTITUENTS IN MALES, CLASSIFIED BY AGE[1]

Age Group (Years) Analysis	20−29	30−39	40−49	50−59	60−69	70−79	Total
Albumin	4.41	4.35	4.29	4.24	4.19	4.13	4.27
g/100 ml	± 0.20	± 0.21	± 0.21	± 0.22	± 0.22	± 0.30	± 0.22
Alkaline phosphatase	9.41	9.50	9.79	9.98	10.21	8.64	9.79
KA units	± 2.34	± 2.65	± 2.69	± 2.92	± 3.25	± 3.31	± 2.85
β-Lipoprotein	7.38	9.81	10.95	11.72	12.23	11.96	11.05
turbidity units	± 2.79	± 3.89	± 4.14	± 4.23	± 4.08	± 4.66	± 4.22
Bilirubin	0.64	0.65	0.63	0.61	0.60	0.68	0.63
mg/100 ml	± 0.31	± 0.33	± 0.28	± 0.28	± 0.30	± 0.52	± 0.30
Calcium	10.03	9.98	9.94	9.91	9.89	9.90	9.93
mg/100 ml	± 0.38	± 0.42	± 0.41	± 0.39	± 0.41	± 0.49	± 0.41
Cholesterol	206.51	235.62	244.56	246.51	248.70	223.16	242.32
mg/100 ml	± 35.30	± 43.06	± 41.11	± 41.74	± 40.64	± 55.90	± 42.70
Creatinine	1.01	1.02	1.04	1.04	1.05	1.10	1.04
mg/100 ml	± 0.16	± 0.17	± 0.17	± 0.19	± 0.18	± 0.22	± 0.18
Globulin	2.89	2.95	2.89	2.89	2.88	2.81	2.90
g/100 ml	± 0.39	± 0.37	± 0.36	± 0.38	± 0.38	± 0.45	± 0.37
Glucose	91.86	91.96	94.14	95.92	96.68	93.63	94.46
mg/100 ml	± 14.68	± 14.50	± 16.50	± 16.13	± 18.26	± 20.89	± 16.41
Inorganic phosphate	3.51	3.56	3.50	3.51	3.56	3.62	3.53
mg/100 ml	± 0.61	± 0.62	± 0.60	± 0.60	± 0.57	± 0.69	± 0.60
Iron	107.70	99.60	99.79	100.35	97.35	96.63	99.75
μg/100 ml	± 31.96	± 28.33	± 29.13	± 30.13	± 30.69	± 31.48	± 29.64
Potassium	4.34	4.38	4.39	4.44	4.49	4.55	4.42
mmole/liter	± 0.34	± 0.37	± 0.37	± 0.38	± 0.41	± 0.52	± 0.38
SGO transaminase	15.16	16.34	16.52	17.07	15.97	17.10	16.57
RF units	± 7.40	± 7.98	± 7.73	± 8.36	± 7.26	± 12.05	± 8.08
Sodium	140.52	140.49	140.45	140.56	140.51	140.28	140.49
mmole/liter	± 2.96	± 2.67	± 2.64	± 2.71	± 2.77	± 3.15	± 2.71
Total lipids	0.85	1.06	1.14	1.17	1.16	0.97	1.12
g/100 ml	± 0.29	± 0.36	± 0.36	± 0.37	± 0.34	± 0.40	± 0.37
Urea	32.53	33.30	33.25	34.17	36.00	36.15	33.91
mg/100 ml	± 6.07	± 5.88	± 5.58	± 6.06	± 6.60	± 7.53	± 6.05
Uric acid	6.29	6.54	6.52	6.53	6.45	6.41	6.51
mg/100 ml	± 1.13	± 1.17	± 1.20	± 1.20	± 1.21	± 1.67	± 1.21
Number in group	96	721	1268	1112	415	105	3717

[1] From Wilding, Rollason, and Robinson (1972). With permission of the author and the Elsevier/North-Holland Press.

TABLE 30.3. MEANS AND STANDARD DEVIATIONS FOR 17 BIOCHEMICAL CONSTITUENTS IN FEMALES, CLASSIFIED BY AGE[1]

Age Group (Years) Analysis	20–29	30–39	40–49	50–59	60–69	70–79	Total
Albumin g/100 ml	4.30 ± 0.22	4.24 ± 0.23	4.20 ± 0.23	4.18 ± 0.20	4.15 ± 0.22	4.13 ± 0.21	4.20 ± 0.22
Alkaline phosphatase KA units	7.28 ± 1.82	7.11 ± 2.22	7.75 ± 2.57	9.87 ± 3.13	10.66 ± 3.47	10.51 ± 3.42	8.65 ± 3.11
β-Lipoprotein turbidity units	9.43 ± 4.58	11.24 ± 4.56	12.22 ± 4.59	13.91 ± 4.79	15.40 ± 4.59	13.82 ± 5.33	12.73 ± 4.93
Bilirubin mg/100 ml	0.55 ± 0.26	0.51 ± 0.22	0.54 ± 0.26	0.52 ± 0.21	0.49 ± 0.24	0.51 ± 0.21	0.52 ± 0.23
Calcium mg/100 ml	9.97 ± 0.42	9.85 ± 0.37	9.85 ± 0.43	9.98 ± 0.40	10.05 ± 0.42	9.88 ± 0.40	9.92 ± 0.41
Cholesterol mg/100 ml	204.04 ± 35.92	221.28 ± 40.45	236.38 ± 38.81	262.99 ± 47.43	273.81 ± 39.85	251.14 ± 50.05	243.81 ± 47.04
Creatinine mg/100 ml	0.79 ± 0.17	0.83 ± 0.14	0.83 ± 0.16	0.84 ± 0.15	0.89 ± 0.17	0.84 ± 0.16	0.84 ± 0.16
Globulin g/100 ml	2.92 ± 0.40	2.87 ± 0.36	2.85 ± 0.41	2.92 ± 0.38	2.92 ± 0.39	2.92 ± 0.40	2.89 ± 0.39
Glucose mg/100 ml	90.06 ± 15.30	92.73 ± 13.72	94.26 ± 14.82	97.90 ± 15.03	96.23 ± 15.97	96.46 ± 19.35	95.01 ± 15.20
Inorganic phosphate mg/100 ml	3.65 ± 0.54	3.62 ± 0.51	3.60 ± 0.61	3.82 ± 0.55	3.85 ± 0.55	3.91 ± 0.61	3.71 ± 0.57
Iron μg/100 ml	99.34 ± 32.22	94.37 ± 37.50	95.20 ± 34.19	90.98 ± 26.58	90.83 ± 26.28	89.84 ± 26.87	93.38 ± 31.61
Potassium mmole/liter	4.31 ± 0.41	4.29 ± 0.39	4.30 ± 0.38	4.37 ± 0.40	4.47 ± 0.43	4.33 ± 0.42	4.34 ± 0.40
SGO transaminase RF units	11.01 ± 5.73	12.07 ± 7.81	11.95 ± 7.43	13.74 ± 5.86	14.68 ± 7.15	15.31 ± 8.66	12.88 ± 7.09
Sodium mmole/liter	139.80 ± 2.67	139.89 ± 2.74	140.02 ± 2.70	140.76 ± 2.60	141.19 ± 2.81	140.02 ± 2.66	140.33 ± 2.72
Total lipids g/100 ml	0.78 ± 0.21	0.93 ± 0.31	1.04 ± 0.32	1.25 ± 0.39	1.35 ± 0.37	1.12 ± 0.32	1.10 ± 0.38
Urea mg/100 ml	29.91 ± 6.82	29.79 ± 5.19	30.90 ± 5.97	33.16 ± 6.34	35.12 ± 6.45	32.86 ± 5.66	31.83 ± 6.29
Uric acid mg/100 ml	4.89 ± 1.00	4.63 ± 1.05	4.66 ± 1.02	5.11 ± 1.13	5.58 ± 1.15	5.22 ± 1.26	4.93 ± 1.13
Number in group	72	193	283	278	229	39	1094

[1] From Wilding, Rollason, and Robinson (1972). With permission of the author and the Elsevier/North-Holland Press.

Research has demonstrated that about 15% of the skeletal mass of males and females is lost due to aging. One finding was that bone loss starts at about age 45 in women and at about age 60 in men. A second was that the degree of loss in bone density in postmenopausal women differed according to whether the menopause was natural or artificial. In the case of the natural menopause, the degree of bone loss was related to age because the menopause is gradual. In the case of artificial menopause, it was related to the number of years that elapsed since the menopause, since it was abrupt. A third finding is that unlike premenopausal women, postmenopausal women cannot adapt to an overnight fast or a low calcium diet—bone resorption occurs in order to maintain circulating levels. A fourth finding is that a low calcium diet aggravates the problem. IF a sufficiently large supplement is ingested, THEN the estrogen deficiency can be offset and Ca balance maintained, thus retarding the development of osteoporosis.

Inorganic Phosphate

Bone resorption and/or increased absorption efficiency results in a circulating level increase of 0.22 mg/100 ml in women between the ages of 50 and 60 years.

Cholesterol

The mean circulating level of cholesterol in premenopausal women is lower than that of men of the same age. The reverse pattern has been observed in postmenopausal women. The postulated reason for this increase is that the fractions of β-lipoprotein and pre-β-lipoprotein formerly used for transport of estrogen are available for and used in increased cholesterol transport. This is unfortunate, as the rate of progression of cholesterol deposition in vascular tissue is greatly increased.

Urea

The blood urea nitrogen level (BUN), which includes uric acid, appears to increase in both sexes between the ages of 50 and 60 years, but the degree of increase is greater in women. Whether this is related to renal cell loss is unclear.

Sodium and Other Constituents

A slight but significant increase in the circulating sodium level occurs with menopause. Fluid retention and increased diastolic blood pressures are also noted. The circulating levels of glucose, potassium, and proteins apparently do not change as a result of menopause. There is limited evidence that suggests that the circulating levels of trace minerals, e.g., Zn, may be altered.

Iron nutriture is not a major concern in middle age. While pregnancy is a possibility for some women almost to the end of middle age, the probability is greatly and progressively reduced. As long as pregnancies continue, the RDA of 18 mg is appropriate. However, after menopause, whether natural or artificial, only a maintenance intake of about 10 mg is necessary.

MIDDLE AGE: DEFICIENT SUPPLY AND INCREASED DEMANDS

A deficient supply of all nutrients is still a possibility. But, except where there is a major intervening variable such as poverty or use of the OCA, the probability is very low. However, there is some evidence that tissue concentrations of Zn and Cr^{+++} are low. The implications and ramifications of this tentative finding are the focus of current research efforts.

MIDDLE AGE: EXCESS SUPPLY OR DECREASED DEMAND

Like deficiency, excess intake of any nutrient is always a possibility. Toxicity due to misuse of dietary supplements can occur. But, as in the previous stage, the only nutrient likely to be ingested by dietary excess is calories.

The cumulative and aggregate effects of a small excess over time is obesity. Bray (1974) testified to the Senate Select Committee on Nutrition and Human Needs:

Between age 20 when the American male completes school, and age 50—a 30-year span—most people will gain about 20 pounds in weight. The proportion of the body which is fat, however, goes up faster than that—rising from 18 to 36 percent. That means that the body's storage of fat has gone up by some 34 pounds while total weight has gone up only 20 pounds.

That means that the lean components of our body have declined some 14 pounds. We are getting fatter and leaner at the same time.

Of the 1 million calories a year we eat, we are storing, on the average, about a quarter of a percent which accounts for our fat accumulation of about 34 pounds.

This is an average excess of only 50 to 75 kcal/day, which is why control is so difficult. See Chapter 24 for preventive diets.

MIDDLE AGE: FOOD ECOLOGY, NUTRITIONAL RISK AND LIFE EXPECTANCY

The middle-aged adult is confronted with the developmental task of resolving the conflict between the need for *generativity* and the natural tendency toward *stagnation* (Erikson 1950) in every domain. The way this conflict is resolved on the job, in the use of leisure time, and in relation to food experiences and food and people interactions determines nutritional risk and may affect life expectancy.

The foodways of the young adult are likely to carry over into middle age. During this stage they may expand and develop in new directions or as a result of continued reinforcement, may become stronger and more resistant to change.

Here again, the degree of resolution of developmental tasks in previous stages as well as whether development or regression occurred has an impact on food ecology. The basic human needs continue to influence food ecology as well. The physiological demand for food is low.

Safety-security needs may reappear as a critical variable. This is especially so for the male. As the insecurities associated with decreased physical prowess develop and one is confronted with major illness/death due to catastrophic disease among one's associates, concern about diet may develop. IF concern is moderate, THEN it may give impetus to improved dietary control. IF it is excessive and the individual feels desperate, THEN overreaction may lead to overcompensation, use of fad diets, dosing with vitamins, etc., accompanied by unwanted side-effects. Thus, unfinished and new business may become intervening variables with extensive ramifications.

Belongingness is not usually a high priority need at this stage, but improvement is always possible. In contrast, the status need may become an overriding factor as one attempts to prop up a sagging ego. IF one lacks status in other domains or feels himself/herself slipping, THEN compensation in this domain may be used as a balancing factor. Unfortunately, consumption of gourmet foods and/or frequent extravagant entertaining by serving rich foods is not consistent with a program for weight control. The hazard is great and many succumb.

Self-actualization is the predominant need in affirming generativity and opposing the tendency toward stagnation. The following points characterize the typical options. IF one is successful in one's social accomplishments AND becomes a leader, THEN demands for innovations provide many opportunities for creating a style associated with one's name. IF one does moderately well AND the leader does not opt to excel in this domain, THEN one may shine by developing a distinctive style, gourmet repertoire, or other specialty. IF one is just a member of the group, THEN although one may develop as much in this domain as the leader, one must not flaunt it. And, IF one does not take a positive action, THEN one will find that "not to decide is to decide."

The food and people interactions of middle-aged people differ from those in other stages of the life cycle. As is true of other age groups, the middle-aged population is heterogeneous with respect to life-style, ethnicity, religion, socioeconomic status, etc. Classification according to composite criteria has lead to development of some "cases" that are models of typicality. These are useful for illustrative purposes, but one must remember that many variations occur. All are associated with nutritional risk and threat to survival. Four common "cases" are sketched briefly to call attention to familiar patterns and their expected outcomes.

Social Eaters

The busy socialite, business executive, or politician is engaged in a highly variable program of daily activities. The individual is busy but expends little physical energy. Frequent social activities center around food/drink and people interactions at meals. At other times, food intake is at irregular intervals and selections are a matter of convenience. In summary, dietary intake is out of control—high in empty calories and low in protective nutrients. Persons in this category are prime candidates for obesity.

Food Lovers

Men and women who like to cook and/or to eat tend to allocate too much time to gratification in this domain. Their social activities involve gourmet cooking groups, groups that eat in the best restaurants weekly, participation in à la mode cooking classes, etc. If they must eat on the fly during the day because of schedule constraints, they more than make up the difference via evening and/or weekend gorging. When overeating is compounded with sedentary living and/or pressure/tension eating to compensate, obesity is a major problem. In summary, dietary intake is too much and obesity is the usual result.

Utilitarian Eaters

Men and women of the "Type A" personality type are hard-driving, consider rest and relaxation a waste of time, and/or have a sedentary life-style. These individuals are work-centered and maintain a continuing urgent-to-frantic pace. They work long hours and get too little sleep. Food is consumed to appease hunger, so they often will eat whatever is convenient. In summary, this often turns out to be high fat, high carbohydrate, high cholesterol, high alcohol, and high caloric. Some aggravate the problem by engaging in heavy social eating/drinking in order to maintain their political position. The expected effect of this life-style is early development of cardiovascular disease.

Compensatory Eaters

Men or women who have reached their level of incompetence do not cope with the frustration, anxiety, and pressure that result, so they work frantically. Most have limited emotional outlets but could not utilize more because they find their work to be emotionally exhausting. This type of individual is so intent on the work that the need for food is scarcely acknowledged. The individual eats whatever, whenever. He/she may bring a lunch as a precaution, make a hurried purchase of pre-packaged snack foods from a mobile truck, or have a sandwich brought in—so that work is minimally disrupted by the need to eat. Coffee is gulped down all day long—16 cups is not uncommon—and the individual is overstimulated and continually wears the mask of fatigue. In summary, this diet tends to be low in protein and high in starch, fat, sugar, and salt. People of this type frequently develop ulcers.

All of these "cases" are at nutritional risk. The obese are likely to develop maturity onset diabetes—a disease in which the pancreas simply cannot produce sufficient insulin to meet needs, although it may produce a normal amount. Aging and progressively inelastic vascular tissue in-filtrated by complex lipid is injured by the high blood pressure, becomes occluded, and fails to supply nutrients to a vital portion of the heart muscle. Heart muscle starvation brings swift death—myocardial infarc-tion—and the hard-driving person is forced to slow down. The ulcer-prone frequently becomes anemic due to chronic blood loss. Thus, the threat appears in all cases.

With so much threat, to say nothing of actual decrease in physical prowess, many initiate a quest for the fountain of youth. Some become food cultists, vitamin cultists in particular, as they strive to prevent, delay, or overcome the manifestations of aging. Bitensky (1973) con-cluded that those who suffer from frustration in achieving a variety of goals in sexual, social, and/or economic spheres and from emotional deprivation and who rejected a religious orientation sought a talisman against aging, a panacea for disease, and an elixir for rejuvenation of body and soul. Vitamins are perceived to meet the needs. The scientific rationale for vitamin use is compatible with areligious beliefs, so when they are invested with magical qualities in preserving youth, they are hailed as the solution by those with a need for insurance.

BIBLIOGRAPHY

BITENSKY, R. 1973. The road to Shangri-la is paved with vitamins. Am. J. Psychiatry *130*, 1253-1256.

BRAY, G.A. 1974. Testimony on Nutrition and Diseases—1974. Part 4, Dia-betes and the Daily Diet, Senate Select Committee on Nutrition and Human Needs. GPO, Washington, D.C.

ERIKSON, E.K. 1950. Childhood and Society. W.W. Norton, New York.

GALLAGHER, J.C., and NORDIN, B.E.C. 1974. Calcium metabolism and the menopause. *In* Biochemistry of Women: Clinical Concepts. A.S. Curry and J.V. Hewitt (Editors). The CRC Press, Cleveland.

WILDING, P. 1974. Biochemical changes at the menopause. *In* Biochemistry of Women: Clinical Concepts. A.S. Curry and J.V. Hewitt (Editors). The CRC Press, Cleveland.

WILDING, P., ROLLASON, J.G., and ROBINSON, D. 1972. Patterns of change for various biochemical constituents detected in a well population screening. Clin. Chim. Acta *41*, 375-387.

31

Nutritional Risk and Life Expectancy: Old Age

The elderly are numerous and nutritionally vulnerable, and their plight is a national concern. Our societal belief is that old age is a time for repose, reflection, and respect but in reality, it is a time of retrenchment and restriction. The result is ruination of ecological balance with respect to food and nutrition; food experiences are reduced and food and people interactions may be almost eliminated.

The proportion of elderly in the American population has increased from 10 to 15% in the last decade but has not peaked yet. This population increase is the natural result of elimination of famine and pestilence that have traditionally decimated populations.

Nutritional vulnerability in old age differs in etiology, nature, and extent from that which occurs in previous stages of the life cycle. The known causes of nutritional vulnerability in the elderly are: (a) the long-term undermining of physical capacity as a result of the cumulative and aggregate effects of physiological insult, i.e., nutrient supply failures, injury, infection, and/or malfunction; (b) poverty, which does not allow for continued purchase of the full array of foods, so because of the deprivation, nutritional quality of the present diet is suboptimal; (c) physical debility and/or disability that often reduces mobility and strength, and so limits ability to obtain exercise and to perform food purchasing and food preparation tasks; (d) emotional-psychological depression that often induces a fatalistic resignation; and (e) mental disintegration that results in inattention, confusion, and/or loss of memory. A large percentage of the under-75-years-old segment is obese and is particularly vulnerable to the immediate onset of degenerative diseases such as diabetes, coronary heart disease, stroke, and cirrhosis. The over-75-years-old segment is more vulnerable to senile starvation or, in less severe forms, to some of the classic deficiency diseases. And, whereas nutritional risk is low among young and middle-aged adults, it is very high among older adults. Among older adults, it appears to increase with age decade.

The older American is confronted with the last of the developmental tasks. At this stage of the life-cycle, the underlying task is to resolve the problem of maintaining *ego integrity* in spite of the natural tendency to *despair* (Erikson 1950). What one has to work with as a result of what has gone on before conditions the way in which one deals with this problem. The nutritional implications and ramifications are profound.

Because our belief is that old age should be a time of reward, the revelation a decade ago that it was often a time of regret, i.e., sorrow, disappointment, and other distressing emotions aroused by circumstances beyond one's power to remedy, was shocking. National concern resulted in a federal mandate for a number of feeding and supplementary income programs.

OLD AGE: NORMAL NUTRITIONAL SUPPLY AND DEMAND

The nutritional requirements of the elderly are unknown (Munro 1980). Differences in mean circulating levels of various nutrients have been documented, but whether these differences are the normal effects of aging or the cumulative and aggregate effects of heredity, cultural setting, food intake, and life-style-related insults is unknown. The RDA for this age group are extrapolations of values for younger adults. Given a combination of medical and dietary assessment, at least 10% of the elderly have been estimated to suffer from nutritional deficiencies.

Noticeable differences in reduced physical capacity begin to surface at some point in early middle age and become progressively greater as one ages. Muscle, nerve, and kidney cell numbers decrease significantly and the collagen content of tendons, ligaments, skin, and blood vessels increases significantly. Thus, by old age, the progressive deterioration in functional capacity is marked. The known effects, implications, and some ramifications are indicated for each class of nutrients.

Energy and Its Sources

The reduction in cell numbers results in decreased energy requirement for and utilization in performance of vital functions as well as in reduced inclination toward physical energy expenditure. So, the total energy needs are less. The best scientific estimate is that between ages 30 and 90 the fixed portion or the BMR is decreased 20%, or approximately 5% per decade. The variable portion, which is related to the nature and extent of physical activity, is probably more variable during this stage of the life cycle than during any other. There are no hard data, but it is reasonable to suppose that since the muscle mass is less, IF an older American performs at the same level as a younger person, THEN the older person had to have had a much higher efficiency and probably used a greater number of calories, all other things being equal.

The weight pattern in old age appears to follow a general pattern. It increases up to about age 65, then it plateaus until about age 75, and then it decreases progressively. During the last stage, both adipose and muscle tissue are used for energy, so that the very oldest usually show marked muscle wasting.

Metabolism of protein, lipids, and carbohydrates differs in old age. The specifics are unknown at this time, but some general trends have been observed.

Protein

The rate of catabolism exceeds the rate of anabolism. Therefore, decreased muscle mass coupled with decreased muscle usage appears to result in a lower set-point for equilibrium between the circulating and labile storage proteins. So, protein is degraded for energy. However, the amino acid requirements for individual amino acids may differ. There is some evidence of increased methionine and lysine requirements; no explanation is available.

Lipids

The circulating levels of cholesterol and triglycerides show a slow but steady increase despite progressive deposition in vascular tissue. In women, this has been attributed to decreased estrogen levels in conjunction with increased transport ability. But, beyond this, little is known.

Carbohydrates

Glucose tolerance is decreased in the majority of individuals over age 70. The circulating levels of glucose may be normal, but the response to a glucose challenge is slower.

Minerals

Little is known about the mineral requirements in old age. Calcium requirements appear to be the same as those for older adults, but because absorption efficiency is decreased due to achlorhydria and excretion may be increased due to impaired renal function and/or the metabolic shifts associated with inactivity, the quantity ingested needs to be greater. Progressive demineralization of bones, called osteoporosis, is commonly observed in older people, especially women. What is known was reviewed in Chapter 30.

Chromium (Cr) has been identified as a critical variable in glucose tolerance. The tissue concentration in middle-aged and older subjects has been demonstrated to be exceptionally low and progressively lower. This is probably the cumulative and aggregate effect of marginal intake over time. At the present time, low Cr^{+++} levels among the elderly are accepted as being normal. However, limited studies have demonstrated that some subjects with low tissue saturation and impaired glucose tolerance can be restored to normal glucose tolerance by Cr^{+++} therapy. As a result of these findings, study of trace mineral nutrition has been intensified. It may turn out that low tissue saturation is non-normal and represents deficiency disease possibilities.

Vitamins

For all vitamins studied so far, there is evidence of a gradual decrease in the mean circulating level with age. The significance of this fact is unknown as are the factors that contribute to the effect. As of 1977, there was no conclusive evidence that supplementation of vitamin intake was beneficial in changing the mean circulating level.

OLD AGE: DEFICIENT NUTRIENT SUPPLY AND INCREASED DEMAND

The limited available information concerning the nutrient intake of the elderly suggests that 85% may ingest less than two-thirds of the RDA of one or more of the following nutrients whose intake has been investigated: protein, calcium, iron, vitamin A, thiamin, riboflavin, and ascorbic acid. In some cases, poor intake at this point in time is only a continuation of a lifetime of poor eating habits. The result is nutritional insult and extensive damage. The cumulative and aggregate effects may become manifest only in old age. In other cases, disorders of structure or function increase demand for particular nutrients or require compensatory adjustment in food intake, which increases the probability of unbalanced intake. In many cases, personal and/or environmental variables, to be discussed in the section on food ecology, intervene and reduce access to food.

So the effects of long-term deficiency are observed in mild to severe form, including all of the classic nutritional deficiency diseases except rickets. Medical conditions with a nutritional component that are very frequently observed are: osteoporosis; simple starvation, especially in those over 75; indigestion; constipation; achlorhydria; and senile glossitis. Medical conditions observed frequently are maturity onset diabetes; chronic starvation with severe emaciation; multiple B vitamin deficiencies; cirrhosis of the liver; and secondary anemia, especially as a result of diseases and/or use of medication that causes chronic blood loss.

In combination, decreased muscle and nerve cell numbers in the gastrointestinal wall—stomach, small, and large intestine—result in decreased muscle tone. The result is a decreased rate of passage and, therefore, increased probability of gas which accounts for the common complaints of constipation and "sour stomach." These are treated by self-medication with antacids. While antacids are relatively harmless, so that they are classified as over-the-counter (OTC) drugs, they do have nutritional side-effects. One-third of the elderly are estimated to have achlorhydria. When coupled with chronic antacid use, the effects are a serious reduction in protein digestion efficiency since protease activity is pH-dependent, destruction of thiamin which is alkaline-sensitive, and decreased absorption of Zn and Fe which are pH-dependent and compete for the same carriers. Pancreatic lipase and/or bile secretion may be reduced; coupled with reduced motility, fat digestion is delayed. So, tolerance to fats is perceived to decrease. Thus, the indigestion is explainable in terms of physiological degeneration.

Reduction in the number of kidney cells results in decreased efficiency in filtration and in controlling reabsorption. Since the rate of protein breakdown exceeds the rate of protein synthesis, the problem is aggravated. The net effect is an increased Blood Urea Nitrogen (BUN) level. When the circulating level of uric acid increases, the probability of attacks of gout becomes significant. Usually, these problems are more prevalent among men, as is nocturia.

The elderly are subject to a variety of minor illnesses. Self-medication with OTC patent remedies is practiced by a great many. Drug-induced malnutrition is a hazard. Common classes of drugs and their expected effects are listed in Table 31.1.

OLD AGE: EXCESS NUTRIENT SUPPLY AND DECREASED DEMAND

In the under-75 age group, obesity is the most prevalent form of malnutrition. But, it decreases in prevalence progressively, since the very obese do not survive long and the incidence in any age group is very low at this stage.

TABLE 31.1. OVER-THE-COUNTER DRUGS USED FREQUENTLY FOR SELF-MEDICATION BY THE ELDERLY

Name[1]	Nutritional Side-Effect
Aspirin (acetylsalicylic acid)	GI irritation and blood loss which may cause anemia; reduced folate absorption; reduced ascorbic acid absorption; reduced production of vitamin K
Castor oil	Increased motility reduces absorption of carotene, vitamins A, D, and E
Coricidin (aspirin, caffeine, phenacetin)	GI irritation and blood loss; may cause anemia
Digel ($Al(OH)_3$, $MgCO_3$, magnesium hydroxides)	Phosphate depletion
Exlax	K loss, hypokalemia, impaired glucose tolerance
Feen-a-mints (phenolphthalein)	Hypo-albuminemia, hypocalcemia, hypokalemia, vitamin D deficiency, electrolyte and fluid loss
Kaopectate	Adsorbs nutrients and coats GI lining, interferes with absorption of all
Metamucil	Reduces appetite and increases motility; interferes with absorption of all
Milk of magnesia	Excessive Mg absorption
Mineral oil	Increased motility reduces absorption of carotene, vitamins A, D, E
Neolid (emulsified castor oil)	Ca and K loss
Ornade decongestant	GI irritation and blood loss
Rolaids (sodium bicarbonate, $Al(OH)_3$)	Raises stomach pH to neutral or alkaline; impairs absorption of protein, thiamin, vitamin A, Fe; causes phosphate depletion

[1] Brand names are used for identification only.

While an aggressive program of weight control is advocated for obese individuals in earlier stages of the life cycle, in order to prevent unwanted outcomes, it is not appropriate at this stage. IF the individual is obese, THEN he/she probably has been obese for some time AND probably has a long history of unsuccessful efforts at weight control or does not value it. THEREFORE, obesity should be accepted as given. A philosophical point is at issue here. IF old age is a time for rest, repose, and respect, THEN is it right to restrict OR, on reflection, is it right to encourage enjoyment of the eating experience, as well as food and people interactions, to the extent possible as long as they do not induce immediate misery by aggravation of a medical condition? In any case, obesity is temporary because after about age 75, weight makes a downturn due to natural decreases in appetite, absorption efficiency, and metabolic efficiency.

The problem of excess intake is most likely to be related to misguided ingestion of megadoses of selected vitamins and/or minerals in a frantic effort to prevent, delay, or overcome the infirmities of old age. To face progressive loss of physical prowess, much less the prospect of disease or mortality, with equanimity is a major challenge. Many panic, i.e., the overpowering fright results in irrational attempts to escape the overwhelming effects. So, they become susceptible to the emotional appeals of food faddists and other health quacks.

Bitensky's reflective analysis (1973) of the beliefs, attitudes, intentions, and behavior of a group of his patients who were vitamin cultists reveals the bases of the problem. He found that in late middle age, those who have not been as successful in all domains as they would like AND whose lack of religious faith precludes any solutions from that quarter, try to prevent, delay, or overcome problems of aging by means of a talisman against infirmity, and use of panaceas for diseases. In this context, vitamins are perceived to be an elixir that rejuvenates body and soul, which causes the exaggerated level of intake.

Among the elderly, one observes those who have followed these cults since late middle age. The cumulative and aggregate effect now becomes manifest as toxicity syndromes. This group is joined by a large number of gullible newcomers who are converted by clever conditioning, coaxing, and cajolery.

OLD AGE: FOOD ECOLOGY, NUTRITIONAL RISK, AND LIFE EXPECTANCY

The degree of importance of food to the elderly is highly variable from unimportant to those who lack appetite and/or have a negative apathetic attitude toward everything to the main topic of conversation in some retirement homes. As of 1960, Beeuwkes, who reviewed the literature on foodways of the elderly, found that the information was meager, in part because sampling was limited largely to those able and willing to participate in the studies. Passage of the Older Americans Act in 1965 resulted in development of social and feeding programs for the elderly; these generated many studies so more information became available at this point.

Two different clusters of foodways are observed in relation to the elderly as a population group. The first set refers to healthy, free-living older individuals and couples; their foodways are indexed under the keyword *gerontology*, i.e., the study of the elderly and the problems of aging. The second set refers to unhealthy, usually institutionalized, older individuals; their foodways are indexed under the keyword *geriatrics*, i.e., the branch of medicine that deals with the medical problems and diseases of the elderly. The factors that create these two patterns of foodways are similar, but a larger subset of reasons and a greater degree of severity usually result in much poorer food and nutrient intakes by geriatric patients.

One group of relatively healthy older people has the means to provide for itself. Members of this group are truly senior citizens, since they continue to be active physically and socially. They may live at home, but often they live in a retirement home or community. These are selected because they provide facilities, food service, and other amenities that enable them to continue to live with a quality of life to which they have been accustomed. A staff or consulting dietitian oversees the aesthetic and nutritional quality of meals provided.

This segment of the elderly is independent—repose, reflection, and respect are theirs to enjoy as the fruits of a good life. They confront the last of the developmental tasks, i.e., to resolve the conflict between *ego integrity* and *despair* (Erikson 1950) from a relatively strong position.

Little is known about the foodways, food ecology, nutritional risk, or life expectancy of members of this group of the elderly. They do not present a problem to society, so they have not been of interest or concern. Study of the techniques of those on a normal positive pathway, in contrast to those on a degenerate pathway, might be illuminating. Identification of the point when some people leave the normal pathway might provide some clues for prevention. Members of this group do not need and do not participate in federal food programs; still, their requirements should be known and their presence acknowledged.

Summarized briefly, the findings of recent studies indicate that the elderly are particularly susceptible to malnutrition for a number of reasons. All result in repression of hunger signals. The array of foods consumed also may be limited to a few low nutrient density items. Lack of dietary diversification reduces the probability of consumption of a nutritionally adequate diet. The causes include, but are not limited to:

(a) Loss of teeth and inadequate dentures result in reduced chewing ability and disinclination to consume foods that require chewing.

(b) Limited food expenditures because of poverty. Inexpensive filler foods rather than nutritious foods are purchased.

(c) Reduced interest in and/or ability to purchase and/or prepare meals because of palsy, little hand strength, limited mobility, etc., result in minimization of these tasks, i.e., to heat and serve or removal of a portion of ready-to-eat items.

(d) Loneliness and lack of social contact, anxiety, or conflict may reduce appetite and result in senile anorexia (see Chapter 16). Lack of appetite reduces the necessity for eating alone. But, they will not necessarily eat with a group, even if an opportunity is available. They are proud. IF they feel that their clothes are not socially acceptable, THEN they may prefer to starve than to face social embarrassment. And, if they perceive that eating companions might not be congenial, they will reject food and people interactions, preferring to go hungry.

(e) Limited food acceptance as a result of early deprivation that closed the food array plus elimination of some accepted foods, especially those containing more than 25% fat or bulk, leaves too few for nutritional adequacy.

(f) Food faddism results in spending scarce resources for expensive but unnecessary vitamins, minerals, and special health foods.

(g) Regression to an ethnic diet enables some to feel some security and to continue to eat. In order to maintain ethnic traditions they spend scarce resources on expensive ethnic delicacies.

The Panel on Aging of the 1969 White House Conference on Food, Nutrition, and Health, the 1970 Task Force on Aging, and testimony in Nutrition and the Elderly—1973 Part I, Feeding the Elderly, which is a transcript of the hearings before the Senate Select Committee on Nutrition and Human Needs, confirmed and expanded on these points. Having identified a problem and created a cause, action programs were conceived to rehabilitate the food ecosystem of the elderly, to resume participation in gratifying food experiences-food and people interactions, to restore ecological balance in the nutritional niche, and to revive respect. The 1972 amendment to Title VII (Public Law 92-258) of the Older Americans Act of 1965 gave program authorization and provided enabling legislation for funding of the Nutrition Program for the Elderly. Justification, according to the Act is:

Many elderly persons do not eat adequately because: (1) they cannot afford to do so; (2) they lack the skills to select and prepare nourishing and well-balanced meals; (3) they have limited mobility which may impair their capacity to shop and cook for themselves; (4) they have feelings of rejection and loneliness which obliterate the incentive necessary to prepare and eat a meal alone. These and other physiological, social, and economic changes that occur with aging result in a pattern of living which causes malnutrition and further physical and mental deterioration.

The last sentence provides the key to reasons for passage of the act. Humanitarianism was involved but cost was the critical variable. The cost of dealing with gerontological problems is much less than the cost of geriatric care. So, the objective is to provide services, including meals, that will enable the elderly to remain free-living as long as possible instead of becoming institutionalized as a result of premature deterioration. Two types of programs are authorized to provide assistance to free-living individuals.

The first involves provision of congregate meals at a centrally located site to ambulatory elderly. This partial solution makes nutritious meals available at low cost and provides eating companions. In small towns where people have been acquainted for many years, this alternative is very successful because the social opportunity to eat with friends without the burden of meal preparation and service is appreciated. In large metropolitan areas where people are unacquainted, this alternative is less successful. Those who always have been outgoing will find congenial eating companions. Others, who are shy, poorly dressed, or who have other social problems may be intimidated and, therefore, may not participate. The major limitation is that for reasons of efficiency in providing this essential service to a large number of people, a set menu is used and the diner has no choice, other than to take or leave what is provided. Still, this program meets the needs of many elderly and the number who would participate far exceeds the number that can be fed, given the funds available.

The second program involves delivery of meals to the homebound. This partial solution makes nutritious meals available at a low cost. While meal companions are not provided, the interactions with the delivery person have been demonstrated to benefit the morale. Here again, the major limitation is that a set menu is provided, so the diner has only two options, i.e., to eat or not eat what is delivered. Still, this program meets the needs of many elderly and enables many to remain in their homes as long as possible.

Other programs not authorized by this act provide supplemental income so that those who can prepare and serve their own meals will have adequate money for food expenditures. This alternative recognizes and respects individual need for control of food choices, eating experiences, and food and people interactions. It is available for those still able to provide their own meals but who lack sufficient money to do so. It is a less costly partial solution since minimum service is provided.

When deterioration has progressed to a point where the individual can no longer care for himself/herself, geriatric care is provided by nursing homes, at private expense, or under medicare. Congregate meals are served in a dining room for those who are ambulatory and room service is provided for those who are bedridden. A staff dietitian or consulting dietitian oversees nutritional quality of the diet and plans modified diets as necessary. Drug therapy and/or secondary psychological problems are intervening variables that frequently interfere with food intake. So, the primary problem is to induce the person to eat. Three continuing challenges are to increase the variety of positive aspects in the eating territory, to increase the value of mealtime in terms of interest and enjoyment, and to increase total intake, perhaps by means of frequent small feedings.

Earlier in this chapter, the developmental task associated with this stage of the life cycle, i.e., resolution of the conflict between ego integrity and despair, was mentioned in relation to senior citizens. However, it applies to other segments of the elderly as well. All are confronted with the conflict as an on-going problem, in one way or another. It surfaces in the food domain in different ways depending on whether one provides one's own food, eats at a congregate meal site, or has room service.

When one provides one's own food, the potential for maintenance of the food-related aspects of ego integrity is good, as long as one has sufficient resources for a decent level of food expenditure. This is because the individual still has some control over all of the variables, i.e., who the eating companions are and how many, what will be consumed (menu planning using preferred foods, purchasing of preferred ingredients and quality, preparation according to preferred method(s), spicing, etc.), when each meal will be consumed—on a fixed or variable schedule, where it will be consumed (the boundaries of the eating territory—dining table, TV tray, etc.)—and how it will be consumed (in courses or all served at the same time). This amount of freedom enables the individual to continue his/her customary patterns without disruption and with a minimum sense of loss since any changes occur gradually rather than abruptly and simultaneously. Relatively speaking, nutritional risk is probably less, since the probability that the individual will continue to eat is high.

In contrast, the institutionalized individual is likely to despair, showing resignation and fatalism. Control of the food ecosystem, i.e., who, what, when, where, and how food is served, is maintained impersonally in the interests of efficiency. As a result, all are continually annoyed with differences in one or more aspects. The resulting disruption of customary habits and sense of loss are demoralizing and demand adjustments many are no longer able to make. So, they despair and become balky—refusing to eat, refusing a specific food, refusing to eat at mealtime and demanding food at other times, etc. Relatively speaking, the nutritional risk is much greater and a life-threatening situation may develop. Thus, the personal and societal costs associated with institutionalization are high. So, institutionalization is to be regarded as a last resort and to be avoided as long as is possible.

When it does occur, family members/friends are well advised to think through the implications of the changed circumstances or relationships. In this domain, food gifts may be an appropriate positive reinforcement to the relationship if carefully selected with the knowledge and consent of the dietitian. It is inappropriate to provide debilitated neglected relatives/friends with sweet and rich (especially forbidden) items as a salve for a guilty conscience. Such food gifts may do more harm than good. (They meet the needs of the donor at the expense of the recipient.)

During the early 1970s, the "McGovern Committee" conducted a series of hearings to focus attention on progress in implementing feeding programs that had been authorized under the Older Americans Act, etc. In 1977, the "McGovern Committee" conducted a hearing entitled "Nutrition: Aging and the Elderly." Testimony revealed that many had been fed, program expansion was needed, nutrition education could be effected and needed to be augmented, etc. Moreover, the Director of the

National Institute of Aging, founded in 1974, stated that the aim of the NIA research program is to expand the knowledge base. Specifically, the nutrition-related portion aims are to determine:

(a) what constitutes an adequate diet for the older person, focusing on the changes that occur with age in the need for nutrients

(b) what older persons eat

(c) the factors that affect eating habits—economic, behavioral, and physiological

(d) changes in the physiology of digestion with age

(e) the assimilation of nutrients into the body tissues in the older person

(f) risk factors for pathology in middle and old age correlated with nutritional status

(g) topics of special significance, such as the interaction of nutrition variables and drugs

In summary, the importance of identifying the dimensions of the nutritional problem of the elderly that are associated with various kinds and levels of food and people interactions that are typical of elderly life-styles is becoming economically more imperative as the proportion of elderly increases. Although recent federally funded projects have fed many people and many studies have contributed baseline data on feeding the elderly, much remains to be done.

At the present time, there has been little or no experimental research applied to the process of rendering a decision with respect to the effectiveness of nutrition education in general (or specific methods in particular) for the elderly. Hence, it is difficult to assign a value to it as a component of the Elderly Nutrition Program. In the absence of such data, there is no valid basis on which to justify or deny its inclusion. (Note: inclusion is based on the assumption that it is probably effective.) A recent paper (Shannon and Smickilas-Wright 1979) discussed this issue and other aspects of nutrition in relation to needs of the elderly.

BIBLIOGRAPHY

BITENSKY, R. 1973. The road to Shangri-la is paved with vitamins. Am. J. Psychiatry *130*, 1253-1256.

BROWN, P.T., BERGAN, J.G., PARSONS, E.P., and KROL, I. 1977. Dietary status of elderly people. Rural, independent-living men and women vs. nursing home residents. J. Am. Dietet. Assoc. *71*, 41-45.

ERIKSON, E.K. 1950. Childhood and Society. W.W. Norton, New York.

GROTKOWSKI, M.L., and SIMS, L.S. 1978. Nutritional knowledge, attitudes, and dietary practices of the elderly. J. Am. Dietet. Assoc. *72*, 499-506.

KOHRS, M.S., O'HANLON, P., and EKLUND, D. 1978. Title VII—Nutrition Program for the Elderly. I. Contribution to one day's dietary intake. J. Am. Dietet. Assoc. 72, 487-492.

MARRS, D.C. 1978. Milk drinking by the elderly of three races. J. Am. Dietet. Assoc. 72, 495-498.

MUNRO, H.N. 1980. Major gap in nutrient allowances. The status of the elderly. J. Am. Dietet. Assoc. 76, 137-141.

ROWE, D. 1978. Aging—a jewel in the mosaic of life. J. Am. Dietet. Assoc. 72, 478-486.

SELECT COMM. ON NUTR. AND HUMAN NEEDS, U.S. SENATE. 1977. Diet Related to Killer Diseases. Vol. VII. Nutrition: Aging and the Elderly. GPO, Washington, D.C.

SHANNON, B., and SMICIKLAS-WRIGHT, H. 1979. Nutrition education in relation to the needs of the elderly. J. Nutr. Educ. 11 (2) 85-89.

32

The Food and Nutrition Delivery System

The basic food delivery system is a complex network for the distribution of foodstuffs, i.e., raw agricultural commodities, partially processed ingredients, and ready-to-eat (RTE) items. The foods are produced and/or processed by one or more groups and ultimately are delivered to another group for consumption. Bigness and complexity create/maintain conditions from which various sets of comtemporary problems arise.

Because the producer of raw agricultural commodities, the processor who manufactures ingredients and RTE items, and the ultimate consumer have different objectives, adjustment of supply and demand is difficult. The producer will supply an item only as long as it is sufficiently profitable. The consumer will demand it only as long as it is a desirable alternative.

Given the uncertainties introduced by these differing objectives, profiteering would be a temptation. In the public interest—to minimize this unwanted outcome—federal planning, monitoring, and coordination are required.

Due to separation between the producer and the consumer, another temptation arises. The past history of any sample of a foodstuff is an unknown and its quality must be estimated from a sample prior to purchase. Deception, with intent to defraud, is an ever present possibility which can be limited by federal monitoring and control. So, a system of standards, inspection, and procedures for redress of grievance become a necessary part of the regulatory function.

Restaurants provide final preparation and deliver food via on-site service to their customers. Here again, because the producer and the consumer differ, problems must be anticipated and controls instituted. The past history of the ingredients and the RTE item after preparation is unknown; wholesomeness, nutritiousness, and aesthetic qualities must be estimated from a sample that is consumed. Deception, with intent to defraud, is a possibility in this situation. To protect the restauranteur's own interests, the food purchasing agent for the restaurant takes precautions with ingredients and food preparation personnel are instructed in sanitary food handling procedures. Systems of inspection by local health departments verify that facilities, equipment, and food handling practices meet the minimum criteria that provide limited control.

Federal food assistance programs also deliver food to consumers. Three methods of delivery have been utilized in recent years: (a) purchasing power is increased via food stamps or WIC vouchers that allow purchase of selected foods at reduced cost; (b) selected surplus foodstuffs have been distributed at predetermined times and places, e.g., via the defunct commodities program; and (c) free or reduced price meals have been provided at established dining sites, e.g., school breakfasts and lunches, elderly feeding programs.

The delivery system is a critical variable. Because of separation between producer and consumer, the potential for abuse is sizeable. The potential for misunderstanding is even greater, and a credibility gap has developed.

Food always has been the major source of nutrients, so the nutrition delivery system traditionally has been viewed as a subsidiary of, i.e., of secondary importance to and/or wholly controlled by, the food delivery system. So, the major systems for control of the nutritive quality of the diet are exercised through federal agencies that monitor and control the food supply. But, food is no longer the only source of nutrients and there is little historical precedent for control as a pharmaceutical product. Moreover, much "food" is not nutritious in the sense that it provides only calories. The task of selecting a nutritionally adequate diet has become more challenging as the number of nutrients to be controlled has increased. Many individuals do not choose a combination of foods that meets their nutritional needs. So, a system of standards, inspections, and education have become a limited but necessary function of the federal government.

Until recently, food industry acceptance of responsibility for the nutritional quality of its products was not as great as that expected by the public. When this was disclosed, a crisis in confidence developed. Still, Americans are comparatively well nourished. What is the problem?

The problem is that economists and/or politicans and nutritionists and/or consumers do not agree on the objectives of food policy decisions (Paarlberg 1977). Therefore, the trade-offs that are made are not wholly satisfactory to any of those interested parties. In fact, nutrition has not been a variable in food policy decisions. According to a report of the Select Committee on Nutrition and Human Needs (1976), the prevailing assumption was that traditional patterns of agricultural production and food marketing could be relied on to provide the quantity and quality of food necessary for consumption of a nutritionally adequate diet by all Americans. However, since 1972, the emphasis has been on conservation of natural resources. An outgrowth of popular interest and governmental concern is the realization that, given limited resources, choices must be made among commodities and among possible production quantities of each. The Committee states, "In times of shortage, health must be the governing factor in the allocation of resources."

THE FOOD DELIVERY SYSTEM: NORMAL SUPPLY AND DEMAND

The food delivery system is comprised of the following components: production, processing, transporting, wholesaling, and retailing. Each component, from point of origin of the basic agricultural commodity to the final product distributed to the consumer, has specified functions with respect to the physical and legal transfer of a shipment of the food from consignor to consignee. And, each component in the series is itself the hub of a complex network whose components interact so as to bring people, places, and things together in a predictable way in performing its functions. The entire system is interactive, responding to internal as well as external pressures from the consumer public, government, and international community.

In the aggregate, the amount of each of the raw agricultural commodities produced determines the basic pattern of buying and selling transactions and the overall level of distribution efficiency for all levels of the food delivery system. The amount of each of the food commodities produced is highly variable at the various production sites within and among years. Still, the demand is relatively fixed. So, the quantity to be delivered from one place to another must be adjusted to rebalance supply and demand. This dynamic state of change is normal, but only limited variation can be tolerated without major economic impact.

To the extent possible, the overall range of variability in agricultural production is controlled by the federal government in the public interest. This is a necessary function in order to ensure that basic levels of production of the various commodities are above the minimum necessary to prevent famine and/or prices above the means of the population. The target food production level is estimated on the basis of the quantity necessary to feed the American people a nutritionally adequate diet, to provide a safety margin, and to allow sales via international trade. By means of monetary policy adjustments with respect to the rate of interest on farm loans, subsidies, price support programs, etc., the federal government, through the USDA, manipulates the incentive to produce each of the agricultural commodities. Thus, the expected volume of food available to be delivered to domestic and foreign markets is controlled to some extent. But, control is imperfect. The observed production level at a particular place or point may differ somewhat from the expected level due to the effects of weather and other uncontrollable factors. So, readjustments must be made throughout the food delivery system.

In their natural state, most agricultural commodities would not be acceptable to or useable by the consumer. So, a variable quantity of a bulky and perishable raw agricultural commodity is formally transported from field to factory, and food processing becomes the second level in the food delivery system. The purposes of food processing are (a) to control the degree of uniformity in sensory attributes, i.e., color, texture, flavor, size and shape, degree of ripeness, and freedom from blemishes, or (b) to transform commodities from basic ingredients to special purpose ingredients or ready-to-eat food items. Depending on the quality and quantity of the raw agricultural commodities delivered and the inventory of each item in the food product array, different proportions are processed one way or another for distribution to various market sectors.

The foods processed for uniformity are fresh milk, eggs, fruits, vegetables, and meats. These are relatively perishable, salable products because processing is limited. Processing targets are adjusted to short-term demands of retailers.

The special purpose ingredients and ready-to-eat food items are engineered foods that have had some processing to preserve. Marketing specialists develop product concepts according to consumer profiles so as to provide salable products, i.e., products that would be acceptable to and meet needs of various segments of the consuming public. A food product development team then produces a prototype product. Next, on-line production capacity and quality control measures are developed. Thereafter, production targets are set and adjusted according to supply of commodities and product demand, as indicated by inventory totals and commitments to wholesalers.

The wholesaler is a middle-man who performs the following functions in the food delivery system:

(a) at the peak of the food production and/or processing season he makes a commitment for or purchases from producers and/or processors a considerable number of units, e.g., carload lots, of particular food products in one or more lines

(b) warehouses them

(c) allots them into smaller units of salable merchandise, e.g., case lots

(d) assembles composite arrays of various food items from among the items and packages sizes according to purchase order specifications

(e) delivers the orders to the retail outlets or institutions according to a mutually agreeable schedule

The amount of a particular food product type available in a specific size of package varies within and among years. For products with an elastic demand, demand varies considerably with price. Otherwise, demand is less variable. Together, supply and demand determine the optimal amount of inventory to be carried by the wholesaler. Since supply and demand of each food is in a dynamic state of change, and the futures market is somewhat unpredictable, market changes must be monitored continually, break-even points recomputed, and the product inventory adjusted accordingly. As long as supply and demand remain within normal ranges, prices will range normally, and normal quantities will be delivered.

The food retailer is a middle-man who sells small quantities of commodities or manufactured foods to the ultimate consumers. A particular retailer offers a subset of the overall array of commodities and manufactured foods for sale; the composition of the subset offered is highly variable among retailers—the types of items are similar but brands and quality differ. Ordinarily, in American retail markets the supply is relatively continuous, but prices of individual foods are raised or lowered to adjust demand to supply potentials. At the same time, since space is at a premium, if the total demand for a food is insufficient to maintain a desired turnover rate, supply is discontinued. Thus, at this level, delivery depends on aggregate preferences; availability is adjusted accordingly.

The restauranteur is a middle-man who sells small quantities of finished foods to ultimate consumers in a public eating place. A wide variety of restaurants exists to meet market demands for a variety of foods and service quality. These include, but are not limited to, (a) table service—table d'hote and à la carte; (b) buffet and cafeteria; (c) short-order, sit-down, e.g., coffee shops, lunch counters, and fast-food; and (d) short-order, take-out. All other things being equal, at a given restaurant the supply of each of the listed menu items is relatively continuous, but prices of individual items are raised or lowered to adjust demand to supply-based profit potential. At the same time, since the number of items offered must be limited for practical reasons, IF the total demand for any item is insufficient to generate a fair portion of total profits, THEN the menu item will be replaced by one with more promise. Thus, at this level, delivery of particular foods depends on aggregate food preferences; availability is adjusted accordingly.

Between each pair of levels in the food delivery system is a transport system. It may be a part of the services provided by the seller to the next level of buyer; a link in a multi-level series of segments of a vertically organized agri-business complex, e.g., Safeway Stores which own all levels from farms to their supermarket chain, or an independent service engaged at a price.

At the lowest level, transport from field to factory, the means of transport of raw agricultural commodities may be a flatbed truck stacked with crates, a dump truck for bulk shipment of a mass of loose, firm, roundish items, or a tank truck for bulk shipment of liquids. At this level, speed, air circulation, evaporation rate, and soil and/or bacterial load are common considerations in controlling loss due to deterioration.

At the next level, bulk transport from processor to wholesaler, the means may be a regular, refrigerator, or freezer truck, but more commonly palletized or containerized loads are transported in semi-trailer trucks, rail cars, airplanes, or ship. At this level, speed, air circulation, temperature, humidity, load stability, and vibration are common considerations in controlling loss during delivery.

At this level, another system is operative in parallel to supply smaller quantities of limited lines of foods to retail outlets and small institutions. The full-service delivery system is used to supply dairy and bakery products on a six-day schedule. Delivery is made in the following way: (a) the route driver loads his truck with each product in the line; quantities are determined by historical usage; (b) at each stop on the route, the driver checks the level of stock on hand, stocks leftovers to the front, replenishes stocks of each item to a predetermined level, removes overage items, and prepares an invoice, listing the quantity stocked and crediting returns.

At the level of supply to retail outlets and small institutions by the processor or wholesaler, two systems are operative. One alternative utilizes drop deliveries, i.e., the shipment is unloaded at a predetermined date. A second alternative is limited service delivery. Specified items and quantities are contracted for in advance by award and acceptance of a formal bid and specifications. Then, if the quantity per purchasing period is open, the purchasing agent notifies the purveyor of the quantity needed and it is delivered on the stipulated day. Or, fixed quantities may be scheduled for routine delivery on a stipulated schedule. Regular flatbed, refrigerated, freezer or semi-trailer trucks may be used depending on the nature and/or quantity of the goods to be delivered.

Nutrient delivery traditionally has been a subsidiary consideration with respect to food delivery. There is some evidence that this is changing. Nutrient contribution *per se* and in relation to dietary intake appears to be a new emphasis. Recently, Johnson (1978), who is a food processing industry spokesman, stated the contemporary position with respect to the food manufacturer's responsibilities in supplying nutrients to promote the nutritional well-being of American consumers. According to Johnson (1978), food manufacturers have taken the position that they will be responsible for the nutrient supply to the American population. Acting responsibly means that in meeting this responsibility, they should emphasize:

(a) Nutritional equivalence in contemporary versions of traditional foods with commonly understood nutrient profiles. This specifically applies to formulated foods that are designed to replace traditional items in the diet.

(b) Definition of and control of nutrient losses during processing and home storage/preparation of each food.

(c) Nutrient information on labels that particular segments of the American population need, e.g., sodium content, ingredients that may evoke an allergic response.

(d) Product safety and value, i.e., by not running dual advertising campaigns for separate lines of junk foods and "natural" foods or creating a false impression of the need for a particular nutrient such as protein.

(e) A positive influence on nutriture of Americans so that necessary nutrients probably will be provided in adequate amounts by the foods consumers are likely to choose—by affecting costs, availability of food, pitch of promotionals, nutrient content, special diet modification, and packaging.

One of the original and continuing purposes of the RDA has been to serve as a guide in planning overall food production. The USDA is legally charged with the responsibility for controlling food production in such a way as to make available the quantity and variety of food necessary for a nutritious diet for the entire population. Usually, actual food disappearance figures, adjusted for population growth in particular age categories, are used as a first approximation to the quantity of each product class that will be necessary in successive reporting periods.

Nutritional status surveys in the 1930s revealed an unacceptable prevalence of multiple B vitamin deficiencies and iron deficiency anemia. Therefore, voluntary programs for fortification and enrichment of white flour, bread, pasta, cornmeal, and rice were promulgated during the 1940s and 1950s. Thus, by fiat and decree, these nutrients were added in stipulated quantities to specified products. This was an effective means to increase delivery of these scarce nutrients since these foods were widely consumed in sufficient quantities to effect the desired change in overall intake. However, no attempt was made to upgrade the natural quantity or the amount retained after processing and storage. Effects of processing on nutrient composition of foods were reviewed in Chapters 2 and 19.

Wholesalers warehouse foods for variable periods—months to years. Foods become inedible because of deteriorative changes in color, flavor, and texture. Such changes cause the food to be unsalable, which is costly. To control costs, wholesalers limit the length of time that they hold foods, according to their estimate of profitability. Deterioration of sensory attributes has been studied extensively and means to retard the rate of such changes have been devised. It turns out that as foods age, these deteriorative reactions use up nutrients in predictable ways. For example, canned goods stored five years have almost no nutritive value—protein is degraded (putrid odor), fat is degraded (rancid odor), carbohydrate is degraded (mushy texture and gas, acid, or alcohol formed), and vitamins A and E are oxidized.

The difficulty for the shopper and consumer is that the age and past history (improper storage at high temperatures results in accelerated aging) of the food are unknown. Cans and frozen food packages are date-coded, but the key to the code is not available to the consumer. As the best alternative to actual age one can make a deduction. During the pre-harvest period, IF there is a good sale, THEN a good crop is expected AND wholesalers are reducing inventories by unloading previous stocks since some degree of age-related deteriorative changes will have occurred. This will make room for future packs and allow prices at a level that is likely to be the peak for this lot of food. IF one is purchasing sale merchandise, although one is tempted to purchase great quantities at bargain prices, THEN one should limit the quantity purchased to an amount that can be consumed in a six- to nine-month period. In this way, one can take advantage of price breaks without compromising nutritive quality. Since at the lower prices, greater than normal amounts can be purchased and consumed, the overall nutritive quality of the diet may be improved.

Retailers also warehouse foods for an indeterminate period. But, on reflection, two different sets of expectations with respect to delivery of nutrients might seem plausible. Large supermarket chain stores usually stock only what sells, so their stock turnover rate is high. Therefore, relative freshness of perishable and preserved items could be expected. So, delivery of nutrients would be high. In contrast, the traditional neighborhood or specialty store often has a low turnover rate for many items stocked, as attested to by the dust on packages. Moreover, these stores are likely to purchase old bargain price packs that wholesalers are unloading. So, their "new" stock is new only to them. Since nutritive quality, like sensory quality, deteriorates progressively with age, purchase of slow moving items from these stores should be avoided.

Deterioration also occurs during transport. It is most obvious in relation to the sensory attributes of fresh and other perishable foods. Deterioration may make the commodity unacceptable. It may result in rejection of a lot of food as substandard. Or, the food still may be acceptable for some other use, but only at a lower price for a downgraded commodity. Since every company is in business to make a profit, the economic incentive operates toward optimality in a trade-off between (a) minimizing losses by controlling the rate of sensory deterioration through appropriate temperature and humidity control and (b) minimizing expenses associated with maintaining such control. Fortunately, the conditions that preserve sensory quality preserve nutritive quality as well. So, to this extent, IF the food delivery system operates to retain sensory quality, THEN it is delivering the nutritional quality.

Quality is a major price determinant, so both buyers and sellers at each level of the food delivery chain have an interest. Raw agricultural commodities are biological materials, so within a given lot attributes are highly variable. But, uniformity and specified attributes are necessary for particular end uses. So, incoming lots are sized and graded and the producer is paid according to the value assigned for the various sizes and grades.

Traditionally, this has had a major effect on what is produced. Because certain grades become desirable to the consumer and sell, the demand increases. This favors production and selling price. To maximize profit, the producer attempts to yield as much of a commodity at the size and grade that are associated with the most favorable price. The aggregate effect is that most of the supply is of the desired quality, all other things such weather being equal.

The federal government, via the USDA, has established grades for most commodity groups, e.g., eggs, milk, butter, classes of poultry, kinds of meat, and for each of the kinds of fruits and vegetables. A graduated series of written descriptions of the sensory attributes and their scores has been devised for use as a standard for comparison. Random samples are drawn from each lot of the commodity. The samples are compared with the standard by inspectors, and a grade is assigned.

Different end uses and/or kinds of processing are associated with the various grades. For example, top grade peaches will be sold for eating out of hand; they are washed, sized mechanically, and packed. Those with a few surface blemishes will be skinned, pitted, halved, and canned. Substandard peaches with many defects will be skinned, pitted, trimmed, sliced or diced, and canned. Those that are green will be held to ripen or if only slightly underripe, processing time will be increased to compensate.

A commodity is graded only once, so its grade accompanies it through the food delivery system. But, its quality can deteriorate as a result of aging and/or poor handling and storage conditions; that is a different situation, and price will be adjusted accordingly. Thus, for example, US No. 1 potatoes that were free from decay would command top prices in October. But, in April the US No. 1 potatoes with 10% decay would not command the top price. So, at this time the wholesaler or retailer must re-sample and make a new price bid on the basis of the proportion of rotten ones to be discarded.

The purchasing agent for the restaurant also requires an extensive knowledge of necessary and sufficient food attributes for each intended end-use. Depending on volume of business, the purchasing agent may utilize a full-service delivery system for one or more commodity classes or may utilize a limited service system based on formal bids for items of stated grades, verified by sampling. The basic quality purchased lays the foundation for final consumption quality.

The household food shopper rarely has either a full-service delivery option, except perhaps for dairy products, or a limited-service option for a home delivery of a telephone order. Instead, self-service is the norm so the household food shopper requires extensive knowledge of appropriate food attributes for intended end-uses. Informal evaluation is commonly based on (a) sensory attributes—color, odor, compression (pinching), etc., and (b) previous experiences with and/or reputation of the retailer, the brand, the grade, the pull-date, etc.

The household food shopping person, who may be the ultimate consumer as well as the purchasing agent, is the link with the food delivery destination. The advent of nutrition labeling resulted in a recent series of FDA-sponsored studies of household food shopper knowledge of food attributes and grades, nutrient composition of foods, effects of food processing on nutrient composition, food substitution on a nutritional basis, etc. From the information available, shoppers appear to have mastered many alternative techniques for controlling food expenditures. But, their mean level of expertise with respect to other considerations is below the desired level, given the sophistication of food technology used in food processing and contemporary food retailing practices used by supermarket chains. Decision quality is poor, so a credibility gap and crisis in confidence have resulted. Efforts to improve competence and confidence are necessary to solve these problems so that the food delivery system can function effectively in supplying the food and nutrients to the ultimate consumer.

THE FOOD DELIVERY SYSTEM: DEFICIENT SUPPLY OR INFLATED DEMAND

For all practical purposes, since the USDA has been charged with assuring the availability of sufficient food to meet the nutritional needs of the American population, the possibility of an absolute supply deficit has not existed. In fact, agricultural production capabilities have not been used to potential. So, the widespread fear of famine that gripped the American population as part of the aftermath of the World Food Conference of 1974 was unwarranted. A catastrophe of the magnitude necessary to produce famine in America is without precedent and is an exceedingly unlikely event.

Individual items and/or particular market forms become unprofitable and disappear from marketing channels. As a result of the Energy Crisis, the economics of producing and/or processing all food items has changed. A number of studies have reported some aspects of food-related energy usage, but as yet little is known. The removal of various foods, even if replaced with alternative items in other market forms, will change the supply and demand relations for many other items. Also, the overall cost of food will increase.

Total food-related energy usage, based on data collected during the 1960s (the latest available), is comprised of the following components (Hirst 1973): agricultural production, 18%; food processing, 13%; food transport, 3%; wholesale/retail food storage, 10%; and home storage/preparation, 30%.

Food processing and related industries ranked sixth highest (1972 data) among industrial energy users. The 14 segments using the most energy were determined (Table 32.1) and in-depth studies of several provide detailed information (Unger 1975).

TABLE 32.1. ENERGY USE BY FOOD-RELATED INDUSTRIES, 1973 DATA[1]

Industry	%
Meat packing	11.9
Commercially prepared animal feeds	10.3
Wet corn milling	10.0
Fluid milk	9.4
Beet sugar processing	9.2
Beer	8.9
Bread and bakery products	8.2
Frozen fruits and vegetables	7.4
Soybean oil extraction/processing	6.7
Canned fruits and vegetables	6.3
Cane sugar refining	5.3
Sausage and meat products	3.0
Animal/marine fats and oils	2.9
Ice production	0.5
	100.0

[1] Adapted from Unger (1975).

Canning is an energy-intensive processing method, particularly when the high costs of producing the cans and the chlorine used in plant sanitization are included. Although canning is not the most energy-intensive processing method, nor necessarily the method most likely to be eliminated, it will be used for illustration.

Canning of low-grade and/or excess commodities such as fruits and vegetables has long been a profitable means of salvage. The food itself, which can be sold profitably in this form especially during the off-season, is saved for the consumers. And, the profit on a portion of the crop that otherwise would be unsalable is saved for the producer. But, to continue, canning must remain profitable to the processor. As energy costs increase, since there is a limit to the price consumers will pay for canned foods, a point will be reached where canning is no longer economically feasible. At this point, foods in this market form will disappear from the market.

Hoarding, speculation, and profiteering in combination are a continually tempting but unethical and illegal pattern of practices. This is because hoarding for speculative purposes would facilitate profiteering, i.e., a supply deficit contrived by withholding food so as to drive prices up. It would allow enormous profit on sales made during the emergency. Obviously, such a situation would not be in the public interest. So, in this regard, the purpose of antitrust legislation is to provide assurance that no combination of individuals/corporations could have enough power over the food delivery system to be able to withhold a necessary and sufficient quantity of the food supply and endanger the lives of the American public. The contemporary political climate of distrust has increased awareness of the potential for abuse and has generated insecurity with respect to the quality of controls employed.

The possibility of a transitory deficiency in supply of a particular commodity in a localized area is a more likely but infrequent occurrence. For example, since the advent of centralized meat cutting and cry-o-vac packaging of retail cuts, on occasion a heavy snowstorm in the midwest has been known to greatly delay rail shipments of fresh meat to the west coast. As a result, supplies of particular items have been exhausted in some cities. This situation may exist for a week or two. During this interval, frozen or otherwise preserved meats or locally grown poultry, etc., are substituted. So, although choice is reduced, substitutions are still possible.

A second example would be the effect of unusually heavy rains on the California lettuce crop in 1978. According to the Western Growers Association, supplies should have been good in the late spring, so prices were expected to range between 39¢ and 65¢/head. Instead, the heavy rains ruined the lettuce and precluded use of mechanical harvesting equipment, so prices quickly soared to $1/head which reduced demand to the small amount available.

Strikes against a particular chain store operation also interfere with the delivery of food. For example, a teamsters' strike involving a dispute in another state may halt outgoing food shipments. Since local warehousing would require a costly duplication of facilities and personnel, many local areas are served by a central warehouse. So, IF there is a strike against the central warehouse, THEN all local communities served from that location will be subjected to supply deficits. Moreover, repeated strikes encourage automation in order to eliminate "people problems." Automated equipment is costly; the cost is passed on to the shoppers and changes the cost relationships among foods, with the result that some foods cease to sell at a competitive level so are eliminated from the line of foods carried. Depending on the substitutions made by consumers in the aggregate, a variety of further adjustments in food delivery would result.

Boycotts also affect the food delivery system, as well as its functional capacity and level of productivity at a particular point in time. Unexpected effects are likely to result. For example, the United Farm Workers' efforts in California in the late 1970s resulted in boycotts of lettuce and grapes. Different effects were observed in each of these cases. Lettuce is a year-round vegetable staple and is used daily in many homes. The boycott disrupted eating practices. This annoyance was endured for the duration of the boycott. Then lettuce consumption rebounded toward normal levels. The fact that grapes are a seasonal item created a different effect. The boycott just eliminated an alternative item from the dietary; it was provoking. Since prices increased as a result of the boycott and did not revert to normal levels, consumption did not rebound.

Another example is the coffee boycott in the late 1970s. Because of a sharp freeze in the producing areas, extensive damage reduced yield for several years. Prices soared immediately in anticipation of a tight supply. The price increase incensed consumers, who boycotted coffee. Substitute beverages were sought, and since the duration was sufficient for new consumption habits to be formed, falling coffee prices did not cause consumption to rebound. Delivery capacity was restored but part of the market had evaporated.

Although food boycotts have been used effectively in the past, there is some evidence that greater understanding of their far-reaching effects decreases the probability of using them to show force. Public education in the complexity of the market situation has emphasized the point that increased costs, which can result from a number of combinations of factors, must be offset by higher prices if the product is to continue to be produced. Thus, the consumer must decide whether the food is worth whatever it costs.

In the short-run, the supply of any commodity is limited. This is because a long lead time is required to grow the raw agricultural commodity, to transform it to a finshed product via processing, and/or to transport it to its final destination. Therefore, any factor that temporarily inflates the demand may cause a supply deficit.

A temporary increase in demand may be natural or contrived. An example of a natural situation would be an unseasonably hot day in late winter or early spring. It would cause a sharp increase in the demand for lemonade and ice cream. Since the continuing demand is low but the seasonal demand is high, the quantity in the food delivery system at that time would be insufficient and would be exhausted by only a fraction of those who would purchase the items. This is an unavoidable deficit. An example of a contrived situation would be the use of advertised specials. These are loss leaders, i.e., necessary or desirable items that are offered at a price that is low enough to entice an extra fraction of the pool of shoppers into the store, where they usually will purchase other items as well. Stores do stock up on the sale merchandise; historical usage provides the best estimate of the amount necessary. However, predictions are not infallible. Demand may be greatly underestimated. When the store cannot deliver the food at the sale price, the shopper will be disappointed if not annoyed. Goodwill is created by issuance of "rain checks."

The short-run deficits have at most a temporary effect on the delivery of nutrients. Usually, the effect is also trivial. This is because the American food supply is abundant, so greater than usual consumption at some other point can more than offset a temporary deficit.

THE FOOD SUPPLY SYSTEM: EXCESS SUPPLY OR DEPRESSED DEMAND

The USDA is also charged with responsibility for disposal of agricultural surpluses. Surpluses occur because adjustments in the amount being produced cannot be made rapidly enough to respond to changing production conditions, given demand. This is because production time for the various commodities varies from a few months to a few years AND mechanisms used to assure that a necessary and sufficient amount will be produced must utilize average yield figures as a basis for actions. When better than usual production conditions occur, a greater than average yield will result. The amount of food consumed by the population as an aggregate is relatively fixed. So, if more is produced than can be consumed, a surplus will result. A small surplus is considered to be good.

Food consumption is considered to be a fixed aggregate demand. It is fixed because:

(a) People can gorge themselves, but there is a physical limit.

(b) People can waste food; the more affluent they are, the less they are concerned with the cost of food waste, all other things being equal. Still, even the affluent do not buy food just to throw it away, so there is a limit.

(c) The demand for agricultural production can be increased to some extent by creating desire for foods that require a large input of feed and forage crops, such as creating a demand for beef in lieu of chicken. The nutritive quality, other than for energy, is approximately the same.

But, 9 lb of feed are necessary to produce 1 lb of beef, and only 2 lb are necessary to produce 1 lb of chicken. Still, there is a limit to the demand for beef.

(d) The demand for agricultural production can be increased to some extent by creating a desire for manufactured food products. Since losses occur at each step of food processing and distribution, despite industry efforts to minimize them, the longer the chain of steps between production of the basic foodstuffs and the final consumer, the greater the fraction that is lost. Therefore, the quantity that must be produced to assure adequacy is greater. Still, there is a limit to the proportion of manufactured foods that can be consumed. In an effort to use byproducts and excesses, new uses are continually being found. Yet, there is a limit to the total amount that will be purchased.

Since there is a practical limit to consumption, given the fact that the economic incentive creates a need for profitability and there is a break-even point for each, large surpluses create a problem. In an effort to sell excesses, the food is offered for sale at progressively lower prices. The greater the surplus, the lower the price necessary to induce more sales. At some point, IF the excess were great enough, THEN the sale price would fall below that necessary to cover the costs of production and some producers would be forced out of business. The USDA cannot permit them to be forced out of business, since their production is usually needed. So, the USDA must act to ensure their business survival. Two kinds of action are taken by the USDA. (1) Surpluses are purchased and disposed of in such a way that they do not interfere with demand or market price. (2) The surpluses are sold on the open market at whatever price they will bring and the producers are compensated for the difference between actual market and average price (price supports). Since situations are complex, a number of other strategies operate for fine adjustment of supply and demand around this basic mechanism for gross control.

Federal food assistance programs, domestic and foreign, provide the mechanism by which the USDA disposes of excess food with minimum interference with demand or market price. Federal food assistance programs minimally interfere because the people served subsist on the periphery of the money-based food delivery system as a consequence of their poverty which severely limits participation.

Food giveaways are the most direct means for disposal of specific surpluses. Unfortunately, people do not eat butter and flour one month, peanut butter and peanuts the next, turkeys and beans the next. They eat a variety of foods that must be supplied. Therefore, an enormous and costly storage and distribution problem results. So, other alternatives have been sought.

Use of food stamps and food vouchers is an indirect and demonstrably effective means for increasing the overall demand for food. It does not aid in disposal of specific surpluses, since people do not purchase just those foods that are in excess supply.

Provision of free or reduced price meals at congregate meal sites is another indirect means for increasing the demand for food. A combination of reimbursement and donated foods has been used. Unfortunately, the food has not always been well accepted, so plate waste is high and some of the donated foods cannot be incorporated in the meals so it is discarded. So, there are outraged charges of abuse. An enormous and costly accountability problem results. So, other alternatives have been sought.

The problem of disposing of excess is essentially reduced to one of how to control the size of the excess at an optimal level. By nature, there are costs associated with each alternative solution and optimality is elusive because the values of the parameters are in a dynamic state of change. Because control is imperfect, the potential for abuse exists. This is because every participant has a vested interest and pursues economic gain. The result is a negative outcome. Everybody can give the minimum and take the maximum, which can bring the entire to the lowest common denominator. The corruptions associated with taking the maximum are the bases for charges of abuse and for the eventual disillusionment with each solution. Obviously, the fundamental problem is one of human nature that cannot be denied. As long as a solution is sought according to morale principles based on materialistic goals, the underlying conflict of interest that leads to charges of abuse cannot be resolved.

The newest solutions involve accountability. Theoretically, the mechanisms for disclosure require true and just dealings at every point in order to be properly accountable. But, this cannot be achieved by fiat and decree any more than by force. It comes from within each individual involved in the process, if at all.

The capacity of a food processing plant is fixed. Because harvest is seasonal, the plant operates at or close to capacity for the duration, often processing a series of commodities. IF the excess quantity of a perishable commodity becomes available during the peak period, THEN it cannot be handled. IF the excess quantity of a perishable commodity becomes available after the peak when the plant is no longer being used to capacity OR IF the commodity can be stored and processing delayed, AND IF other ingredients/supplies necessary to the processing can be procured, THEN the processor usually will purchase and process some portion of the excess because he can make higher profits per unit on the excess portion. This is because (a) fixed operating costs have been covered by the regular run and (b) cost per unit of the commodity has been decreased. So, even if he should be forced to sell his processed food at a somewhat lower than normal price, if he can sell the entire quantity, his total profit will be greater, up to the point of diminishing returns.

At the wholesale and retail levels of the food delivery chain, some of the excess will be purchased outright. Since they purchase the item at a reduced per unit price, they can sell it at a somewhat reduced price and still make a profit. As long as the market holds, they will continue to purchase and sell because the more they sell, the greater their total profits. Thus, when more is available, the food delivery system will deliver it until the market is glutted, the point of diminishing returns.

Since transport is a support service business, the necessary units to handle peak needs will be available by prior arrangement. Whether transport of excess quantities is feasible will depend on timing of the excess in relation to the peak and overall transport capacity. IF capacity can be arranged, THEN the excess will be transported, since total profit increases up to the point of diminishing returns.

FOOD ECOLOGY, NUTRITIONAL RISK, AND LIFE EXPECTANCY

The food delivery system is big and complex, operating effectively and simultaneously on multiple levels to supply food and nutrients to the ultimate consumer. Until recent years, relationships between the consumer and the food delivery system, although imperfect, were on a normal pathway and the environment was characterized by mutual trust and goodwill.

Then, negative attitudes infiltrated from other domains and adversely affected the quality of existing relationships. Disillusionment, erosion, detachment, and separation followed in turn. The resultant irresponsibility, should it become general, could create nutritional vulnerability to say nothing of a threat to life expectancy.

Consumers and the food delivery system are mutually dependent so a facilitating relationship needs to be strengthened. Both sides need to take an objective look and give credit where credit is due and not punish all for the misdeeds of a few.

At the present time, the negative impact of food advertising is regarded by some Americans as outrageous. Legitimately, the purposes of advertising are to inform, notify, and/or to call public attention to product X. A food, usually a processed item, is advertised by emphasizing positive qualities to arouse a desire to buy. There is some evidence that advertising has gone too far; both the nature and extent of food ads are questioned.

The nature of food advertising is known to everybody in general as a result of casual observation. The cumulative and aggregate effects have become public knowledge only as a result of a few documented studies. The samples appear unbiased and in harmony with casual observations. So, findings are regarded as representative.

Masover (1977) reported that 85% of the weekend food ads were for low nutrient density foods. From the advertising view, the strategy of pairing snack food ads with leisure time makes sense. From the health view, active physical pursuits are sought to increase energy expenditure so consumption of appealing snacks of high caloric density as part of the activity would be counter-productive.

The same study reported the weekday distribution of food ads as follows:

(a) non-nutritive and low nutrient density food classes (approximately 70%)—Foods advertised were: beverages including beer and wine, 40%; sweets, 11%; high fat foods, 16%; and relishes, condiments, etc., 3%.

(b) high nutrient density food classes (25% of the food ads)—Foods advertised were bread and cereal products, 13%; meat and meat substitutes, 6%; dairy products, 3%; and fruits and vegetables, 3%.

The extent of food advertising on television is documented by figures from Leading Advertisers, Inc. Their 1975 figures indicate that about $1.15 billion were spent on food advertisements. This was aproximately 28% of the total amount of money spent on television advertisements that year. Figures for radio and newspaper advertisements were not cited.

The U.S. Senate Select Committee on Nutrition and Human Needs conducted several hearings on the effects of television advertisements on children's choice of foods. And, much testimony on the negative effects on health was submitted. So, in the "Dietary Goals for the United States" there is a statement that is thought provoking.

It is important to point out that the amounts of advertising for various kinds of foods are not dictated by any overall plan for the achievement of a healthful diet but by needs of various firms at any given moment. Furthermore, those foods most heavily advertised are predominantly processed foods since it is difficult to develop brand loyalties for relatively undifferentiated raw staples.[1]

The "needs" referred to above are general, yet they apply to each and every food product. They are to (a) optimize profits, i.e., maximize sales subject to cost-effectiveness, (b) maintain, if not expand, the firm's position in the market by means of effective competition, and (c) increase the volume of sales to the extent possible. Basic competition involves the efforts of two or more firms to secure the consumer's business by offering

---

[1] From Select Comm. on Nutrition and Human Needs, U.S. Senate (1977).

the most favorable terms; in this case, advertising is the interfacing medium.

However, the differences among major brands may be trivial. So, the struggle for a superior position in the market becomes the objective. The goal is to obtain/maintain the top market position. Because only one firm can have this position, the struggle intensifies.

There is no advertising conspiracy against the health of Americans. The problem is simply the end result (i.e., the cumulative and aggregate effect) of the individual action(s) of persons in various capacities working toward company objectives. Each pursues the goal in relation to his/her part, without knowledge or responsibility for what others are doing even though it is parallel. Since the corporate officials have overview and coordination functions, and presumably know what is going on, IF they create/maintain the conditions under which counter-productive nutrition messages are approved, THEN they should be called to account.

As a result of the negative impact of the adverse publicity accompanying the hearings on the effects of food ads on television, the food processing industry has had to revaluate message content and programming strategies. Industry spokesmen are assuming leadership roles. IF effective, THEN control will come from the industry. The alternative is federal regulatory action; this has been proposed and advocated. To regulate by fiat and decree is a last resort since advertising is not that enforceable and a further deterioration in consumer-industry relations would be the likely result.

The vulnerability of the food delivery system to and challenges resulting from the Energy Crisis have even greater potential implications for the system and consumers. As a result of other than agricultural production energy inputs, the net ratio of energy expended per food calorie produced is negative. It has been estimated variously as 5—7:1. So, a revaluation of the relative value of various alternative sources of energy is occurring.

Food is power and food costs are personal, so politics is vigorous. Like other industrial segments, the food processing industry must control energy usage to some acceptable level. To fail would be unthinkable since once such failure were exposed, little could be done to avert natural outcomes. As a protection, an immediate response to the Energy Crisis resulted in exploration of alternatives, selection of the most promising, and rapid implementation. Still, the pressure has and probably will continue to grow. Neither short run nor long run effects are clear.

Use of convenience foods, which are energy-intensive in processing, transportation, and storage phases, has increased dramatically. This trend is expected to continue in the short run. This trend is unfortunate and accounts for the fact that household energy requirements are the second highest usage, as noted by Unger (1975). Public service announcements on television and mailing inserts by power companies have created public awareness of the waste and high cost of frequent opening of refrigerator and oven doors. Some reduction is possible in this area with no unwanted effects. A pilot Energy Extension Service was instituted in ten states in 1978 to provide information and advice to consumers on methods of energy conservation. Whether food storage/preparation energy usage can be contained is unclear.

BIBLIOGRAPHY

HIRST, E. 1973. Energy use for food in the United States. Rept. ORNL-NSF-EP 57, Oak Ridge National Laboratory, Oak Ridge, Tenn.

JOHNSON, O.C. 1978. The food manufacturer's responsibility for the consumer's nutritional well-being. Food Processing *39* (1) 43-44.

MASOVER, R. 1977. *Cited in* Select Comm. on Nutrition and Human Needs, U.S. Senate. 1977. Dietary Goals for the United States. Second edition. (Committee Print). GPO, Washington, D.C.

PAARLBERG, D. 1977. Food and economics. J. Am. Dietet. Assoc. *71*, 107-110.

SELECT COMM. ON NUTRITION AND HUMAN NEEDS, U.S. SENATE. 1976. Nutrition and Health II. Nutrition and Health Revised with a Study of the Impact of Nutritional Health Considerations on Food Policy. (Committee Print). GPO, Washington, D.C.

SELECT COMM. ON NUTRITION AND HUMAN NEEDS, U.S. SENATE. 1977. Dietary Goals for the United States. Second edition (Committee Print). GPO, Washington, D.C.

UNGER, S.G. 1975. Energy utilization in the leading energy-consuming food processing industries. Food Technol. *29* (12) 33-36, 38-41, 43, 45.

WITTWER, S.H. 1975. Food production: technology and the resource base. Science *188* (4188) 579-584.

33

Frame Shift Problems

Frame shift problems are neither new nor unusual, even in the food and nutrition domain. For centuries, the popular notion was that a good diet was one that was filling. This concept was valid in times and places where the usual problem was to obtain enough food. Later, the general roles of protein, fat, and CHO were acknowledged, and as detailed information became available, the frame of reference shifted from the general to the specific. With each discovery of the nutritional requirement for another vitamin or mineral, the frame of reference with respect to what is a good diet changed again and again.

Dietary surveys then "discovered" new nutritional problems, i.e., certain groups in the American population presented an abnormally low biochemical index and/or habitually consumed diets that were somewhat lacking in one or more of the known nutrients. As knowledge of nutrient requirements and the effects of variation in supply and demand have expanded, new frame shifts have caused other nutrition-related problems to become apparent, especially those related to life expectancy. This process is to be expected as is the continued discovery of new problems with each frame shift.

Each set of problems is expected to challenge professionals anew, and demands new approaches and strategies in working toward solutions. The challenges to professionals are commonly perceived at three levels, namely:

(a) to create public awareness of the discovery of new problems that have become apparent because of a frame shift

(b) to develop public understanding of, and individual judgment with respect to, the probable need for personal dietary adjustment

(c) to develop public appreciation of the implications of problems that require public assistance

PERSPECTIVES

Pursuit of truth is a common objective. Nutritional truth is multi-faceted and truths are found at many levels of food and nutritional knowledge. The human condition is such that we cannot know all. And, what we do know has been revealed only gradually as when we have adopted new foodways that caused new nutritional requirements to come to light. Since adoption of new foodways is a diffuse process, fragments of nutritional truth are revealed in kaleidoscopic patterns. Ideally, prior to introduction of new foods the truth with respect to their nutritional effects could be predicted and evaluated. In practice, tools have proved to be inadequate and we have been, and continue to be, somewhat in the dark. However, the glimpses that we have had have been somewhat disquieting to many. This has been reflected in the common urge to guard against the dark. Hence, nutritional specifications have been in-corporated into the food product development process as a security measure. Widely practiced, these specifications would stabilize compo-sition values and improve the quality of predictions. Perhaps more ac-ceptable truths would emerge.

A frame shift should not be a cause for alarm. It should be regarded as a signal alerting one to the need for assessment to determine whether compensatory changes would be beneficial. It is natural and normal for food consumption patterns to change for many reasons, among them new food item alternatives, altered circumstances and/or resources, different food exposure, and influence and suasion on philosophy and values. And, it is natural and normal for different nutrient intake patterns to be associated with different threats to life expectancy.

A person does not routinely pay that much attention to his/her nutri-ent intake, since in our time nutritional status is ordinarily not that pressing. One consumes his/her "customary" diet that is in a dynamic state of change. The main disadvantage of this mode is that the individu-al is likely to be unaware that nutrient intake has changed until a strong signal is perceived that commands attention. Then attention is focused on nutrient intake and a "discovery" of inappropriate intake is made. The individual discovers that the frame of reference has shifted; either the food sources or nutritional needs have changed, or both. Intake of some nutrients may be high enough or low enough to warrant deliberate change so as to rebalance intake. While such changes are in process, full attention is given to nutrient intake. Then, when the signal shuts off, priorities are likely to shift. Then, attention wanes and is redirected to other pressing needs. Another disadvantage is that given competition for attention, only major problems are addressed and these evoke a cor-respondingly greater response.

THE CONTEMPORARY TWIST

A major theme running through previous discussions is that in the United States, in this century, two major types of frame shifts have occurred. These have involved the relationships between food and nutrition on one hand and nutrition and life expectancy on the other. In summary:

(a) Food sources of nutrients have changed. Basic foodstuffs still provide nutrients in amounts that approximate the expected, but the level of consumption of most of these has changed. Moreover, consumption of highly processed ready-to-eat foods has increased. These items contain different amounts of the various nutrients, i.e., some in reduced quantities due to processing losses and others in augmented quantities due to enrichment or fortification. As a result, traditional expectations of nutrient contributions from items in particular food classes are no longer reliable.

(b) Nutrient availability has changed, especially since World War II. Malnutrition is frequently an oversupply problem rather than the traditional undersupply problem. However, the undersupply problem does continue to afflict small population segments, especially when most vulnerable, as during a growth phase. Oversupply of protein, fat, and CHO has created/contributed to widespread energy storage problems and/or early onset of degenerative killer diseases. Oversupply of other nutrients by non-need-related use of supplements can and does result in development of harmful, if not usually fatal, toxicity syndromes.

The complex and far-reaching food and nutrient consumption changes underlying the first type of frame shift occurred gradually and without prior public awareness of associated implications and ramifications. Then, after the changes in food and nutrient consumption patterns were well established, dietary survey data began to reflect the cumulative and aggregate effects. New food and nutrient intake patterns were reported. As these patterns were noticeably different from previous ones, public explanations became necessary and desirable. Ostensibly, the purpose was to induce those whose diets were extreme to moderate their intakes.

Unfortunately, the common level of nutrition knowledge is not adequate to enable most individuals to understand the importance of such changes in intake and/or determine personal applicability with respect to need for a dietary intake correction. And, lack of necessary and sufficient nutrient composition data added to the problem of those who needed such data and created anxiety. So, not surprisingly, an emotional rather than a reasoned response was the most frequent outcome. However, responses probably ranged from skepticism regarding the nature and extent of dietary intake pattern changes to indifference to alarm and panic.

Given the variability in human nature, this range of responses should have been anticipated. Response by a vocal minority was to call for a return to "former" eating patterns. Of course, this was not generally feasible, given the changes in other aspects of life-style that had created/ maintained the dietary changes. In reality, the frame had shifted for all time. So, the only option has been to accept the frame shift and to make additional compensatory changes.

The complex and far-reaching life-style changes underlying the second type of frame shift occurred recently and without prior public awareness of the physical fitness implications. Obesity, high blood pressure, anemia, and missing/decayed teeth are frequent manifestations documented as lack of physical fitness. A rising incidence of degenerative killer diseases attracted additional attention. In an effort to identify factors in the etiology of the latter, factor analysis of all available kinds of data became a common procedure. In some cases, intakes of specific nutrients were implicated as primary factors (not proven causes). Consequently, new speculations arose and were misinterpreted as causes, and waves of popular confusion, anxiety, and suspicion resulted. Widespread, if transitory, adoption of particular dietary regimens followed. Unfortunately, the common level of health maintenance knowledge is not adequate for most people to understand the importance of obesity or other manifestations of lack of physical fitness and/or to determine personal applicability with respect to need for dietary intake correction. Hence, they are not motivated even when uneasy.

So, here again when the frame shift occurred, the general population was vulnerable. The full range of responses was observed. Rather than an appropriate correctional response, many responded with emotion rather than reason.

THE CONTEMPORARY SOLUTION

Frame shifts are bound to occur intermittently. These must be acknowledged by professionals and the public must be informed. As of now, professionals seem to be in a quandary with respect to the most effective mode for accomplishing their objectives in meeting the tri-level challenges without alarming the public.

The root concern is that individuals remain open to the possibility that gradual change in nutrient intake/needs has occurred which necessitates compensatory intake adjustments. IF a person could remain open to this possibility, THEN the individual probably would be receptive to messages reporting common dietary changes and effects that signal need for revaluation of personal nutrient intake. At the same time, acknowledgement of such national changes as the natural outcome of other changes would reduce the probability of overreaction. While small national changes in dietary intake can be ignored, a national nutritional surveillance system that identifies trends sooner would reduce the hazard of unwanted changes of an important magnitude. This would reduce the necessity for major dietary change and the accompanying disruption in personal feeding practices.

Appendix

NUTRITIVE VALUE OF FOODS

USDA Home and Garden Bull. 72
(Prepared by Agricultural Research Service)

CONTENTS

United States Department of Agriculture Home and Garden Bulletin 72 is reproduced here in its entirety as a supplementary reference for this text.

NUTRITIVE VALUE OF FOODS

By Catherine F. Adams and Martha Richardson[1]
Consumer and Food Economics Institute

A glass of milk . . . a slice of cooked meat . . . an apple . ,. . a slice of bread . . . What food values does each contain? How much cooked meat will a pound of raw meat yield? How much daily protein is recommended for a healthy 14-year-old boy?

Ready answers to questions like these are helpful to homemakers who need the information to plan nutritionally adequate diets and to nutritionists, dietitians, physicians, and other consumers.

The answers will be found in the tables in this publication.

EXPLANATION OF THE TABLES

Nutritive value of foods—Table 2

Table 2 shows the food values in 730 foods commonly used.

Foods listed.—Foods are grouped under the following main headings:

- Dairy products
- Eggs
- Fats and oils
- Fish, shellfish, meat, and poultry
- Fruits and fruit products
- Grain products
- Legumes (dry), nuts, and seeds
- Sugars and sweets
- Vegetables and vegetable products
- Miscellaneous items

Most of the foods listed are in ready-to-eat form. Some are basic products widely used in food preparation, such as flour, fat, and cornmeal.

The weight in grams for an approximate measure of each food is shown. A footnote indicates if inedible parts are included in the description and the weight. For example, item 246 is half a grapefruit with peel having a weight of 241 grams. A footnote to this item explains that the 241 grams include the weight of the peel.

The approximate measure shown for each food is in cups, ounces, pounds, some other well-known unit, or a piece of certain size. The cup measure refers to the standard measuring cup of 8 fluid ounces or one-half liquid pint. The ounce refers to one-sixteenth of a pound avoirdupois, unless fluid ounce is indicated. The weight of a fluid ounce varies according to the food measured. Some helpful volume and weight equivalents are shown in table 1.

[1] The authors gratefully acknowledge the assistance of Ruth G. Bowman of this Institute in compiling the data on the subject matter printed here.

Table 1.—Equivalents by volume and weight

Volume

Level measure	Equivalent
1 gallon (3.786 liters; 3,786 milliliters)	4 quarts
1 quart (0.946 liter; 946 milliliters)	4 cups
1 cup (237 milliliters)	8 fluid ounces ½ pint 16 tablespoons
2 tablespoons (30 milliliters)	1 fluid ounce
1 tablespoon (15 milliliters)	3 teaspoons
1 pound regular butter or margarine	4 sticks 2 cups
1 pound whipped butter or margarine	6 sticks 2 8-ounce containers 3 cups

Weight

Avoirdupois weight	Equivalent
1 pound (16 ounces)	453.6 grams
1 ounce	28.35 grams
3½ ounces	100 grams

Food values.—Table 2 also shows values for protein, fat, total saturated acids, two unsaturated fatty acids (oleic acid and linoleic acid), total carbohydrates, four minerals (calcium, iron, phosphorus, and potassium), and five vitamins (vitamin A, thiamin, riboflavin, niacin, and ascorbic acid or vitamin C). Food energy is in calories. The calorie is the unit of measure for the energy furnished the body by protein, fat, and carbohydrate.

These values can be used to compare kinds and amounts of nutrients in different foods. They sometimes can be used to compare different forms of the same food.

Water content is included because the percentage of moisture present is needed for identification and comparison of many food items.

The values for food energy (calories) and nutrients shown in table 2 are the amounts present in the edible part of the item, that is, in only that portion customarily eaten—corn without cob, meat without bone, potatoes without skin, European-type grapes without seeds. If additional parts are eaten—the potato skin, for example—amounts of some nutrients obtained will be somewhat greater than those shown.

Values for thiamin, riboflavin, and niacin in white flours and white bread and rolls are based on the increased enrichment levels put into effect for those products by the Food and Drug Administration in 1974. Iron values for these products and the values for enriched cornmeals, pastas, farina, and rice (except riboflavin) represent the minimum levels of enrichment promulgated under the Federal Food, Drug, and Cosmetic Act of 1955. Riboflavin values of rice for unenriched rice, as the levels for riboflavin have been stayed. Thiamin, riboflavin, and niacin values for products prepared with white flours represent the use of flours enriched at the 1974 levels and iron at the 1955 levels. Enriched flour is predominantly used in home-prepared and commercially prepared baked goods.

New fatty acid values are given for dairy products, eggs, meats, some grain products, nuts, and soups. The values are based on recent comprehensive research by USDA to update and extend tables for fatty acid content of foods.

Niacin values are for preformed niacin occurring naturally in foods. The values do not include additional niacin that the body may form from tryptophan, an essential amino acid in the protein of most foods. Among the better sources of tryptophan are milk, meats, eggs, legumes, and nuts.

Values have been calculated from the ingredients in typical recipes for many of the prepared items such as biscuits, corn muffins, macaroni and cheese, custard, and many dessert-type items.

Values for toast and cooked vegetables are without fat added, either during preparation or at the table. Some destruction of vitamins, especially ascorbic acid, may occur when vegetables are cut or shredded. Since such losses are variable, no deduction has been made.

For meat, values are for meat cooked and drained of the drippings. For many cuts, two sets of values are shown: meat including fat and meat from which the fat has been removed either in the kitchen or on the plate.

A variety of manufactured items—some of the milk products, ready-to-eat breakfast cereals, imitation cream products, fruit drinks, and various mixes—are included in table 2. Frequently these foods are fortified with one or more nutrients. If nutrients are added, this information is on the label. Values shown here for these foods are usually based on products from several manufacturers and may differ somewhat from the values provided by any one source.

Yield of cooked meat—Table 3

Meat undergoes certain losses from the time it is purchased to the time it is served. Among these losses are those from evaporation of moisture, loss of fat in the drippings, and removal of bone and various trimmings.

Table 3 shows, for several retail cuts, the yield of cooked meat from 1 pound of raw meat. Yield is given as ounces of

Cooked meat with bone and fat
Cooked lean and fat
Cooked lean only.

Among the factors influencing the yield of meat is the proportion of fat and lean in the piece. Many cuts have a layer of fat extending all or part way around. The thickness of this fat varies because cutting and trimming practices for retail distribution differ widely. The information on yield in table 3 and on nutritive value in table 2 applies to retail cuts trimmed according to typical market practice. Deposits of fat within a cut may be extensive and usually are not affected by retail trimming but may be discarded at the table.

Recommended Daily Dietary Allowances—Table 4

Table 4 shows Recommended Daily Dietary Allowances (RDA's) for calories and for several nutrients essential for maintenance of good nutrition in healthy, normally active persons. This table is an abbreviated version adapted from more extensive material published by the Food and Nutrition Board, National Academy of Sciences—National Research Council in 1974.

Additional nutrients for which the Food and Nutrition Board published RDA's are the B-vitamins (vitamins B_6 and B_{12} and folacin), vitamins D and E, magnesium, iodine, and zinc.

Data for these nutrients are not shown in tables 2 or 4. However, table 5 lists foods that are of special value in supplying these eight nutrients (either because they are high in the nutrient or because quantities generally eaten supply **relatively** large amounts).

Recommended iron allowances for infants, children 1 to 3 years old, and females of childbearing age are almost impossible to obtain through ordinary foods. Choosing foods rich in iron—lean meats, shellfish, liver, heart, kidney, dry beans and peas, dark-green vegetables, dried fruit, cereals with added iron, and molasses—can help to meet iron allowances.

More detailed information about RDA's may be obtained from the publication from which table 4 is adapted.

FURTHER INFORMATION

A number of other publications of the Agricultural Research Service, U.S. Department of Agriculture, give helpful information about nutrients and where they are found in foods.

Single copies of the following bulletins are free from the Office of Communication, U.S. Department of Agriculture, Washington, D.C. 20250. Send your requests including ZIP code, on a post card.

Family Fare: A Guide to Good Nutrition .... G 1
Food and Your Weight .... G 74
Conserving the Nutritive Values in Foods .... G 90

Agriculture Handbook No. 8, "Composition of Foods . . . Raw, Processed, Prepared," is a more technical publication with data for a much more extensive list of foods. In it data are presented for the nutrients in 100 grams of edible portion and 1 pound of food as purchased. Nutrients in household measures and market units for many foods are in Agriculture Handbook No. 456, "Nutritive Value of American Foods in Common Units."

Information about nutrition labeling and the percent of the U.S. RDA's of eight nutrients furnished by several household measures of foods may be found in Agriculture Information Bulletin No. 382, "Nutrition Labeling—Tools for Its Use."

The handbooks may be purchased from the Superintendent of Documents, U.S. Government Printing Office, Washington, D.C. 20402: the Consumer Information Center, Pueblo, Colorado 81009; or any U.S. Government Printing Office bookstore.

TABLE 2.— NUTRITIVE VALUES OF THE EDIBLE PART OF FOODS

(Dashes (—) denote lack of reliable data for a constituent believed to be present in measurable amount)

NUTRIENTS IN INDICATED QUANTITY

Item No. (A)	Foods, approximate measures, units, and weight (edible part unless footnotes indicate otherwise) (B)	Weight Grams	Water (C) Per cent	Food energy (D) Cal- ories	Pro- tein (E) Grams	Fat (F) Grams	Satu- rated (total) (G) Grams	Oleic (H) Grams	Lino- leic (I) Grams	Carbo- hydrate (J) Grams	Calcium (K) Milli- grams	Phos- phorus (L) Milli- grams	Iron (M) Milli- grams	Potas- sium (N) Milli- grams	Vitamin A value (O) Inter- national units	Thiamin (P) Milli- grams	Ribo- flavin (Q) Milli- grams	Niacin (R) Milli- grams	Ascorbic acid (S) Milli- grams
	DAIRY PRODUCTS (CHEESE, CREAM, IMITATION CREAM, MILK, RELATED PRODUCTS)																		
	Butter. See Fats, oils; related products, items 103-108.																		
	Cheese:																		
	Natural:																		
1	Blue---- 1 oz----	28	42	100	6	8	5.3	1.9	0.2	1	150	110	0.1	73	200	0.01	0.11	0.3	0
2	Camembert (3 wedges per 4-oz container). 1 wedge----	38	52	115	8	9	5.8	2.2	.2	Trace	147	132	.1	71	350	.01	.19	.2	0
	Cheddar:																		
3	Cut pieces---- 1 oz----	28	37	115	7	9	6.1	2.1	.2	Trace	204	145	.2	28	300	.01	.11	Trace	0
4	Shredded---- 1 cu in----	17.2	37	70	4	6	3.7	1.3	.1	Trace	124	88	.1	17	180	Trace	.06	Trace	0
5	Cottage (curd not pressed down)---- 1 cup----	113	37	455	28	37	24.2	8.5	.7	1	815	579	.8	111	1,200	.03	.42	.1	0
	Creamed (cottage cheese, 4% fat):																		
6	Large curd---- 1 cup----	225	79	235	28	10	6.4	2.4	.2	6	135	297	.3	190	370	.05	.37	.3	Trace
7	Small curd---- 1 cup----	210	79	220	26	9	6.0	2.2	.2	6	126	277	.3	177	340	.04	.34	.3	Trace
8	Low fat (2%)---- 1 cup----	226	79	205	31	4	2.8	1.0	.1	8	155	340	.4	217	160	.05	.42	.3	Trace
9	Low fat (1%)---- 1 cup----	226	82	165	28	2	1.5	.5	.1	6	138	302	.3	193	80	.05	.37	.3	Trace
10	Uncreamed (cottage cheese dry curd, less than 1/2% fat). 1 cup----	145	80	125	25	1	.4	.1	Trace	3	46	151	.3	47	40	.04	.21	.2	0
11	Cream---- 1 oz----	28	54	100	2	10	6.2	2.4	.2	1	23	30	.3	34	400	Trace	.06	Trace	0
	Mozzarella, made with—																		
12	Whole milk---- 1 oz----	28	48	90	6	7	4.4	1.7	.2	1	163	117	.1	21	260	Trace	.08	Trace	0
13	Part skim milk---- 1 oz----	28	49	80	8	5	3.1	1.2	.1	1	207	149	.1	27	180	.01	.10	Trace	0
	Parmesan, grated:																		
14	Cup, not pressed down---- 1 cup----	100	18	455	42	30	19.1	7.7	.3	4	1,376	807	1.0	107	700	.05	.39	.3	0
15	Tablespoon---- 1 tbsp----	5	18	25	2	2	1.0	.4	Trace	Trace	69	40	Trace	5	40	Trace	.02	Trace	0
16	Ounce---- 1 oz----	28	18	130	12	9	5.4	2.2	.1	1	390	229	.3	30	200	.01	.11	.1	0
17	Provolone---- 1 oz----	28	41	100	7	8	4.8	1.7	.1	1	214	141	.1	39	230	.01	.09	Trace	0
	Ricotta, made with—																		
18	Whole milk---- 1 cup----	246	72	428	28	32	20.4	7.1	.7	7	509	389	.9	257	1,210	.03	.48	.3	0
19	Part skim milk---- 1 cup----	246	74	340	28	19	12.1	4.7	.5	13	669	449	1.1	308	1,060	.05	.46	.2	0
20	Romano---- 1 oz----	28	31	110	9	8			.2	1	302	215	Trace	160	160		.11	Trace	0
21	Swiss---- 1 oz----	28	37	105	8	8	5.0	1.7	.2	1	272	171	Trace	31	240	.01	.10	Trace	0
	Pasteurized process cheese:																		
22	American---- 1 oz----	28	39	105	6	9	5.6	2.1	.2	Trace	174	211	.1	46	340	.01	.10	Trace	0
23	Swiss---- 1 oz----	28	42	95	7	7	4.5	1.7	.1	1	219	216	.2	61	230	Trace	.08	Trace	0
24	Pasteurized process cheese food, American. 1 oz----	28	43	95	6	7	4.4	1.7	.1	2	163	130	.2	79	260	.01	.13	Trace	0
25	Pasteurized process cheese spread, American. 1 oz----	28	48	82	5	6	3.8	1.5	.1	2	159	202	.1	69	220	.01	.12	Trace	0
	Cream, sweet:																		
26	Half-and-half (cream and milk)---- 1 cup----	242	81	315	7	28	17.3	7.0	.6	10	254	230	.2	314	260	.08	.36	.2	2
27	1 tbsp----	15	81	20	Trace	2	1.1	.4	Trace	1	16	14	Trace	19	20	.01	.02	Trace	Trace
28	Light, coffee, or table---- 1 cup----	240	74	470	6	46	28.8	11.7	1.0	9	231	192	.1	292	1,730	.08	.36	.1	2
29	1 tbsp----	15	74	30	Trace	3	1.8	.7	.1	1	14	12	Trace	18	110	Trace	.02	Trace	Trace

(A)	(B)	(grams)	(C)	(D)	(E)	(F)	(G)	(H)	(I)	(J)	(K)	(L)	(M)	(N)	(O)	(P)	(Q)	(R)	(S)
	Whipping, unwhipped (volume about double when whipped):																		
	Light:																		
30	1 cup	239	64	700	5	74	46.2	18.3	1.5	7	166	146	0.1	231	2,690	0.06	0.30	0.1	1
31	1 tbsp	15	64	45	Trace	5	2.9	1.1	Trace	Trace	10	9	Trace	15	170	Trace	.02	Trace	Trace
	Heavy:																		
32	1 cup	238	58	820	5	88	54.8	22.2	2.0	7	154	149	Trace	179	3,500	.05	.26	.1	Trace
33	1 tbsp	15	58	80	Trace	6	3.5	1.4	.1	Trace	10	9	Trace	11	220	Trace	.02	Trace	Trace
	Whipped topping, (pressurized):																		
34	1 cup	60	61	155	2	13	8.3	3.4	.3	7	61	54	Trace	88	550	Trace	.04	Trace	0
35	1 tbsp	3	61	10	Trace	1	.4	.2	Trace	Trace	3	3	Trace	4	30	Trace	Trace	Trace	0
	Cream, sour:																		
36	1 cup	230	71	495	7	48	30.0	12.1	1.1	10	268	195	.1	331	1,820	.08	.34	.2	2
37	1 tbsp	12	71	25	Trace	3	1.6	.6	.1	1	14	10	Trace	17	90	Trace	.02	Trace	Trace
	Cream products, imitation (made with vegetable fat):																		
	Sweet:																		
	Creamers:																		
	Liquid (frozen):																		
38	1 cup	245	77	335	2	24	22.8	.3	0	28	23	157	.1	467	220[1]	0	0	0	0
39	1 tbsp	15	77	20	Trace	1	1.4	Trace	0	2	1	10	Trace	29	10[1]	0	0	0	0
	Powdered:																		
40	1 cup	94	2	515	5	33	30.6	.9	Trace	52	21	397	.1	763	190[1]	0	.16[1]	0	0
41	1 tsp	2	2	10	Trace	1	.7	Trace	0	1	Trace	8	Trace	16	Trace[1]	0	Trace[1]	0	0
	Whipped topping:																		
	Frozen:																		
42	1 cup	75	50	240	1	19	16.3	1.0	.2	17	5	6	.1	14	650[1]	0	0	0	0
43	1 tbsp	4	50	15	Trace	1	.9	.1	Trace	1	Trace	Trace	Trace	1	30[1]	0	0	0	0
	Powdered, made with whole milk.																		
44	1 cup	80	67	150	3	10	8.5	.6	.2	13	72	69	Trace	121	290[1]	.02	.09	Trace	1
45	1 tbsp	4	67	10	Trace	Trace	.4	Trace	Trace	1	4	3	Trace	6	10[1]	Trace	Trace	Trace	Trace
	Pressurized:																		
46	1 cup	70	60	185	1	16	13.2	1.4	.2	11	4	13	Trace	13	330[1]	0	0	0	0
47	1 tbsp	4	60	10	Trace	1	.8	.1	Trace	1	Trace	1	Trace	1	20[1]	0	0	0	0
	Sour dressing (imitation sour cream) made with nonfat dry milk.																		
48	1 cup	235	75	415	8	39	31.2	4.4	1.1	11	266	205	.1	380	20[1]	.09	.38	.2	2
49	1 tbsp	12	75	20	Trace	2	1.6	.2	.1	1	14	10	Trace	19	Trace[1]	.01	.02	Trace	Trace
	Ice cream. See Milk desserts, frozen (items 75–80).																		
	Ice milk. See Milk desserts, frozen (items 81–83).																		
	Milk:																		
	Fluid:																		
50	Whole (3.3% fat)— 1 cup	244	88	150	8	8	5.1	2.1	.2	11	291	228	.1	370	310[2]	.09	.40	.2	2
	Lowfat (2%):																		
51	No milk solids added— 1 cup	244	89	120	8	5	2.9	1.2	.1	12	297	232	.1	377	500	.10	.40	.2	2
	Milk solids added:																		
52	Label claim less than 10 g of protein per cup. 1 cup	245	89	125	9	5	2.9	1.2	.1	12	313	245	.1	397	500	.10	.42	.2	2
53	Label claim 10 or more grams of protein per cup (protein fortified). 1 cup	246	88	135	10	5	3.0	1.2	.1	14	352	276	.1	447	500	.11	.48	.2	3
	Lowfat (1%):																		
54	No milk solids added— 1 cup	244	90	100	8	3	1.6	.7	.1	12	300	235	.1	381	500	.10	.41	.2	2
	Milk solids added:																		
55	Label claim less than 10 g of protein per cup. 1 cup	245	90	105	9	2	1.5	.6	.1	12	313	245	.1	397	500	.10	.42	.2	2
56	Label claim 10 or more grams of protein per cup (protein fortified). 1 cup	246	89	120	10	3	1.8	.7	.1	14	349	273	.1	444	500	.11	.47	.2	3
	Nonfat (skim):																		
57	No milk solids added— 1 cup	245	91	85	8	Trace	.3	.1	Trace	12	302	247	.1	406	500	.09	.37	.2	2

[1]Vitamin A value is largely from beta-carotene used for coloring. Riboflavin value for items 40–41 apply to products with added riboflavin.

[2]Applies to product without added vitamin A. With added vitamin A, value is 500 International Units (I.U.).

TABLE 2.—NUTRITIVE VALUES OF THE EDIBLE PART OF FOODS - Continued

(Dashes (—) denote lack of reliable data for a constituent believed to be present in measurable amount)

Item No. (A)	Foods, approximate measures, units, and weight (edible part unless footnotes indicate otherwise) (B)	Water (C) Per cent	Food energy (D) Calories	Pro-tein (E) Grams	Fat (F) Grams	Fatty Acids: Saturated (total) (G) Grams	Unsaturated: Oleic (H) Grams	Linoleic (I) Grams	Carbo-hydrate (J) Grams	Calcium (K) Milligrams	Phos-phorus (L) Milligrams	Iron (M) Milligrams	Potas-sium (N) Milligrams	Vitamin A value (O) International units	Thiamin (P) Milligrams	Ribo-flavin (Q) Milligrams	Niacin (R) Milligrams	Ascorbic acid (S) Milligrams
	DAIRY PRODUCTS (CHEESE, CREAM, IMITATION CREAM, MILK; RELATED PRODUCTS)—Con.																	
	Milk—Continued																	
	Fluid—Continued																	
	Nonfat (skim)—Continued																	
	Milk solids added:																	
58	Label claim less than 10 g of protein per cup. 1 cup	90	90	9	1	0.4	0.1	Trace	12	316	255	0.1	416	500	0.10	0.43	0.2	2
59	Label claim 10 or more grams of protein per cup (protein forti-fied). 1 cup	89	100	10	1	.4	.1	Trace	14	352	275	.1	446	500	.11	.48	.2	3
60	Buttermilk 1 cup	90	100	8	2	1.3	.5	Trace	12	285	219	.1	371	[3]80	.08	.38	.1	2
	Canned:																	
61	Whole milk 1 cup	74	340	17	19	11.6	5.3	0.4	25	657	510	.5	764	[4]610	.12	.80	.5	5
62	Skim milk 1 cup	79	200	19	1	.3	.1	Trace	29	738	497	.7	845	[4]1,000	.11	.79	.4	3
63	Sweetened, condensed 1 cup	27	980	24	27	16.8	6.7	.7	166	868	775	.6	1,136	[3]1,000	.28	1.27	.6	8
	Dried:																	
64	Buttermilk 1 cup	3	465	41	7	4.3	1.7	.2	59	1,421	1,119	.4	1,910	[5]260	.47	1.90	1.1	7
	Nonfat instant:																	
65	Envelope, net wt., 3.2 oz[2] 1 envelope	4	325	32	1	.4	.1	Trace	47	1,120	896	.3	1,552	[6]2,160	.38	1.59	.8	5
66	Cup[2] 1 cup	4	245	24	Trace	.3	.1	Trace	35	837	670	.2	1,160	[6]1,610	.28	1.19	.6	4
	Milk beverages:																	
	Chocolate milk (commercial):																	
67	Regular 1 cup	82	210	8	8	5.3	2.2	.2	26	280	251	.6	417	300	.09	.41	.3	2
68	Lowfat (2%) 1 cup	84	180	8	5	3.1	1.3	.1	26	284	254	.6	422	500	.10	.42	.3	2
69	Lowfat (1%) 1 cup	85	160	8	3	1.5	.7	.1	26	287	257	.6	426	500	.10	.40	.2	2
70	Eggnog (commercial) 1 cup	74	340	10	19	11.3	5.0	.6	34	330	278	.5	420	890	.09	.48	.3	4
	Malted milk, home-prepared with 1 cup of whole milk and 2 to 3 heaping tsp of malted milk powder (about 3/4 oz):																	
71	Chocolate 1 cup of milk plus 3/4 oz of powder.	81	235	9	9	5.5	—	—	29	304	265	.5	500	330	.14	.43	.7	2
72	Natural 1 cup of milk plus 3/4 oz of powder.	81	235	11	10	6.0	—	—	27	347	307	.3	529	380	.20	.54	1.3	2
	Shakes, thick:[8]																	
73	Chocolate, container, net wt., 10.6 oz. 1 container	72	355	9	8	5.0	2.0	.2	63	396	378	.9	672	260	.14	.67	.4	0
74	Vanilla, container, net wt., 11 oz. 1 container	74	350	12	9	5.9	2.4	.2	56	457	361	.3	572	360	.09	.61	.5	0
	Milk desserts, frozen:																	
	Ice cream:																	
	Regular (about 11% fat):																	
75	Hardened 1/2 gal	61	2,155	38	115	71.3	28.8	2.6	254	1,406	1,075	1.0	2,052	4,340	.42	2.63	1.1	[6]
76	1 cup	61	270	5	14	8.9	3.6	.3	32	176	134	.1	257	540	.05	.33	.1	1
77	3-fl oz container	61	100	2	5	3.4	1.4	.1	12	66	51	Trace	96	200	.02	.12	.1	Trace
78	Soft serve (frozen custard) 1 cup	60	375	7	23	13.5	5.9	.6	38	236	199	.4	338	790	.08	.45	.2	1
79	Rich (about 16% fat), hardened. 1/2 gal	59	2,805	33	190	118.3	47.8	4.3	256	1,213	927	.8	1,771	7,200	.36	2.27	.9	5
80	1 cup	59	350	4	24	14.7	6.0	.5	32	151	115	.1	221	900	.04	.28	.1	1
	Ice milk:																	
81	Hardened (about 4.3% fat) 1/2 gal	69	1,470	41	45	28.1	11.3	1.0	232	1,409	1,035	1.5	2,117	1,710	.61	2.78	.9	6
82	1 cup	69	185	5	6	3.5	1.4	.1	29	176	129	.1	265	210	.08	.35	.1	1

(A)	(B)	(C)	(D)	(E)	(F)	(G)	(H)	(I)	(J)	(K)	(L)	(M)	(N)	(O)	(P)	(O)	(R)	(S)
83	Soft serve (about 2.6% fat)------- 1 cup	70	225	8	5	2.9	1.2	0.1	38	274	202	0.3	412	180	0.12	0.54	0.2	1
84	Sherbet (about 2% fat)------- 1/2 gal	66	2,160	17	31	19.0	7.7	.7	469	827	594	2.5	1,585	1,480	.26	.71	1.0	31
85	------- 1 cup	66	270	2	4	2.4	1.0	.1	59	103	74	.3	198	190	.03	.09	.1	1
86	Milk desserts, other: Custard, baked------- 1 cup	77	305	14	15	6.8	5.4	.7	29	297	310	1.1	387	930	.11	.50	.3	1
	Puddings: From home recipe: Starch base:																	
87	Chocolate------- 1 cup	66	385	8	12	7.6	3.3	.2	67	250	255	1.3	445	390	.05	.36	.3	1
88	Vanilla (blancmange)------- 1 cup	76	285	9	10	6.2	2.5	.2	41	298	232	Trace	352	410	.08	.41	.3	2
89	Tapioca cream------- 1 cup	72	220	8	8	4.1	2.5	.5	28	173	180	.7	223	480	.07	.30	.2	2
	From mix (chocolate) and milk:																	
90	Regular (cooked)------- 1 cup	70	320	9	8	4.3	2.6	.2	59	265	247	.8	354	340	.05	.39	.3	2
91	Instant------- 1 cup	69	325	8	7	3.6	2.2	.3	63	374	237	1.3	335	340	.08	.39	.3	2
	Yogurt: With added milk solids: Made with lowfat milk:																	
92	Fruit-flavored------- 1 container, net wt., 8 oz	75	230	10	3	1.8	.6	.1	42	343	269	.2	439	[10]120	.08	.40	.2	1
93	Plain------- 1 container, net wt., 8 oz	85	145	12	4	2.3	.8	.1	16	415	326	.2	531	[10]150	.10	.49	.3	2
94	Made with nonfat milk------- 1 container, net wt., 8 oz	85	125	13	Trace	.3	.1	Trace	17	452	355	.2	579	[10]20	.11	.53	.3	2
	Without added milk solids:																	
95	Made with whole milk------- 1 container, net wt., 8 oz	88	140	8	7	4.8	1.7	.1	11	274	215	.1	351	280	.07	.32	.2	1

EGGS

(A)	(B)	(C)	(D)	(E)	(F)	(G)	(H)	(I)	(J)	(K)	(L)	(M)	(N)	(O)	(P)	(O)	(R)	(S)
	Eggs, large (24 oz per dozen): Raw:																		
96	Whole, without shell------- 1 egg	75	80	6	6	1.7	2.0	.6	Trace	28	90	1.0	65	260	.04	.15	Trace	0
97	White------- 1 white	88	15	3	Trace	0	0	0	Trace	4	4	Trace	45	0	Trace	.09	Trace	0
98	Yolk------- 1 yolk	49	65	3	6	1.7	2.1	.6	Trace	26	86	.9	15	310	.04	.07	Trace	0
	Cooked:																		
99	Fried in butter------- 1 egg	72	85	5	6	2.4	2.2	.6	1	26	80	.9	58	290	.03	.13	Trace	0
100	Hard-cooked, shell removed------- 1 egg	75	80	6	6	1.7	2.0	.6	1	28	90	1.0	65	260	.04	.14	Trace	0
101	Poached------- 1 egg	74	80	6	6	1.7	2.0	.6	1	28	90	1.0	65	260	.04	.13	Trace	0
102	Scrambled (milk added) in butter. Also omelet------- 1 egg	76	95	6	7	2.8	2.3	.6	1	47	97	.9	85	310	.04	.16	Trace	0

FATS, OILS; RELATED PRODUCTS

(A)	(B)	(C)	(D)	(E)	(F)	(G)	(H)	(I)	(J)	(K)	(L)	(M)	(N)	(O)	(P)	(O)	(R)	(S)
	Butter: Regular (1 brick or 4 sticks per lb):																		
103	Stick (1/2 cup)------- 1 stick	16	815	1	92	57.3	23.1	2.1	Trace	27	26	.2	29	[11]3,470	.01	.04	Trace	0
104	Tablespoon (about 1/8 stick)------- 1 tbsp	16	100	Trace	12	7.2	2.9	.3	Trace	3	3	Trace	4	[11]430	Trace	Trace	Trace	0
105	Pat (1 in square, 1/3 in high; 90 per lb)------- 1 pat	16	35	Trace	4	2.5	1.0	.1	Trace	1	1	Trace	1	[11]150	Trace	Trace	Trace	0
	Whipped (6 sticks or two 8-oz containers per lb):																		
106	Stick (1/2 cup)------- 1 stick	16	540	1	61	38.2	15.4	1.4	Trace	18	17	.1	20	[12]2,310	Trace	.03	Trace	0
107	Tablespoon (about 1/8 stick)------- 1 tbsp	16	65	Trace	8	4.7	1.9	.2	Trace	2	2	Trace	2	[11]290	Trace	Trace	Trace	0
108	Pat (1 1/4 in square, 1/3 in high; 120 per lb)------- 1 pat	16	25	Trace	3	1.9	.8	.1	Trace	1	1	Trace	1	[11]120	0	Trace	Trace	0

3 Applies to product without vitamin A added.
4 Applies to product with added vitamin A. Without added vitamin A, value is 20 International Units (I.U.).
5 Yields 1 qt of fluid milk when reconstituted according to package directions.
6 Applies to product with added vitamin A.
7 Weight applies to product with label claim of 1 1/3 cups equal 3.2 oz.
8 Applies to products made from thick shake mixes and that do not contain added ice cream. Products made from milk shake mixes are higher in fat and usually contain added ice cream.
9 Content of fat, vitamin A, and carbohydrate varies. Consult the label when precise values are needed for special diets.
10 Applies to product made with milk containing no added vitamin A.
11 Based on year-round average.

TABLE 2.—NUTRITIVE VALUES OF THE EDIBLE PART OF FOODS - Continued

(Dashes (—) denote lack of reliable data for a constituent believed to be present in measurable amount)

NUTRIENTS IN INDICATED QUANTITY

(A) Item No.	(B) Foods, approximate measures, units, and weight (edible part unless footnotes indicate otherwise)	Grams (weight)	(C) Water Percent	(D) Food energy Calories	(E) Protein Grams	(F) Fat Grams	(G) Saturated (total) Grams	(H) Oleic Grams	(I) Linoleic Grams	(J) Carbohydrate Grams	(K) Calcium Milligrams	(L) Phosphorus Milligrams	(M) Iron Milligrams	(N) Potassium Milligrams	(O) Vitamin A value International units	(P) Thiamin Milligrams	(Q) Riboflavin Milligrams	(R) Niacin Milligrams	(S) Ascorbic acid Milligrams
	FATS, OILS, RELATED PRODUCTS—Con.																		
109	Fats, cooking (vegetable shortenings) 1 cup	200	0	1,770	0	200	48.8	88.2	48.4	0	0	0	0	0	—	0	0	0	0
110	1 tbsp	13	0	110	0	13	3.2	5.7	3.1	0	0	0	0	0	—	0	0	0	0
111	Lard 1 cup	205	0	1,850	0	205	81.0	83.8	20.5	0	0	0	0	0	0	0	0	0	0
112	1 tbsp	13	0	115	0	13	5.1	5.3	1.3	0	0	0	0	0	0	0	0	0	0
	Margarine: Regular (1 brick or 4 sticks per lb):																		
113	Stick (1/2 cup) 1 stick	113	16	815	1	92	16.7	42.9	24.9	Trace	27	26	.2	29	[12]3,750	.01	.04	Trace	0
114	Tablespoon (about 1/8 stick) 1 tbsp	14	16	100	Trace	12	2.1	5.7	3.1	Trace	3	3	Trace	4	[12]470	Trace	Trace	Trace	0
115	Pat (1 in square, 1/3 in high; 90 per lb) 1 pat	5	16	35	Trace	4	.7	1.9	1.1	Trace	1	1	Trace	1	[12]170	Trace	Trace	Trace	0
116	Soft, two 8-oz containers per lb 1 container	227	16	1,635	1	184	32.5	71.5	65.4	Trace	53	52	.4	59	[12]7,500	.01	.08	.1	0
117	1 tbsp	14	16	100	Trace	12	2.0	4.5	4.1	Trace	3	3	Trace	4	[12]470	Trace	Trace	Trace	0
	Whipped (6 sticks per lb):																		
118	Stick (1/2 cup) 1 stick	76	16	545	Trace	61	11.2	28.7	16.7	Trace	18	17	.1	20	[12]2,500	Trace	.03	Trace	0
119	Tablespoon (about 1/8 stick) 1 tbsp	9	16	70	Trace	8	1.4	3.6	2.1	Trace	2	2	Trace	2	[12]310	Trace	Trace	Trace	0
	Oils, salad or cooking:																		
120	Corn 1 cup	218	0	1,925	0	218	27.7	53.6	125.1	0	0	0	0	0	—	0	0	0	0
121	1 tbsp	14	0	120	0	14	1.7	3.3	7.8	0	0	0	0	0	—	0	0	0	0
122	Olive 1 cup	216	0	1,910	0	216	30.7	154.4	17.7	0	0	0	0	0	—	0	0	0	0
123	1 tbsp	14	0	120	0	14	1.9	9.7	1.1	0	0	0	0	0	—	0	0	0	0
124	Peanut 1 cup	216	0	1,910	0	216	37.4	98.5	67.0	0	0	0	0	0	—	0	0	0	0
125	1 tbsp	14	0	120	0	14	2.3	6.2	4.2	0	0	0	0	0	—	0	0	0	0
126	Safflower 1 cup	218	0	1,925	0	218	20.5	25.9	159.8	0	0	0	0	0	—	0	0	0	0
127	1 tbsp	14	0	120	0	14	1.3	1.6	10.0	0	0	0	0	0	—	0	0	0	0
128	Soybean oil, hydrogenated (partially hardened) 1 cup	218	0	1,925	0	218	31.8	93.1	75.6	0	0	0	0	0	—	0	0	0	0
129	1 tbsp	14	0	120	0	14	2.0	5.8	4.7	0	0	0	0	0	—	0	0	0	0
130	Soybean-cottonseed oil blend, hydrogenated 1 cup	218	0	1,925	0	218	38.2	63.0	99.6	0	0	0	0	0	—	0	0	0	0
131	1 tbsp	14	0	120	0	14	2.4	3.9	6.2	0	0	0	0	0	—	0	0	0	0
	Salad dressings: Commercial: Blue cheese:																		
132	Regular 1 tbsp	15	32	75	1	8	1.6	1.7	3.8	1	12	11	Trace	6	30	Trace	.02	Trace	Trace
133	Low calorie (5 Cal per tsp) 1 tbsp	16	84	10	Trace	1	.5	.3	Trace	1	10	8	Trace	5	30	Trace	.01	Trace	Trace
	French:																		
134	Regular 1 tbsp	16	39	65	Trace	6	1.1	1.3	3.2	3	2	2	.1	13	—	—	—	—	—
135	Low calorie (5 Cal per tsp) 1 tbsp	16	77	15	Trace	1	.1	.1	.4	2	2	2	.1	13	—	—	—	—	—
	Italian:																		
136	Regular 1 tbsp	15	28	85	Trace	9	1.6	1.9	4.7	1	2	1	Trace	2	Trace	Trace	Trace	Trace	—
137	Low calorie (2 Cal per tsp) 1 tbsp	15	90	10	Trace	1	.1	.1	.4	Trace	Trace	1	Trace	2	Trace	Trace	Trace	Trace	—
138	Mayonnaise 1 tbsp	14	15	100	Trace	11	2.0	2.4	5.6	Trace	3	4	.1	5	40	Trace	.01	Trace	—
	Mayonnaise type:																		
139	Regular 1 tbsp	15	41	65	Trace	6	1.1	1.4	3.2	2	2	4	Trace	1	30	Trace	Trace	Trace	—
140	Low calorie (8 Cal per tsp) 1 tbsp	16	81	20	Trace	2	.4	.4	1.0	2	3	4	Trace	1	40	Trace	Trace	Trace	—
141	Tartar sauce, regular 1 tbsp	14	34	75	Trace	8	1.5	1.8	4.1	1	3	4	.1	11	30	Trace	Trace	Trace	Trace
	Thousand Island:																		
142	Regular 1 tbsp	16	32	80	Trace	8	1.4	1.7	4.0	2	2	3	.1	18	50	Trace	Trace	Trace	Trace
143	Low calorie (10 Cal per tsp) 1 tbsp	15	68	25	Trace	2	.4	.4	1.0	2	2	3	.1	17	50	Trace	Trace	Trace	Trace
	From home recipe:																		
144	Cooked type 1 tbsp	16	68	25	1	2	.5	.6	.3	2	14	15	.1	19	80	.01	.03	Trace	Trace

FISH, SHELLFISH, MEAT, POULTRY: RELATED PRODUCTS

(A)	(B)		(C)	(D)	(E)	(F)	(G)	(H)	(I)	(J)	(K)	(L)	(M)	(N)	(O)	(P)	(Q)	(R)	(S)
145	Fish and shellfish: Bluefish, baked with butter or margarine.	3 oz	85	68	135	22	4	—	—	—	0	25	244	0.6	—	40	0.09	0.08	1.6	—
	Clams:																			
146	Raw, meat only	3 oz	85	82	65	11	1	0.2	Trace	Trace	2	59	138	5.2	154	90	.08	.15	1.1	8
147	Canned, solids and liquid	3 oz	85	86	45	7	1	.6	Trace	0.1	1	47	116	3.5	119	—	.01	.09	.9	—
148	Crabmeat (white or king), canned, not pressed down.	1 cup	135	77	135	24	3		0.4			61	246	1.1	149	—	.11	.11	2.6	—
149	Fish sticks, breaded, cooked, frozen (stick, 4 by 1 by 1/2 in).	1 fish stick or 1 oz	28	66	50	5	3				2	3	47	.1	—	0	.01	.02	.5	—
150	Haddock, breaded, fried[14]	3 oz	85	66	140	17	5	1.4	2.2	1.2	5	34	210	1.0	296	—	.03	.06	2.7	2
151	Ocean perch, breaded, fried[14]	1 fillet	85	59	195	16	11	2.7	4.4	2.3	6	28	192	1.1	242	—	.10	.10	1.6	—
152	Oysters, raw, meat only (13-19 medium Selects).	1 cup	240	85	160	20	4	1.3	.2	.1	8	226	343	13.2	290	740	.34	.43	6.0	—
153	Salmon, pink, canned, solids and liquid.	3 oz	85	71	120	17	5	.9	.8	.1	0	[15]167	243	.7	307	60	.03	.16	6.8	—
154	Sardines, Atlantic, canned in oil, drained solids.	3 oz	85	62	175	20	9	3.0	2.5	.5	0	372	424	2.5	502	190	.02	.17	4.6	—
155	Scallops, frozen, breaded, fried, reheated.	6 scallops	90	60	175	16	8				9									
156	Shad, baked with butter or margarine, bacon.	3 oz	85	64	170	20	10				0	20	266	.5	320	30	.11	.22	7.3	—
	Shrimp:																			
157	Canned meat	3 oz	85	70	100	21	1	.1	.1	Trace	1	98	224	2.6	104	50	.01	.03	1.5	—
158	French fried[16]	3 oz	85	57	190	17	9	2.3	3.7	2.0	9	61	162	1.7	195	70	.03	.07	2.3	—
159	Tuna, canned in oil, drained solids.	3 oz	85	61	170	24	7	1.7	1.7	.7	0	7	199	1.6	—	70	.04	.10	10.1	—
160	Tuna salad[17]	1 cup	205	70	350	30	22	4.3	6.3	6.7	7	41	291	2.7	—	590	.08	.23	10.3	2
161	Meat and meat products: Bacon, (20 slices per lb, raw), broiled or fried, crisp.	2 slices	15	8	85	4	8	2.5	3.7	.7	Trace	2	34	.5	35	0	.08	.05	.8	—
	Beef, cooked: Cuts braised, simmered or pot roasted:																			
162	Lean and fat (piece, 2 1/2 by 2 1/2 by 3/4 in).	3 oz	85	53	245	23	16	6.8	6.5	.4	0	10	114	2.9	184	30	.04	.18	3.6	—
163	Lean only from item 162	2.5 oz	72	62	140	22	5	2.1	1.8	.2	0	10	108	2.7	176	10	.04	.17	3.3	—
	Ground beef, broiled:																			
164	Lean with 10% fat	3 oz or patty 3 by 5/8 in	85	60	185	23	10	4.0	3.9	.3	0	10	196	3.0	261	20	.08	.20	5.1	—
165	Lean with 21% fat	2.9 oz or patty 3 by 5/8 in	82	54	235	20	17	7.0	6.7	.4	0	9	159	2.6	221	30	.07	.17	4.4	—
	Roast, oven cooked, no liquid added: Relatively fat, such as rib:																			
166	Lean and fat (2 pieces, 4 1/8 by 2 1/4 by 1/4 in).	3 oz	85	40	375	17	33	14.0	13.6	.8	0	8	158	2.2	189	70	.05	.13	3.1	—
167	Lean only from item 166[18]	1.8 oz	51	57	125	14	7	3.0	2.5	.3	0	6	131	1.8	161	10	.04	.11	2.6	—
	Relatively lean, such as heel of round:																			
168	Lean and fat (2 pieces, 4 1/8 by 2 1/4 by 1/4 in).	3 oz	85	62	165	25	7	2.8	2.7	.2	0	11	208	3.2	279	10	.06	.19	4.5	—

[12] Based on average vitamin A content of fortified margarine. Federal specifications for fortified margarine require a minimum of 15,000 International Units (I.U.) of vitamin A per pound.
[13] Fatty acid values apply to product made with regular-type margarine.
[14] Dipped in egg, milk or water, and breadcrumbs; fried in vegetable shortening.
[15] If bones are discarded, value for calcium will be greatly reduced.
[16] Dipped in egg, breadcrumbs, and flour or batter.
[17] Prepared with tuna, celery, salad dressing (mayonnaise type), pickle, onion, and egg.
[18] Outer layer of fat on the cut was removed to within approximately 1/2 in of the lean. Deposits of fat within the cut were not removed.

TABLE 2.— NUTRITIVE VALUES OF THE EDIBLE PART OF FOODS - Continued

(Dashes (—) denote lack of reliable data for a constituent believed to be present in measurable amount)

Item No.	Foods, approximate measure, units, and weight (edible part unless footnotes indicate otherwise)		Water	Food energy	Protein	Fat	Fatty Acids Saturated (total)	Unsaturated Oleic	Linoleic	Carbohydrate	Calcium	Phosphorus	Iron	Potassium	Vitamin A value	Thiamin	Riboflavin	Niacin	Ascorbic acid
(A)	(B)	Grams	(C) Per cent	(D) Calories	(E) Grams	(F) Grams	(G) Grams	(H) Grams	(I) Grams	(J) Grams	(K) Milligrams	(L) Milligrams	(M) Milligrams	(N) Milligrams	(O) International units	(P) Milligrams	(Q) Milligrams	(R) Milligrams	(S) Milligrams
	FISH, SHELLFISH, MEAT, POULTRY; RELATED PRODUCTS—Con.																		
	Meat and meat products—Continued																		
	Beef,[1] cooked—Continued																		
	Roast, oven cooked, no liquid added—Continued																		
	Relatively lean such as heel of round—Continued																		
169	Lean only from item 168-- 2.8 oz	78	65	125	24	3	1.2	1.0	0.1	0	10	199	3.0	268	Trace	0.06	0.18	4.3	—
	Steak:																		
	Relatively fat-sirloin, broiled:																		
170	Lean and fat (piece, 2 1/2 by 2 1/2 by 3/4 in.) 3 oz	85	44	330	20	27	11.3	11.1	.6	0	9	162	2.5	220	50	.05	.15	4.0	—
171	Lean only from item 170-- 2.0 oz	56	59	115	18	4	1.8	1.6	.2	0	7	146	2.2	202	10	.05	.14	3.6	—
	Relatively lean-round, braised:																		
172	Lean and fat (piece, 4 1/8 by 2 1/4 by 1/2 in.) 3 oz	85	55	220	24	13	5.5	5.2	.4	0	10	213	3.0	272	20	.07	.19	4.8	—
173	Lean only from item 172-- 2.4 oz	68	61	130	21	4	1.7	1.5	.2	0	9	182	2.5	238	10	.05	.16	4.1	—
	Beef, canned:																		
174	Corned beef-- 3 oz	85	59	185	22	10	4.9	4.5	.2	0	17	90	3.7	—	—	.01	.20	2.9	—
175	Corned beef hash-- 1 cup	220	67	400	19	25	11.9	10.9	.5	24	29	147	4.4	440	—	.02	.20	4.6	—
176	Beef, dried, chipped-- 2 1/2-oz jar	71	48	145	24	4	2.1	2.0	.1	0	14	287	3.6	142	—	.05	.23	2.7	0
177	Beef and vegetable stew-- 1 cup	245	82	220	16	11	4.9	4.5	.2	15	29	184	2.9	613	2,400	.15	.17	4.7	17
178	Beef potpie (home recipe), baked[13] (piece, 1/3 of 9-in diam. pie)-- 1 piece	210	55	515	21	30	7.9	12.8	6.7	39	29	149	3.8	334	1,720	.30	.30	5.5	6
179	Chili con carne with beans, canned-- 1 cup	255	72	340	19	16	7.5	6.8	.3	31	82	321	4.3	594	150	.08	.18	3.3	—
180	Chop suey with beef and pork (home recipe)-- 1 cup	250	75	300	26	17	8.5	6.2	.7	13	60	248	4.8	425	600	.28	.38	5.0	33
181	Heart, beef, lean, braised-- 3 oz	85	61	160	27	5	1.5	1.1	.6	1	5	154	5.0	197	20	.21	1.04	6.5	1
	Lamb, cooked:																		
	Chop, rib (cut 3 per lb with bone), broiled:																		
182	Lean and fat-- 3.1 oz	89	43	360	18	32	14.8	12.1	1.2	0	8	139	1.0	200	—	.11	.19	4.1	—
183	Lean only from item 182-- 2 oz	57	60	120	16	6	2.5	2.1	.2	0	6	121	1.1	174	—	.09	.15	3.4	—
	Leg, roasted:																		
184	Lean and fat (2 pieces, 4 1/8 by 2 1/4 by 1/4 in.)-- 3 oz	85	54	235	22	16	7.3	6.0	.6	0	9	177	1.4	241	—	.13	.23	4.7	—
185	Lean only from item 184-- 2.5 oz	71	62	130	20	5	2.1	1.8	.2	0	9	169	1.4	227	—	.12	.21	4.4	—
	Shoulder, roasted:																		
186	Lean and fat (3 pieces, 2 1/2 by 2 1/2 by 1/4 in.)-- 3 oz	85	50	285	18	23	10.8	8.8	.9	0	9	146	1.0	206	—	.11	.20	4.0	—
187	Lean only from item 186-- 2.3 oz	64	61	130	17	6	3.6	2.3	.2	0	8	140	1.0	193	—	.10	.18	3.7	—
188	Liver, beef, fried[15] (slice, 6 1/2 by 2 3/8 by 3/8 in.),[22] 3 oz	85	56	195	22	9	2.5	3.5	.9	5	9	405	7.5	323	[21]45,390	.22	3.56	14.0	23
	Pork, cured, cooked:																		
189	Ham, light cure, lean and fat, roasted (2 pieces, 4 1/8 by 2 1/4 by 1/4 in.)[22] 3 oz	85	54	245	18	19	6.8	7.9	1.7	0	8	146	2.2	199	0	.40	.15	3.1	—
	Luncheon meat:																		
190	Boiled ham, slice (8 per 8-oz pkg.)-- 1 oz	28	59	65	5	5	1.7	2.0	.4	0	3	47	.8	—	0	.12	.04	.7	—
191	Canned, spiced or unspiced: Slice, approx. 3 by 2 by 1/2 in.-- 1 slice	60	55	175	9	15	5.4	6.7	1.0	1	5	65	1.3	133	0	.19	.13	1.8	—

(A)	(B)		(C)	(D)	(E)	(F)	(G)	(H)	(I)	(J)	(K)	(L)	(M)	(N)	(O)	(P)	(Q)	(R)	(S)
	Pork, fresh,[18] cooked: Chop, loin (cut 3 per lb with bone), broiled:																		
192	Lean and fat	2.7 oz	78	42	305	19	25	8.9	10.4	2.2	0	9	209	2.7	216	0	0.75	0.22	4.5	—
193	Lean only from item 192	2 oz	56	53	150	17	9	3.1	3.6	.8	0	7	181	2.2	192	0	.63	.18	3.8	—
	Roast, oven cooked, no liquid added:																			
194	Lean and fat (piece, 2 1/2 by 2 1/2 by 3/4 in)	3 oz	85	46	310	21	24	8.7	10.2	2.2	0	9	218	2.7	233	0	.78	.22	4.8	—
195	Lean only from item 194	2.4 oz	68	55	175	20	10	3.5	4.1	.8	0	9	211	2.6	224	0	.73	.21	4.4	—
	Shoulder cut, simmered:																			
196	Lean and fat (3 pieces, 2 1/2 by 2 1/2 by 1/4 in)	3 oz	85	45	320	20	26	9.3	10.9	2.3	0	9	118	2.6	158	0	.46	.21	4.1	—
197	Lean only from item 196	2.2 oz	63	60	135	18	6	2.2	2.6	.6	0	8	111	2.3	146	0	.42	.19	3.7	—
	Sausages (see also Luncheon meat (items 190-191)):																			
198	Bologna, slice (8 per 8-oz pkg.)	1 slice	28	56	85	3	8	3.0	3.4	.5	Trace	2	36	.5	65	—	.05	.06	.7	—
199	Braunschweiger, slice (6 per 6-oz pkg.)	1 slice	28	53	90	4	8	2.6	3.4	.8	1	3	69	1.7	—	1,850	.05	.41	2.3	—
200	Brown and serve (10-11 per 8-oz pkg.), browned	1 link	17	40	70	3	6	2.3	2.8	.7	Trace										—
201	Deviled ham, canned	1 tbsp	13	51	45	2	4	1.5	1.8	.4	0	1	12	.3	—	0	.02	.01	.2	—
202	Frankfurter (8 per 1-lb pkg.), cooked (reheated)	1 frankfurter	56	57	170	7	15	5.6	6.5	1.2	1	3	57	.8	—	0	.08	.11	1.4	—
203	Meat, potted (beef, chicken, turkey), canned	1 tbsp	13	61	30	2	2	—	—	—	0				35	—	Trace	.03	.2	—
204	Pork link (16 per 1-lb pkg.), cooked	1 link	13	35	60	2	6	2.1	2.4	.5	Trace	1	21	.3	35	0	.10	.04	.5	—
	Salami:																			
205	Dry type, slice (12 per 4-oz pkg.)	1 slice	10	30	45	2	4	1.6	1.6	.1	Trace	1	28	.4	—	—	.04	.03	.5	—
206	Cooked type, slice (8 per 8-oz pkg.)	1 slice	28	51	90	5	7	3.1	3.0	.2	Trace	3	57	.7	—	—	.07	.07	1.2	—
207	Vienna sausage (7 per 4-oz can)	1 sausage	16	63	40	2	3	1.2	1.4	.2	Trace	1	24	.3	—	—	.01	.02	.4	—
	Veal, medium fat, cooked, bone removed:																			
208	Cutlet (4 1/8 by 2 1/4 by 1/2 in), braised or broiled	3 oz	85	60	185	23	9	4.0	3.4	.4	0	9	196	2.7	258	—	.06	.21	4.6	—
209	Rib (2 pieces, 4 1/8 by 2 1/4 by 1/4 in), roasted	3 oz	85	55	230	23	14	6.1	5.1	.6	0	10	211	2.9	259	—	.11	.26	6.6	—
	Poultry and poultry products: Chicken, cooked:																			
210	Breast, fried,[23] bones removed, 1/2 breast (3.3 oz with bones)	2.8 oz	79	58	160	26	5	1.4	1.8	1.1	1	9	218	1.3	—	70	.04	.17	11.6	—
211	Drumstick, fried,[23] bones removed (2 oz with bones)	1.3 oz	38	55	90	12	4	1.1	1.3	.9	Trace	6	89	.9	—	50	.03	.15	2.7	—
212	Half broiler, broiled, bones removed (10.4 oz with bones)	6.2 oz	176	71	240	42	7	2.2	2.5	1.3	0	16	355	3.0	483	160	.09	.34	15.5	—
213	Chicken, canned, boneless	3 oz	85	65	170	18	10	3.2	3.8	2.0	0	18	210	1.3	117	200	.03	.11	3.7	3
214	Chicken a la king, cooked (home recipe)	1 cup	245	68	470	27	34	12.7	14.3	3.3	12	127	358	2.5	404	1,130	.10	.42	5.4	12
215	Chicken and noodles, cooked (home recipe)	1 cup	240	71	365	22	18	5.9	7.1	3.5	26	26	247	2.2	149	430	.05	.17	4.3	Trace

[18] Outer layer of fat on the cut was removed to within approximately 1/2 in of the lean. Deposits of fat within the cut were not removed.
[19] Crust made with vegetable shortening and enriched flour.
[20] Regular-type margarine used.
[21] Value varies widely.
[22] Outer layer of fat on the cut was removed. Deposits of fat within the cut were not removed.
[23] About one-fourth of the outer layer of fat on the cut was removed. Deposits of fat within the cut were not removed.
[25] Vegetable shortening used.

11

TABLE 2.—NUTRITIVE VALUES OF THE EDIBLE PART OF FOODS - Continued

(Dashes (—) denote lack of reliable data for a constituent believed to be present in measurable amount)

Item No. (A)	Foods, approximate measures, units, and weight (edible part unless footnotes indicate otherwise) (B)	Water (C) Per cent	Food energy (D) Calories	Protein (E) Grams	Fat (F) Grams	Saturated (total) (G) Grams	Unsaturated Oleic (H) Grams	Linoleic (I) Grams	Carbohydrate (J) Grams	Calcium (K) Milligrams	Phosphorus (L) Milligrams	Iron (M) Milligrams	Potassium (N) Milligrams	Vitamin A value (O) International units	Thiamin (P) Milligrams	Riboflavin (Q) Milligrams	Niacin (R) Milligrams	Ascorbic acid (S) Milligrams
	FISH, SHELLFISH, MEAT, POULTRY, RELATED PRODUCTS—Con.																	
	Poultry and poultry products—Continued																	
	Chicken chow mein:																	
216	Canned -- 1 cup	89	95	7	Trace	—	—	—	18	45	85	1.3	418	150	0.05	0.10	1.0	13
217	From home recipe -- 1 cup	78	255	31	10	2.4	3.4	3.1	10	58	293	2.5	473	280	.08	.23	4.3	10
218	Chicken potpie (home recipe), baked, 1/3 piece (1/3 of 9-in diam. pie). -- 1 piece	57	545	23	31	11.3	10.9	5.6	42	70	232	3.0	343	3,090	.34	.31	5.5	5
	Turkey, roasted, flesh without skin:																	
219	Dark meat, piece, 2 1/2 by 1 5/8 by 1/4 in. -- 4 pieces	61	175	26	7	2.1	1.5	1.5	0	—	—	2.0	338	—	.03	.20	3.6	—
220	Light meat, piece, 4 by 2 by 1/4 in. -- 2 pieces	62	150	28	3	.9	.6	.7	0	—	—	1.0	349	—	.04	.12	9.4	—
	Light and dark meat:																	
221	Chopped or diced -- 1 cup	61	265	44	9	2.5	1.7	1.8	0	11	351	2.5	514	—	.07	.25	10.8	—
222	Pieces (1 slice white meat, 4 by 2 by 1/4 in with 2 slices dark meat, 2 1/2 by 1 5/8 by 1/4 in). -- 3 pieces	61	160	27	5	1.5	1.0	1.1	0	7	213	1.5	312	—	.04	.15	6.5	—
	FRUITS AND FRUIT PRODUCTS																	
	Apples, raw, unpeeled, without cores:																	
223	2 3/4-in diam. (about 3 per lb with cores) -- 1 apple	84	80	Trace	1	—	—	—	20	10	14	.4	152	120	.04	.03	.1	6
224	3 1/4-in diam. (about 2 per lb with cores). -- 1 apple	84	125	Trace	1	—	—	—	31	15	21	.6	233	190	.06	.04	.2	8
225	Applejuice, bottled or canned[24] -- 1 cup	88	120	Trace	Trace	—	—	—	30	15	22	1.5	250	—	.02	.05	.2	2[52]
	Applesauce, canned:																	
226	Sweetened -- 1 cup	76	230	1	Trace	—	—	—	61	10	13	1.3	166	100	.05	.03	.1	3[53]
227	Unsweetened -- 1 cup	89	100	Trace	Trace	—	—	—	26	10	12	1.2	190	100	.05	.02	.1	2[53]
	Apricots:																	
228	Raw, without pits (about 12 per lb with pits). -- 3 apricots	85	55	1	Trace	—	—	—	14	18	25	.5	301	2,890	.03	.04	.6	11
229	Canned in heavy sirup (halves and sirup). -- 1 cup	77	220	2	Trace	—	—	—	57	28	39	.8	604	4,490	.05	.05	1.0	10
	Dried:																	
230	Uncooked (28 large or 37 medium halves per cup). -- 1 cup	25	340	7	1	—	—	—	86	87	140	7.2	1,273	14,170	.01	.21	4.3	16
231	Cooked, unsweetened, fruit and liquid. -- 1 cup	76	215	4	1	—	—	—	54	55	88	4.5	795	7,500	.01	.13	2.5	8
232	Apricot nectar, canned -- 1 cup	85	145	1	Trace	—	—	—	37	23	30	.5	379	2,380	.03	.03	.5	2[36]
	Avocados, raw, whole, without skins and seeds:																	
233	California, mid- and late-winter (with skin and seed, 3 1/8-in diam.; wt., 10 oz). -- 1 avocado	74	370	5	37	5.5	22.0	3.7	13	22	91	1.3	1,303	630	.24	.43	3.5	30
234	Florida, late summer and fall (with skin and seed, 3 5/8-in diam.; wt., 1 lb). -- 1 avocado	78	390	4	33	6.7	15.7	5.3	27	30	128	1.8	1,836	880	.33	.61	4.9	43
235	Banana without peel (about 2.6 per lb with peel). -- 1 banana	76	100	1	Trace	—	—	—	26	10	31	.8	440	230	.06	.07	.8	12
236	Banana flakes -- 1 tbsp	3	20	Trace	Trace	—	—	—	5	2	6	.2	92	50	.01	.01	.2	Trace

(A)	(B)	(C)	(D)	(E)	(F)	(G)	(H)	(I)	(J)	(K)	(L)	(M)	(N)	(O)	(P)	(Q)	(R)	(S)
237	Blackberries, raw------------- 1 cup	85	85	2	1	—	—	—	19	46	27	1.3	245	290	0.04	0.06	0.6	30
238	Blueberries, raw------------- 1 cup	83	90	1	1	—	—	—	22	22	19	1.5	117	150	.04	.09	.7	20
	Cantaloup. See Muskmelons (item 271)																	
	Cherries:																	
239	Sour (tart), red, pitted, canned, water pack. 1 cup	88	105	2	Trace	—	—	—	26	37	32	.7	317	1,660	.07	.05	.5	12
240	Sweet, raw, without pits and stems. 10 cherries	80	45	1	Trace	—	—	—	12	15	13	.3	129	70	.03	.04	.3	7
241	Cranberry juice cocktail, bottled, sweetened. 1 cup	83	165	Trace	Trace	—	—	—	42	13	8	.8	25	Trace	.03	.03	.1	[28]81
242	Cranberry sauce, sweetened, canned, strained. 1 cup	62	405	Trace	1	—	—	—	104	17	11	.6	83	60	.03	.03	.1	6
	Dates:																	
243	Whole, without pits------------- 10 dates	23	220	2	Trace	—	—	—	58	47	50	2.4	518	40	.07	.08	1.8	0
244	Chopped------------- 1 cup	23	490	4	1	—	—	—	130	105	112	5.3	1,153	90	.16	.18	3.9	0
245	Fruit cocktail, canned, in heavy sirup. 1 cup	80	195	1	Trace	—	—	—	50	23	31	1.0	411	360	.05	.03	1.0	5
	Grapefruit:																	
	Raw, medium, 3 3/4-in diam. (about 1 lb 1 oz):																	
246	Pink or red------ 1/2 grapefruit with peel[28]	89	50	1	Trace	—	—	—	13	20	20	.5	166	540	.05	.02	.2	44
247	White------ 1/2 grapefruit with peel[28]	89	45	1	Trace	—	—	—	12	19	19	.5	159	10	.05	.02	.2	44
248	Canned, sections with sirup------ 1 cup	81	180	2	Trace	—	—	—	45	33	36	.8	343	30	.08	.05	.5	76
	Grapefruit juice:																	
249	Raw, pink, red, or white------ 1 cup	90	95	1	Trace	—	—	—	23	22	37	.5	399	([29])	.10	.05	.5	93
	Canned, white:																	
250	Unsweetened------ 1 cup	89	100	1	Trace	—	—	—	24	20	35	1.0	400	20	.07	.05	.5	84
251	Sweetened------ 1 cup	86	135	1	Trace	—	—	—	32	20	35	1.0	405	30	.08	.05	.5	78
	Frozen, concentrate, unsweetened:																	
252	Undiluted, 6-fl oz can------ 1 can	62	300	4	1	—	—	—	72	70	124	.8	1,250	60	.29	.12	1.4	286
253	Diluted with 3 parts water by volume. 1 cup	89	100	1	Trace	—	—	—	24	25	42	.2	420	20	.10	.04	.5	96
254	Dehydrated crystals, prepared with water (1 lb yields about 1 gal). 1 cup	90	100	1	Trace	—	—	—	24	22	40	.2	412	20	.10	.05	.5	91
	Grapes, European type (adherent skin), raw:																	
255	Thompson Seedless------------- 10 grapes	81	35	Trace	Trace	—	—	—	9	6	10	.2	87	50	.03	.02	.2	2
256	Tokay and Emperor, seeded types------ 10 grapes[30]	81	40	Trace	Trace	—	—	—	10	7	11	.2	99	60	.03	.02	.2	2
	Grapejuice:																	
257	Canned or bottled------------- 1 cup	83	165	1	Trace	—	—	—	42	28	30	.8	293	—	.10	.05	.5	[25]Trace
	Frozen concentrate, sweetened:																	
258	Undiluted, 6-fl oz can------ 1 can	53	395	1	Trace	—	—	—	100	22	32	.9	255	40	.13	.22	1.5	[31]32
259	Diluted with 3 parts water by volume. 1 cup	86	135	1	Trace	—	—	—	33	8	10	.3	85	10	.05	.08	.5	[31]10
260	Grape drink, canned------ 1 cup	86	135	Trace	Trace	—	—	—	35	8	10	.3	88	[32] 10	.03	[32].03	.3	[32]
261	Lemon, raw, size 165, without peel and seeds (about 4 per lb with peels and seeds). 1 lemon	90	20	1	Trace	—	—	—	6	19	12	.4	102	10	.03	.01	.1	39
	Lemon juice:																	
262	Raw------------- 1 cup	91	60	1	Trace	—	—	—	20	17	24	.5	344	50	.07	.02	.2	112
263	Canned, or bottled, unsweetened------ 1 cup	92	55	1	Trace	—	—	—	19	17	24	.5	344	50	.07	.02	.2	102
264	Frozen, single strength, unsweetened, 6-fl oz can. 1 can	92	40	1	Trace	—	—	—	13	13	16	.5	258	40	.05	.02	.2	81
	Lemonade concentrate, frozen:																	
265	Undiluted, 6-fl oz can------ 1 can	49	425	Trace	Trace	—	—	—	112	9	13	.4	153	40	.05	.06	.7	66
266	Diluted with 4 1/3 parts water by volume. 1 cup	89	105	Trace	Trace	—	—	—	28	2	3	.1	40	10	.01	.02	.2	17

[19] Crust made with vegetable shortening and enriched flour.
[24] Also applies to pasteurized apple cider.
[25] Applies to product without added ascorbic acid. For value of product with added ascorbic acid, refer to label.
[26] Based on product without added ascorbic acid.
[28] Based on product with label claim of 45% of U.S. RDA in 6 fl oz.
[29] Based on product with label claim of 100% of U.S. RDA in 6 fl oz.
[28] Weight includes peel and membranes between sections. Without these parts, the weight of the edible portion is 123 g for item 246 and 118 g for item 247.
[29] For white-fleshed varieties, value is about 20 International Units (I.U.) per cup; for red-fleshed varieties, 1,080 I.U.
[30] Weight includes seeds. Without seeds, weight of the edible portion is 57 g.
[31] Applies to product with added ascorbic acid. Without added ascorbic acid, based on claim that 6 fl oz of reconstituted juice contain 45% or 50% of the U.S. RDA, value in milligrams is 108 or 120 for a whole carton (item 258), 36 or 40 for 1 cup of diluted juice (item 259).
[32] Applies to product with added ascorbic acid. Without added ascorbic acid, values in milligrams would be 0.60 for thiamin, 0.80 for riboflavin, and trace for ascorbic acid. For products with only ascorbic acid added, value varies with the brand. Consult the label.

13

TABLE 2.—NUTRITIVE VALUES OF THE EDIBLE PART OF FOODS - Continued

(Dashes (—) denote lack of reliable data for a constituent believed to be present in measurable amount)

Item No. (A)	Foods, approximate measures, units, and weight (edible part unless footnotes indicate otherwise) (B)	Grams	Water (C) Per cent	Food energy (D) Calories	Protein (E) Grams	Fat (F) Grams	Saturated (total) (G) Grams	Oleic (H) Grams	Linoleic (I) Grams	Carbohydrate (I) Grams	Calcium (K) Milligrams	Phosphorus (L) Milligrams	Iron (M) Milligrams	Potassium (N) Milligrams	Vitamin A value (O) International units	Thiamin (P) Milligrams	Riboflavin (Q) Milligrams	Niacin (R) Milligrams	Ascorbic acid (S) Milligrams
	FRUITS AND FRUIT PRODUCTS—Con.																		
	Limeade concentrate, frozen:																		
267	Undiluted, 6-fl oz can ----- 1 can	218	50	410	Trace	Trace	—	—	—	108	11	13	0.2	129	Trace	0.02	0.02	0.2	26
268	Diluted with 4 1/3 parts water by volume. ----- 1 cup	247	89	100	Trace	Trace	—	—	—	27	3	3	Trace	32	Trace	Trace	Trace	Trace	6
	Limejuice:																		
269	Canned, unsweetened ----- 1 cup	246	90	65	1	Trace	—	—	—	22	22	27	.5	256	20	.05	.02	.2	79
270	----- 1 cup	246	90	65	1	Trace	—	—	—	22	22	27	.5	256	20	.05	.02	.2	52
	Muskmelons, raw, with rind, without seed cavity:																		
271	Cantaloup, orange-fleshed (with rind and seed cavity, 5-in diam., 2 1/3 lb). ----- 1/2 melon with rind[33]	477	91	80	2	Trace	—	—	—	20	38	44	1.1	682	9,240	.11	.08	1.6	90
272	Honeydew (with rind and seed cavity, 6 1/2-in diam., 5 1/4 lb). ----- 1/10 melon with rind[33]	226	91	50	1	Trace	—	—	—	11	21	24	.6	374	60	.06	.04	.9	34
	Oranges, all commercial varieties, raw:																		
273	Whole, 2 5/8-in diam., without peel and seeds (about 2 1/2 per lb with peel and seeds). ----- 1 orange	131	86	65	1	Trace	—	—	—	16	54	26	.5	263	260	.13	.05	.5	66
274	Sections without membranes ----- 1 cup	180	86	90	2	Trace	—	—	—	22	74	36	.7	360	360	.18	.07	.7	90
	Orange juice:																		
275	Raw, all varieties ----- 1 cup	248	88	110	2	Trace	—	—	—	26	27	42	.5	496	500	.22	.07	1.0	124
276	Canned, unsweetened ----- 1 cup	249	87	120	2	Trace	—	—	—	28	25	45	1.0	496	500	.17	.05	.7	100
	Frozen concentrate:																		
277	Undiluted, 6-fl oz can ----- 1 can	213	55	360	5	Trace	—	—	—	87	75	126	.9	1,500	1,620	.68	.11	2.8	360
278	Diluted with 3 parts water by volume. ----- 1 cup	249	87	120	2	Trace	—	—	—	29	25	42	.2	503	540	.23	.03	.9	120
279	Dehydrated crystals, prepared with water (1 lb yields about 1 gal). ----- 1 cup	248	88	115	1	Trace	—	—	—	27	25	40	.5	518	500	.20	.07	1.0	109
	Orange and grapefruit juice: Frozen concentrate:																		
280	Undiluted, 6-fl oz can ----- 1 can	210	59	330	4	1	—	—	—	78	61	99	.8	1,308	800	.48	.06	2.3	302
281	Diluted with 3 parts water by volume. ----- 1 cup	248	88	110	1	Trace	—	—	—	26	20	32	.2	439	270	.15	.02	.7	102
282	Papayas, raw, 1/2-in cubes ----- 1 cup	140	89	55	1	Trace	—	—	—	14	28	22	.4	328	2,450	.06	.06	.4	78
	Peaches: Raw:																		
283	Whole, 2 1/2-in diam., peeled, pitted (about 4 per lb with peels and pits). ----- 1 peach	100	89	40	1	Trace	—	—	—	10	9	19	.5	202	[34]1,330	.02	.05	1.0	7
284	Sliced ----- 1 cup	170	89	65	1	Trace	—	—	—	16	15	32	.9	343	[34]2,260	.03	.09	1.7	12
	Canned, yellow-fleshed, solids and liquid (halves or slices):																		
285	Syrup pack ----- 1 cup	256	79	200	1	Trace	—	—	—	51	10	31	.8	333	1,100	.03	.05	1.5	8
286	Water pack ----- 1 cup	244	91	75	1	Trace	—	—	—	20	10	32	.7	334	1,100	.02	.07	1.5	7
	Dried:																		
287	Uncooked ----- 1 cup	160	25	420	5	1	—	—	—	109	77	187	9.6	1,520	6,240	.02	.30	8.5	29
288	Cooked, unsweetened, halves and juice. ----- 1 cup	250	77	205	3	1	—	—	—	54	38	93	4.8	743	3,050	.01	.15	3.8	5

(A)	(B)	(C)	(D)	(E)	(F)	(G)	(H)	(I)	(J)	(K)	(L)	(M)	(N)	(O)	(P)	(Q)	(R)	(S)
	Frozen, sliced, sweetened:																	
289	10-oz container -- 284	77	250	1	Trace	---	---	---	64	11	37	1.4	352	1,850	0.03	0.11	2.0	³³116
290	Cup -- 250	77	220	1	Trace	---	---	---	57	10	33	1.3	310	1,630	.03	.10	1.8	³³103
	Pears: Raw, with skin, cored:																	
291	Bartlett, 2 1/2-in diam. (about 2 1/2 per lb with cores and stems) -- 1 pear -- 164	83	100	1	1	---	---	---	25	13	18	.5	213	30	.03	.07	.2	7
292	Bosc, 2 1/2-in diam. (about 3 per lb with cores and stems) -- 1 pear -- 141	83	85	1	1	---	---	---	22	11	16	.4	83	30	.03	.06	.1	6
293	D'Anjou, 3-in diam. (about 2 per lb with cores and stems) -- 1 pear -- 200	83	120	1	1	---	---	---	31	16	22	.6	260	40	.04	.08	.2	8
294	Canned, solids and liquid, syrup pack, heavy (halves or slices) -- 1 cup -- 255	80	195	1	1	---	---	---	50	13	18	.5	214	10	.03	.05	.3	3
	Pineapple:																	
295	Raw, diced -- 1 cup -- 155	85	80	1	Trace	---	---	---	21	26	12	.8	226	110	.14	.05	.3	26
	Canned, heavy syrup pack, solids and liquid:																	
296	Crushed, chunks, tidbits -- 1 cup -- 255	80	190	1	Trace	---	---	---	49	28	13	.8	245	130	.20	.05	.5	18
297	Slices and liquid: Large -- 1 slice; 2 1/4 tbsp liquid. -- 105	80	80	Trace	Trace	---	---	---	20	12	5	.3	101	50	.08	.02	.2	7
298	Medium -- 1 slice; 1 1/4 tbsp liquid. -- 58	80	45	Trace	Trace	---	---	---	11	6	3	.2	56	30	.05	.01	.1	4
299	Pineapple juice, unsweetened, canned. -- 1 cup -- 250	86	140	1	Trace	---	---	---	34	38	23	.8	373	130	.13	.05	.5	²⁷80
	Plums: Raw, without pits:																	
300	Japanese and hybrid (2 1/8-in diam., about 6 1/2 per lb with pits) -- 1 plum -- 66	87	30	Trace	Trace	---	---	---	8	8	12	.3	112	160	.02	.02	.3	4
301	Prune-type (1 1/2-in diam., about 15 per lb with pits) -- 1 plum -- 28	79	20	Trace	Trace	---	---	---	6	3	5	.1	48	80	.01	.01	.1	1
	Canned, heavy syrup pack (Italian prunes) with pits and liquid:																	
302	Cup³⁶ -- 272	77	215	1	Trace	---	---	---	56	23	26	2.3	367	3,130	.05	.05	1.0	5
303	Portion³⁶ -- 3 plums; 2 3/4 tbsp liquid.³⁶ -- 140	77	110	1	Trace	---	---	---	29	12	13	1.2	189	1,610	.03	.03	.5	3
	Prunes, dried, "softenized," with pits:																	
304	Uncooked -- 4 extra large or 5 large prunes.³⁶ -- 49	28	110	1	Trace	---	---	---	29	22	34	1.7	298	590	.04	.07	.7	1
305	Cooked, unsweetened, all sizes, fruit and liquid. -- 1 cup³⁶ -- 250	66	255	2	1	---	---	---	67	51	79	3.8	695	1,590	.07	.15	1.5	2
306	Prune juice, canned or bottled -- 1 cup -- 256	80	195	1	Trace	---	---	---	49	36	51	1.8	602	—	.03	.03	1.0	5
	Raisins, seedless:																	
307	Cup, not pressed down -- 1 cup -- 145	18	420	4	Trace	---	---	---	112	90	146	5.1	1,106	30	.16	.12	.7	1
308	Packet, 1/2 oz (1 1/2 tbsp) -- 1 packet -- 14	18	40	Trace	Trace	---	---	---	11	9	14	.5	107	Trace	.02	.01	.1	Trace
	Raspberries, red:																	
309	Raw, capped, whole -- 1 cup -- 123	84	70	1	1	---	---	---	17	27	27	1.1	207	160	.04	.11	1.1	31
310	Frozen, sweetened, 10-oz container -- 1 container -- 284	74	280	2	1	---	---	---	70	37	48	1.7	284	200	.06	.17	1.7	60
	Rhubarb, cooked, added sugar:																	
311	From raw -- 1 cup -- 270	63	380	1	Trace	---	---	---	27	211	41	1.6	548	220	.05	.14	.8	16
312	From frozen, sweetened -- 1 cup -- 270	63	385	1	1	---	---	---	90	211	32	1.9	475	190	.05	.11	.5	16

²⁷Based on product with label claim of 100% of U.S. RDA in 6 fl oz.
³³Weight includes rind. Without rind, the weight of the edible portion is 272 g for item 271 and 149 g for item 272.
³⁴Represents yellow-fleshed varieties. For white-fleshed varieties, value is 50 International Units (I.U.) for 1 peach, 90 I.U. for 1 cup of slices.
³⁵Value represents products without added ascorbic acid. For products with added ascorbic acid, value in milligrams is 116 for a 10-oz container, 103 for 1 cup.
³⁶Weight includes pits. After removal of the pits, the weight of the edible portion is 258 g for item 302, 133 g for item 303, 43 g for item 304, and 213 g for item 305.

15

TABLE 2.— NUTRITIVE VALUES OF THE EDIBLE PART OF FOODS—Continued

(Dashes (—) denote lack of reliable data for a constituent believed to be present in measurable amount)

Item No.	Foods, approximate measure, units, and weight (edible part unless footnotes indicate otherwise)		Water	Food energy	Protein	Fat	Fatty Acids Saturated (total)	Unsaturated Oleic	Linoleic	Carbohydrate	Calcium	Phosphorus	Iron	Potassium	Vitamin A value	Thiamin	Riboflavin	Niacin	Ascorbic acid
(A)	(B)	Grams	(C) Percent	(D) Calories	(E) Grams	(F) Grams	(G) Grams	(H) Grams	(I) Grams	(J) Grams	(K) Milligrams	(L) Milligrams	(M) Milligrams	(N) Milligrams	(O) International units	(P) Milligrams	(Q) Milligrams	(R) Milligrams	(S) Milligrams
	FRUITS AND FRUIT PRODUCTS—Con.																		
	Strawberries:																		
313	Raw, whole berries, capped — 1 cup	149	90	55	1	1	—	—	—	13	31	31	1.5	244	90	0.04	0.10	0.9	88
	Frozen, sweetened:																		
314	Sliced, 10-oz container — 1 container	284	71	310	1	1	—	—	—	79	40	48	2.0	318	90	.06	.17	1.4	151
315	Whole, 1-lb container (about 1 3/4 cups) — 1 container	454	76	415	2	1	—	—	—	107	59	73	2.7	472	140	.09	.27	2.3	249
316	Tangerine, raw, 2 3/8-in diam., size 176, without peel (about 4 per lb with peels and seeds). — 1 tangerine	86	87	40	1	Trace	—	—	—	10	34	15	.3	108	360	.05	.02	.1	27
317	Tangerine juice, canned, sweetened. — 1 cup	249	87	125	1	Trace	—	—	—	30	44	35	.5	440	1,040	.15	.05	.2	54
318	Watermelon, raw, 4 by 8 in wedge with rind and seeds (1/16 of 32 2/3-lb melon, 10 by 16 in). — 1 wedge with rind and seeds[17]	926	93	110	2	1	—	—	—	27	30	43	2.1	426	2,510	.13	.13	.9	30
	GRAIN PRODUCTS																		
	Bagel, 3-in diam.:																		
319	Egg — 1 bagel	55	32	165	6	2	0.5	0.9	0.8	28	9	43	1.2	41	30	.14	.10	1.2	0
320	Water — 1 bagel	55	29	165	6	2	.2	.4	.6	30	8	41	1.2	42	0	.15	.11	1.4	0
321	Barley, pearled, light, uncooked — 1 cup	200	11	700	16	2	.3	.2	.8	158	32	378	4.0	320	0	.24	.10	6.2	0
	Biscuits, baking powder, 2-in diam. (enriched flour, vegetable shortening):																		
322	From home recipe — 1 biscuit	28	27	105	2	5	1.2	2.0	1.2	13	34	49	.4	33	Trace	.08	.08	.7	Trace
323	From mix[38] — 1 biscuit	28	29	90	2	3	.6	1.1	.7	15	19	65	.6	32	Trace	.09	.08	.8	Trace
324	Breadcrumbs (enriched):[38] Dry, grated — 1 cup	100	7	390	13	5	1.0	1.6	1.4	73	122	141	3.6	152	Trace	.35	.35	4.8	Trace
	Breads:																		
325	Boston brown bread, canned, slice 3 1/4 by 1/2 in.[38] Soft. See White bread (items 349-350). — 1 slice	45	45	95	2	1	.1	.2	.2	21	41	72	.9	131	[39]0	.06	.04	.7	0
	Cracked-wheat bread (3/4 enriched wheat flour, 1/4 cracked wheat):[38]																		
326	Loaf, 1 lb — 1 loaf	454	35	1,195	39	10	2.2	3.0	3.9	236	399	581	9.5	608	Trace	1.52	1.13	14.4	Trace
327	Slice (18 per loaf) — 1 slice	25	35	65	2	1	.1	.2	.2	13	22	32	.5	34	Trace	.08	.06	.8	Trace
	French or Vienna bread, enriched:[38]																		
328	Loaf, 1 lb — 1 loaf	454	31	1,315	41	14	3.2	4.7	4.6	251	195	386	10.0	408	Trace	1.80	1.10	15.0	Trace
	Slice:																		
329	French (5 by 2 1/2 by 1 in) — 1 slice	35	31	100	3	1	.2	.4	.4	19	15	30	.8	32	Trace	.14	.08	1.2	Trace
330	Vienna (4 3/4 by 4 by 1/2 in). — 1 slice	25	31	75	2	1	.2	.3	.3	14	11	21	.6	23	Trace	.10	.06	.8	Trace
	Italian bread, enriched:																		
331	Loaf, 1 lb — 1 loaf	454	32	1,250	41	4	.6	.3	1.5	256	77	349	10.0	336	0	1.80	1.10	15.0	0
332	Slice, 4 1/2 by 3 1/4 by 3/4 in. — 1 slice	30	32	85	3	Trace	Trace	Trace	.1	17	5	23	.7	22	0	.12	.07	1.0	0
	Raisin bread, enriched:[38]																		
333	Loaf, 1 lb — 1 loaf	454	35	1,190	30	13	3.0	4.7	3.9	243	322	395	10.0	1,057	Trace	1.70	1.07	10.7	Trace
334	Slice (18 per loaf) — 1 slice	25	35	65	2	1	.2	.3	.2	13	18	22	.6	58	Trace	.09	.06	.6	Trace

(A)	(B)	(C)	(D)	(E)	(F)	(G)	(H)	(I)	(J)	(K)	(L)	(M)	(N)	(O)	(P)	(Q)	(R)	(S)
	Rye Bread:																	
	American, light (2/3 enriched wheat flour, 1/3 rye flour):																	
335	Loaf, 1 lb---- 1 loaf (454)	36	1,100	41	5	0.7	0.5	2.2	236	340	667	9.1	658	0	1.35	0.98	12.9	0
336	Slice (4 3/4 by 3 3/4 by 7/16 in)---- 1 slice (25)	36	60	2	Trace	Trace	Trace	.1	13	19	37	.5	36	0	.07	.05	.7	0
	Pumpernickel (2/3 rye flour, 1/3 enriched wheat flour):																	
337	Loaf, 1 lb---- 1 loaf (454)	34	1,115	41	5	.7	.5	2.4	241	381	1,039	11.8	2,059	0	1.30	.93	8.5	0
338	Slice (5 by 4 by 3/8 in)³⁸---- 1 slice (32)	34	80	3	Trace	Trace	Trace	.2	13	27	73	.8	145	0	.09	.07	.6	0
	White bread, enriched:³⁸																	
	Soft-crumb type:³⁸																	
339	Loaf, 1 lb---- 1 loaf (454)	36	1,225	39	15	3.4	5.3	4.6	229	381	440	11.3	476	Trace	1.80	1.10	15.0	Trace
340	Slice (18 per loaf)---- 1 slice (25)	36	70	2	1	.2	.3	.3	13	21	24	.6	26	Trace	.10	.06	.8	Trace
341	Slice, toasted---- 1 slice (22)	25	70	2	1	.2	.3	.3	13	21	24	.6	26	Trace	.08	.05	.8	Trace
342	Slice (22 per loaf)---- 1 slice (20)	36	55	2	1	.2	.2	.2	10	17	19	.5	21	Trace	.08	.05	.7	Trace
343	Slice, toasted---- 1 slice (17)	25	55	2	1	.2	.2	.2	10	17	19	.5	21	Trace	.06	.05	.7	Trace
344	Loaf, 1 1/2 lb---- 1 loaf (680)	36	1,835	59	22	5.2	7.9	6.9	343	571	660	17.0	714	Trace	2.70	1.65	22.5	Trace
345	Slice (24 per loaf)---- 1 slice (28)	36	75	2	1	.2	.3	.3	14	24	27	.7	29	Trace	.11	.07	.9	Trace
346	Slice, toasted---- 1 slice (24)	25	75	2	1	.2	.3	.2	14	24	27	.7	29	Trace	.09	.07	.9	Trace
347	Slice (28 per loaf)---- 1 slice (24)	36	65	2	1	.2	.3	.2	12	20	23	.6	25	Trace	.10	.06	.8	Trace
348	Slice, toasted---- 1 slice (21)	25	65	2	1	.2	.2	.2	12	20	23	.6	25	Trace	.08	.06	.8	Trace
349	Cubes---- 1 cup (30)	36	80	3	1	.2	.4	.3	15	25	29	.8	32	Trace	.12	.07	1.0	Trace
350	Crumbs---- 1 cup (45)	36	120	4	1	.3	.5	.5	23	38	44	1.1	47	Trace	.18	.11	1.5	Trace
	Firm-crumb type:³⁸																	
351	Loaf, 1 lb---- 1 loaf (454)	35	1,245	41	17	3.9	5.9	5.2	228	435	463	11.3	549	Trace	1.80	1.10	15.0	Trace
352	Slice (20 per loaf)---- 1 slice (23)	35	65	2	1	.2	.3	.3	12	22	23	.6	28	Trace	.09	.06	.8	Trace
353	Slice, toasted---- 1 slice (20)	24	65	2	1	.2	.3	.3	12	22	23	.6	28	Trace	.07	.06	.8	Trace
354	Loaf, 2 lb---- 1 loaf (907)	35	2,495	82	34	7.7	11.8	10.4	455	871	925	22.7	1,097	Trace	3.60	2.20	30.9	Trace
355	Slice (34 per loaf)---- 1 slice (27)	35	75	2	1	.2	.3	.3	14	26	28	.7	33	Trace	.11	.06	.9	Trace
356	Slice, toasted---- 1 slice (23)	24	75	2	1	.2	.3	.3	14	26	28	.7	33	Trace	.09	.06	.9	Trace
	Whole-wheat bread:																	
	Soft-crumb type:³⁸																	
357	Loaf, 1 lb---- 1 loaf (454)	36	1,095	41	12	2.2	2.9	4.2	224	381	1,152	13.6	1,161	Trace	1.37	.45	12.7	Trace
358	Slice (16 per loaf)---- 1 slice (28)	36	65	3	1	.1	.2	.3	14	24	71	.8	72	Trace	.09	.03	.8	Trace
359	Slice, toasted---- 1 slice (24)	24	65	3	1	.1	.2	.2	14	24	71	.8	72	Trace	.07	.03	.8	Trace
	Firm-crumb type:³⁸																	
360	Loaf, 1 lb---- 1 loaf (454)	36	1,100	48	14	2.5	3.3	4.9	216	449	1,034	13.6	1,238	Trace	1.17	.54	12.7	Trace
361	Slice (18 per loaf)---- 1 slice (25)	36	60	3	1	.1	.2	.3	12	25	57	.8	68	Trace	.06	.03	.7	Trace
362	Slice, toasted---- 1 slice (21)	24	60	3	1	.1	.2	.2	12	25	57	.8	68	Trace	.05	.03	.7	Trace
	Breakfast cereals:																	
	Hot type, cooked:																	
	Corn (hominy) grits, degermed:																	
363	Enriched---- 1 cup (245)	87	125	3	Trace	Trace	Trace	Trace	27	2	25	.7	27	⁴⁰Trace	.10	.07	1.0	0
364	Unenriched---- 1 cup (245)	87	125	3	Trace	Trace	Trace	Trace	27	2	25	.2	27	⁴⁰Trace	.05	.05	.5	0
365	Farina, quick-cooking, enriched---- 1 cup (245)	89	105	3	Trace	Trace	Trace	Trace	22	⁴⁷147	⁴¹113	(⁴⁷)	25	0	.12	.07	1.0	0
366	Oatmeal or rolled oats---- 1 cup (240)	87	130	5	2	.4	.8	.9	23	22	137	1.4	146	0	.19	.05	.2	0
367	Wheat, rolled---- 1 cup (240)	80	180	5	1	—	—	—	41	19	182	1.7	202	0	.17	.07	2.2	0
368	Wheat, whole-meal---- 1 cup (245)	88	110	4	1	—	—	—	23	17	127	1.2	118	0	.15	.05	1.5	0
	Ready-to-eat:																	
369	Bran flakes (40% bran), added sugar, salt, iron, vitamins---- 1 cup (35)	3	105	4	1				28	19	125	12.4	137	1,650	.41	.49	4.1	12
370	Bran flakes with raisins, added sugar, salt, iron, vitamins---- 1 cup (50)	7	145	4	1				40	28	146	17.7	154	2,350	.58	.71	5.8	18

³⁷Weight includes rind and seeds. Without rind and seeds, weight of the edible portion is 426 g.

³⁸Made with vegetable shortening.

³⁹Applies to product made with white cornmeal. With yellow cornmeal, value is 30 International units (I.U.).

⁴⁰Applies to white varieties. For yellow varieties, value is 150 International units (I.U.).

⁴¹Applies to products that do not contain di-sodium phosphate. If di-sodium phosphate is an ingredient, value is 162 mg.

⁴⁵Value may range from less than 1 mg to about 8 mg depending on the brand. Consult the label.

TABLE 2.– NUTRITIVE VALUES OF THE EDIBLE PART OF FOODS - Continued

(Dashes (—) denote lack of reliable data for a constituent believed to be present in measurable amount)

Item No. (A)	Foods, approximate measure, units, and weight (edible part unless footnotes indicate otherwise) (B)		Water (C) Per cent	Food energy (D) Calories	Protein (E) Grams	Fat (F) Grams	Fatty Acids			Carbo-hydrate (J) Grams	Calcium (K) Milligrams	Phos-phorus (L) Milligrams	Iron (M) Milligrams	Potas-sium (N) Milligrams	Vitamin A value (O) International units	Thiamin (P) Milligrams	Ribo-flavin (Q) Milligrams	Niacin (R) Milligrams	Ascorbic acid (S) Milligrams
		Grams					Satu-rated (total) (G) Grams	Unsaturated Oleic (H) Grams	Lino-leic (I) Grams										
	GRAIN PRODUCTS—Con.																		
	Breakfast cereals—Continued																		
	Ready-to-eat—Continued																		
	Corn flakes:																		
371	Plain, added sugar, salt, iron, vitamins. 1 cup-----	25	4	95	2	Trace	—	—	—	21	(*3)	9	0.6	30	1,180	0.29	0.35	2.9	9
372	Sugar-coated, added salt, vitamins. 1 cup-----	40	2	155	2	Trace	—	—	—	37	1	10	1.0	27	1,880	.46	.56	4.6	14
373	Corn, puffed, plain, added sugar, salt, iron, vita-mins. 1 cup-----	20	4	80	2	1	—	—	—	16	4	18	2.3	—	940	.23	.28	2.3	7
374	Corn, shredded, added sugar, salt, iron, thiamin, niacin. 1 cup-----	25	3	95	2	Trace	—	—	—	22	1	10	.6	—	0	.11	.05	.5	0
375	Oats, puffed, added sugar, salt, minerals, vitamins. 1 cup-----	25	3	100	3	1	—	—	—	19	44	102	2.9	—	1,180	.29	.35	2.9	9
	Rice, puffed:																		
376	Plain, added iron, thiamin, niacin. 1 cup-----	15	4	60	1	Trace	—	—	—	13	3	14	.3	15	0	.07	.01	.7	0
377	Presweetened, added salt, iron, vitamins. 1 cup-----	28	3	115	1	0	—	—	—	26	3	14	*1.1	43	1,250	.38	.43	5.0	*515
378	Wheat flakes, added sugar, salt, iron, vitamins. 1 cup-----	30	4	105	3	Trace	—	—	—	24	12	83	(*3)	81	1,410	.35	.42	3.5	11
	Wheat, puffed:																		
379	Plain, added iron, thiamin, niacin. 1 cup-----	15	3	55	2	Trace	—	—	—	12	4	48	.6	51	0	.08	.03	1.2	0
380	Presweetened, added salt, iron, vitamins. 1 cup-----	38	3	140	3	Trace	—	—	—	33	7	52	*1.6	63	1,680	.50	.57	6.7	*520
381	Wheat, shredded, plain------ 1 oblong biscuit or 1/2 cup spoon-size biscuits.	25	7	90	2	1	—	—	—	20	11	97	.9	87	0	.06	.03	1.1	0
382	Wheat germ, without salt and sugar, toasted. 1 tbsp-----	6	4	25	2	1	—	—	—	3	3	70	.5	57	10	.11	.05	.3	1
383	Buckwheat flour, light, sifted 1 cup-----	98	12	340	6	1	—	—	—	78	11	86	1.0	314	0	.08	.04	.4	0
384	Bulgur, canned, seasoned----- 1 cup-----	135	56	245	8	4	0.2	0.4	0.4	44	27	263	1.9	151	0	.08	.05	4.1	0
	Cake icings. See Sugars and Sweets (items 532-536).																		
	Cakes made from cake mixes with enriched flour:[6]																		
	Angelfood:																		
385	Whole cake (9 3/4-in diam. tube cake). 1 cake-----	635	34	1,645	36	1	—	—	—	377	603	756	2.5	381	0	.37	.95	3.6	0
386	Piece, 1/12 of cake------- 1 piece-----	53	34	135	3	Trace	—	—	—	32	50	63	.2	32	0	.03	.08	.3	0
	Coffeecake:																		
387	Whole cake (7 3/4 by 5 5/8 by 1 1/4 in). 1 cake-----	430	30	1,385	27	41	11.7	16.3	8.8	225	262	748	6.9	469	690	.82	.91	7.7	1
388	Piece, 1/6 of cake------- 1 piece-----	72	30	230	5	7	2.0	2.7	1.5	38	44	125	1.2	78	120	.14	.15	1.3	Trace
	Cupcakes, made with egg, milk, 2 1/2-in diam.:																		
389	Without icing-------- 1 cupcake-----	25	26	90	1	3	.8	1.2	.7	14	40	59	.3	21	40	.05	.05	.4	Trace
390	With chocolate icing----- 1 cupcake-----	36	22	130	2	5	2.0	1.6	.6	21	47	71	.4	42	60	.05	.06	.4	Trace
	Devil's food with chocolate icing:																		
391	Whole, 2 layer cake (8- or 9-in diam.). 1 cake-----	1,107	24	3,755	49	136	50.0	44.9	17.0	645	653	1,162	16.6	1,439	1,660	1.06	1.65	10.1	1
392	Piece, 1/16 of cake------- 1 piece-----	69	24	235	3	8	3.1	2.8	1.1	40	41	72	1.0	90	100	.07	.10	.6	Trace
393	Cupcake, 2 1/2-in diam----- 1 cupcake-----	35	24	120	2	4	1.6	1.4	.5	20	21	37	.5	46	50	.03	.05	.3	Trace

(A)	(B)	(grams)	(C)	(D)	(E)	(F)	(G)	(H)	(I)	(J)	(K)	(L)	(M)	(N)	(O)	(P)	(Q)	(R)	(S)
	Gingerbread:																		
394	Whole cake (8-in square)------ 1 cake	570	37	1,575	18	39	9.7	16.6	10.0	291	513	570	8.6	1,562	Trace	0.84	1.00	7.4	Trace
395	Piece, 1/9 of cake------ 1 piece	63	37	175	2	4	1.1	1.8	1.1	32	57	63	.9	173	Trace	.09	.11	.8	Trace
	White, 2 layer with chocolate icing:																		
396	Whole cake (8- or 9-in diam.)-- 1 cake	1,140	21	4,000	44	122	48.2	46.4	20.0	716	1,129	2,041	11.4	1,322	680	1.50	1.77	12.5	.8
397	Piece, 1/16 of cake------ 1 piece	71	21	250	3	8	3.0	2.9	1.2	45	70	127	.7	82	40	.09	.11	.8	Trace
	Yellow, 2 layer with chocolate icing:																		
398	Whole cake (8- or 9-in diam.)-- 1 cake	1,108	26	3,735	45	125	47.8	47.8	20.3	638	1,008	2,017	12.2	1,208	1,550	1.24	1.67	10.6	Trace
399	Piece, 1/16 of cake------ 1 piece	69	26	235	3	8	3.0	3.0	1.3	40	63	126	.8	75	100	.08	.10	.7	Trace
	Cakes made from home recipes using enriched flour:[47]																		
	Boston cream pie with custard filling:																		
400	Whole cake (8-in diam.)------ 1 cake	825	35	2,490	41	78	23.0	30.1	15.2	412	553	833	8.2	[49]734	1,730	1.04	1.27	9.6	2
401	Piece, 1/12 of cake------ 1 piece	69	35	210	3	6	1.9	2.5	1.3	34	46	70	.7	[49]61	140	.09	.11	.8	Trace
	Fruitcake, dark:																		
402	Loaf, 1-lb (7 1/2 by 2 by 1 1/2 in)------ 1 loaf	454	18	1,720	22	69	14.4	33.5	14.8	271	327	513	11.8	2,250	540	.72	.73	4.9	2
403	Slice, 1/30 of loaf------ 1 slice	15	18	55	1	2	.5	1.1	.5	9	11	17	.4	74	20	.02	.02	.2	Trace
	Plain, sheet cake:																		
	Without icing:																		
404	Whole cake (9-in square)------ 1 cake	777	25	2,830	35	108	29.5	44.4	23.9	434	497	793	8.5	[49]614	1,320	1.21	1.40	10.2	2
405	Piece, 1/9 of cake------ 1 piece	86	25	315	4	12	3.3	4.9	2.6	48	55	88	.9	[49]68	150	.13	.15	1.1	Trace
	With uncooked white icing:																		
406	Whole cake (9-in square)------ 1 cake	1,096	21	4,020	37	129	42.2	49.5	24.4	694	548	822	8.2	[49]669	2,190	1.22	1.47	10.2	2
407	Piece, 1/9 of cake------ 1 piece	121	21	445	4	14	4.7	5.5	2.7	77	61	91	.8	[49]74	240	.14	.16	1.1	Trace
	Pound:[50]																		
408	Loaf, 8 1/2 by 3 1/2 by 3 1/4 in. 1 loaf	565	16	2,725	31	170	42.9	73.1	39.6	273	107	418	7.9	345	1,410	.90	.99	7.3	0
409	Slice, 1/17 of loaf------ 1 slice	33	16	160	2	10	2.5	4.3	2.3	16	6	24	.5	20	80	.05	.06	.4	0
	Spongecake:																		
410	Whole cake (9 3/4-in diam. tube cake)------ 1 cake	790	32	2,345	60	45	13.1	15.8	5.7	427	237	885	13.4	687	3,560	1.10	1.64	7.4	Trace
411	Piece, 1/12 of cake------ 1 piece	66	32	195	5	4	1.1	1.3	.5	36	20	74	1.1	57	300	.09	.14	.6	Trace
	Cookies made with enriched flour:[50][51]																		
	Brownies with nuts:																		
	Home-prepared, 1 3/4 by 1 3/4 by 7/8 in.:																		
412	From home recipe------ 1 brownie	20	10	95	1	6	1.5	3.0	1.2	10	8	30	.4	38	40	.04	.03	.2	Trace
413	From commercial recipe------ 1 brownie	20	11	85	1	4	.9	1.4	1.3	13	9	27	.4	34	20	.03	.02	.2	Trace
414	Frozen, with chocolate icing,[52] 1 1/2 by 1 3/4 by 7/8 in.-- 1 brownie	25	13	105	1	5	2.0	2.2	.7	15	10	31	.4	44	50	.03	.03	.2	Trace
	Chocolate chip:																		
415	Commercial, 2 1/4-in diam., 3/8 in thick. 4 cookies	42	3	200	2	9	2.8	2.9	2.2	29	16	48	1.0	56	50	.10	.17	.9	Trace
416	From home recipe, 2 1/3-in diam. 4 cookies	40	3	205	2	12	3.5	4.5	2.9	24	14	40	.8	47	40	.06	.06	.5	Trace
417	Fig bars, square (1 5/8 by 1 5/8 by 3/8 in) or rectangular (1 1/2 by 1 3/4 by 1/2 in). 4 cookies	56	14	200	2	3	.8	1.2	.7	42	44	34	1.0	111	60	.04	.14	.9	Trace
418	Gingersnaps, 2-in diam., 1/4 in thick. 4 cookies	28	3	90	2	2	.7	1.0	.6	22	20	13	.7	129	20	.08	.06	.7	0
419	Macaroons, 2 3/4-in diam., 1/4 in thick. 2 cookies	38	4	180	2	9	—	—	—	25	10	32	.3	176	0	.02	.06	.2	0
420	Oatmeal with raisins, 2 5/8-in diam., 1/4 in thick. 4 cookies	52	3	235	3	8	2.0	3.3	2.0	38	11	53	1.4	192	30	.15	.10	1.0	Trace

[44] Value varies with the brand. Consult the label.
[45] Value varies with the brand. Consult the label.
[46] Applies to product with added ascorbic acid. Without added ascorbic acid, value is trace.
[47] Excepting angelfood cake, cakes were made from mixes containing vegetable shortening; icings, with butter.
[48] Excepting spongecake, made with vegetable shortening used for cake portion; butter, for icing. If butter or margarine used for cake portion, vitamin A values would be higher.
[49] Applies to product made with a sodium aluminum-sulfate type baking powder. With a low-sodium type baking powder containing potassium, value would be about twice the amount shown.
[50] Equal weights of flour, sugar, eggs, and vegetable shortening.
[51] Products are commercial unless otherwise specified.
[52] Made with enriched flour and vegetable shortening except for macaroons which do not contain flour or shortening.
[53] Icing made with butter.

19

TABLE 2.— NUTRITIVE VALUES OF THE EDIBLE PART OF FOODS - Continued

(Dashes (—) denote lack of reliable data for a constituent believed to be present in measurable amount)

Item No. (A)	Foods, approximate measures, units, and weight (edible part unless footnotes indicate otherwise) (B)	Grams	Water (C) Percent	Food energy (D) Calories	Protein (E) Grams	Fat (F) Grams	Saturated (total) (G) Grams	Oleic (H) Grams	Linoleic (I) Grams	Carbohydrate (J) Grams	Calcium (K) Milligrams	Phosphorus (L) Milligrams	Iron (M) Milligrams	Potassium (N) Milligrams	Vitamin A value (O) International units	Thiamin (P) Milligrams	Riboflavin (Q) Milligrams	Niacin (R) Milligrams	Ascorbic acid (S) Milligrams
	GRAIN PRODUCTS—Con.																		
	Cookies made with enriched flour[50][51]—Continued																		
421	Plain, prepared from commercial chilled dough, 2 1/2-in diam., 1/4 in thick. 4 cookies	48	5	240	2	12	3.0	5.2	2.9	31	17	35	0.6	23	30	0.10	0.08	0.9	0
422	Sandwich type (chocolate or vanilla), 1 3/4-in diam., 3/8 in thick. 4 cookies	40	2	200	2	9	2.2	3.9	2.2	28	10	96	.7	15	0	.06	.10	.7	0
423	Vanilla wafers, 1 3/4-in diam., 1/4 in thick. 10 cookies	40	3	185	2	6	—	—	—	30	16	25	.6	29	50	.10	.09	.8	0
	Cornmeal:																		
424	Whole-ground, unbolted, dry form. 1 cup	122	12	435	11	5	.5	1.0	2.5	90	24	312	2.9	346	[5]620	.46	.13	2.4	0
425	Bolted (nearly whole-grain), dry form. 1 cup	122	12	440	11	4	.5	.9	2.1	91	21	272	2.2	303	[5]590	.37	.10	2.3	0
	Degermed, enriched:																		
426	Dry form. 1 cup	138	12	500	11	2	.2	.4	.9	108	8	137	4.0	166	[5]610	.61	.36	4.8	0
427	Cooked. 1 cup	240	88	120	3	Trace	Trace	.1	.2	26	2	34	1.0	38	[5]140	.14	.10	1.2	0
	Degermed, unenriched:																		
428	Dry form. 1 cup	138	12	500	11	2	.2	.4	.9	108	8	137	1.5	166	[5]610	.19	.07	1.4	0
429	Cooked. 1 cup	240	88	120	3	Trace	Trace	.1	.2	26	2	34	.5	38	[5]140	.05	.02	.2	0
	Crackers:[43]																		
430	Graham, plain, 2 1/2-in square. 2 crackers	14	6	55	1	1	.3	.5	.3	10	6	21	.5	55	0	.02	.08	.5	0
431	Rye wafers, whole-grain, 1 7/8 by 3 1/2 in. 2 wafers	13	6	45	2	Trace	—	—	—	10	7	50	.5	78	0	.04	.03	.2	0
432	Saltines, made with enriched flour. 4 crackers or 1 packet	11	4	50	1	1	.3	.5	.4	8	2	10	.5	13	0	.05	.05	.4	0
	Danish pastry (enriched flour), plain without fruit or nuts:[54]																		
433	Packaged ring, 12 oz. 1 ring	340	22	1,435	25	80	24.3	31.7	16.5	155	170	371	6.1	381	1,050	.97	1.01	8.6	Trace
434	Round piece, about 4 1/4-in diam. by 1 in. 1 pastry	65	22	275	5	15	4.7	6.1	3.2	30	33	71	1.2	73	200	.18	.19	1.7	Trace
435	Ounce. 1 oz	28	22	120	2	7	2.0	2.7	1.4	13	14	31	.5	32	90	.08	.08	.7	Trace
	Doughnuts, made with enriched flour:[38]																		
436	Cake type, plain, 2 1/2-in diam., 1 in high. 1 doughnut	25	24	100	1	5	1.2	2.0	1.1	13	10	48	.4	23	20	.05	.05	.4	Trace
437	Yeast-leavened, glazed, 3 3/4-in diam., 1 1/4 in high. 1 doughnut	50	26	205	3	11	3.3	5.8	3.3	22	16	33	.6	34	25	.10	.10	.8	0
	Macaroni, enriched, cooked (cut lengths, elbows, shells):																		
438	Firm stage (hot). 1 cup	130	64	190	7	1	—	—	—	39	14	85	1.4	103	0	.23	.13	1.8	0
	Tender stage:																		
439	Cold macaroni. 1 cup	105	73	115	4	Trace	—	—	—	24	8	53	.9	64	0	.15	.08	1.2	0
440	Hot macaroni. 1 cup	140	73	155	5	Trace	—	—	—	32	11	70	1.3	85	0	.20	.11	1.5	0
	Macaroni (enriched) and cheese:																		
441	Canned[56]. 1 cup	240	80	230	9	10	4.2	3.1	1.4	26	199	182	1.0	139	260	.12	.24	1.0	Trace
442	From home recipe (served hot)[56]. 1 cup	200	58	430	17	22	8.9	8.8	2.9	40	362	322	1.8	240	860	.20	.40	1.8	Trace
	Muffins made with enriched flour:[38]																		
	From home recipe:																		
443	Blueberry, 2 3/8-in diam., 1 1/2 in high. 1 muffin	40	39	110	3	4	1.1	1.4	.7	17	34	53	.6	46	90	.09	.10	.7	Trace
444	Bran. 1 muffin	40	35	105	3	4	1.2	1.4	.8	17	57	162	1.5	172	90	.07	.10	1.7	Trace
445	Corn (enriched degermed cornmeal and flour), 2 3/8-in diam., 1 1/2 in high. 1 muffin	40	33	125	3	4	1.2	1.6	.9	19	42	68	.7	54	[57]120	.10	.10	.7	Trace

(A)	(B)	Grams	(C)	(D)	(E)	(F)	(G)	(H)	(I)	(J)	(K)	(L)	(M)	(N)	(O)	(P)	(Q)	(R)	(S)
446	Plain, 3-in diam., 1 1/2 in high. — 1 muffin	40	38	120	3	4	1.0	1.7	1.0	17	42	60	0.6	50	40	0.09	0.12	0.9	Trace
	From mix, egg, milk:																		
447	Corn, 2 3/8-in diam., 1 1/2 in high.[56] — 1 muffin	40	30	130	3	4	1.2	1.7	.9	20	96	152	.6	44	[57]100	.08	.09	.7	Trace
448	Noodles (egg noodles), enriched, cooked. — 1 cup	160	71	200	7	2	—	—	—	37	16	94	1.4	70	110	.22	.13	1.9	0
449	Noodles, chow mein, canned. — 1 cup	45	1	220	6	11	—	—	—	26	—	—	—	—	0	—	—	—	—
450	Pancakes, (4-in diam.):[55][56] Buckwheat, made from mix (with buckwheat and enriched flours), egg and milk added. — 1 cake	27	58	55	2	2	.8	.9	.4	6	59	91	.4	66	60	.04	.05	.2	Trace
	Plain:																		
451	Made from home recipe using enriched flour. — 1 cake	27	50	60	2	2	.5	.8	.4	9	27	38	.4	33	30	.06	.07	.5	Trace
452	Made from mix with enriched flour, egg and milk added. — 1 cake	27	51	60	2	2	.7	.7	.3	9	58	70	.3	42	70	.04	.06	.2	Trace
	Pies, piecrust made with enriched flour, vegetable shortening (9-in diam.):																		
	Apple:																		
453	Whole — 1 pie	945	48	2,420	21	105	27.0	44.5	25.2	360	76	208	6.6	756	280	1.06	.79	9.3	9
454	Sector, 1/7 of pie — 1 sector	135	48	345	3	15	3.9	6.4	3.6	51	11	30	.9	108	40	.15	.11	1.3	2
	Banana cream:																		
455	Whole — 1 pie	910	54	2,010	41	85	26.7	33.2	16.2	279	601	746	7.3	1,847	2,280	.77	1.51	7.0	9
456	Sector, 1/7 of pie — 1 sector	130	54	285	6	12	3.8	4.7	2.3	40	86	107	1.0	264	333	.11	.22	1.0	1
	Blueberry:																		
457	Whole — 1 pie	945	51	2,285	23	102	24.8	43.7	25.1	330	104	217	9.5	614	280	1.03	.80	10.0	28
458	Sector, 1/7 of pie — 1 sector	135	51	325	3	15	3.5	6.2	3.6	47	15	31	1.4	88	40	.15	.11	1.4	4
	Cherry:																		
459	Whole — 1 pie	945	47	2,465	25	107	28.2	45.0	25.3	363	132	236	6.6	992	4,160	1.09	.84	9.8	Trace
460	Sector, 1/7 of pie — 1 sector	135	47	350	4	15	4.0	6.4	3.6	52	19	34	.9	142	590	.16	.12	1.4	Trace
	Custard:																		
461	Whole — 1 pie	910	58	1,985	56	101	33.9	38.5	17.5	213	874	1,028	8.2	1,247	2,090	.79	1.92	5.6	0
462	Sector, 1/7 of pie — 1 sector	130	58	285	8	14	4.8	5.5	2.5	30	125	147	1.2	178	300	.11	.27	.8	0
	Lemon meringue:																		
463	Whole — 1 pie	840	47	2,140	31	86	26.1	33.8	16.4	317	118	412	6.7	420	1,430	.61	.84	5.2	25
464	Sector, 1/7 of pie — 1 sector	120	47	305	4	12	3.7	4.8	2.3	45	17	59	1.0	60	200	.09	.12	.7	4
	Mince:																		
465	Whole — 1 pie	945	43	2,560	24	109	28.0	45.9	25.2	389	265	359	13.3	1,682	20	.96	.86	9.8	9
466	Sector, 1/7 of pie — 1 sector	135	43	365	3	16	4.0	6.6	3.6	56	38	51	1.9	240	Trace	.14	.12	1.4	1
	Peach:																		
467	Whole — 1 pie	945	48	2,410	24	101	24.8	43.7	25.1	361	95	274	8.5	1,408	6,900	1.04	.97	14.0	28
468	Sector, 1/7 of pie — 1 sector	135	48	345	3	14	3.5	6.2	3.6	52	14	39	1.2	201	990	.15	.14	2.0	4
	Pecan:																		
469	Whole — 1 pie	825	20	3,450	42	189	27.8	101.0	44.2	423	388	850	25.6	1,015	1,320	1.80	.95	6.9	Trace
470	Sector, 1/7 of pie — 1 sector	118	20	495	6	27	4.0	14.4	6.3	61	55	122	3.7	145	190	.26	.14	1.0	Trace
	Pumpkin:																		
471	Whole — 1 pie	910	59	1,920	36	102	37.4	37.5	16.6	223	464	628	7.3	1,456	22,480	.78	1.27	7.0	Trace
472	Sector, 1/7 of pie — 1 sector	130	59	275	5	15	5.4	5.4	2.4	32	66	90	1.1	208	3,210	.11	.18	1.0	Trace
473	Piecrust (home recipe) made with enriched flour and vegetable shortening, baked. — 1 pie shell, 9-in diam.	180	15	900	11	60	14.8	26.1	14.9	79	25	90	3.1	89	0	.47	.40	5.0	0
474	Piecrust mix with enriched flour and vegetable shortening, 10-oz pkg. prepared and baked. — Piecrust for 2-crust pie, 9-in diam.	320	19	1,485	20	93	22.7	39.7	23.4	141	131	272	6.1	179	0	1.07	.79	9.9	0

[53] Made with vegetable shortening.
[54] Products are commercial unless otherwise specified.
[55] Made with enriched flour and vegetable shortening except for macaroons which do not contain flour or shortening.
[56] Applies to yellow varieties; white varieties contain only a trace.
[57] Contains vegetable shortening and butter.
[58] Made with corn oil.
[59] Made with regular margarine.
[60] Applies to product made with yellow cornmeal.
[61] Made with enriched degermed cornmeal and enriched flour.

TABLE 2.— NUTRITIVE VALUES OF THE EDIBLE PART OF FOODS - Continued

(Dashes (—) denote lack of reliable data for a constituent believed to be present in measurable amount)

Item No. (A)	Foods, approximate measures, units, and weight (edible part unless footnotes indicate otherwise) (B)	Grams	Water (C) Percent	Food energy (D) Calories	Protein (E) Grams	Fat (F) Grams	Saturated (total) (G) Grams	Oleic (H) Grams	Linoleic (I) Grams	Carbohydrate Grams	Calcium (K) Milligrams	Phosphorus (L) Milligrams	Iron (M) Milligrams	Potassium (N) Milligrams	Vitamin A value (O) International units	Thiamin (P) Milligrams	Riboflavin (Q) Milligrams	Niacin (R) Milligrams	Ascorbic acid (S) Milligrams
	GRAIN PRODUCTS—Con.																		
475	Pizza (cheese) baked, 4 3/4-in sector; 1/8 of 12-in pie.[19] 1 sector	60	45	145	6	4	1.7	1.5	0.6	22	86	89	1.1	67	230	0.16	0.18	1.6	4
	Popcorn, popped:																		
476	Plain, large kernel. 1 cup	6	4	25	1	Trace	Trace	.1	.2	5	1	17	.2	—	—	—	.01	.1	0
477	With oil (coconut) and salt added, large kernel. 1 cup	9	3	40	1	2	1.5	.2	.2	5	1	19	.2	—	—	—	.01	.2	0
478	Sugar coated. 1 cup	35	4	135	2	1	.5	.2	.4	30	2	47	.5	—	—	—	.02	.4	0
	Pretzels, made with enriched flour:																		
479	Dutch, twisted, 2 3/4 by 2 5/8 in. 1 pretzel	16	5	60	2	1	—	—	—	12	4	21	.2	21	0	.05	.04	.7	0
480	Thin, twisted, 3 1/4 by 2 1/4 by 1/4 in. 10 pretzels	60	5	235	6	3	—	—	—	46	13	79	.9	78	0	.20	.15	2.5	0
481	Stick, 2 1/4 in long. 10 pretzels	3	5	10	Trace	Trace	—	—	—	2	1	4	Trace	4	0	.01	.01	.1	0
	Rice, white, enriched: Instant, ready-to-serve, hot:																		
482	1 cup	165	73	180	4	Trace	Trace	Trace	Trace	40	5	31	1.3	—	0	.21	(55)	1.7	0
	Long grain:																		
483	Raw. 1 cup	185	12	670	12	1	.2	.2	.1	149	44	174	5.4	170	0	.81	.06	6.5	0
484	Cooked, served hot. 1 cup	205	73	225	4	Trace	.1	.1	.1	50	21	57	1.8	57	0	.23	.02	2.1	0
	Parboiled:																		
485	Raw. 1 cup	185	10	685	14	1	.2	.1	.1	150	111	370	5.4	278	0	.81	.07	6.5	0
486	Cooked, served hot. 1 cup	175	73	185	4	Trace	.1	.1	.1	41	33	100	1.4	75	0	.19	.02	2.1	0
	Rolls, enriched:[19] Commercial:																		
487	Brown-and-serve (12 per 12-oz pkg.), browned. 1 roll	26	27	85	2	2	.4	.7	.5	14	20	23	.5	25	Trace	.10	.06	.9	Trace
488	Cloverleaf or pan, 2 1/2-in diam., 2 in high. 1 roll	28	31	85	2	2	.4	.6	.4	15	21	24	.5	27	Trace	.11	.07	.9	Trace
489	Frankfurter and hamburger (8 per 11 1/2-oz pkg.). 1 roll	40	31	120	3	2	.5	.8	.6	21	30	34	.8	38	Trace	.15	.10	1.3	Trace
490	Hard, 3 3/4-in diam., 2 in high. 1 roll	50	25	155	5	2	.4	.6	.5	30	24	46	1.2	49	Trace	.20	.12	1.7	Trace
491	Hoagie or submarine, 11 1/2 by 3 by 2 1/2 in. 1 roll	135	31	390	12	4	.9	1.4	1.4	75	58	115	3.0	122	Trace	.54	.32	4.5	Trace
	From home recipe:																		
492	Cloverleaf, 2 1/2-in diam., 2 in high. 1 roll	35	26	120	3	3	.8	1.1	.7	20	16	36	.7	41	30	.12	.12	1.2	Trace
	Spaghetti, enriched, cooked:																		
493	Firm stage, "al dente," served hot. 1 cup	130	64	190	7	1	—	—	—	39	14	85	1.4	103	0	.23	.13	1.8	0
494	Tender stage, served hot. 1 cup	140	73	155	5	1	—	—	—	32	11	70	1.3	85	0	.20	.11	1.5	0
	Spaghetti (enriched) in tomato sauce with cheese:																		
495	From home recipe. 1 cup	250	77	260	9	9	2.0	5.4	.7	37	80	135	2.3	408	1,080	.25	.18	2.3	13
496	Canned. 1 cup	250	80	190	6	2	.5	.3	.4	39	40	88	2.8	303	930	.35	.28	4.5	10
	Spaghetti (enriched) with meat balls and tomato sauce:																		
497	From home recipe. 1 cup	248	70	330	19	12	3.3	6.3	.9	39	124	236	3.7	665	1,590	.25	.30	4.0	22
498	Canned. 1 cup	250	78	260	12	10	2.2	3.3	3.9	29	53	113	3.3	245	1,000	.15	.18	2.3	5
499	Toaster pastries. 1 pastry	50	12	200	3	6	—	—	—	36	(54)	(67)	1.9	(74)	500	.16	.17	2.1	(60)
	Waffles, made with enriched flour, 7-in diam.:[19]																		
500	From home recipe. 1 waffle	75	41	210	7	7	2.3	2.8	1.4	28	85	130	1.3	109	250	.17	.23	1.4	Trace
501	From mix, egg and milk added. 1 waffle	75	42	205	7	8	2.8	2.9	1.2	27	179	257	1.0	146	170	.14	.22	.9	Trace

(A)	(B)	(C)	(D)	(E)	(F)	(G)	(H)	(I)	(J)	(K)	(L)	(M)	(N)	(O)	(P)	(Q)	(R)	(S)
	Wheat flours:																	
	All-purpose or family flour, enriched:																	
502	Sifted, spooned — 1 cup	115	420	12	1	0.2	0.1	0.5	88	18	100	3.3	109	0	0.74	0.46	6.1	0
503	Unsifted, spooned — 1 cup	125	455	13	1	.2	.1	.5	95	20	109	3.6	119	0	.80	.50	6.6	0
504	Cake or pastry flour, enriched, sifted, spooned 1 cup	96	350	7	1	.1	.1	.3	76	16	70	2.8	91	0	.61	.38	5.1	0
505	Self-rising, enriched, unsifted, spooned. 1 cup	125	440	12	1	.2	.1	.5	93	331	583	3.6	—	0	.80	.50	6.6	0
506	Whole-wheat, from hard wheats, stirred. 1 cup	120	400	16	2	.4	.2	1.0	85	49	446	4.0	444	0	.66	.14	5.2	0
	LEGUMES (DRY), NUTS, SEEDS; RELATED PRODUCTS																	
	Almonds, shelled:																	
507	Chopped (about 130 almonds) 1 cup	130	775	24	70	5.6	47.7	12.8	25	304	655	6.1	1,005	0	.31	1.20	4.6	Trace
508	Slivered, not pressed down (about 115 almonds). 1 cup	115	690	21	62	5.0	42.2	11.3	22	269	590	5.4	889	0	.28	1.06	4.0	Trace
	Beans, dry: Common varieties as Great Northern, and others: Cooked, drained:																	
509	Great Northern 1 cup	180	210	14	1	—	—	—	38	90	266	4.9	749	0	.25	.13	1.3	0
510	Pea (navy) 1 cup	190	225	15	1	—	—	—	40	95	281	5.1	790	0	.27	.13	1.3	0
	Canned, solids and liquid: White with—																	
511	Frankfurters (sliced) 1 cup	255	365	19	18	2.4	2.8	.6	32	94	303	4.8	668	330	.18	.15	3.3	Trace
512	Pork and tomato sauce 1 cup	255	310	16	7	—	—	—	48	138	235	4.6	536	330	.20	.08	1.5	5
513	Pork and sweet sauce 1 cup	255	385	16	12	4.3	5.0	1.1	54	161	291	5.9	—	10	.15	.10	1.3	—
514	Red kidney 1 cup	255	230	15	1	—	—	—	42	74	278	4.6	673	10	.13	.10	1.5	—
515	Lima, cooked, drained 1 cup	190	260	16	1	—	—	—	49	55	293	5.9	1,163	30	.25	.11	1.3	—
516	Blackeye peas, dry, cooked (with residual cooking liquid). 1 cup	250	190	13	1	—	—	—	35	43	238	3.3	573	30	.40	.10	1.0	—
517	Brazil nuts, shelled (6-8 large kernels). 1 oz	28	185	4	19	4.8	6.2	7.1	3	53	196	1.0	203	Trace	.27	.03	.5	—
518	Cashew nuts, roasted in oil 1 cup	140	785	24	64	12.9	36.8	10.2	41	53	522	5.3	650	140	.60	.35	2.5	—
	Coconut meat, fresh:																	
519	Piece, about 2 by 2 by 1/2 in 1 piece	45	155	2	16	14.0	.9	.3	4	6	43	.8	115	0	.02	.01	.2	1
520	Shredded or grated, not pressed down. 1 cup	80	275	3	28	24.8	1.6	.5	8	10	76	1.4	205	0	.04	.02	.4	2
521	Filberts (hazelnuts), chopped (about 80 kernels). 1 cup	115	730	14	72	5.1	55.2	7.3	19	240	388	3.9	810	—	.53	—	1.0	Trace
522	Lentils, whole, cooked 1 cup	200	210	16	Trace	—	—	—	37	50	238	4.2	498	40	.14	.12	1.2	0
523	Peanuts, roasted in oil, salted (whole halves, chopped). 1 cup	144	840	37	72	13.7	33.0	20.7	27	107	577	3.0	971	—	.46	.19	24.8	0
524	Peanut butter 1 tbsp	16	95	4	8	1.5	3.7	2.3	3	9	61	.3	100	—	.02	.02	2.4	0
525	Peas, split, dry, cooked 1 cup	200	230	16	1	—	—	—	42	22	178	3.4	592	80	.30	.18	1.8	—
526	Pecans, chopped or pieces (about 120 large halves). 1 cup	118	810	11	84	7.2	50.5	20.0	17	86	341	2.8	712	150	1.01	.15	1.1	2
527	Pumpkin and squash kernels, dry, hulled. 1 cup	140	775	41	65	11.8	23.5	27.5	21	71	1,602	15.7	1,386	100	.34	.27	3.4	—
528	Sunflower seeds, dry, hulled 1 cup	145	810	35	69	8.2	13.7	43.2	29	174	1,214	10.3	1,334	70	2.84	.33	7.8	—
	Walnuts: Black:																	
529	Chopped or broken kernels 1 cup	125	785	26	74	6.3	13.3	45.7	19	Trace	713	7.5	575	380	.28	.14	.9	—
530	Ground (finely) 1 cup	80	500	16	47	4.0	8.5	29.2	12	Trace	455	4.8	368	240	.18	.09	.6	—
531	Persian or English, chopped (about 60 halves). 1 cup	120	780	18	77	8.4	11.8	42.2	19	119	455	3.7	540	40	.40	.16	1.1	2

[1] Crust made with vegetable shortening and enriched flour.
[3] Made with vegetable shortening.
[5] Product may or may not be enriched with riboflavin. Consult the label.
[6] Value varies with the brand. Consult the label.

23

TABLE 2.— NUTRITIVE VALUES OF THE EDIBLE PART OF FOODS - Continued

(Dashes (—) denote lack of reliable data for a constituent believed to be present in measurable amount)

Item No.	Foods, approximate measures, units, and weight (edible part unless footnotes indicate otherwise)	Grams	Water Per cent	Food energy Calories	Protein Grams	Fat Grams	Fatty Acids Saturated (total) Grams	Unsaturated Oleic Grams	Linoleic Grams	Carbohydrate Grams	Calcium Milligrams	Phosphorus Milligrams	Iron Milligrams	Potassium Milligrams	Vitamin A value International units	Thiamin Milligrams	Riboflavin Milligrams	Niacin Milligrams	Ascorbic acid Milligrams
(A)	(B)		(C)	(D)	(E)	(F)	(G)	(H)	(I)	(J)	(K)	(L)	(M)	(N)	(O)	(P)	(Q)	(R)	(S)
	SUGARS AND SWEETS																		
	Cake icings:																		
	Boiled, white:																		
532	Plain----------- 1 cup	94	18	295	1	0	0	0	0	75	2	2	Trace	17	0	Trace	0.03	Trace	0
533	With coconut----- 1 cup	166	15	605	3	13	11.0	.9	Trace	124	10	50	0.8	277	0	0.02	.07	0.3	1
	Uncooked:																		
534	Chocolate made with milk and butter----- 1 cup	275	14	1,035	9	38	23.4	11.7	1.0	185	165	305	3.3	536	580	.06	.28	.6	1
535	Creamy fudge from mix and water----- 1 cup	245	15	830	7	16	5.1	6.7	3.1	183	96	218	2.7	238	Trace	.05	.20	.7	Trace
536	White----- 1 cup	319	11	1,200	2	21	12.7	5.1	.5	260	48	38	Trace	57	860	Trace	.06	Trace	Trace
	Candy:																		
537	Caramels, plain or chocolate----- 1 oz	28	8	115	1	3	1.6	1.1	.1	22	42	35	.4	54	Trace	.01	.05	.1	Trace
	Chocolate:																		
538	Milk, plain----- 1 oz	28	1	145	2	9	5.5	3.0	.3	16	65	65	.3	109	80	.02	.10	.1	Trace
539	Semisweet, small pieces (60 per oz)--- 1 cup or 6-oz pkg	170	1	860	7	61	36.2	19.8	1.7	97	51	255	4.4	553	30	.02	.14	.9	0
540	Chocolate-coated peanuts--- 1 oz	28	1	160	5	12	4.0	4.7	2.1	11	33	84	.4	143	Trace	.10	.05	2.1	Trace
541	Fondant; uncoated (mints, candy corn, other)--- 1 oz	28	8	105	Trace	1	.1	.3	.1	25	4	2	.3	1	0	Trace	Trace	Trace	0
542	Fudge, chocolate, plain--- 1 oz	28	8	115	1	3	1.3	1.4	.6	21	22	24	.3	42	Trace	.01	.03	.1	Trace
543	Gum drops--- 1 oz	28	12	100	Trace	Trace	—	—	—	25	2	Trace	.1	1	0	0	Trace	0	0
544	Hard--- 1 oz	28	1	110	0	Trace	—	—	—	28	6	2	.5	1	0	0	0	0	0
545	Marshmallows--- 1 oz	28	17	90	1	Trace	—	—	—	23	5	2	.5	2	0	0	Trace	Trace	0
	Chocolate-flavored beverage powders (about 4 heaping tsp per oz):																		
546	With nonfat dry milk--- 1 oz	28	2	100	5	1	.5	.3	Trace	20	167	155	.5	227	10	.04	.21	.2	1
547	Without milk--- 1 oz	28	1	100	2	1	.4	.2	Trace	25	9	48	.6	142	—	.01	.03	.1	0
548	Honey, strained or extracted--- 1 tbsp	21	17	65	Trace	0	0	0	0	17	1	1	.1	11	0	Trace	.01	.1	Trace
549	Jams and preserves--- 1 tbsp	20	29	55	Trace	Trace	—	—	—	14	4	2	.2	18	Trace	Trace	.01	Trace	Trace
550	--- 1 packet	14	29	40	Trace	Trace	—	—	—	10	3	1	.1	12	Trace	Trace	.01	Trace	Trace
551	Jellies--- 1 tbsp	18	29	50	Trace	Trace	—	—	—	13	4	1	.3	14	Trace	Trace	.01	Trace	1
552	--- 1 packet	14	29	40	Trace	Trace	—	—	—	10	3	1	.2	11	Trace	Trace	Trace	Trace	1
	Sirups:																		
	Chocolate-flavored sirup or topping:																		
553	Thin type--- 1 fl oz or 2 tbsp	38	32	90	1	1	.5	.3	Trace	24	6	35	.6	106	Trace	.01	.03	.2	0
554	Fudge type--- 1 fl oz or 2 tbsp	38	25	125	2	5	3.1	1.6	.1	20	48	60	.5	107	60	.02	.08	.2	Trace
	Molasses, cane:																		
555	Light (first extraction)--- 1 tbsp	20	24	50	—	—	—	—	—	13	33	9	.9	183	—	.01	.01	Trace	—
556	Blackstrap (third extraction)--- 1 tbsp	20	24	45	—	—	—	—	—	11	137	17	3.2	585	—	.02	.04	Trace	—
557	Sorghum--- 1 tbsp	21	23	55	—	—	—	—	—	14	35	5	2.6	—	—	—	—	—	—
558	Table blends, chiefly corn, light and dark--- 1 tbsp	21	24	60	0	0	0	0	0	15	9	3	.8	1	0	0	0	0	0
	Sugars:																		
559	Brown, pressed down--- 1 cup	220	2	820	0	0	0	0	0	212	187	42	7.5	757	0	.02	.07	.4	0
	White:																		
560	Granulated--- 1 cup	200	1	770	0	0	0	0	0	199	0	0	.2	6	0	0	0	0	0
561	--- 1 tbsp	12	1	45	0	0	0	0	0	12	0	0	Trace	Trace	0	0	0	0	0
562	--- 1 packet	6	1	23	0	0	0	0	0	6	0	0	Trace	Trace	0	0	0	0	0
563	Powdered, sifted, spooned into cup--- 1 cup	100	1	385	0	0	0	0	0	100	0	0	.1	3	0	0	0	0	0

VEGETABLE AND VEGETABLE PRODUCTS

(A)	(B)	(C)	(D)	(E)	(F)	(G)	(H)	(I)	(J)	(K)	(L)	(M)	(N)	(O)	(P)	(Q)	(R)	(S)
	Asparagus, green: Cooked, drained: Cuts and tips, 1 1/2- to 2-in lengths:																	
564	From raw — 1 cup — 145	94	30	3	Trace	—	—	—	5	30	73	0.9	265	1,310	0.23	0.26	2.0	38
565	From frozen — 1 cup — 180	93	40	6	Trace	—	—	—	6	40	115	2.2	396	1,530	.25	.23	1.8	41
	Spears, 1/2-in diam. at base:																	
566	From raw — 4 spears — 60	94	10	1	Trace	—	—	—	2	13	30	.4	110	540	.10	.11	.8	16
567	From frozen — 4 spears — 60	92	15	2	Trace	—	—	—	2	13	40	.7	143	470	.10	.08	.7	16
568	Canned, spears, 1/2-in diam. at base. — 4 spears — 80	93	15	2	Trace	—	—	—	3	15	42	1.5	133	640	.05	.08	.6	12
	Beans: Lima, immature seeds, frozen, cooked, drained:																	
569	Thick-seeded types (Fordhooks) — 1 cup — 170	74	170	10	Trace	—	—	—	32	34	153	2.9	724	390	.12	.09	1.7	29
570	Thin-seeded types (baby limas) — 1 cup — 180	69	210	13	Trace	—	—	—	40	63	227	4.7	709	400	.16	.09	2.2	22
	Snap: Green:																	
571	Cooked, drained: From raw (cuts and French style). — 1 cup — 125	92	30	2	Trace	—	—	—	7	63	46	.8	189	580	.09	.11	.6	15
	From frozen:																	
572	Cuts — 1 cup — 135	92	35	2	Trace	—	—	—	8	54	43	.9	205	780	.09	.12	.5	7
573	French style — 1 cup — 130	92	35	2	Trace	—	—	—	8	49	39	1.2	177	590	.08	.10	.4	9
574	Canned, drained solids (cuts). — 1 cup — 135	92	30	2	Trace	—	—	—	7	61	34	2.0	128	530	.04	.07	.4	5
	Yellow or wax:																	
575	Cooked, drained: From raw (cuts and French style). — 1 cup — 125	93	30	2	Trace	—	—	—	6	63	46	.8	189	290	.09	.11	.6	16
576	From frozen (cuts) — 1 cup — 135	92	35	2	Trace	—	—	—	8	47	42	.9	221	140	.09	.11	.5	8
577	Canned, drained solids (cuts). — 1 cup — 135	92	30	2	Trace	—	—	—	7	61	34	2.0	128	140	.04	.07	.4	7
	Beans, mature. See Beans, dry (items 509-515) and Blackeye peas, dry (item 516).																	
	Bean sprouts (mung):																	
578	Raw — 1 cup — 105	89	35	4	Trace	—	—	—	7	20	67	1.4	234	20	.14	.14	.8	20
579	Cooked, drained — 1 cup — 125	91	35	4	Trace	—	—	—	7	21	60	1.1	195	30	.11	.13	.9	8
	Beets: Cooked, drained, peeled:																	
580	Whole beets, 2-in diam. — 2 beets — 100	91	30	1	Trace	—	—	—	7	14	23	.5	208	20	.03	.04	.3	6
581	Diced or sliced — 1 cup — 170	91	55	2	Trace	—	—	—	12	24	39	.9	354	30	.05	.07	.5	10
	Canned, drained solids:																	
582	Whole beets, small — 1 cup — 160	89	60	2	Trace	—	—	—	14	30	29	1.1	267	30	.02	.05	.2	5
583	Diced or sliced — 1 cup — 170	89	65	2	Trace	—	—	—	15	32	31	1.2	284	30	.02	.05	.2	5
584	Beet greens, leaves and stems, cooked and drained. — 1 cup — 145	94	25	2	Trace	—	—	—	5	144	36	2.8	481	7,400	.10	.22	.4	22
	Blackeye peas, immature seeds, cooked and drained: From raw:																	
585	From raw — 1 cup — 165	72	180	13	1	—	—	—	30	40	241	3.5	625	580	.50	.18	2.3	28
586	From frozen — 1 cup — 170	66	220	15	1	—	—	—	40	43	286	4.8	573	290	.68	.19	2.4	15
	Broccoli, cooked, drained: From raw:																	
587	Stalk, medium size — 1 stalk — 180	91	45	6	1	—	—	—	8	158	112	1.4	481	4,500	.16	.36	1.4	162
588	Stalks cut into 1/2-in pieces — 1 cup — 155	91	40	5	Trace	—	—	—	7	136	96	1.2	414	3,880	.14	.31	1.2	140
	From frozen:																	
589	Stalk, 4 1/2 to 5 in long — 1 stalk — 30	91	10	1	Trace	—	—	—	1	12	17	.2	66	570	.02	.03	.2	22
590	Chopped — 1 cup — 185	92	50	5	1	—	—	—	9	100	104	1.3	392	4,810	.11	.22	.9	105
591	**Brussels sprouts,** cooked, drained: From raw, 7-8 sprouts (1 1/4- to 1 1/2-in diam.). — 1 cup — 155	88	55	7	1	—	—	—	10	50	112	1.7	423	810	.12	.22	1.2	135
592	From frozen — 1 cup — 155	89	50	5	Trace	—	—	—	10	33	95	1.2	457	880	.12	.16	.9	126

25

TABLE 2.— NUTRITIVE VALUES OF THE EDIBLE PART OF FOODS Continued

(Dashes (—) denote lack of reliable data for a constituent believed to be present in measurable amount)

Item No. (A)	Foods, approximate measures, units, and weight (edible part unless footnotes indicate otherwise) (B)	Water (C) Per-cent	Food energy (D) Cal-ories	Pro-tein (E) Grams	Fat (F) Grams	Fatty Acids Satu-rated (total) (G) Grams	Unsaturated Oleic (H) Grams	Unsaturated Lino-leic (I) Grams	Carbo-hydrate (J) Grams	Calcium (K) Milli-grams	Phos-phorus (L) Milli-grams	Iron (M) Milli-grams	Potas-sium (N) Milli-grams	Vitamin A value (O) Inter-national units	Thiamin (P) Milli-gram	Ribo-flavin (Q) Milli-grams	Niacin (R) Milli-grams	Ascorbic acid (S) Milli-grams
	VEGETABLE AND VEGETABLE PRODUCTS—Con.																	
	Cabbage:																	
	Common varieties:																	
	Raw:																	
593	Coarsely shredded or sliced-- 1 cup	70	92	15	1	Trace	—	—	4	34	20	0.3	163	90	0.04	0.04	0.02	33
594	Finely shredded or chopped-- 1 cup	90	92	20	1	Trace	—	—	5	44	26	.4	210	120	.05	.05	.3	42
595	Cooked, drained-- 1 cup	145	94	30	2	Trace	—	—	6	64	29	.4	236	190	.06	.06	.4	48
596	Red, raw, coarsely shredded or sliced. 1 cup	70	90	20	1	Trace	—	—	5	29	25	.6	188	30	.06	.04	.3	43
597	Savoy, raw, coarsely shredded or sliced. 1 cup	75	92	15	2	Trace	—	—	3	47	38	.6	188	140	.04	.06	.2	39
598	Cabbage, celery (also called pe-tsai or wongbok), raw, 1-in pieces. 1 cup	75	95	10	1	Trace	—	—	2	32	30	.5	190	110	.04	.03	.5	19
599	Cabbage, white mustard (also called bokchoy or pakchoy), cooked, drained. 1 cup	170	95	25	2	Trace	—	—	4	252	56	1.0	364	5,270	.07	.14	1.2	26
	Carrots:																	
	Raw, without crowns and tips, scraped:																	
600	Whole, 7 1/2 by 1 1/8 in, or strips, 2 1/2 to 3 in long. 1 carrot or 18 strips	72	88	30	1	Trace	—	—	7	27	26	.5	246	7,930	.04	.04	.4	6
601	Grated-- 1 cup	110	88	45	1	Trace	—	—	11	41	40	.8	375	12,100	.07	.06	.7	9
602	Cooked (crosswise cuts), drained 1 cup	155	91	50	1	Trace	—	—	11	51	48	.9	344	16,280	.08	.08	.8	9
	Canned:																	
603	Sliced, drained solids-- 1 cup	155	91	45	1	Trace	—	—	10	47	34	1.1	186	23,250	.03	.05	.6	3
604	Strained or junior (baby food) 1 oz (1 3/4 to 2 tbsp)--	28	92	10	Trace	Trace	—	—	2	7	6	.1	51	3,690	.01	.01	.1	1
605	Cauliflower: Raw, chopped-- 1 cup	115	91	31	3	Trace	—	—	6	29	64	1.3	339	70	.13	.12	.8	90
	Cooked, drained:																	
606	From raw (flower buds)-- 1 cup	125	93	30	3	Trace	—	—	5	26	53	.9	258	80	.11	.10	.8	69
607	From frozen (flowerets)-- 1 cup	180	94	30	3	Trace	—	—	6	31	68	.9	373	50	.07	.09	.7	74
	Celery, Pascal type, raw:																	
608	Stalk, large outer, 8 by 1 1/2 in, at root end. 1 stalk	40	94	5	Trace	Trace	—	—	2	16	11	.1	136	110	.01	.01	.1	4
609	Pieces, diced-- 1 cup	120	94	20	1	Trace	—	—	5	47	34	.4	409	320	.04	.04	.4	11
	Collards, cooked, drained:																	
610	From raw (leaves without stems)- 1 cup	190	90	65	7	1	—	—	10	357	99	1.5	498	14,820	.21	.38	2.3	144
611	From frozen (chopped)-- 1 cup	170	90	50	5	1	—	—	10	299	87	1.7	401	11,560	.10	.24	1.0	56
	Corn, sweet:																	
	Cooked, drained:																	
612	From raw, ear 5 by 1 3/4 in-- 1 ear[61]	140	74	70	2	1	—	—	16	2	69	.5	151	[62]310	.09	.08	1.1	7
	From frozen:																	
613	Ear, 5 in long-- 1 ear[61]	229	73	120	4	1	—	—	27	4	121	1.0	291	[62]440	.18	.10	2.1	9
614	Kernels-- 1 cup	165	77	130	5	1	—	—	31	5	120	1.3	304	[62]580	.15	.10	2.5	8
	Canned:																	
615	Cream style-- 1 cup	256	76	210	5	2	—	—	51	8	143	1.5	248	[62]840	.08	.13	2.6	13
	Whole kernel:																	
616	Vacuum pack-- 1 cup	210	76	175	5	1	—	—	43	6	153	1.1	204	[62]740	.06	.13	2.3	11
617	Wet pack, drained solids-- 1 cup	165	76	140	4	1	—	—	33	8	81	.8	160	[62]580	.05	.08	1.5	7
	Cowpeas. See Blackeye peas. (Items 585-586).																	
	Cucumber slices, 1/8 in thick (large, 2 1/8-in diam.; small, 1 3/4-in diam.):																	
618	With peel-- 6 large or 8 small slices	28	95	5	Trace	Trace	—	—	1	7	8	.3	45	70	.01	.01	.1	3

(A)	(B)			(C)	(D)	(E)	(F)	(G)	(H)	(I)	(J)	(K)	(L)	(M)	(N)	(O)	(P)	(Q)	(R)	(S)
619	Without peel	6 1/2 large or 9 small pieces	28	96	5	Trace	Trace	—	—	—	1	5	5	0.1	45	Trace	0.01	0.01	0.1	3
620	Dandelion greens, cooked, drained	1 cup	105	90	35	2	1	—	—	—	7	147	44	1.9	244	12,290	.14	.17	1.6	19
621	Endive, curly (including escarole), raw, small pieces	1 cup	50	93	10	1	Trace	—	—	—	2	41	27	.9	147	1,650	.04	.07	.3	5
622	Kale, cooked, drained: From raw (leaves without stems and midribs)	1 cup	110	88	45	5	1	—	—	—	7	206	64	1.8	243	9,130	.11	.20	1.8	102
623	From frozen (leaf style)	1 cup	130	91	40	4	1	—	—	—	7	157	62	1.3	251	10,660	.08	.20	.9	49
	Lettuce, raw: Butterhead, as Boston types:																			
624	Head, 5-in diam	1 head[3]	220	95	25	2	Trace	—	—	—	4	57	42	3.3	430	1,580	.10	.10	.5	13
625	Leaves	1 outer or 2 inner or 3 heart leaves	15	95	Trace	Trace	Trace	—	—	—	Trace	5	4	.3	40	150	.01	.01	Trace	1
	Crisphead, as Iceberg:																			
626	Head, 6-in diam	1 head[4]	567	96	70	5	1	—	—	—	16	108	118	2.7	943	1,780	.32	.32	1.6	32
627	Wedge, 1/4 of head	1 wedge	135	96	20	1	Trace	—	—	—	4	27	30	.7	236	450	.08	.08	.4	8
628	Pieces, chopped or shredded	1 cup	55	96	5	Trace	Trace	—	—	—	2	11	12	.3	96	180	.03	.03	.2	3
629	Looseleaf (bunching varieties including romaine or cos), chopped or shredded pieces	1 cup	55	94	10	1	Trace	—	—	—	2	37	14	.8	145	1,050	.03	.04	.2	10
630	Mushrooms, raw, sliced or chopped	1 cup	70	90	20	2	Trace	—	—	—	3	4	81	.6	290	Trace	.07	.32	2.9	2
631	Mustard greens, without stems and midribs, cooked, drained	1 cup	140	93	30	3	1	—	—	—	6	193	45	2.5	308	8,120	.11	.20	.8	67
632	Okra pods, 3 by 5/8 in, cooked	10 pods	106	91	30	2	Trace	—	—	—	6	98	43	.5	184	520	.14	.19	1.0	21
	Onions: Mature: Raw:																			
633	Chopped	1 cup	170	89	65	3	Trace	—	—	—	15	46	61	.9	267	[5]Trace	.05	.07	.3	17
634	Sliced	1 cup	115	89	45	2	Trace	—	—	—	10	31	41	.6	181	[5]Trace	.03	.05	.2	12
635	Cooked (whole or sliced), drained	1 cup	210	92	60	3	Trace	—	—	—	14	50	61	.8	231	[5]Trace	.06	.06	.4	15
636	Young green, bulb (3/8 in diam.) and white portion of top	6 onions	30	88	15	Trace	Trace	—	—	—	3	12	12	.2	69	Trace	.02	.01	.1	8
637	Parsley, raw, chopped	1 tbsp	4	85	Trace	Trace	Trace	—	—	—	Trace	7	2	.2	25	300	Trace	.01	Trace	6
638	Parsnips, cooked (diced or 2-in lengths)	1 cup	155	82	100	2	1	—	—	—	23	70	96	.9	587	50	.11	.12	.2	16
	Peas, green: Canned:																			
639	Whole, drained solids	1 cup	170	77	150	8	1	—	—	—	29	44	129	3.2	163	1,170	.15	.10	1.4	14
640	Strained (baby food)	1 oz (1 3/4 to 2 tbsp)	28	86	15	1	Trace	—	—	—	3	3	18	.3	28	140	.02	.03	.3	3
641	Frozen, cooked, drained	1 cup	160	82	110	8	Trace	—	—	—	19	30	138	3.0	216	960	.43	.14	2.7	21
642	Peppers, hot, red, without seeds, dried (ground chili powder, added seasonings)	1 tsp	2	9	5	Trace	Trace	—	—	—	1	5	4	.3	20	1,300	Trace	.02	.2	Trace
	Peppers, sweet (about 5 per lb., whole), stem and seeds removed:																			
643	Raw	1 pod	74	93	15	1	Trace	—	—	—	4	7	16	.5	157	310	.06	.06	.4	94
644	Cooked, boiled, drained	1 pod	73	95	15	1	Trace	—	—	—	3	7	12	.4	109	310	.05	.05	.4	70
645	Potatoes, cooked: Baked, peeled after baking (about 2 per lb., raw)	1 potato	156	75	145	4	Trace	—	—	—	33	14	101	1.1	782	Trace	.15	.07	2.7	31
	Boiled (about 3 per lb., raw):																			
646	Peeled after boiling	1 potato	137	80	105	3	Trace	—	—	—	23	10	72	.8	556	Trace	.12	.05	2.0	22
647	Peeled before boiling	1 potato	135	83	90	3	Trace	—	—	—	20	8	57	.7	385	Trace	.12	.05	1.6	22
	French-fried, strip, 2 to 3 1/2 in long:																			
648	Prepared from raw	10 strips	50	45	135	2	7	1.7	1.2	3.3	18	8	56	.7	427	Trace	.07	.04	1.6	11
649	Frozen, oven heated	10 strips	50	53	110	2	4	1.1	.8	2.1	17	5	43	.9	326	Trace	.07	.01	1.3	11
650	Hashed brown, prepared from frozen	1 cup	155	56	345	3	18	4.6	3.2	9.0	45	28	78	1.9	439	Trace	.11	.03	1.6	12
	Mashed, prepared from— Raw:																			
651	Milk added	1 cup	210	83	135	4	2	.7	.4	Trace	27	50	103	.8	548	40	.17	.11	2.1	21

[1] Weight includes cob. Without cob, weight is 77 g for item 612, 126 g for item 613.
[2] Based on yellow varieties. For white varieties, value is trace.
[3] Weight includes refuse of outer leaves and core. Without these parts, weight is 163 g.
[4] Weight includes core. Without core, weight is 539 g.
[5] Value based on white-fleshed varieties. For yellow-fleshed varieties, value in International Units (I.U.) is 70 for item 633, 50 for item 634, and 80 for item 635.

TABLE 2.—NUTRITIVE VALUES OF THE EDIBLE PART OF FOODS - Continued

(Dashes (—) denote lack of reliable data for a constituent believed to be present in measurable amount)

Item No. (A)	Foods, approximate measures, units, and weight (edible part unless footnotes indicate otherwise) (B)	Measure	Grams	Water (C) Per cent	Food energy (D) Cal.	Protein (E) Grams	Fat (F) Grams	Saturated (total) (G) Grams	Oleic (H) Grams	Linoleic (I) Grams	Carbohydrate (J) Grams	Calcium (K) Milligrams	Phosphorus (L) Milligrams	Iron (M) Milligrams	Potassium (N) Milligrams	Vitamin A value (O) International units	Thiamin (P) Milligrams	Riboflavin (Q) Milligrams	Niacin (R) Milligrams	Ascorbic acid (S) Milligrams
	VEGETABLE AND VEGETABLE PRODUCTS—Con.																			
	Potatoes, cooked—Continued																			
	Mashed, prepared from—Continued																			
	Raw—Continued																			
652	Milk and butter added	1 cup	210	80	195	4	9	5.6	2.3	0.2	26	50	101	0.8	525	360	0.17	0.11	2.1	19
653	Dehydrated flakes (without milk), water, milk, butter, and salt added	1 cup	210	79	195	4	7	3.6	2.1	.2	30	65	99	.6	601	270	.08	.08	1.9	11
654	Potato chips, 1 3/4 by 2 1/2 in oval cross section.	10 chips	20	2	115	1	8	2.1	1.4	4.0	10	8	28	.4	226	Trace	.04	.01	1.0	3
655	Potato salad, made with cooked salad dressing.	1 cup	250	76	250	7	7	2.0	2.7	1.3	41	80	160	1.5	798	350	.20	.18	2.8	28
656	Pumpkin, canned	1 cup	245	90	80	2	1	—	—	—	19	61	64	1.0	588	15,680	.07	.12	1.5	12
657	Radishes, raw (prepackaged) stem ends, rootlets cut off.	4 radishes	18	95	5	Trace	Trace	—	—	—	1	5	6	.2	58	Trace	.01	.01	.1	5
658	Sauerkraut, canned, solids and liquid.	1 cup	235	93	40	2	Trace	—	—	—	9	85	42	1.2	329	120	.07	.09	.5	33
	Southern peas. See Blackeye peas (items 585-586).																			
	Spinach:																			
659	Raw, chopped	1 cup	55	91	15	2	Trace	—	—	—	2	51	28	1.7	259	4,460	.06	.11	.3	28
660	Cooked, drained: From raw	1 cup	180	92	40	5	1	—	—	—	6	167	68	4.0	583	14,580	.13	.25	.9	50
	From frozen:																			
661	Chopped	1 cup	205	92	45	6	1	—	—	—	8	232	90	4.3	683	16,200	.14	.31	.8	39
662	Leaf	1 cup	190	92	45	6	1	—	—	—	7	200	84	4.8	688	15,390	.15	.27	1.0	53
663	Canned, drained solids	1 cup	205	91	50	6	1	—	—	—	7	242	53	5.3	513	16,400	.04	.25	.6	29
	Squash, cooked:																			
664	Summer (all varieties), diced, drained.	1 cup	210	96	30	2	Trace	—	—	—	7	53	53	.8	296	820	.11	.17	1.7	21
665	Winter (all varieties), baked, mashed.	1 cup	205	81	130	4	1	—	—	—	32	57	98	1.6	945	8,610	.10	.27	1.4	27
	Sweetpotatoes:																			
	Cooked (raw, 5 by 2 in; about 2 1/2 per lb):																			
666	Baked in skin, peeled	1 potato	114	64	160	2	1	—	—	—	37	46	66	1.0	342	9,230	.10	.08	.8	25
667	Boiled in skin, peeled	1 potato	151	71	170	3	1	—	—	—	40	48	71	1.1	367	11,940	.14	.09	.9	26
668	Candied, 2 1/2 by 2-in piece	1 piece	105	60	175	1	3	2.0	.8	.1	36	39	45	.9	200	6,620	.06	.04	.4	11
	Canned:																			
669	Solid pack (mashed)	1 cup	255	72	275	5	1	—	—	—	63	64	105	2.0	510	19,890	.13	.10	1.5	36
670	Vacuum pack, piece 2 3/4 by 1 in.	1 piece	40	72	45	1	Trace	—	—	—	10	10	16	.3	80	3,120	.02	.02	.6	6
	Tomatoes:																			
671	Raw, 2 3/5-in diam. (3 per 12 oz pkg.).	1 tomato[6]	135	94	25	1	Trace	—	—	—	6	16	33	.6	300	1,110	.07	.05	.9	[6]28
672	Canned, solids and liquid	1 cup	241	94	50	2	Trace	—	—	—	10	[6]14	46	1.2	523	2,170	.12	.07	1.7	41
673	Tomato catsup	1 cup	273	69	290	5	1	—	—	—	69	60	137	2.2	991	3,820	.25	.19	4.4	41
674		1 tbsp	15	69	15	Trace	Trace	—	—	—	4	3	8	.1	54	210	.01	.01	.2	2
	Tomato juice, canned:																			
675	Cup	1 cup	243	94	45	2	Trace	—	—	—	10	17	44	2.2	552	1,940	.12	.07	1.9	39
676	Glass: (6 fl oz)	1 glass	182	94	35	2	Trace	—	—	—	8	13	33	1.6	413	1,460	.09	.05	1.5	29
677	Turnips, cooked, diced	1 cup	155	94	35	1	Trace	—	—	—	8	54	37	.6	291	Trace	.06	.08	.5	34
	Turnip greens, cooked, drained:																			
678	From raw (leaves and stems)	1 cup	145	94	30	3	Trace	—	—	—	5	252	49	1.5	246	8,270	.15	.33	.7	68
679	From frozen (chopped)	1 cup	165	93	40	4	Trace	—	—	—	6	195	64	2.6	—	11,390	.08	.15	.7	31
680	Vegetables, mixed, frozen, cooked	1 cup	182	83	115	6	1	—	—	—	24	46	115	2.4	348	9,010	.22	.13	2.0	15

28

MISCELLANEOUS ITEMS

(A)	(B)	(C)	(D)	(E)	(F)	(G)	(H)	(I)	(J)	(K)	(L)	(M)	(N)	(O)	(P)	(Q)	(R)	(S)
	Baking powders for home use:																	
	Sodium aluminum sulfate:																	
681	With monocalcium phosphate monohydrate. 1 tsp — 3.0	2	5	Trace	Trace	0	0	0	1	58	87	—	5	0	0	0	0	0
682	With monocalcium phosphate monohydrate, calcium sulfate. 1 tsp — 2.9	1	5	Trace	Trace	0	0	0	1	183	45	—		0	0	0	0	0
683	Straight phosphate — 1 tsp — 3.8	2	5	Trace	Trace	0	0	0	1	239	359	—	6	0	0	0	0	0
684	Low sodium — 1 tsp — 4.3	2	5	Trace	Trace	0	0	0	2	207	314	—	471	0	0	0	0	0
685	Barbecue sauce — 1 cup — 250	81	230	4	17	2.2	4.3	10.0	20	53	50	2.0	435	900	.03	.03	.8	13
686	Beverages, alcoholic: Beer — 12 fl oz — 360	92	150	1	0	0	0	0	14	18	108	Trace	90	—	.01	.11	2.2	—
	Gin, rum, vodka, whisky:																	
687	80-proof — 1 1/2-fl oz jigger — 42	67	95	—	—	0	0	0	Trace	—	—	—	1	—	—	—	—	—
688	86-proof — 1 1/2-fl oz jigger — 42	64	105	—	—	0	0	0	Trace	—	—	—	1	—	—	—	—	—
689	90-proof — 1 1/2-fl oz jigger — 42	62	110	—	—	0	0	0	Trace	—	—	—	1	—	—	—	—	—
	Wines:																	
690	Dessert — 3 1/2-fl oz glass — 103	77	140	Trace	0	0	0	0	8	8	10	.4	77	—	.01	.02	.2	—
691	Table — 3 1/2-fl oz glass — 102	86	85	Trace	0	0	0	0	4	9	10	.4	94	—	Trace	.01	.1	—
	Beverages, carbonated, sweetened, nonalcoholic:																	
692	Carbonated water — 12 fl oz — 366	92	115	0	0	0	0	0	29	—	—	—	—	0	0	0	0	0
693	Cola type — 12 fl oz — 369	90	145	0	0	0	0	0	37	—	—	—	—	0	0	0	0	0
694	Fruit-flavored sodas and Tom Collins mixer — 12 fl oz — 372	88	170	0	0	0	0	0	45	—	—	—	—	0	0	0	0	0
695	Ginger ale — 12 fl oz — 366	92	115	0	0	0	0	0	29	—	—	—	0	0	0	0	0	0
696	Root beer — 12 fl oz — 370	90	150	0	0	0	0	0	39	—	—	—	0	0	0	0	0	0
	Chili powder. See Peppers, hot, red (item 642).																	
	Chocolate:																	
697	Bitter or baking — 1 oz — 28	2	145	3	15	8.9	4.9	.4	8	22	109	1.9	235	20	.01	.07	.4	0
	Semisweet, see Candy, chocolate (item 539).																	
698	Gelatin, dry — 1 7-g envelope — 7	13	25	6	Trace	0	0	0	0	—	—	—	—	—	—	—	—	—
699	Gelatin dessert prepared with gelatin dessert powder and water — 1 cup — 240	84	140	4	0	0	0	0	34	—	—	—	—	—	—	—	—	—
700	Mustard, prepared, yellow — 1 tsp or individual serving pouch or cup — 5	80	5	Trace	Trace	—	—	Trace	Trace	4	4	.1	7	—	—	—	—	—
	Olives, pickled, canned:																	
701	Green — 4 medium or 3 extra large or 2 giant[69] — 16	78	15	Trace	2	.2	1.2	.1	Trace	8	2	.2	7	40	—	—	—	—
702	Ripe, Mission — 3 small or 2 large[69] — 10	73	15	Trace	2	.2	1.2	.1	Trace	9	1	.1	2	10	Trace	Trace	Trace	—
	Pickles, cucumber:																	
703	Dill, medium, whole, 3 3/4 in long, 1 1/4-in diam. — 1 pickle — 65	93	5	Trace	Trace	—	—	—	1	17	14	.7	130	70	Trace	.01	Trace	4
704	Fresh-pack, slices 1 1/2-in diam, 1/4 in thick — 2 slices — 15	79	10	Trace	Trace	—	—	—	3	5	4	.3	—	20	Trace	Trace	Trace	1
705	Sweet, gherkin, small, whole, about 2 1/2 in long, 3/4-in diam. — 1 pickle — 15	61	20	Trace	Trace	—	—	—	5	2	2	.2	—	10	Trace	Trace	Trace	1
706	Relish, finely chopped, sweet — 1 tbsp — 15	63	20	Trace	Trace	—	—	—	5	3	2	.1	—	—	—	—	—	—
	Popcorn. See items 476-478.																	
707	Popsicle, 3-fl oz size — 1 popsicle — 95	80	70	0	0	0	0	0	18	0	—	Trace	—	0	0	0	0	0

[66] Weight includes cores and stem ends. Without these parts, weight is 123 g.
[67] Based on year-round average. For tomatoes marketed from November through May, value is about 12 mg; from June through October, 32 mg.
[68] Applies to product without calcium salts added. Value for products with calcium salts added may be as much as 63 mg for whole tomatoes, 241 mg for cut forms.
[69] Weight includes pits. Without pits, weight is 13 g for item 701, 9 g for item 702.

29

TABLE 2.— NUTRITIVE VALUES OF THE EDIBLE PART OF FOODS - Continued

(Dashes (—) denote lack of reliable data for a constituent believed to be present in measurable amount)

Item No. (A)	Foods, approximate measures, units, and weight (edible part unless footnotes indicate otherwise) (B)	Grams	Water (C) Per cent	Food energy (D) Cal ories	Pro tein (E) Grams	Fat (F) Grams	Fatty Acids Satu rated (total) (G) Grams	Unsaturated Oleic (H) Grams	Lino leic (I) Grams	Carbo hydrate (J) Grams	Calcium (K) Milli grams	Phos phorus (L) Milli grams	Iron (M) Milli grams	Potas sium (N) Milli grams	Vitamin A value (O) Inter national units	Thiamin (P) Milli grams	Ribo flavin (Q) Milli grams	Niacin (R) Milli grams	Ascorbic acid (S) Milli grams
	MISCELLANEOUS ITEMS—Con.																		
	Soups:																		
	Canned, condensed:																		
	Prepared with equal volume of milk:																		
708	Cream of chicken---------1 cup	245	85	180	7	10	4.2	3.6	1.3	15	172	152	0.5	260	610	0.05	0.27	0.7	2
709	Cream of mushroom-------1 cup	245	83	215	7	14	5.4	2.9	4.6	16	191	169	.5	279	250	.10	.34	.7	1
710	Tomato------------------1 cup	250	84	175	7	7	3.4	1.7	1.0	23	168	155	.8	418	1,200	.10	.25	1.3	15
	Prepared with equal volume of water:																		
711	Bean with pork----------1 cup	250	84	170	8	6	1.2	1.8	2.4	22	63	128	2.3	395	650	.13	.08	1.0	3
712	Beef broth, bouillon, consomme.-----1 cup	240	96	30	5	0	0	0	0	3	Trace	31	.5	130	Trace	Trace	.02	1.2	—
713	Beef noodle-------------1 cup	240	93	65	4	3	.6	.7	.8	7	7	48	1.0	77	50	.05	.07	1.0	Trace
714	Clam chowder, Manhattan type (with tomatoes, without milk).--1 cup	245	92	80	2	3	.5	.4	1.3	12	34	47	1.0	184	880	.02	.02	1.0	Trace
715	Cream of chicken--------1 cup	240	92	95	3	6	1.6	2.3	1.1	8	24	34	.5	79	410	.02	.05	.5	Trace
716	Cream of mushroom-------1 cup	245	90	135	2	10	2.6	1.7	4.5	10	41	50	.5	98	70	.02	.12	.7	Trace
717	Minestrone--------------1 cup	245	90	105	5	3	.7	.9	1.3	14	37	59	1.0	314	2,350	.07	.05	1.0	—
718	Split pea---------------1 cup	245	85	145	9	3	1.1	1.2	.4	21	29	149	1.5	270	440	.25	.15	1.5	1
719	Tomato------------------1 cup	245	91	90	2	2	.5	.5	1.0	16	15	34	.7	230	1,000	.05	.05	1.2	12
720	Vegetable beef----------1 cup	245	92	80	5	2	—	—	—	10	12	49	.7	162	2,700	.05	.05	1.0	—
721	Vegetarian--------------1 cup	245	92	80	2	2	—	—	—	13	20	39	1.0	172	2,940	.05	.05	1.0	—
	Dehydrated:																		
722	Bouillon cube, 1/2 in---1 cube	4	4	5	1	Trace	—	—	—	Trace	—	—	—	4	—	—	—	—	—
	Mixes:																		
	Unprepared:																		
723	Onion-----------1 1/2-oz pkg	43	3	150	6	5	1.1	2.3	1.0	23	42	49	.6	238	30	.05	.03	.3	6
	Prepared with water:																		
724	Chicken noodle----------1 cup	240	95	55	2	1	—	—	—	8	7	19	.2	19	50	.07	.05	.5	Trace
725	Onion-------------------1 cup	240	96	35	1	1	—	—	—	6	10	12	.2	58	Trace	Trace	Trace	Trace	2
726	Tomato vegetable with noodles.-----1 cup	240	93	65	2	1	—	—	—	12	7	19	.2	29	480	.05	.02	.5	5
727	Vinegar, cider----------1 tbsp	15	94	Trace	Trace	0	0	0	0	1	1	1	.1	15	—	—	—	—	—
728	White sauce, medium, with enriched flour.---1 cup	250	73	405	10	31	19.3	7.8	.8	22	288	233	.5	348	1,150	.12	.43	.7	2
	Yeast:																		
729	Baker's, dry, active----1 pkg	7	5	20	3	Trace	—	—	—	3	3	90	1.1	140	Trace	.16	.38	2.6	Trace
730	Brewer's, dry-----------1 tbsp	8	5	25	3	Trace	—	—	—	3	[79]17	140	1.4	152	Trace	1.25	.34	3.0	Trace

[79]Value may vary from 6 to 60 mg.

Table 3.—Yield of cooked meat per pound of raw meat as purchased

Retail cut and method of cooking	Yield after cooking (less dripping)	
	Parts weighed	Weight
		Ounces
Chops or steaks for broiling or frying:		
With bone and relatively large amount of fat, such as pork or lamb chops; beef rib, sirloin, or porterhouse steaks.	Lean, bone, fat	10-12
	Lean and fat	7-10
	Lean only	5-7
Without bone and with very little fat, such as round of beef, veal steaks.	Lean and fat	12-13
	Lean only	9-12
Ground meat for broiling or frying, such as beef, lamb, or pork patties.	Patties	9-13
Roast for oven cooking (no liquid added):		
With bone and relatively large amount of fat, such as beef rib, loin, chuck; lamb shoulder, leg; pork, fresh or cured.	Lean, bone, fat	10-12
	Lean and fat	8-10
	Lean only	6-9
Without bone	Lean and fat	10-12
	Lean only	7-10
Cuts for pot roasting, simmering, braising, stewing:		
With bone and relatively large amount of fat, such as beef chuck, pork shoulder.	Lean, bone, fat	10-11
	Lean and fat	8-9
	Lean only	6-8
Without bone and with relatively small amount of fat, such as trimmed beef, veal.	Lean with adhering fat	9-11

31

TABLE 4.—RECOMMENDED DAILY DIETARY ALLOWANCES (RDA'S)[1]

(Designed for the maintenance of good nutrition of practically all healthy persons in the United States.)

Sex-age category	Age Years From	Age Years To	Weight Kilograms	Weight Pounds	Height Centimeters	Height Inches	Food energy Calories	Protein Grams	Minerals Calcium Milligrams	Minerals Phosphorus Milligrams	Minerals Iron Milligrams	Vitamin A International units	Thiamin Milligrams	Riboflavin Milligrams	Niacin Milligrams	Ascorbic acid Milligrams
Infants ...	0	0.5	6	14	60	24	kg x 117 / lb x 53.2	kg x 2.2 / lb x 1.0	360	240	10	1,400	0.3	0.4	5	35
	0.5	1	9	20	71	28	kg x 108 / lb x 49.1	kg x 2.0 / lb x 0.9	540	400	15	2,000	.5	.6	8	35
Children ..	1	3	13	28	86	34	1,300	23	800	800	15	2,000	.7	.8	9	40
	4	6	20	44	110	44	1,800	30	800	800	10	2,500	.9	1.1	12	40
	7	10	30	66	135	54	2,400	36	800	800	10	3,300	1.2	1.2	16	40
Males......	11	14	44	97	158	63	2,800	44	1,200	1,200	18	5,000	1.4	1.5	18	45
	15	18	61	134	172	69	3,000	54	1,200	1,200	18	5,000	1.5	1.8	20	45
	19	22	67	147	172	69	3,000	54	800	800	10	5,000	1.5	1.8	20	45
	23	50	70	154	172	69	2,700	56	800	800	10	5,000	1.4	1.6	18	45
	51+		70	154	172	69	2,400	56	800	800	10	5,000	1.2	1.5	16	45
Females...	11	14	44	97	155	62	2,400	44	1,200	1,200	18	4,000	1.2	1.3	16	45
	15	18	54	119	162	65	2,100	48	1,200	1,200	18	4,000	1.1	1.4	14	45
	19	22	58	128	162	65	2,100	46	800	800	18	4,000	1.1	1.4	14	45
	23	50	58	128	162	65	2,000	46	800	800	18	4,000	1.0	1.2	13	45
	51+		58	128	162	65	1,800	46	800	800	10	4,000	1.0	1.2	12	45
Pregnant .							+300	+30	1,200	1,200	[2]+18	5,000	+.3	+.3	+2	60
Lactating							+500	+20	1,200	1,200	18	6,000	+.3	+.5	+4	80

32

[1] Source: Adapted from Recommended Dietary Allowances, 8th ed., 1974, 128 pp. Washington, D.C. 20418: National Academy of Sciences–National Research Council. Also available in libraries. This publication tabulates the RDA's for 8 more nutrients, discusses the basis for all the RDA's, and reviews current knowledge of the dietary needs for other nutrients.

[2] This increased requirement cannot be met by ordinary diets; therefore, the use of supplemental iron is recommended.

NOTE.–The Recommended Daily Dietary Allowances (RDA's) should not be confused with the U.S. Recommended Daily Allowances (U.S. RDA's). The RDA's are amounts of nutrients recommended by the Food and Nutrition Board of the National Research Council and are considered adequate for maintenance of good nutrition in healthy persons in the United States. The allowances are revised from time to time in accordance with newer knowledge of nutritional needs.

The U.S. RDA's are the amounts of protein, vitamins, and minerals established by the Food and Drug Administration as standards for nutrition labeling. These allowances were derived from the RDA's set by the Food and Nutrition Board. The U.S. RDA for most nutrients approximates the highest RDA of the sex-age categories in this table, excluding the allowances for pregnant and lactating females. Therefore, a diet that furnishes the U.S. RDA for a nutrient will furnish the RDA for most people and more than the RDA for many. U.S. RDA's are protein, 45 grams (eggs, fish, meat, milk, poultry), 65 grams (other foods); vitamin A, 5,000 International Units; thiamin, 1.5 milligrams; riboflavin, 1.7 milligrams; niacin, 20 milligrams; ascorbic acid, 60 milligrams; calcium, 1 gram; phosphorus, 1 gram; iron, 18 milligrams. For additional information on U.S. RDA's, see the Federal Register, vol. 38, no. 49 (Mar. 14, 1973), pp. 6959-6960, and Agriculture Information Bulletin 382, "Nutrition Labeling–tools for its use" (described on p. 8).

Table 5.—Food sources of additional nutrients

Vitamins

Vitamin B$_6$	Vitamin B$_{12}$	Vitamin E
Bananas	(present in foods of animal origin only)	Vegetable oils
Whole-grain cereals		Margarine
Chicken	Kidney	Whole-grain cereals
Dry legumes	Liver	Peanuts
Egg yolk	Meat	
Most dark-green leafy vegetables	Milk	**Folacin**
	Most cheese	
Most fish and shellfish	Most fish	Liver
Muscle meats, liver and kidney	Shellfish	Dark-green vegetables
Peanuts, walnuts, filberts, and peanut butter	Whole egg and egg yolk	Dry beans
Potatoes and sweet potatoes		Peanuts
Prunes and raisins	**Vitamin D**	Wheat germ
Yeast	Vitamin D milks	
	Egg yolk	
	Saltwater fish	
	Liver	

Minerals

Iodine	Magnesium	Zinc
Iodized salt	Bananas	Shellfish
Seafood	Whole-grain cereals	Meat
	Dry beans	Cheese
	Milk	Whole-grain cereals
	Most dark-green vegetables	Dry beans
	Nuts	Cocoa
	Peanuts and peanut butter	Nuts

Index to the Appendix

☆ U.S. GOVERNMENT PRINTING OFFICE : 1977 O—245-966

Index

Other AVI Books

ALCOHOL AND THE DIET
  Roe

CARBOHYDRATES AND HEALTH
  Hood, Wardrip and Bollenback

DIETARY NUTRIENT GUIDE
  Pennington

DRUG-INDUCED NUTRITIONAL DEFICIENCIES
  Roe

EVALUATION OF PROTEINS FOR HUMANS
  Bodwell

FOOD AND YOUR WELL-BEING
  Labuza

FOOD FOR THOUGHT
  2nd Edition   *Labuza and Sloan*

FOOD PROTEINS
  Whitaker and Tannenbaum

IMMUNOLOGICAL ASPECTS OF FOODS
  Catsimpoolas

MENU PLANNING
  2nd Edition   *Eckstein*

NUTRITIONAL EVALUATION OF FOOD PROCESSING
  2nd Edition   *Harris and Karmas*

NUTRITIONAL QUALITY INDEX OF FOODS
  Hansen, Wyse and Sorenson

PROGRESS IN HUMAN NUTRITION
  Vol. 1   *Margen*
  Vol. 2   *Margen and Ogar*

SCHOOL FOODSERVICE
  Van Egmond